DIAGNOSTIC CYTOLOGY OF THE URINARY TRACT

with Histopathologic and Clinical Correlations

DIAGNOSTIC CYTOLOGY OF THE URINARY TRACT

with Histopathologic and Clinical Correlations

LEOPOLD G. KOSS, M.D.
Professor and Chairman Emeritus
Department of Pathology
Albert Einstein College of Medicine, Montefiore Medical Center,
New York, New York

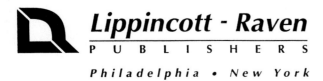

Lippincott - Raven
PUBLISHERS

Philadelphia • New York

Acquisitions Editor: Richard Winters
Sponsoring Editor: Mary Beth Murphy
Production Editor: Virginia Barishek
Cover Designer: Richard Spencer
Production: Caslon, Inc.

Compositor: The Composing Room of Michigan, Inc.
Prepress: Jay's Publishers Services, Inc.
Printer/Binder: Quebecor/Kingsport
Color Separator: Princeton Polychrome Press
Color Insert Printer: Walsworth Publishing

Library of Congress Cataloging-in-Publication Data

Koss, Leopold G.
    Diagnostic cytology of the urinary tract : with histopathologic
and clinical correlations / Leopold G. Koss
        p.   cm.
    Includes bibliographical references and index.
ISBN 0-397-51475-1
    1. Urinary organs—Diseases—Cytodiagnosis.   2. Urinary organs—
Histopathology.   I. Title.
    [DNLM: 1. Urologic Neoplasms—diagnosis.   2. Cytodiagnosis.
3. Urinary Tract—pathology.   WJ 160 K86d 1995]
RC874.K67   1995
616.6'07582—dc20
DNLM/DLC
for Library of Congress   95-15499
                                                              CIP

9   8   7   6   5   4   3   2   1

To Lydia with thanks

Contributors

Bogdan Czerniak, M.D.
Assistant Professor of Pathology, University of Texas
M.D. Anderson Cancer Center, Houston, Texas
Chapter 11: Molecular Biology of Common
Tumors of the Urinary Tract

Fritz Herz, Ph.D.
Associate Professor of Pathology, Albert Einstein
College of Medicine/Montefiore Medical Center,
Bronx, New York
Chapter 11: Molecular Biology of Common
Tumors of the Urinary Tract

Walter Nathrath, M.D.
Professor of Pathology, Technical University of
Munich, Germany
Chapter 10: Immunochemistry

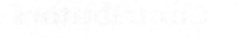

Preface

The writing of this book was prompted by the numerous consultations on the cytology and histology of urinary tract lesions that have reached my desk within the last 25 years. This experience has made it clear that interpretation of cytology of the urinary sediment, washings, brushings, needle aspirations, and tissue biopsies from the organs of the urinary tract can be a source of considerable diagnostic difficulty. Although I have treated the topics in several published books,* the information was widely dispersed. It therefore appeared reasonable to consolidate and summarize the existing knowledge pertaining to all organs of the urinary tract and to complete it by adding new data that would update the published information. Thus, in addition to the chapters describing diagnostic cytologic, histologic, and, when needed, clinical findings in various organs of the urinary tract, several chapters have been added: a chapter on quantitative cytology; a chapter on the current status of molecular biology by two of my long-term co-workers, Drs. Bogdan Czerniak and Fritz Herz; and a chapter on immunochemistry, kindly contributed by Professor Walter Nathrath from Munich, Germany.

_____

*Tumors of the Urinary Bladder, Atlas of Tumor Pathology, Second Series, Fascicle 11, Washington, D.C., The Armed Forces Institute of Pathology, 1974; Supplement, 1985; Diagnostic Cytology and its Histopathologic Bases, 4th Ed., Philadelphia, J.B. Lippincott, 1992; Aspiration Biopsy: Cytologic Interpretation and Histopathologic Bases, with Stanisław Woyke and Włodzimierz Olszewski, 2nd Ed., New York and Tokyo, Igaku Shoin, 1992.

My former co-worker of many years, Ms. Carol Bales, helped in updating the chapter on techniques. My deep thanks go to these contributors, who completed the work on time in spite of many conflicting duties and obligations, and my apologies to them for the numerous phone calls and letters reminding them of the deadlines to meet.

I thank the many colleagues who kindly allowed the use of old and new illustrations, particularly Professors Stanisław Woyke (currently in Kuwait) and Włodzimierz Olszewski (Warsaw, Poland) who generously allowed the use of several photographs from our book, *Aspiration Biopsy* (Igaku-Shoin, 1992), in Chapter 8.

My thanks also go to Mr. Richard Winters, my Medical Editor at J.B. Lippincott Company, who became my friend, and who was very accommodating of my many requests, documenting, to my surprise, that there are publishers who have a heart and a soul.

An author always hopes that a book will be well received because it meets the needs and the requirements of his colleagues, in this case pathologists, cytopathologists, cytotechnologists, nephrologists, and urologists. Needless to say, no book is perfect: the task of writing is so demanding and time-consuming that a certain amount of built-in obsolescence is unavoidable. I would be grateful for any comments from readers that could improve future editions of this work.

Leopold G. Koss, M.D.

Acknowledgments

Dr. Mark Suhrland, the Chief of the Cytology Service at Montefiore Medical Center, took upon himself the onerous task of serving as the principal reviewer of the written text. He was joined in this task by Drs. Norwin Becker, Kathie Schlesinger, and Antonio Cajigas, who reviewed selected chapters. Kathie also provided data on flow cytometry and image analysis from the departmental file. My secretary, Mrs. Cordelia Silvestri, played a key role in the preparation of the manuscript. Without her help, the book would have never been completed. The cytopathology fellows at Montefiore Medical Center for 1994/1995, Drs. Joan Cangiarella, Aaron Feliz, and Rana Hoda, spent many hours reviewing the galleys and provided invaluable help in updating the bibliography.

My sincere thanks go to all of them.

L.G.K.

Contents

Chapter 4

Cytologic Manifestations of Benign Disorders Affecting Cells of the Lower Urinary Tract   45

Chapter 5

Tumors of the Bladder   71

Chapter 6

The Urethra, Ureters, Renal Pelves, and Ileal Conduit   141

PART II

The Prostate, Kidney, Adrenal, Pararenal, and Retroperitoneal Spaces

Chapter 7

The Prostate   163

Contents

Chapter 11
Molecular Biology of Common Tumors of the Urinary Tract   345
Bogdan Czerniak, M.D.
Fritz Herz, Ph.D.

Introduction

HISTORICAL NOTE

Examination of urine as a means of diagnosing human illness was known to ancient Egyptians. Badr noted that hematuria, as evidence of infection with *Schistosoma haematobium,* was recorded in the papyrus of Kahun (1900 B.C.) (Fig. 1). The famous Ebers papyrus (1550 B.C.) suggests that hematuria was due to "worms in the belly." The ancient Egyptians were also aware of the relationship between water (in their cases, through agricultural activities in the fields irrigated by the river Nile) and bloody urine, a relationship that was clarified only in 1852 with the discovery of *Schistosoma heamatobium* by Theodore Bilharz. The relationship of schistosomiasis to bladder cancer was established by Ferguson in 1911.

From the time of Hippocrates into the 19th century, the gross examination of urine was thought to be an important diagnostic procedure. The smell, color, and transparency of the urine and the amount and nature of the sediment, often examined in specially constructed glass containers, were considered a guide to diagnosis and treatment of the underlying disorder (Fig. 2). There are several 16th- and 17th-century paintings of physicians examining urine at the bedside or practicing "uroscopy." Perhaps the epitome of this "science" was a pamphlet published in London in 1637 by Thomas Brian, Member of Parliament, entitled *The Pisse-prophet or certaine pisse pot lectures. Wherein are newly discovered the old fallacies, deceit, and juggling of the Pisse-pot Science, used by all those (whether Quacks and Empirics, or other methodicall Physicians) who pretend knowledge of Diseases, by the Urine, in giving judgment of the same.*

In his remarkable article on the subject of uroscopy (*i.e.,* the science of diagnosis and treatment of diseases based on visual examination or urine samples) Fisman (1993) commented on the work of Brian and his contemporaries in 17th-century England.* Brian exposed the practice of uroscopy, which was often based on the examination of urine alone, in the absence of the patient. Samples were often brought to the practitioner's office by servants or family members; sometimes the same sample was taken to several practitioners until the most pleasing diagnostic conclusion was obtained. Brian's pamphlet describes various ruses used by 17th-century physicians to obtain from the messengers helpful information about the patient. It is of interest that the vestiges of these fraudulent practices persisted until the early days of the 20th century. Fisman cited and illustrated a 1911 advertisement by a company in Grand Rapids, Michigan, that claimed to be able to establish a diagnosis and prescribe treatment based on analysis of mailed urine samples.

The 19th century brought major changes in the

---

*I am grateful to Dr. William W. Johnston of Duke University Medical School, who brought Fisman's article to my attention, and to Mr. Fisman for additional comments.

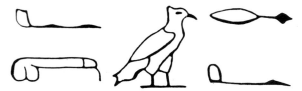

Figure 1. Hematuria, as recorded in the papyrus of Kahun (1900 B.C.), with reference to schistosomiasis (Badr, M.: Schistosomiasis in Ancient Egypt. *In* El-Bolkainy, M., and Chu, E.W., Eds.: Detection of Bladder Cancer Associated with Schistosomiasis. Cairo, Egypt: The National Cancer Institute, 1981. Reproduced with permission).

examination of urine. Besides the progress in organic chemistry that allowed the study of the major chemical constituents of urine and their correlation with disease states, microscopic examination of the urinary sediment slowly entered into the medical armamentarium. The ordinary "urinanalysis," persisting until today, calls for a casual microscopic examination of unstained urinary sediment for the presence of erythrocytes, leukocytes, casts, and epithelial cells. Staining of the urinary sediment, which allows a more detailed examination of the cells, was introduced only in the 20th century.

Still, careful microscopic analysis of cells began in the middle of the 19th century. In 1856 Wilhelm Duschan Lambl (also known as Vilem Dušan Lambl), a Czech physician from Prague, wrote an article entitled "Ueber Harnblasenkrebs. Ein Beitrag zur mikroskopischen Diagnostik am Krankenbette" [On cancer of the bladder. A contribution to microscopic diagnosis at bedside], in which he said the following: "The diagnosis of cancer of the bladder by microscopy of the urinary sediment has received no thorough treatment in the available literature—or rather has not

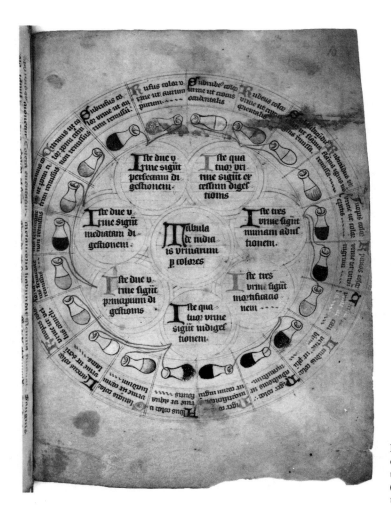

Figure 2. Medieval uroscopy chart used in diagnosis. Note the appearance of the glass urinals surrounding the diagnostic options. (Manuscript Ashmole 391 [V], fol. 10r, courtesy of Bodleian Library, Oxford, U.K.)

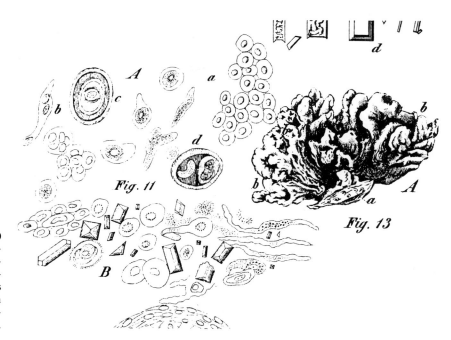

Figure 3. Figure 11 (*left*) from Lambl's 1856 paper, illustrating various cells and crystals observed in the urinary sediment. Figure 13 (*right*) shows a "papillary pseudoplasma from the urethra of a girl"—undoubtedly a condyloma acuminatum.

been mentioned at all." He then proceeded to describe in considerable detail the cytologic findings in six tumors of the bladder, one uterine carcinoma involving the bladder, one "benign papilloma" of the urethra observed in a girl (presumably a condyloma acuminatum), and two inflammatory conditions serving as controls (Fig. 3). Lambl's life story and contributions have been described in some detail by two meritorious historians of human cytology, Heinz Grunze and Arthur Spriggs. It is of incidental interest that Lambl's contributions were not limited to bladder cancer. He was immortalized in the name of the parasite *Giardia lamblia*.

Other 19th century observers reported on the diagnostic value of cytology in tumors of the urinary tract. The great British microscopist Beale, who in 1854 published one of the most comprehensive and astute books on the subject of clinical microscopy, subsequently wrote extensively on urinary cytology and in 1864 described cancer cells in the urine. In the same year, a Scottish physician named Sanders described in the Edinburgh Medical Journal a patient in whose urinary sediment fragments of cancerous tissue were observed. Shortly thereafter, in 1869, a British physician, Dickinson, reported a similar observation. While there may have been other sporadic reports on this subject that are not known to me, it is noteworthy that in 1892, a New York pathologist, Frank Ferguson, stated at a meeting of the New York Pathological Society that the microscopic examination of histo-

logic sections of paraffin-embedded urinary sediment is one of the most important diagnostic procedures in bladder cancer.

The circumstances of Ferguson's presentation are of personal interest to me: the New York Pathological Society, founded in 1844 and incorporated in 1887, is the oldest pathology society in continuing existence in the world, and as a past president of this Society, I am pleased that Ferguson should have chosen this forum for his presentation. Regretfully, however, there is no evidence that Ferguson's observations were noted by the medical community: I do not know of any records of cytologic diagnosis of cancer of the lower urinary tract before 1945. In that year Papanicolaou and the urologist Marshall reported on cytologic examination of the urinary sediment in 83 patients. The diagnostic results were reported as 88.8% correct "positive" and 60% correct "negative," thus hardly worthy of note, were it not for the illustrious authors and the fact that the article appeared in the exclusive scientific journal *Science*. In the 1950s, Geoffrey Crabbe, a British cytopathologist, published several papers on the application of voided urine cytology to the surveillance of workers at high risk for bladder cancer who were employed in the dyestuff industries in England, where carcinogenic aromatic amines were produced in open systems. Crabbe's contributions proved to be of seminal value, as they led to a series of observations of workers exposed to a potent bladder carcinogen, para-aminodiphenyl, in the United States. A series of pub-

Principal
Diagnostic
Approach

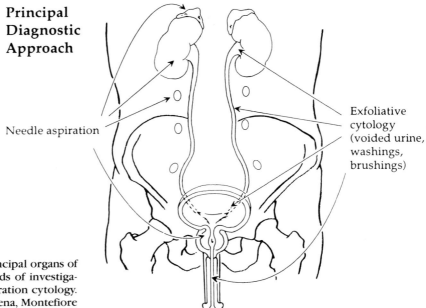

Needle aspiration

Exfoliative
cytology
(voided urine,
washings,
brushings)

Figure 4. A diagram of the principal organs of the urinary tract and the methods of investigation by either exfoliative or aspiration cytology. (Diagram by Dr. Diane Hamele-Bena, Montefiore Medical Center, Bronx, N.Y.)

lications from my laboratory in 1960, 1965, and 1969, defined the diagnostic limits and achievements of cytology of voided urine and introduced the concept of *nonpapillary carcinoma in situ* as the principal precursor lesions of invasive cancer of the urinary bladder. These observations have completely modified the approach to the diagnosis and treatment of tumors of the bladder (for further comments see Chapter 5).

CURRENT STATUS

It is of interest that 130 years after the publication of Lambl's fundamental contribution on the cytology of bladder cancer, the benefits and limitations of urinary tract cytology are still poorly understood by urologists and by pathologists. There is no recorded recent survey of practicing urologists on the subject of cytology of the urinary tract. It would be a safe bet that the expectations of individual practitioners would vary from total indifference to the method as worthless in clinical practice, to the rare enthusiastic endorsement, with the majority expressing a moderate degree of interest in a method of occasional value. Yet there is excellent evidence that cytology of the urinary tract is one of the most important diagnostic methods in urologic oncology, provided that: (1) it is used properly by the urologist under well-defined circumstances and for well-defined reasons; (2) it is per-

formed by a laboratory competent in processing and interpreting such specimens; and (3) the urologist and the pathologist understand the limitations of the method and are familiar with the possible sources of error.

The primary purpose of cytologic examination of the urinary tract is detection and diagnosis of malignant tumors, nearly all of which are of epithelial origin. The examination of voided urine is an efficient method of diagnosis of some diseases of the lower urinary tract, *i.e.,* the bladder, urethra, ureters, and renal pelves. With the passage of time, examination of urine has been supplemented by other methods of securing cell samples. Thus, lavage (washings) and brushing techniques have been applied to these organs. With the increasing acceptance of thin needle aspiration biopsy, organs hitherto inaccessible, such as the prostate, the kidneys, the adrenals, and the lymph nodes, can now be sampled by cytologic techniques. Figure 4 summarizes the targets of cytologic diagnosis of organs of interest to the urologist.

In this work, I discuss the fundamental principles underlying the cytologic diagnosis and differential diagnosis of cancer of the lower urinary tract in various types of samples. The various methods of collecting and processing specimens are described. Other cytologic techniques, such as thin needle aspiration biopsy of the kidney, the prostate, and other organs of interest to the urologist are discussed in later chapters. The use and value of new contemporary approaches to urinary cytology and the diagnosis and monitoring of tumors, namely flow cytometry, image analysis, immunocytochemistry, and molecular biology are briefly discussed in the closing chapters.

BIBLIOGRAPHY

Adams, F.: The genuine work of Hippocrates. New York, William Wood & Co., 1886.

Badr, M.: Schistosomiasis in ancient Egypt. *In* El-Bolkainy, M.N., and Chu, E.W., Eds.: Detection of Bladder Cancer Associated with Schistosomiasis. Cairo, Egypt: The National Cancer Institute, Cairo University, Al-Ahram Press, 1981, pp. 1–8.

Beale, L.S.: The Microscope and Its Application to Clinical Medicine. London, Highley, 1854.

Beale, L.S.: Urine, urinary deposits and calculi and on the treatment of urinary diseases. 2nd Ed. London, J. Churchill and Sons, 1864.

Bilharz, T.: Ein Beitrag zur Helminthographia humana aus brieflichen Mittheilungen des Dr. Bilhartz in Cairo, nebst Bermerkungen von C.T.V. Siebolt. Z. Wissenschaftl Zool. *4:* 53–76, 1852.

Brian, T.: The Pisse-Prophet or certaine pissepot lectures. Wherein are newly discovered the old fallacies, deceit, and juggling of the Pisse-pot Science, used by all those (whether Quacks and Empiricks, or other methodicall Physicians) who pretend knowledge of Diseases, by the Urine, in giving judgement of the same. London, R. Thrale, 1637.

Crabbe, J.G.S.: Cytological methods of control for bladder tumours of occupational origin. *In* Wallace, D.M., Ed.: Tumours of the Bladder. Edinburgh, Livingstone, 1959, pp. 56–76.

Crabbe, J.G.S.: Cytology of voided urine with special reference to "benign" papilloma and some of the problems encountered in the preparation of the smears. Acta Cytol., *5:* 233–240, 1961.

Crabbe, J.G.S., Cresdee, W.C., Scott, T.S., and Williams, M.H.C.: Cytological diagnosis of bladder tumours among dyestuff workers. Brit. J. Industr. Med., *13:* 270–276, 1956.

Dickinson, W.H.: Portions of cancerous growth passed by the urethra. Tr. Path. Soc. London, *20:* 233–237, 1869.

Ferguson, A.R.: Associated bilharziasis and primary malignant diseases of the urinary bladder with observations on a series of forty cases. J. Pathol. Bacteriol., *16:* 76–94, 1911.

Ferguson, F.: The diagnosis of tumors of the bladder by microscopical examination. N.Y. Path. Soc. Meeting of April 27, 1892, pp. 71–73.

Fisman, D.: Pisse-prophets and puritans: Thomas Brian, uroscopy and seventeenth-century English medicine. Pharos, *56:* 6–11, 1993.

Grunze, H., and Spriggs, A.I.: What did Dr. Lambl say in 1856 about cancer cells in urine? Zeiss Inform. Oberkochen, *28:* 44–46, 1986.

Koss, L.G., Melamed, M.R., and Kelly, R.E.: Further cytologic and histologic studies of bladder lesions in workers exposed to *para-aminodiphenyl.* JNCI, *46:* 585–595, 1969.

Koss, L.G., Melamed, M.R., Ricci, A., Melick, W.F., and Kelly, R.E.: Carcinogensis in the human urinary bladder. Observations after exposure to *para-aminodiphenyl.* N. Engl. J. Med. *272:* 767–770, 1965.

Lambl, W.: Uber Harnblasenkrebs. Ein Beitrag zur mikroskopischen Diagnostic am Krankenbette. Prager Vierteljahreshrift f. Heilkunde *49:* 1–15, 1856.

Melamed, M.R., Koss, L.G., Ricci, A., and Whitmore, W.F., Jr.: Cytohistological observations on developing carcinoma of urinary bladder in men. Cancer, *13:* 67–74, 1960.

Papanicolaou, G.N., Marshall, V.F.: Urine sediment smears: A diagnostic procedure in cancers of the urinary tract. Science, *101:* 519–521, 1945.

Sanders, W.K.: Cancer of the bladder. Edinburgh M.J., *111:* 273–274, 1864.

PART I

The Lower Urinary Tract

CHAPTER 1

Indications, Collection, and Laboratory Processing of Cytologic Samples

PRINCIPAL INDICATIONS

Cytologic examination of the lower urinary tract may be of value in the diagnosis of a broad variety of benign and malignant diseases of the bladder, urethra, ureters and renal pelves, described in this book. However, the method has important limitations in reference to the diagnosis of well-differentiated (low-grade) papillary tumors which, as a general rule, cannot be reliably identified in cytologic material. On the other hand, the method yields excellent results in the identification of high-grade tumors, flat carcinomas in situ, and related abnormalities, occurring either as a primary event or as a secondary lesion, accompanying papillary tumors in a synchronous or metachronous fashion. Because of the major diagnostic and prognostic significance of carcinoma in situ and related states, their discovery is the primary target of cytologic examination of the lower urinary tract (see Chap. 5).

Therefore, the principal indications for use of cytology in disorders of the *lower urinary tract* are as follows:

1. The diagnosis of high-grade urothelial (transitional cell) carcinomas, most importantly flat carcinoma in situ and related lesions
2. Follow-up of patients with urothelial (transitional cell) tumors, regardless of grade
3. Monitoring of patients with urothelial tumors undergoing or following treatment.

Carol Bales, CT(ASCP), CT(IAC) made significant contributions to this chapter.

COLLECTION TECHNIQUES

Several collection techniques are available for cytologic investigation of disorders of the lower urinary tract. All of these techniques have advantages, limitations, and sources of error, which will be discussed in this and subsequent chapters. The simplest of these techniques is the collection of voided urine.

Voided Urine

Voided urine, if appropriately collected and processed in the laboratory, *provides reliable information on the status of the epithelium of the urinary bladder, urethra, ureters, and renal pelves, particularly in reference to high-grade tumors of the urinary tract, and flat (nonpapillary) carcinoma in situ and related lesions* (see Chap. 5).

Methods of Collection

Optimal results are obtained if three samples of urine are collected on three consecutive days. In our experience, the first morning urine contains the richest population of cells which, unfortunately, are often poorly preserved. Therefore, we recommend that the second morning voiding be used. Suitable glass or plastic containers with a capacity of about 250 to 300 milliliters, about one-third to one-half filled with a fixative, should be prepared in advance and handed to the patient. The containers should have a wide opening to facilitate direct voiding. Larger amounts of urine are not useful. In our experience the optimal universal fixative is a solution of 50% ethanol, preferably with 2% Carbowax (polyethylene glycol) added. The preparation of the fixative and processing methods are described on p. 6.

Specimens collected in fixative do not require refrigeration. Fresh urine samples that are delivered to the laboratory for processing within 6 to 12 hours of voiding do not require fixation because the pH of the sample is usually low and the high osmolality caused by urea does not affect the epithelial cells to any significant degree. Unfixed polymorphonuclear leukocytes, on the other hand, may become enlarged and lose their segmentation.

The principal advantage of voided urine is the ease with which multiple specimens may be obtained. However, the urine often contains degenerating epithelial cells with cytoplasmic vacuolization and nuclear pyknosis or breakdown that are sometimes difficult to interpret. Voided urine may also harbor cells with benign abnormalities, described in Chapter 4, that may lead to an erroneous diagnosis of cancer.

Some investigators have suggested that hydrating the patient before the collection of voided urine samples improves the desquamation of well-preserved epithelial cells. A procedure proposed by the late John K. Frost, M.D., was as follows: make the patient drink a glass of water every 15 minutes for 2 hours. Discard the first voided urine specimen. The second voided urine specimen, obtained approximately 1 hour after cessation of hydration, is processed for cytologic analysis. This approach significantly reduces the proportion of degenerated and poorly preserved cells, but is time-consuming and, therefore, is rarely used.

Pearson et al. (1981) observed that optimal preservation of cells occurs at pH of 4.5, whereas at higher pH levels cell degeneration and loss occur rapidly. These authors suggest that the ingestion of 1 g of ascorbic acid (vitamin C) at bedtime results in a better preservation of cells in voided urine samples obtained on the following morning.

Catheterized Bladder Urine

There are certain advantages in securing catheterized urine, more so in female patients than in male patients. Urine thus obtained is free of contaminants that sometimes tend to obscure the cytologic picture, particularly cells from the cervix and vagina. The urothelial cells are often better preserved than in voided urine. The make-up of catheterized urine is similar to that of voided urine, except that large urothelial cells (umbrella cells) and clusters of urothelial cells are

very common (see Chaps. 2 and 3). The principal disadvantage of catheterized urine is the need for an intervention that may be painful to some patients, particularly males, and it is not without dangers of infection, even of a Gram-negative septicemia.

As with voided urine, catheterized specimens promptly delivered to the laboratory for processing do not require fixation. If a long delay before laboratory processing is anticipated, fixation in 50% ethyl alcohol with or without 2% Carbowax (polyethylene glycol) is advisable.

Retrograde Catheterization

Retrograde catheterization of the ureters and renal pelves is often used to identify the nature of space-occupying lesions of these organs. The procedure is occasionally useful in the identification and localization of high grade tumors of the ureters and renal pelves (see Chap. 6). In such cases care must be exercised to use separate catheters for each side in order to avoid cross-contamination of the specimens. Most often, however, the procedure *fails* in the differential diagnosis of space-occupying lesions, particularly in the identification of low-grade tumors or lithiasis, because the cytologic presentation of these lesions cannot be distinguished from that of normal urothelium.

The use of a fixative is the same as recommended for catheterized urine samples.

Collection of Urine From the Ureters

A far more useful procedure in the cytologic examination of the ureters and the renal pelves is collection of urine using a shallowly-inserted catheter. In this procedure the epithelium of the ureters is not damaged and the spontaneously desquamated cells are much easier to examine and to interpret than the cell population resulting from a retrograde catheterization. Admittedly, the procedure may be time-consuming because of the slow drip of urine. Patience on the part of the patient and the urologist is required for a collection of a sample of 5 or more ml needed for an adequate cytologic examination. The use of containers with a fixative is recommended.

Bladder Washings (Barbotage)

This technique may be applied during cystoscopic examination or via a catheter. During cystoscopy, from 50 to 100 ml of normal saline or Ringer's solution are instilled into the bladder and repeatedly aspirated, reinjected, and reaspirated (5 to 10 times) to secure the largest possible number of cells. The material may be forwarded fresh to the laboratory for immediate processing or fixed in ethanol or in Carbowax–alcohol fixative, preferably in a container prepared in advance of the procedure.

Obtaining bladder washings through a catheter is much more difficult, particularly in male patients. Although some observers claim success with this method of collection, in our experience the procedure is poorly tolerated by patients, who complain of considerable discomfort. The procedure consists of instilling 50 ml of normal saline or Ringer's solution into the bladder through a catheter or a similar instrument. Optimally, the fluid should be repeatedly aspirated and reinstilled. In practice, one or two instillations and aspirations constitute the limit of the patient's tolerance. The use of a container with a fixative is recommended.

This technique has been extensively used to obtain cell samples for DNA analysis. The results of DNA analysis are not affected by the recommended fixatives (see Chap. 9).

Brushings

The use of small brushes to secure cell samples from defined areas of the urinary tract has become quite widespread. Brushings of the renal pelves and ureters are often used in the differential diagnosis of space-occupying lesions of these two organs—for example, stones and papillary tumors. In most cases this procedure fails to provide the desired information, particularly with low-grade tumors and is, in my experience, the most important source of diagnostic errors.

If the urologist wishes to perform the procedure, clean microscopic glass slides and a jar with 50% ethanol to be used as a fixative should be prepared in advance. Upon completion of the procedure, the brush should be cut off and placed on a slide. The brush should be rolled on the slide in a small circle, not larger than 2 to 3 cm in diameter. Care should be taken to smear as much of the material collected by the brush as possible, by exercising a *slight* pressure on the brush. The slide must be placed immediately in fixative to avoid drying. The brush itself, which often contains residual cells, may be placed in a separate small bottle with 70% alcohol to be forwarded to the laboratory for further processing.

If the urologist is not comfortable with the technique of smear preparation, the brush can be placed in the alcohol fixative and forwarded to the laboratory. *Do not use* formalin or Bouin's fixative, as these harden the cells and make their removal from the brush very difficult. The methods of laboratory processing of brush specimens are described on p. 12.

Ileal Bladder Urine

After cystectomy for malignant tumors of the urinary bladder, an artificial bladder is often constructed from segments of the small intestine, notably the ileum. Because of the propensity of urothelial tumors to sequentially affect various segments of the lower urinary tract, the status of the ureters and the renal pelves must be monitored after a cystectomy. Collection of urine from the ileal bladder serves this purpose well. The fixation procedure is the same as for catheterized urine, given earlier in this chapter.

Aspiration biopsy technique is described in Chapters 7 and 8.

LABORATORY PROCESSING OF SAMPLES

Basic Principles

Microscopic examination of cells must be performed on cell spreads or smears on glass slides or filters. Unfixed and unstained cells may be examined under a *phase microscope*. This method rarely allows an accurate morphologic analysis, although it can be used as a rapid, preliminary assessment of the sample in terms of cellularity and the presence or absence of various cell types, sometimes including cancer cells (de Voogt et al., 1977).

Another preliminary method of cell analysis, using a light microscope, is based on air-dried smears, stained with rapid stains, such as toluidine blue or Diff-Quik.*

However, a detailed analysis of cells requires fixation and permanent staining of the sample. Several methods of cell processing are described below; all require fixation of cells.

Fixatives

As mentioned on p. 4, the most common universal primary fixative for urine or washing samples is 50% ethyl alcohol, preferably supplemented with 2% Carbowax, which infiltrates and preserves cells. Methods of preparation are described below.

---

*Baxter Diagnostics, P.O. Box 520672, Miami, FL 33152-0672.

Preparation of Carbowax (polyethylene glycol 1500) Stock Solution.

Polyethylene glycol 1500* is solid at room temperature, with a melting point of 43° to 46°C. A stock solution of Carbowax can be prepared as follows: Pour 500 ml of water into a 1,000-ml graduated cylinder. Melt polyethylene glycol (Carbowax) in an incubator or hot-air oven at 50° to 100°C. Add 500 ml of the melted Carbowax to the water. This mixture will not solidify and can be stored in a 1-liter screw-cap bottle.

Preparation of 2% Carbowax (polyethylene glycol) solution in 50% ethanol (Universal primary fixative for urine samples).

A liter of 2% Carbowax solution in 50% ethanol is prepared by mixing 435 ml of water, 525 ml of 95% ethyl alcohol, and 40 ml of the water-based stock solution of Carbowax. (Preparation of the stock solution is described above).

Note: This solution may be used as a universal fixative, replacing 50% ethanol. This is *not to be used for laboratory processing of the samples* by the Bales' method, which requires a 2% Carbowax solution in 70% ethanol, described below.

Processing of Urine and Washings of Bladder or Renal Pelvis

A variety of methods of processing of cytologic samples have been developed to deal with the unique characteristics of fluids with low cellularity and low protein content such as voided urine or bladder washings. Direct smears from the sediment, cytocentrifuge preparations, membrane filters, reverse filtration, and cell-block techniques yield adequate preparations if specimens are handled with care. Prevention of cell loss and satisfactory preservation of morphologic detail are the two goals of the procedure.

Smears of Sediment

After centrifugation of the specimen for 10 to 15 minutes at 600*g* (500 to 1,000 revolutions per minute, depending on the type of the centrifuge), the supernatant can be discarded and the sediment smeared on clean glass slides. Because of the very low protein content of urine and washings of the urinary tract, it is advisable to prepare slides coated with an adhesive substance in advance (see p. 11) to improve cell attachment prior to fixation and staining. Even under

these circumstances, cell loss may be substantial. The method has the advantage of simplicity; it is, however, much inferior to the preparation technique described by Bales.

Dhundee and Rigby (1990) proposed that smears of the sediment should be prepared from fresh centrifuged urine samples, followed by alcohol fixation. They claimed an increased sensitivity of this method when compared with smear preparations of fixed sediment. It should be noted that the use of the Carbowax (polyethylene glycol) fixative, as described in the Bales' method, prevents to some extent the loss of cells that is commonly experienced with alcohol fixation alone.

Semiautomated Bales' Method

The semiautomated technique developed in our laboratory (Bales, 1981), results in smears or cytocentrifuge preparations that are rich in cells of excellent morphologic quality, arranged in a monolayer. The method is applicable to urines, washings, and other specimens with a low cell content. The principle of the method is the processing of a predetermined amount of sediment, measured with micropipettes and fixed in 70% ethanol with 2% Carbowax added. We recommend this method as the optimal way of processing urine samples.

Materials Required

The following materials are required for the procedure:

1. Carbowax (polyethylene glycol 1500)*
2. Ethanol (95% solution)
3. Oxford Series P-700 Micro-pipetting system† with one pipette each of capacities 3 μl (catalog no. 21-180-23), 50 μl (catalog no. 21-180-38), and 200 μl (catalog no. 21-180-42) and plastic disposable tips (catalog no. 21-240-10)
4. Standard Repipet Dispenser of 1-ml capacity (Fisher Scientific, catalog no. 13-687053)
5. Repipet Jrs. Variable Volume Dispenser of 5-ml capacity (Fisher Scientific, catalog no. 13-687-59A)
6. Vortex-Genie Mixer (Fisher Scientific, catalog no. 12-812)
7. Plastic test tubes of 50-ml capacity
8. Clean glass slides

---

*Spectrum Chemical Mfg. Corp. 14422 S. San Pedro St., Gardena, CA 90248; or Sigma Chem. Co., P.O. Box 14508, St. Louis, MO 63178.

*Spectrum Chemical Mfg. Corp., 14422 S. San Pedro St., Gardena, CA 90248; or Sigma Chem. Co., P.O. Box 14508, St. Louis, MO 63178.

†Fisher Scientific Company, 50 Fadem Rd., Springfield, NJ 07081.

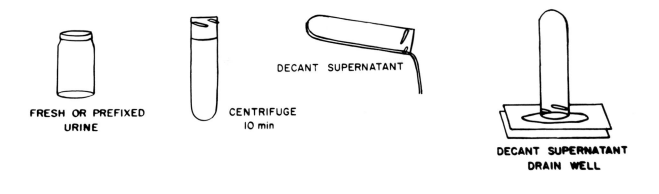

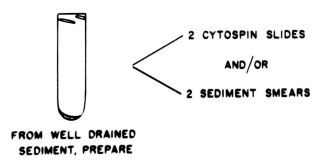

FIGURE 1-1. Initial steps in Bales' method of preparation of urinary sediment for cytologic examination (see also Figs. 1-2 and 1-3). For details, see text.

Procedure

PREPARATION OF 2% CARBOWAX (POLYETHYLENE GLYCOL) SOLUTION IN 70% ETHANOL (FOR LABORATORY PROCESSING OF SAMPLES)

A liter of 2% Carbowax fixative in 70% ethanol is prepared by mixing 223 ml of water, 737 ml of 95% ethyl alcohol, and 40 ml of the water-based stock solution of Carbowax. The preparation of the stock solution of Carbowax is described on p. 6.

PRELIMINARY PREPARATION OF SAMPLE

The preliminary preparation of a sample is carried out in the following steps (Fig. 1-1), using fresh urine or bladder washings.

1. Centrifuge 50 ml of the sample for 10 minutes at 600g (500 to 1,500 rpm, depending on the length of the arm of the centrifuge).
2. Pour off the supernatant and invert the centrifuge tube on paper toweling to drain the sediment well.
3. Using a Vortex mixer, briefly agitate the well-drained sediment.
4. Proceed to cytocentrifuge or smear preparations as desired.

PREPARATION OF CYTOCENTRIFUGE SLIDES

To prepare slides by cytocentrifugation, use the following steps (Fig. 1-2):

1. Aspirate precisely 3 μl of the sediment obtained in the preliminary preparation of the sample.
2. If using Cytospin I cytocentrifuge,‡ expel the sediment into a test tube containing 400 μl of 2% solution of Carbowax in 70% ethyl alcohol. (Test tubes can be filled in advance using a repipette set to dispense 400 μl of fixative. These tubes must be stored in the refrigerator until needed.) If the more efficient Cytospin II or III cytocentrifuge‡ is used, particularly if the sediment is cell-rich, (a

‡Shandon, Inc., 171 Industry Drive, Pittsburgh, PA 15275.

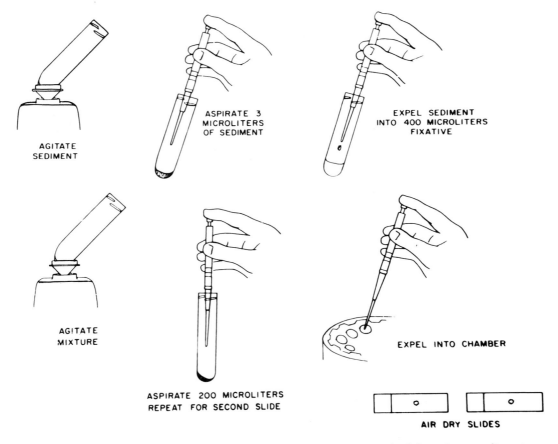

AGITATE
SEDIMENT

ASPIRATE 3
MICROLITERS
OF SEDIMENT

EXPEL SEDIMENT
INTO 400 MICROLITERS
FIXATIVE

AGITATE
MIXTURE

ASPIRATE 200 MICROLITERS
REPEAT FOR SECOND SLIDE

EXPEL INTO CHAMBER

AIR DRY SLIDES

FIGURE 1-2. Preparation of cytocentrifuge slides by Bales' method for urinary sediment (see also Figs. 1-1 and 1-3). For details, see text.

layer of sediment 1- to 2-mm thick is seen at the bottom of the centrifuge tube after preliminary preparation of the sample), dilute the sediment further by placing 3 μl of the sediment in 800 μl of the 2% solution of Carbowax in 70% alcohol. For further comments on cytocentrifugation, see p. 9.

3. Briefly agitate the mixture on a Vortex mixer to prevent formation of cell aggregates.
4. Aspirate 200 μl of the suspension with an automatic pipette and place in a cytocentrifuge chamber.
5. Repeat step 4 and place 200 μl of the cell suspension in the opposite cytocentrifuge chamber.
6. Spin for 5 minutes, remove slides, and allow them to air-dry for 10 to 30 minutes in a dust-free environment.
7. Rinse slides in 95% alcohol for 10 minutes prior to staining.

PREPARATION OF SMEARS

Smears may be prepared from the sediment as follows (Fig. 1-3):

1. Add 3 to 5 ml of the 2% Carbowax solution in 70% ethanol to the sediment obtained in the preliminary preparation of the sample and agitate on a Vortex mixer.
2. Let stand in a vertical position for 10 minutes, and thereafter centrifuge at 600g for 10 minutes.
3. Pour off the supernatant and drain the sediment as described in step 3 of the preliminary preparation of sample. Agitate the sediment on the Vortex mixer.
4. Aspirate 50 μl of the sediment by means of an automatic pipette and place on a clean glass slide. Lay a second clean slide on top of the sediment

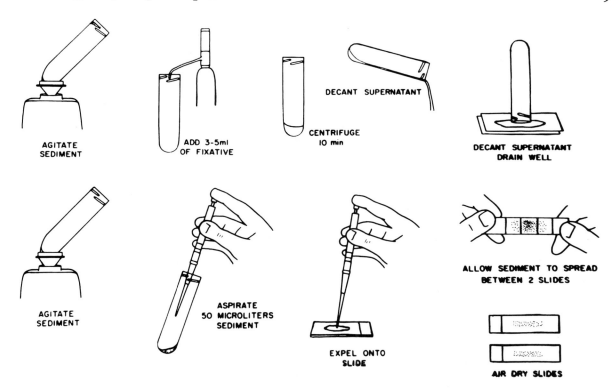

FIGURE 1-3. AGITATE SEDIMENT · ADD 3-5ml OF FIXATIVE · CENTRIFUGE 10 min · DECANT SUPERNATANT · DECANT SUPERNATANT DRAIN WELL · AGITATE SEDIMENT · ASPIRATE 50 MICROLITERS SEDIMENT · EXPEL ONTO SLIDE · ALLOW SEDIMENT TO SPREAD BETWEEN 2 SLIDES · AIR DRY SLIDES

FIGURE 1-3. Preparation of urinary sediment smears by Bales' method (see also Figs. 1-1 and 1-2). For details, see text.

and let the sediment spread spontaneously between the two slides. Pull the slides apart with a gentle gliding motion. Place the two slides with the gray sediment face up, and let them air-dry for 10 to 30 minutes in a dust-free location.

5. Rinse the dry slides for 10 minutes in 95% ethanol prior to staining.

RESULTS

Cell-rich, yet flat, monolayer cytocentrifuge preparations of urine are routinely obtained by the use of this method. The epithelial cells, whether benign or malignant, are exceptionally well preserved. There is virtually no overlapping of cells. Minimal drying artifacts are occasionally observed in polymorphonuclear leukocytes. The method provides sufficient detail for it to be used routinely in image analysis of sediments of voided urine with excellent results.

The method is highly recommended and can be executed by technical personnel with minimal training and experience.

COMMENT

Major objections to the use of the cytocentrifuge include distortion of cellular morphology due to air-drying artifact and loss of cells by absorption of fluid into the filter card. Both of these difficulties have been overcome with the technique described. Our procedure was initially developed for the Shandon Cytospin I cytocentrifuge. In 1981, Shandon introduced the Cytospin II cytocentrifuge with somewhat different features, one of which is the automatic formation of an air bubble between the cell suspension and the slide. Recovery rates from the Cytospin II or III are consistently higher than those with the Cytospin I. As described, the use of Cytospin II or III requires an adjustment of cell concentration in cell-rich samples to prevent overlapping. The cell-rich samples are recognized in the test tube, following the preliminary preparation, because they form a visible milky residue in the bottom of the test tube. Such samples must be diluted to provide monolayer preparation (see p. 7). The volume of sediment used remains the same.

Precaution: After processing of Carbowax-treated samples, the sample chambers of the cytocentrifuge should be thoroughly washed. Chambers that are merely rinsed and allowed to dry can contaminate new specimens with cells from previous runs. Washing the chambers with a small brush or soaking them in a bleach solution usually prevents this from occurring. Alternatively, the chambers can be sterilized with boiling water or autoclaved at 120°C, or they can be cleaned with a chemical sterilizing agent such as Decon 90.* Disposable cytocentrifuge chambers with attached filter cards are available from Shandon. Such chambers eliminate the possibility of cross contamination and, more importantly, limit exposure to infectious material.

Excellent cytocentrifuge preparations can also be obtained by the method described by Gill in the Cytospin Manual from Shandon Instruments, Inc.[†]

Use of Membrane Filters

Membrane filters with small pore size have been used for many years to capture cells in fluid specimens, particularly those fluids with sparse cell content, including urine and bladder washings. Although such filters effectively retain the cells, they also have significant disadvantages:

- The preparations dry out rapidly and cannot be effectively stored.
- The cells are often distorted by pores.
- The cells are often placed in several planes of vision and focusing may be time-consuming.
- The optimal preparations require a great deal of laboratory expertise.

I believe that filter preparations are inferior to the preparations obtained by the method developed by Bales, described above. Nonetheless, a brief description of this technique is provided.

Three principal filter types are available for cytologic work: Gelman,[‡] Millipore,[§] and Nuclepore.[‖]

Gelman and Millipore filters are made of cellulose, are approximately 140 μm thick, and are opaque white in appearance until cleared in xylene and mounted in a mounting medium with a similar refrac-

tive index. The Nuclepore is a colorless, transparent membrane, 10 μm thick, made of polycarbonate. Rectangular sheets (19 × 42 mm Millipore and Nuclepore, 17 × 42 mm Gelman), 25-mm disks, and 47-mm disks that can be cut in half to make two slides are available. The pore diameter most frequently used for cytologic preparation is 5 μm.

The materials needed, specimen requirements, and method of filtration are essentially the same for all three types of filters. The major differences are related to staining and mounting of the filters.

Materials Needed

1. Membrane filters
2. Filter holder to fit membrane to be used[§]
3. Vacuum flask, tubing, and a three-way stopcock[§]
4. Vacuum source with regulator and gauge[§]
5. Forceps (nonserrated)
6. Balanced salt (electrolyte) solution, such as Hanks' balanced salt solution. Normal saline solution is frequently used, but it may cause nuclear and cytoplasmic distortion.
7. Petri dishes
8. 95% Ethyl alcohol

Specimen Collection

For best results, specimens should be collected fresh. Prefixation coagulates proteins that may clog the filters and harden the cells into spherical shapes, preventing flattening of the cells on the membrane's surface.

Special care must be used in processing urine samples. Voided urine contains salts that are in solution at body temperature but that may precipitate when the urine cools to room temperature. Even though the urine appears grossly clear, these salts may clog the filters. Therefore, urine samples should be centrifuged for 10 minutes, the supernatant poured off, and the sediment resuspended in a balanced salt solution. Centrifuge this sample again and carefully pour off the supernatant. Once washed, cells do not adhere well to the centrifuge tube. Mix sediment with the small amount of balanced salt solution that runs down the side of the tube. The sample is now ready for filtration.

Methods of Filtration

1. Label filters with indelible ink or hard lead pencil.
2. Pre-expand Millipore and Gelman filters in a Petri dish filled with 95% ethyl alcohol for 10 to 15 seconds. This prevents wrinkling of the filter when it is refixed in alcohol. Moisten Nuclepore filters in a Petri dish filled with a balanced salt solution.
3. Moisten the grid of the filter setup with balanced salt solution. Using nonserrated forceps, lay the pre-expanded or premoistened filter on the grid, label side up.

---

*Markson Scientific, Inc., Box 767, Del Mar, CA 92014.

[†]Shandon Instruments, Inc., 171 Industry Drive, Pittsburgh, PA 15275.

[‡]Baxter Diagnostics, MC., Scientific Products, McGraw Park, IL 60085-6787.

[§]Millipore Filter Corp., Bedford, MA 01730-9903.

[‖]VWR Scientific, P.O. Box 7900, San Francisco, CA 94120.

4. Place the funnel on top of the filter. Do not clamp the funnel to base. Add 15 to 20 ml of balanced salt solution to the funnel and start the vacuum. The filter will be flattened by allowing a portion of the salt solution to pass through the filter. Stop the vacuum at this point and clamp the funnel to the grid.

5. Add 50 to 100 ml of balanced salt solution to the funnel. By means of a disposable pipette, add one to two drops of the sediment to the solution in the funnel.

6. Start vacuum (up to 100 mm Hg for Millipore and Gelman filters and up to 20 mm Hg for Nuclepore filters). As the specimen filters, add balanced salt solution from a squeeze bottle to rinse the filter well. The stream of the squeeze bottle should be directed against the sides of the funnel to minimize aerosol sprays and to prevent disturbance of the cells on the surface of the filter. Stop the vacuum as soon as the flow of liquid begins to slow down. The filter should appear to be clean. Red blood cells will give the filter a reddish hue. To lyse these red blood cells, add a few milliliters of 50% ethanol. If the filter is not overloaded, it will change from red to white. The surface of the filter should always be covered with fluid. *Never permit the filter to dry.*

7. Add 20 to 30 ml of 95% ethanol to fix the cells in situ. After 1 minute, carefully restart the vacuum to pull the fixative through the filter. Stop the vacuum when a small amount of alcohol still remains to cover the filter.

8. Unclamp the funnel, remove the wet filter with a nonserrated forceps, and place the filter, cell side up, in a Petri dish with 95% ethanol. The filter is ready for staining after remaining in fixative for one half hour.

9. Place funnel, forceps, and grid in disinfectant solution. For comments on staining of filters, see p. 14.

Transferring Cells from a Membrane Filter to a Glass Slide (Reverse Filtration): The Use of Adhesives

A variety of imprint techniques, in which a filter is pressed cell side down against a glass slide to transfer cells, have been reported. The method, which may give excellent results, should be used with glass slides coated with an *adhesive substance* to minimize the loss of cells. In 1983 Nielsen et al. compared cell recovery rates from Millipore filters, using plain glass slides or slides coated with *egg albumin-glycerine, Apathy's syrup,* and *gelatin-chrome alum.* Filter preparations were made from urine preserved in Esposti's fixative (50 ml of glacial acetic acid, 225 ml of distilled water, and 225 ml of methanol) and pressed against the slides. Egg albumin–glycerine and Apathy's syrup did not increase the transfer of cells when compared with slides without adhesives. The percentage of cells recovered varied from less than 10% to slightly more than 70%. However, gelatin–chrome alum (1 g gelatin, 0.1 g chromalum, 100 ml H_2O; add 1 ml of thymol in ethanol as a preservative) had a pronounced adhesive effect. In every instance, at least 94% and sometimes as many as 99% of the cells were transferred (see reference for details of the procedure). The slides may be processed as smears. Another cell adhesive is Poly-L-lysine,* in dilution of 1:10 or 1:20 in deionized water (Domagala et al., 1979). Clean slides are placed in the solution for 5 minutes and air-dried. The cells adhere well to the coated slides. Another excellent adhesive is 3-aminopropyl-triethoxysilane (3-APTES).* The compound adheres to glass and binds to cells. A 2% solution of 3-APTES in acetone is prepared for coating clean glass slides. The adhesive can be used in reverse filtration but also for purposes of in situ hybridization of archival material (Liang et al., 1991).

Mounting the Filter Preparations

The selection of the appropriate mounting medium for filters is important. The refractive index of the medium must match the refractive index of the stained filter and of the glass slide on which the filter is placed. A detailed analysis of the problem is provided in Koss, 1992, pages 1486–1487.

Coverslipping the Cell Sample

Practice is necessary to achieve well-mounted slides, free of air bubbles and artifacts. A minimum of mounting medium should be used, because too much mounting medium interferes with microscopic detail, making the cell film appear hazy or milky when examined with the high dry objective. If the mounting medium and coverslip are applied too slowly to Papanicolaou stained slides, a common artifact appears as a brown, refractile pigment-like substance on the surface of the cells. This artifact is caused by air trapped on the surface of the cell when xylene is allowed to evaporate. If this artifact occurs, the slide may be soaked in xylene, absolute alcohol, and 95% alcohol, rinsed in running tap water, and restained in OG and EA (see page 12). In stubborn cases, after the running water rinse, the slide may be placed in glycerine for half an hour and rinsed well in tap water prior to reapplication of the counterstains.

Special precautions are necessary in coverslipping

---

*Sigma Diagnostics, 3050 Spruce St., St. Louis, MO 63103.

Gelman and Millipore filters. For details, see Koss, 1992, pages 1487–1488.

Preparation of Smears From Brushes

For microscopic examination, brushings may be processed as smears prepared by the urologist in the cystoscopy suite. *The smears require immediate fixation in ethyl alcohol (50% or, preferably, 70% solution).* In my experience urologists may have problems with the preparation of adequate, well-spread smears. It is, therefore, preferable to cut off the brush and place it in a bottle with alcohol or alcohol-Carbowax fixative. *Formalin fixative should not be used for brushes,* because it causes precipitates that may obscure the cells. In the laboratory the cell content of the brushes is best secured by transferring the brush with the fixative into a centrifuge tube and agitating the specimen on a Vortex mixer for 10 minutes. The sediment is then centrifuged and prepared as any other fluid specimen (see p. 6).

Cell Block Techniques

Cell block techniques are based on the principle of embedding in paraffin the urinary sediment obtained by centrifugation. The method, applicable to cytologic samples with abundant sediment, allows for cutting multiple sections, suitable for routine stains, special stains and immunocytochemistry. Several variants of this method exist. Perhaps the most popular one consists of adding a few drops of melted agar to the drained sediment in the centrifuge tube, allowing agar to gel at room temperature. The gelled agar is easily removed by a metal spoon, placed in tissue paper, and processed for paraffin embedding (for further details, see Bales and Durfee, 1992). The method is very useful in aspiration biopsies.

Duarte (1991) introduced a modification of this method, applicable to specimens with scanty cellularity: the cell pellet is fixed, frozen, and embedded in plastic. This allows for cutting of multiple 2 μm sections (often of the same cells) using an ultramicrotome. Multiple stains and immunostains may be performed on the sediment.

New Apparatus for Processing of Urine Sediments

A recently introduced machine, ThinPrep 2000,* can be used for processing of urine and other body

*Cytyc Corp., 237 Cedar Hill St., Marlborough, MA 01752.

fluids. The machine, which is expensive, automatically disperses the cells in the sample. The cells are deposited on a filter and transferred to glass slides. Special solutions for cell suspension and preservation must be purchased from the company.

Although we have had no personal experience with the apparatus, we have seen some of the preparations that were of good quality. The yield of epithelial cells from a few urine samples was apparently significantly higher with this machine than with the cytocentrifuge (Papillo and Lapen, 1994).

Stains

A number of stains, some very simple and some complicated, may be used for staining the samples from the urinary tract. Some observers use rapid *hematologic stains* or their variants such as toluidine blue or May-Gruenwald-Giemsa. These stains have the advantage of simplicity and speed and, with experience, may yield satisfactory diagnostic results. The clear disadvantage of these stains in reference to epithelial cells is the difficulty of assessing nuclear abnormalities. We recommend that such stains be used only as a preliminary stain to assess the cellularity of the sample but not for diagnostic purposes.

Papanicolaou stain of fixed samples offers the best option of judging the fine details of cell structure. All illustrations in this book are stained with this method, unless indicated otherwise in the text or legends to illustrations.

Papanicolaou stain is a polychrome stain utilizing hematoxylin for nuclear stain and a special eosin formula (EA) and Orange G (OG) as counterstains. The stain has the advantage of excellent nuclear morphology and differential staining of cytoplasm that is very helpful in identifying urothelial cells, squamous cells, glandular cells, and a variety of nonepithelial cell types.

The procedures for the most commonly used stains are listed below. For further information on preparation procedures and a detailed analysis of these stains and other technical data, the reader is referred to Bales and Durfee (1992).

Toluidine Blue Stain

Product name: toluidine blue 0 (Fisher Scientific, catalog no. SP107-10).

PREPARATION OF STAIN

- 0.05 g toluidine blue powder
- 20 ml 95% ethanol
- 80 ml distilled water

Mix and filter before use.

Use toluidine blue as a rapid stain to verify the presence of satisfactory material:

1. Fix the smear for at least 15 seconds in 70–95% ethanol or methanol.
2. Remove the slide from the fixative and place it on a paper towel.
3. Apply 1 or 2 drops of toluidine blue stain to the smear.
4. Cover the slide with a coverslip. After 10 to 15 seconds, blot out the excess stain by turning the coverslipped slide over on paper towels and pressing gently.
5. Examine the slide for adequacy of the specimen while it is still wet and, before it dries, return it to the fixative. The coverslip will easily fall off, and the smear can be submitted for Papanicolaou stain without further preparation (see below).

Diff-Quik Stain

The Diff-Quik staining procedure is a rapid modification of Wright's stain. The fixative and the two staining solutions are purchased in 1-gallon (3.78-liter) containers.* The staining procedure involves the following steps:

1. Fixative—20 seconds
2. Staining solution I—20 seconds
3. Staining solution II—3 or 4 dips, no more than 10 seconds
4. Distilled water—10 seconds
5. Ethanol 95%—10 seconds
6. Absolute ethanol—15 seconds
   Fixative—20 seconds
7. Xylene—15—20 seconds
8. Mount in Coverbond†

The results produced with Diff-Quik stain are similar to those obtained with Wright-Giemsa. Smears stained with Diff-Quik may be restained with Papanicolaou stain, without destaining. Better results, however, are obtained after destaining in 95% ethanol for 15 minutes. The Diff-Quik-stained smear is processed using one-half the timing for the routine Papanicolaou stain.

May-Gruenwald-Giemsa Stain for Air-Dried Smears

May-Gruenwald-Giemsa stain is best used on air-dried smears. The stain is prepared as follows:

STOCK SOLUTION

- May-Gruenwald stock‡: Dissolve 1.0 g eosin-methylene blue in 100 ml methyl alcohol (does not require refrigeration)
- Giemsa stock§: Add 1.0 g Giemsa powder to 66 ml glycerine. Incubate at 37°C for 3 hours, mixing occasionally. To the incubated stain, add 66 ml methyl alcohol. Store in the refrigerator (good for 6 months).

WORKING STAINS

- May-Gruenwald working stain: Add 20 ml methyl alcohol to 40 ml stock stain (prepare weekly).
- Giemsa working stain: Add 5 ml Giemsa stock stain to 45 ml distilled water (prepare daily).

STAINING PROCEDURE

1. May-Gruenwald working stain—15 minutes
2. Rinse in tap water
3. Giemsa working stain—15 minutes
4. Rinse in tap water
5. Air-dry
6. Xylene—10 seconds (twice)
7. Mount

Papanicolaou Stain

The following procedure results in excellent, crisp staining of smears or filter preparations:

1. Running water—10 seconds
2. Hematoxylin—2 minutes
3. Running water—10 seconds
4. Bluing solution‖—1 minute
5. Running water—10 seconds
6,7. Ethanol 95%—10 seconds each (two changes)
8. OG-6¶—2 minutes
9,10. Ethanol 95%—10 seconds each (two changes)
11. EA-65¶—2 minutes
12–14. Ethanol 95%—10 seconds each (three changes)
15,16. Absolute ethanol—10 seconds each (two changes)
17–19. Xylene 10 seconds each (three changes)
20. Mount as described for Diff-Quik

---

*Baxter Diagnostics, P.O. Box 520672, Miami, FL 33152-0672.

†Baxter Healthcare Corp., Scientific Div., 1430 Waukegan Rd., McGow Park, IL 60085.

---

‡Purchase as Jenner stain from Paragon C & C Co., Inc., 190 Willow Ave., Bronx, NY 10454; or Harleco, EM Diagnostic Systems, 480 Democrat Rd., Gibbstown, NJ 08027.

§Any commercially available Giemsa stain powder is satisfactory. We use Giemsa stain SO-G-28 from Fisher Scientific, Fair Lawn, NJ 07410.

‖Scott solution: 40 g $MgSO_4$ (anhydrous), 20 g $NaHCO_3$, 10 liters H_2O mixed until dissolved.

¶Harleco, EM Diagnostic Systems, 480 Democrat Rd., Gibbstown, NJ 08027.

For restaining Diff-Quik-stained smears, the timing of each step is cut in half.

Important Factors Influencing the Staining Results of Filters by the Papanicolaou Method

Millipore and Gelman filters should not be attached to a glass slide for staining. Clamp-style paper clips that allow filters to hang freely during the staining process may be used. Nuclepore filters may be clipped to a glass slide for staining.

For the Papanicolaou staining sequence, see p. 13. During the staining sequence, Nuclepore filters behave similarly to glass slides with the exception of clearing in xylene. The time in xylene should be limited to 10 to 15 minutes to prevent the filters from curling and rolling up tightly. The background of Millipore and Gelman filters will stain with hematoxylin and the cytoplasmic stains. If the background is too heavily stained, cytologic detail and cellular contrast are obscured. After the water rinse following hematoxylin, the filter is slowly dipped approximately 30 times in an 0.025% or 0.05% solution of hydrochloric acid (HCl). The filter should appear pale yellow at this point. The extremely low concentration of HCl does not decolorize the cells but is sufficient to partially decolorize the background of the filter.

As with hematoxylin, the background of the Millipore and Gelman filters is stained by EA and OG cytoplasmic stains. To minimize stain retention, the filters should be rinsed for a longer period. Following OG the slides must remain in three sequential 95% alcohol rinses, 1 minute each, with minimal dipping. The filters are stained for a longer period in EA and are rinsed for 4 minutes, 2 minutes, and 1 minute, respectively, in three sequential 95% alcohol rinses. It is important that no dipping occur during this sequence. Dipping will cause the stain to be removed from the cells as well as the filter background.

Absolute isopropyl alcohol must be substituted for the three final absolute ethanol rinses when staining Millipore filters. Absolute ethyl alcohol can soften and dissolve these filters. The Nucleopore filters can be dissolved either before or after staining. For details, see Bales and Durfee (1992), pages 1484–1486.

The Feulgen Stain for DNA

The Feulgen stain, a specific stain of double-stranded deoxyribonucleic acid, is extensively used for DNA measurements by image analysis (see Chap. 9). The two strands of DNA are hydrolyzed (separated) by HCl, exposing sugar-aldehyde residues. These are captured by the Schiff reagent and result in a deep purple stain of nuclear DNA.

1. *Smears:* Smears fixed in alcohol or air dried are suitable for staining without any further steps. Stained smears may be destained and rehydrated in a descending series of alcohols (100%→80%→25%→water).
   Tissue sections: Histologic sections of tissues fixed in 4% to 10% buffered formalin (and related fixatives that preserve DNA) may be stained after deparaffinization and rehydration in a descending series of alcohols (see above). Tissues fixed in mercury-containing fixatives are not suitable for DNA staining, unless mercury salts are removed with iodine thiosulfate first. The results are of questionable value.
2. Place smears or tissues in the 1N (normal) hydrochloric acid (preheated) at 60°C for 10 minutes.
3. Immerse in Schiff's reagent for 10 minutes (see below).
4. Wash 2 minutes in each of three successive baths of 0.05 M metabisulfite (see below). The sulfite baths should be discarded daily.
5. Wash for 5 minutes in running water.
6. Counterstain a few seconds in 0.01% fast-green FCF, C.I. No. 42053 in 95% alcohol. The stain does not wash out in alcohol, but if it is too intense, it may be removed promptly in water.
7. Complete the dehydration with 100% alcohol; clear through one change of alcohol and xylene (50:50) and two of xylene. Mount in polystyrene, ester gum, Permount, HSR, or other synthetic resin or in balsam.

Periodic Acid-Schiff Reaction Reagent (PAS)

PREPARATION OF SOLUTIONS

Periodic Acid. Prepare a 1% aqueous solution.

Schiff Reagent

Distilled water	100 ml
Basic fuchsin, C.I. No. 42500	1 g
Sodium or potassium metabisulfite	2 g
NHCl	20 ml
Activated charcoal	0.3 g

Bring the water to a boil and remove from the heat. When the solution cools to 60°C add the basic fuchsin. Filter the solution and then add the sodium or potassium metabisulfate and HCl. Pour this solution into a stoppered, dark bottle and keep at room temperature for 18 to 24 hours. Add the charcoal and vigorously shake the mixture for 1 minute. Filter this solution and store at 0° to 5°C. Discard this reagent when a pink color develops.

Sodium Metabisulfite Solution

Stock solution: Prepare a 10% aqueous solution.

Working solution: 5 ml of stock mixed with 100 ml of distilled water.

There are several Feulgen staining kits available from commercial sources.* Follow the manufacturer's instructions in using these kits.

BIBLIOGRAPHY

Adler, C.: Gelatin-chrome alum: A better section adhesive. Histologic, *8,* 115–116, 1978.

Affandi, M. Z.: Use of hairspray as a smear fixative. Acta Cytol., *33,* 419, 1989.

Bales, C. E.: A semi-automated method for preparation of urine sediment for cytologic evaluation. Acta Cytol., *25,* 323–326, 1981.

Bales, C. E., and Durfee, G. R.: Cytologic Techniques. Chapter 33 *In* Koss, L. G. (Ed.): Diagnostic Cytology and Its Histopathologic Bases. 4th Ed. Philadelphia, J. B. Lippincott, 1992, 1451–1531.

Barrett, D. L., and King, E. B.: Comparison of cellular recovery rates and morphological detail obtained using membrane filter and cytocentrifuge technique. Acta Cytol., *20,* 174–180, 1976.

Beyer-Boon, M. E.: The efficacy of urinary cytology. Dissertation, Univ. of Leiden, the Netherlands, 1977.

Beyer-Boon, M. E., and Voorn-den Hollander, M. J. A.: Cell yield with various cytopreparatory techniques for urinary cytology. Acta Cytol., *22,* 589–594, 1978.

Boon, M. E., Wickel, A. F., Ruth, A. M., and Davoren, M. B.: Role of the air bubble in increasing cell recovery using cytospin I and II. Acta Cytol., *27,* 699–702, 1983.

Borgstrom, E., Wahren, B., and Gustafson, H.: Fluorescence methods for measuring the A, B, and H isoantigens on cytological material from bladder carcinoma. Urol. Res., *13,* 43–45, 1985.

Coon, J. S., and Weinstein, R. S.: Detection of A,B,H tissue isoantigens by immunoperoxidase methods in normal and neoplastic urothelium. Comparison with the erythorocyte adherence method. Am. J. Clin. Pathol., *76,* 163–171, 1981.

Crabtree, W. N., and Murphy, W. M.: The value of ethanol as a fixative in urinary cytology. Acta Cytol., *24,* 452–455, 1980.

deVoogt, H. J., Beyer-Boon, M. E., and Brussec, J. A. M.:

The value of phase contrast microscopy for urinary cytology. Reliability and pitfalls. Acta Cytol., *19,* 542–546, 1975.

deVoogt, H. J., Rathert, P., and Beyer-Boon, M. E.: Urinary Cytology. New York, Springer-Verlag, 1977.

Dhundee, J., and Rigby, H. S.: Comparison of two preparatory techniques for urine cytology. J. Clin. Path., *43,* 1034–1035, 1990.

Domagala, W., Kahan, A. V., and Koss, L. G.: A simple method of preparation and identification of cells for scanning electron microscopy. Acta Cytol., *23,* 140–146, 1979.

Duarte, L.: A new technique facilitating studies of scant cell specimens. Biotechnic and Histochem., *66,* 200–202, 1991.

Failde, M., Eckert, W. G., and Patterson, J. N.: A comparison of a simple centrifuge method and the Millipore filter technic in urinary cytology. Acta Cytol., *7,* 199–206, 1963.

Keebler, C. M., Reagan, J. W., and Wied, G. L.: Compendium on Cytopreparatory Techniques. 4th Ed. Chicago, Tutorials of Cytology, 1976.

Koss, L. G.: Diagnostic Cytology and Its Histopathologic Bases. 4th Ed. Philadelphia, J. B. Lippincott, 1992.

Liang, X. M., Wieczorek, R. L., and Koss, L. G.: In situ hybridization with human papillomavirus using biotinylated DNA probes on archival cervical smears. J. Histochem. Cytochem., *39,* 771–775, 1991.

Lindberg, L. G., and Ohlin, B.: Specimen fixation in urinary cytology. Acta Cytol., *22,* 142–145, 1978.

Luzzatto, R., and Teloken, C.: Use of the cytobrush in the diagnosis of male urethral herpesvirus infection. Acta Cytol., *33,* 417–418, 1989.

Marwah, S., Devlin, D., and Dekker, A.: A comparative cytologic study of 100 urine specimens processed by the slide centrifuge and membrane filter techniques. Acta Cytol., *22,* 431–434, 1978.

McLennan, B. L., Oertel, Y. C., Malmgren, R. A., and Mendoza, M.: The effect of water soluable contrast material on urine cytology. Acta Cytol., *22,* 230–233, 1978.

Nielsen, M. L., Fischer, S., Hogsborg, E., and Therkelsen, K.: Adhesives for retaining prefixed urothelial cells on slides after imprinting from cellulosic filters. Acta Cytol., *27,* 371–375, 1983.

Ocklind, G.: Optically eliminating the visible outlines of pores in intact polycarbonate (Nuclepore) filters. Acta Cytol., *31,* 946–949, 1987.

Papillo, J. L., and Lapen, D.: Cell yield. ThinPrep vs. cytocentrifuge. Acta Cytol., *38,* 33–36, 1994.

Pearson, J. C., Kromhout, L., and King, E. B.: Evaluation of collection and preservation techniques for urinary cytology. Acta Cytol., *25,* 327–333, 1981.

Sternheimer, R.: A supravital cytodiagnostic stain for urinary sediments. J.A.M.A. *231,* 826–832, 1975.

---

*For example from Cell Analysis Systems, Inc., 909 South Route 83, Elmhurst, IL 60126-4944.

CHAPTER 2

The Cellular and Acellular Components of the Urinary Sediment

The cells that are the subject of morphologic analysis of the urinary sediment are derived from several different sources. The most important source is the urothelium (transitional epithelium) lining the urinary bladder, ureters, renal pelves and, in part, the urethra. Other epithelial variants, such as the squamous epithelium, glandular epithelium of the intestinal type, and renal tubular epithelium also contribute to the diversity of the epithelial cells. Blood cells, macrophages, and other cells extraneous to the urinary tract are commonly observed. The urinary sediment often contains crystals, contaminants, and renal casts. All these microscopic structures will be described in this chapter.

NORMAL UROTHELIUM (TRANSITIONAL EPITHELIUM) AND ITS CELLS

Histology and Ultrastructure

The urine is a toxic substance that must be contained within the bladder. There exists, therefore, a protective mechanism or a *urine–blood barrier* that effectively prevents the seepage of urine into the bloodstream. The bladder wall is composed of an epithelium, the underlying connective tissue (lamina propria), two layers of smooth muscle, and a serosa, derived from the peritoneum, all being richly vascularized.

It has been reported by Ro et al. (1987) that a muscularis mucosae as a continuous layer may be observed in the lamina propria in a few bladders (3 of 100). In most bladders (91 of 100), however, only a "dispersed" layer of muscle fibers was noted. In 6 bladders, no muscle fibers were found in this location. Although occasional muscle fibers may be observed in the lamina propria, I am not sure that they deserve to be identified as a "layer" or that they play a significant role either in physiology or pathology of the bladder.

Although it is likely that several of the components of the bladder wall act in unison to constitute the urine–blood barrier, the first line of defense is the epithelium, which also lines the ureters and the renal pelves. The highly specialized epithelium is unique to the lower urinary tract and, therefore, deserves a separate designation as the *urothelium,* a term that corresponds much better to the current state of knowledge than the widely used term "transitional epithelium."

In histologic sections, the epithelium lining the human urinary bladder, ureters, and renal pelves is normally composed of 7 to 8 layers of cells, provided with a unique superficial layer (Fig. 2-1). The number of cell layers appears to be constant in the ureter but is highly variable in the urinary bladder, depending on the state of dilatation or contraction of this organ: fewer cell layers are visible in a dilated bladder than in a contracted bladder (Fig. 2-2). The variability in the number of cell layers is accounted for by the presumed mechanism of cell movements in the contract-

17

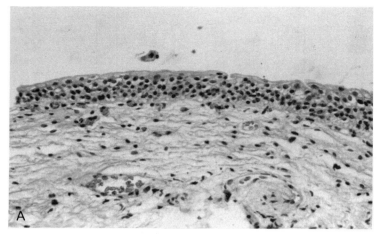

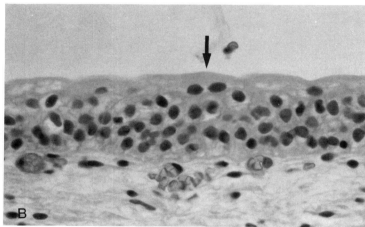

FIGURE 2-1. (*A*) Low- and (*B*) high-power view of normal human urothelium (distended bladder). Note the 6 to 7 layers of cells and the presence of the very large superficial cells (umbrella cells) on the surface. One umbrella cell has two nuclei (*arrow*). Small capillary vessels are present immediately beneath the epithelium in the lamina propria. (*A* × 150; *B* × 350.)

ed and dilated bladder. It is assumed that the epithelial cells are capable of "sliding" against each other, thus adjusting to the volume requirements without breaking the continuity of the urine–blood barrier.

An important feature of the urothelium is the presence of a superficial layer composed of very large, often multinucleated cells that may measure from 20 to 50 μm in diameter. The superficial cells are also known as *"umbrella cells"* because each one of them extends over several smaller cells of the underlying layer in umbrella-like fashion (see Fig. 2-2).

The cells of the deeper layers of the urothelium resemble parabasal cells from the deeper layers of the squamous epithelium: they measure from 7 to 10 μm in diameter that increases towards the surface, and are bound to each other by numerous solid cell junctions, the desmosomes. Their nuclei are spherical and open or vesicular. The basal layer of the epithelium, composed of the smallest cells, is bound to the lamina densa of the basement membrane by specialized structures known as hemidesmosomes.

It is of note that there are also immunologic differences between the deeper layers of the urothelium and the superficial umbrella cell layer (Cordon-Cardo et al., 1984, 1987). As discussed in detail in Chapter 11 and shown in Table 11-2, the umbrella cells contain certain types of keratin filaments that are common to simple epithelia and are not found in the deeper layers of the urothelium. Normal urothelial cells can easily be cultured from voided urine (Herz et al., 1979, 1985).

Ultrastructure of the Umbrella Cells

On the surface, facing the lumen of the organ, the lateral membranes of adjacent umbrella cells are bound to each other by tight junctions (Fig. 2-3A), cell devices preventing the seepage of urine across the epithelium. The surface membrane of the epithelial cells has unique ultrastructural characteristics. The principal feature of the membrane is the rigid segments known as plaques. The plaques are composed of two electron opaque layers, with an electron-lucent layer sandwiched in between. Because of the unequal

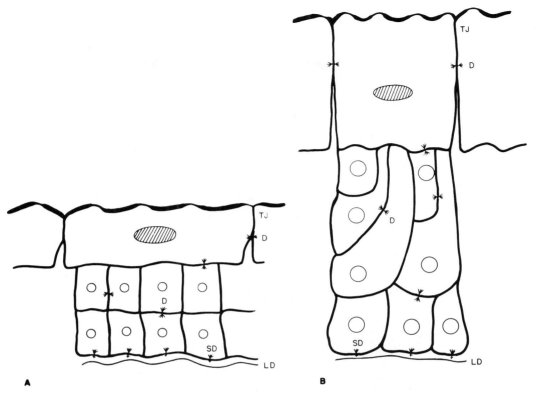

FIGURE 2-2. Schematic drawing of the structure of the urothelium in a dilated (*A*) and contracted (*B*) bladder. The cells are bound to each other by desmosomes; the epithelium is bound to the lamina densa (LD) of the basement membrane by hemidesmosomes. The superficial umbrella cells are bound to each other by tight junctions (TJ). The surface of the umbrella cells is lined by plaques of the asymmetric unit membrane (see also Fig. 2-3). The nuclei of the umbrella cells are larger than those of the deeper cell layers and may be multiple.

thickness of the electron opaque layers this membrane is known as the *asymmetric unit membrane* (AUM) (Fig. 2-3*A, inset*). The asymmetric unit membrane is formed in the Golgi apparatus of the superficial cells and is packaged in the form of oblong vesicles that travel to the surface, replacing the worn or damaged membrane (Hicks, 1966; Koss, 1969). Several recently characterized structural proteins known as uroplakins are the principal components of the plaques, as documented by immunochemistry (Yu et al., 1990; Wu et al., 1990; Lin et al., 1994). It is of interest that the cultured normal human urothelial cells retain the ability to form AUM (Shokri-Tabibzadeh et al., 1982).

The plaques are separated from each other by short segments of ordinary, flexible cell membrane that does not have any special morphologic features, but is characterized by a specific glycoprotein (Yu et al., 1992). The apparent role of these segments is to confer flexibility to the plaques so that the superficial cells can adapt to the changing volume of the organ. This is

particularly important in reference to the urinary bladder, which may be either distended or contracted, depending on the volume of urine. In distended bladder studied by scanning electron microscopy, the umbrella cells are rather flat and their surface is characterized by ridges formed by AUM (Fig. 2-3*B*); in contracted bladder they are more cuboidal in shape. In the contracted bladder the asymmetric unit membrane is stored in the form of invaginations or canals, leading from the surface to the depth of the cell. In the dilated bladder the canals either disappear or become very shallow, the asymmetric unit membrane being used to form the surface of the umbrella cells.

The Significance of Umbrella Cells in Tissue Sections

In tissue sections, the structure of the umbrella cells cannot be fully appreciated. Their characteristic features are better seen in exfoliated material (see p. 21).

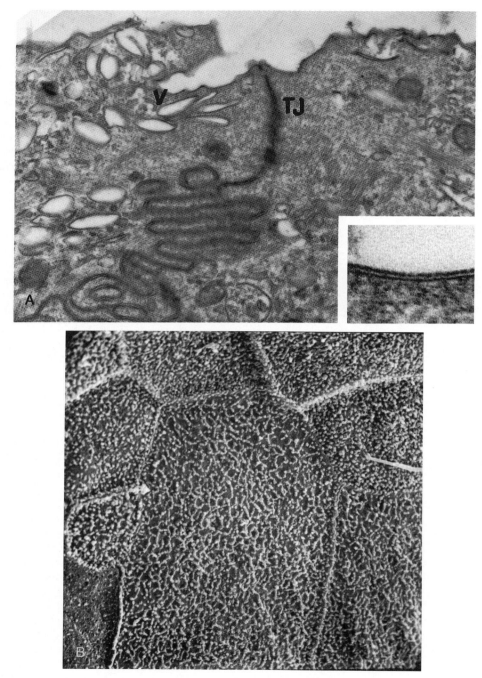

FIGURE 2-3. (*A*) Electron microscopic structure of normal human urothelium. The two adjacent superficial cells are bound by a tight junction (TJ). Numerous oblong vesicles (V) may be noted. The angulated surface reflects the presence of the asymmetric unit membrane shown in *inset.* (*A* approx. × 24,000; *inset* approx. × 150,000). (*B*) Scanning electron micrograph of superficial urothelial cells in a distended human bladder. The surface is covered by uniform, stubby microridges (approx × 5,000). (From Hicks, R.M., and Newman, J. Scanning electron microscopy of urinary sediment. In: Koss, L.G., and Coleman, D.V. (Eds.): Advances in Clinical Cytology. vol. 2. New York, Masson, 1984.)

The presence of the superficial cells in histologic material, such as bladder biopsies, reflects the integrity of the epithelium. Their absence indicates that the epithelium has been damaged, either because of a pathologic process or because the tissue has not been carefully handled during processing.

Variants of Normal Urothelium

In a congenital abnormality known as exstrophy, wherein the bladder is located outside the abdominal wall, the epithelium shows a great variety of types, such as normal urothelium, squamous epithelium, and mucus-producing colonic epithelium. In this rare condition, the epithelial variants are fully displayed, reflecting the embryonal origin of the bladder from the cloaca, *i.e.,* the terminal portion of the embryonal intestinal tract, and the genital tubercle (Koss, 1975).

Careful mapping studies of normal urinary bladders obtained at autopsies of people dying of unrelated causes have shown that several epithelial variants may be observed in the lower urinary tract (Wiener et al., 1979; Ito et al., 1981). The most common variants are the nests of von Brunn (commonly known as Brunn's nests) and cystitis cystica and glandularis (Fig. 2-4*A*). *Brunn's nests* are button-like dips of urothelium into the lamina propria. The nests either are solid structures, composed of urothelial cells, or may show central cysts that may be lined by mucus-producing columnar, glandular cells. The center of the cystic nests may contain mucus. The frequency of distribution and the location of the Brunn's nests in 61 bladders from males and 39 bladders from females is shown in Fig. 2-4*B*. It may be noted that Brunn's nests may be found with a high degree of frequency in all parts of the bladder in both sexes.

Cystitis cystica and glandularis is a term attached to cystic structures lined by cuboidal or columnar mucus-producing cells. The cysts may be small, limited to lamina propria, or quite large, sometimes involving the epithelium, the lamina propria, and even the muscularis of the bladder (Fig. 2-4*C*). Contrary to the name attached to them, the cysts are not of inflammatory origin but represent a variant of the epithelium. The distribution of cystitis cystica in the normal bladders is shown in Figure 2-4*D*. This variant is most commonly observed in the area of the trigone.

The presence of *squamous epithelium of vaginal type* in the trigone of the bladder is yet another epithelial variant, observed mainly in women and rarely in men (Fig. 2-5). The term "squamous metaplasia" or "pseudomembranous trigonitis" sometimes has been applied to this entity, although there is no evidence whatever that the squamous epithelium is related to an inflammatory process. It appears likely that the squamous epithelium in women follows the hormonal cyclic changes of the vaginal epithelium (see p. 30).

Areas of *mucus-producing epithelium,* often resembling the epithelium of the small or large bowel, may also line areas of bladder surface, replacing the urothelium. In such epithelial areas, specialized enteric cells, such as Paneth cells, may be observed (Fig. 2-6). Exceptionally, ciliated columnar epithelium may be seen.

The urothelial variants have no pathologic significance in normal individuals with the exception of cystitis cystica composed of large cysts that may be symptomatic. However, in tumors of the urothelium, especially carcinomas, these variants may be represented either as a subsidiary or as the dominant feature of these tumors.

Cells Derived From Normal Urothelium

The fundamental principles underlying the interpretation of the cytologic samples derived from the bladder, ureters, and renal pelves are vested in the histologic structure of normal urothelium.

In cytologic preparations there are two principal characteristics of cells derived from normal urothelium that set them apart from other epithelial structures:

1. *The marked variability in the size and structure of the component cells reflecting the differences between the superficial cells, umbrella cells, and cells derived from the deeper epithelial layers*
2. *The tendency of these cells to desquamate in clusters* (Fig. 2-7). These features are directly related to the structure of the urothelium, described above.

Superficial (Umbrella) Cells

Regardless of the type of sample and collection technique used, the superficial urothelial cells are a common component of the urine sediment. Such cells may have single or multiple nuclei, the latter feature being much better appreciated in exfoliated material than in tissue sections. The umbrella cells with single nuclei are large, measuring from 20 to 30 μm in diameter, hence somewhat similar in size to superficial squamous cells. The umbrella cells are characterized by the configuration of their membrane and their nuclei (Figs. 2-7*A* and 2-8*A,B*). One or two surfaces of such cells are often flat or slightly curved and sharply demarcated. The membranes may form sharp angles with each other (see Fig. 2-7*A*). Under favorable conditions of cell preservation and under high-dry power of the microscope, one may observe that

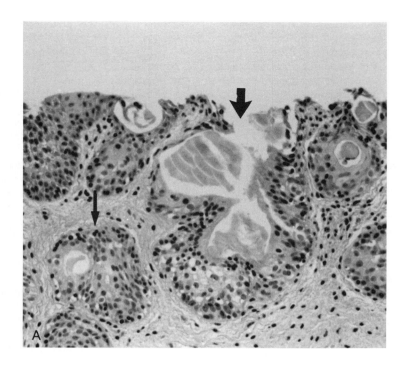

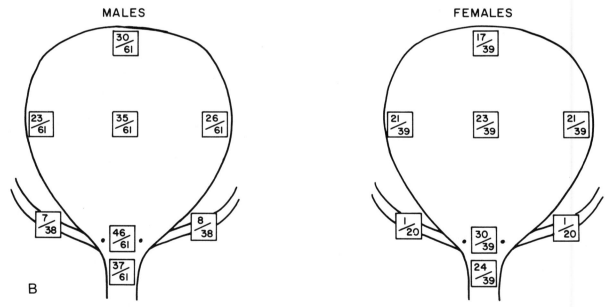

MALES   FEMALES

B

FIGURE 2-4. (*A*) Brunn's nests and a focus of "cystitis glandularis." Note the nests of urothelial cells in the lamina propria (*small arrow*). One open focus of cystitis glandularis is shown (*large arrow*). The latter structure is lined by mucus-producing columnar cells; the lumen is filled with mucus (× 350). (*C*) See opposite page. Bladder with "cystitis glandularis." The cysts, located in the lamina propria, are quite large (× 150). (*B,D*) Diagrams showing the frequency and sites of occurrence of these two variants of the urothelium in 61 males and 39 females with normal bladders. (*B* and *D* from Wiener, D. P., Koss, L. G., Sablay, B., and Freed, S. Z.: The prevalence and significance of Brunn's nests, cystitis cystica and squamous metaplasia in normal bladders. J. Urol., *122,* 317–321, 1979, with permission).

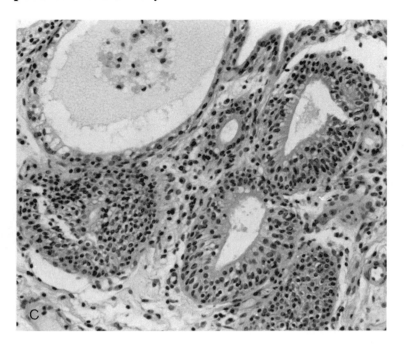

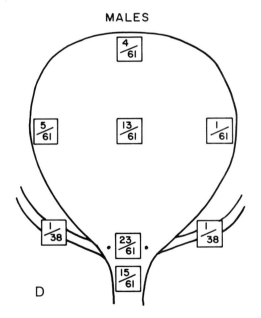

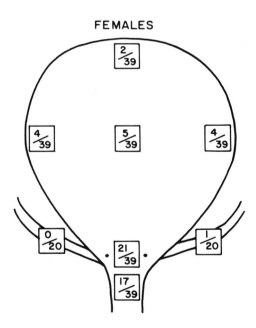

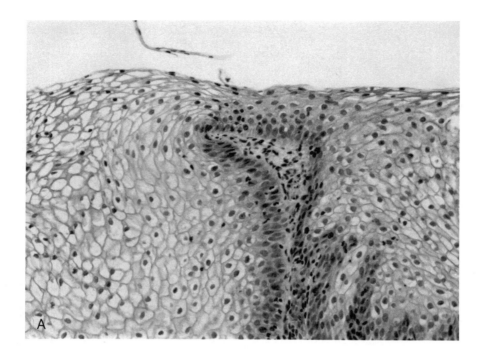

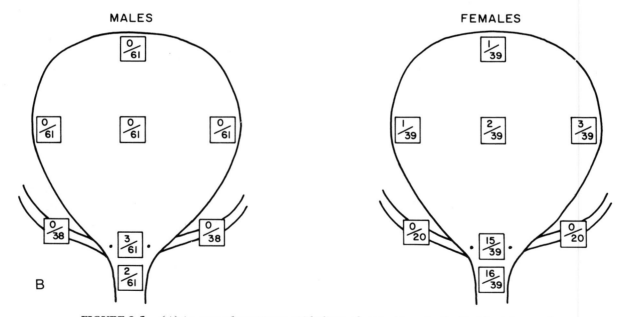

FIGURE 2-5.   (*A*) An area of squamous epithelium of vaginal type in the bladder trigone of a young woman (× 350). (*B*) A diagram showing the distribution of this variant in 61 males and 39 females: this variant is much more common in the trigone area of women than in men.

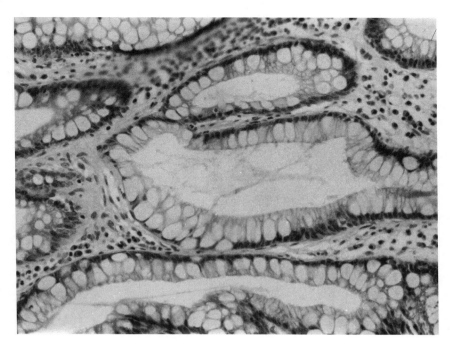

FIGURE 2-6. Mucus-producing epithelium of colonic type in an exstrophic bladder. Similar findings, usually confined to a small area of the bladder epithelium, may occur in otherwise normal people. A malignant transformation of this type of epithelium may occur, resulting in carcinomas of intestinal types (× 350).

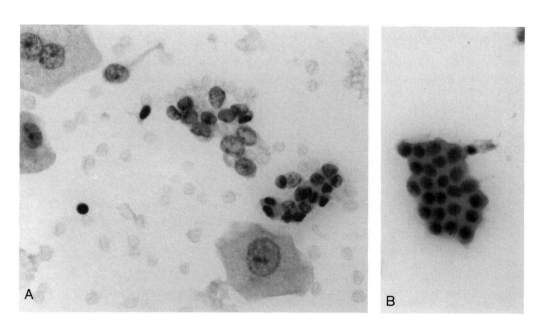

FIGURE 2-7. Bladder washings. (*A*) The two types of urothelial cells, large and small, are seen in the same field. The larger cells are the superficial umbrella cells. The smaller cells are derived from the deeper layers of the urothelium and often desquamate in clusters. Note the angulated thick membrane of the superficial cell and the large nucleus with two chromocenters. (*B*) A tight cluster of cells from the deeper epithelial layers (*A,B* × 560).

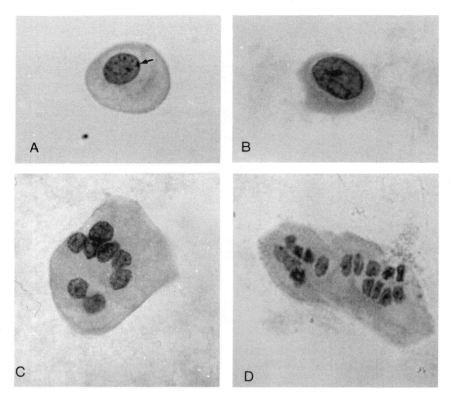

FIGURE 2-8. (*A* and *B*) Voided urine. Superficial urothelial cells (umbrella cells) with single nuclei. Note the thick, sharply demarcated cell membrane on cell surface. The nuclei are finely granular ("salt and pepper" appearance). Note the presence of sex chromatin in *A* (*arrow*). (*C* and *D*) Multinucleated umbrella cells in a sample obtained by retrograde catheterization. Note the sharply demarcated cell membrane in *C.* (*A,B* × 1,000; *C,D* × 560.)

the flat cell membrane, corresponding to the asymmetric unit membrane (see p. 19), is not only thick but also refractile. The remaining cell membrane may show cytoplasmic extensions. Multinucleated umbrella cells are much larger, sometimes forming true giant cells (see below and Figs. 2-8C,D and 2-9). The cytoplasm is usually eosinophilic, often finely granular, and sometimes vacuolated. In an occasional umbrella cell there are larger cytoplasmic vacuoles, sometimes containing fragments of amorphous material or inspissated mucus (Dorfman and Monis, 1964). Exceptionally, umbrella cells may contain an inclusion of inspissated mucus (see Fig. 2-11D). The significance of this finding is not known.

The nuclei of the umbrella cells are either single or multiple and may vary in size. The single nuclei are very large, measuring 10 or more μm in diameter, and are spherical or slightly ovoid in configuration. Not surprisingly, the DNA content of the nuclei of the umbrella cells may be the double of other normal cells (tetraploid nuclei, see Chapter 9). The nuclear membrane is heavy and sharply demarcated (see Figs. 2-7A and 2-8A,B). The nucleoplasm is finely granular, has a "salt-and-pepper" appearance, and often contains one or more prominent chromocenters (see Fig. 2-7A). The structure of the nucleus is much better seen in bladder washings than in voided urine (com-

pare Figs. 2-7A and 2-8A). In females, a sex chromatin body attached to the nuclear membrane may be seen (see Fig. 2-8A). Binucleated cells are common. Such cells are often larger than the mononucleated umbrella cells and their nuclei are somewhat smaller.

Large, multinucleated umbrella cells are by far the most striking component of the urinary sediment, particularly in washings or brushings of bladder or ureter (see Figs. 2-8C,D and 2-9). The size of these cells may vary from 20 to 50 μm or more in the largest diameter. The number of nuclei may vary from 3 to 50 and sometimes even more. The shape of these cells is often polygonal, and their outline is scalloped. One flat or convex thick surface, corresponding to the luminal face of the urothelium is often recognized (Fig. 2-9A). The nuclei may be oval or spherical and are usually of approximately equal sizes. It is not uncommon, however, to encounter such giant cells with nuclei of extremely variable sizes, some very small and some very large, with a diameter 3 or 4 times larger than average (Fig. 2-9B). In the nuclei of umbrella cells, the presence of one or more large, irregular granules of condensed chromatin (chromocenters) may be striking (Fig. 2-9). True nucleoli, characterized by an eosinophilic center, may sometimes be observed. In some umbrella cells, the nuclei may be pyknotic and poorly preserved (Fig. 2-9C). Common

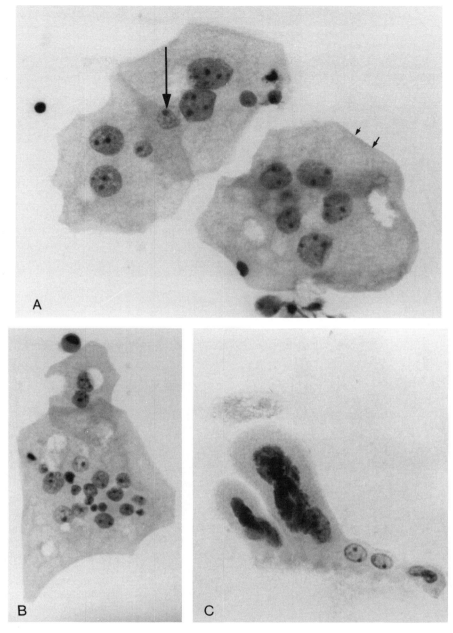

FIGURE 2-9. Multinucleated umbrella cells in bladder washings. (*A*) Three large multi-nucleated cells with scalloped membrane. A thickened flat surface (*small arrows*) is seen in the cell on the right. The nuclei are large and vary in size. All nuclei contain single or multiple prominent chromocenters (*large arrow*), against a background of finely granular chromatin. Cytoplasmic vacuoles are common in such cells. (*B*) An umbrella cell with numerous small nuclei of variable sizes (left), overlaying a cell with two nuclei. Two mononucleated umbrella cells are seen on right. (*C*) Two umbrella cells with pyknotic, degenerated nuclei, mimicking hyperchromasia. Note the two attached normal nuclei (*A,B,C* × 560).

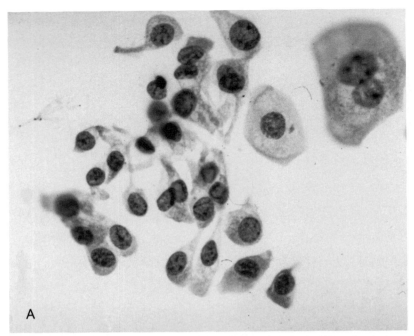

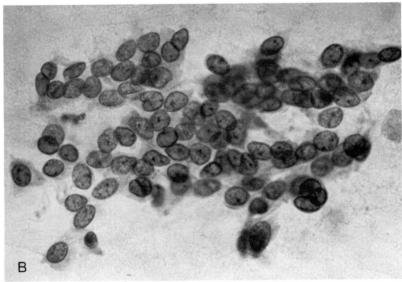

FIGURE 2-10. (*A* and *B*) Cells originating from the deeper layers of the urothelium (bladder washings). In *A,* the deeper cells are polygonal. Their size can be compared with that of the two umbrella cells in the same field (one, not in focus, is binucleated). In *B,* the nuclear structure is well shown. Note the "salt and pepper" bland chromatin structure and the small chromocenters (× 560). (*A* from Koss, L. G.: Diagnostic Cytology and Its Histopathologic Bases. 4th Ed. Philadelphia, J. B. Lippincott, 1992.)

errors in diagnosis are based on the presence of the giant umbrella cells that are mistaken for giant tumor cells or for large multinucleated macrophages, sometimes seen in inflammatory processes.

The mechanism of formation of the multinucleated umbrella cells is not clear. Cell fusion, which accounts for the formation of foreign body giant cells and Langhans' giant cells from epithelioid cells or immobilized small macrophages, is extremely unlikely to occur in the epithelium. Hence the best explanation for the occurrence of these cells is endomitosis, a

nuclear division taking place without cytoplasmic division. The functional role of the multinucleated cells also remains a mystery. It is not known at this time what role, if any, these cells play in the function of the urine–blood barrier.

Cells Originating From the Deeper Layers of the Urothelium

Small epithelial cells derived from the deeper layers of the urothelium often desquamate in clusters, particularly if the specimen was obtained with the

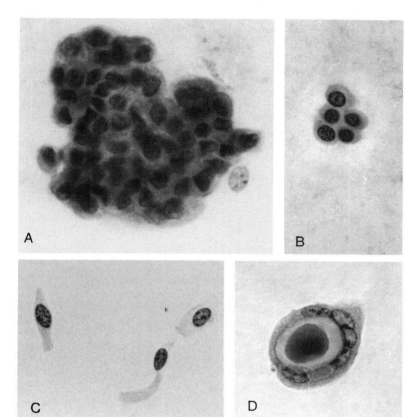

FIGURE 2-11. (*A* and *B*) Voided urine. Clusters of small urothelial cells from deeper epithelial layers. In *A,* the large cluster is approximately spherical or "papillary." Note in *B* the perfectly spherical dark nuclei. Such cells *do not* represent a pathologic process. (*C*) Columnar epithelial cells, bladder washings. (*D*) A multinucleated cell, containing a large mucus inclusion of unknown significance (*A* × 350; *B, C* and *D* × 560).

help of an instrument (see Fig. 2-7*B* and Fig. 2-10). Single small urothelial cells are observed in voided urine, usually in the presence of an inflammatory process with destruction of the superficial layer.

The clusters of the deeper cells may be tightly packed and may assume a spherical "papillary" configuration with sharp borders (see Fig. 2-7*B* and Fig. 2-11*A*). Such clusters are often misinterpreted as reflecting papillary tumors (see Chap. 5). When the deep cells are removed from their setting by an instrument, they often appear in loose clusters wherein the structure of the individual cells may be better appreciated (Fig. 2-10). Such cells are often polygonal or elongated, sometimes columnar in shape, and nearly always show cytoplasmic extensions, often forming contacts among cells. The cytoplasmic extensions are the result of the tough desmosomal junctions that exercise a pull on the cytoplasm. The amount of the basophilic cytoplasm in such cells depends on the layer of origin. It is more abundant in cells derived from the more superficial layers. Single cells resemble parabasal squamous cells in size and configuration. These cells are often spherical or round, particularly in voided urine, but may also show cytoplasmic extensions.

Regardless of the variability in shape, the nuclei of the smaller urothelial cells are of approximately the same size, measuring about 5 μm in diameter. They are usually finely granular and bland and contain one, rarely two, small chromocenters. In voided urine, the nuclei may be either pale or opaque and occasionally somewhat darker staining (Fig. 2-11*B*).

Other Cells of Urothelial Origin

Occasionally mucus-containing columnar epithelial cells, characterized by a peripheral nucleus and distended, clear cytoplasm (Fig. 2-11*C*) are observed. Such cells are derived from cystitis cystica and other mucus-producing variants of the urothelium, described on p. 21. Sometimes such cells are ciliated.

Unusual Findings

MITOTIC ACTIVITY IN NORMAL UROTHELIAL CELLS

Occasionally mitotic figures may be observed in small urothelial cells, particularly after a cystoscopy or a transurethral resection (TUR) of the anterior prostate (Fig. 2-12*A*). In the absence of other obvious abnormalities, the mitoses reflect a regenerating urothelium and do not indicate the presence of a tumor.

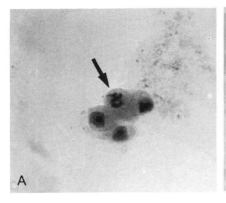
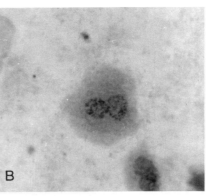

FIGURE 2-12. (*A*) A mitosis in a urothelial cell (*arrow*), 3 days after transurethral resection (TUR) of the prostate. There was no evidence of bladder disease. (*B*) Urothelial umbrella cell with finely condensed chromatin in both nuclei. The significance of this rare finding is unknown (*A,B* × 560).

Chromatin Condensation in Urothelial Cell Nuclei

For reasons unknown, perhaps related to some drugs or fixatives, a peculiar condensation of chromatin, resembling mitotic prophase, sometimes may be observed in superficial umbrella cells (Fig. 2-12*B*). So far as one can tell, this very rare finding is of no diagnostic significance.

OTHER BENIGN CELLS

Squamous Cells

Squamous cells of various sizes and degrees of maturation are a common component of the urinary sediment, particularly in voided urine (Fig. 2-13). Such cells are much more abundant in female than in male patients, although there are some males who shed numerous squamous cells. In women, these cells originate in the squamous epithelium of vaginal type that is commonly observed in the trigone of the urinary bladder (see p. 21); voided urine sediment may also contain squamous cells derived from the vulva, vagina, or even the uterine cervix. Such cells may be benign or malignant (see Chap. 5). In men, the origin of the squamous cells is in the terminal portion of the urethra. Among the benign squamous cells one may distinguish superficial cells, characterized by a small, pyknotic nucleus and abundant cytoplasm, intermediate cells with somewhat larger, open or vesicular nuclei (Fig. 2-13*A*), and still smaller parabasal cells. Navicular cells are intermediate squamous cells with large cytoplasmic deposits of glycogen (staining yellow in Papanicolaou stain), and peripheral nuclei (Fig. 2-13*B*). Such cells may be observed during pregnancy, early menopause, and sometimes in women receiving hormonal therapy. Such cells may also be observed in male patients receiving therapy with

estrogenic compounds for prostate cancer (see Chap. 7). Squamous cells may also be anucleated and fully keratinized, *i.e.*, represented by keratinized shells of the size and shape of squamous cells, in which the nucleus has been obliterated by accumulated keratin (see Chap. 4). The presence of these "ghost" cells may be of diagnostic significance as representing leukoplakia (see p. 57) or squamous carcinoma of the bladder (see p. 97).

The Urocytogram

In women the population of squamous cells in the urinary sediment may be used to determine the level of estrogenic activity (the so-called urocytogram). The urocytogram is based on cells derived from the squamous epithelium of the genital tract that are often observed in the urinary sediment. It appears likely that the squamous epithelium in the trigone of the bladder is yet another source of cycling squamous cells (Tyler, 1962). The basic assumption of the urocytogram is the dependence of the maturation of the squamous epithelium of the female genital tract on estrogens, or other hormones with similar activity. It is known from studies of cyclic changes in the female genital tract that the mature superficial squamous cells usually (although not always) are formed under the impact of estrogens. In the absence of estrogenic activity the squamous epithelium does not reach full maturity and its surface is formed by intermediate or parabasal cells. Thus, it has been proposed that the numerical relationship of the mature, superficial squamous cells to less mature squamous cells (intermediate and parabasal varieties) in the urinary sediment reflects the level of estrogen activity (Lencioni, 1972). The assumption is only partially correct because other factors, such as inflammatory events, may also cause squamous epithelium to mature. Urocytograms may also be used to study endocrine disorders (Lencioni et al., 1973), but have now been replaced by better and more precise methods of hormonal as-

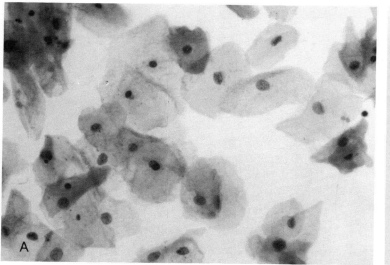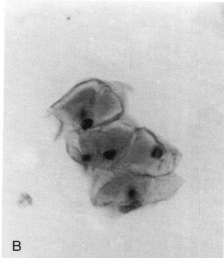

FIGURE 2-13. (*A*) Squamous cells of superficial and intermediate type in voided urine sediment. (*B*) Navicular cells from the voided urine sediment of a pregnant woman. Note the large, cytoplasmic deposits of glycogen, pushing the nucleus to the periphery (*A,B* × 560).

sessment and the value of the procedure is questionable (Koss, 1992).

Renal Tubular Cells

Cells derived from renal tubules sometimes may be recognized in the urinary sediment. These are small, usually poorly preserved cells with pyknotic, dark, condensed spherical nuclei and granular eosinophilic cytoplasm (Fig. 2-14). The tubular cells are easier to recognize when they form small clusters or casts (see Fig. 2-16A). The significance of the renal tubular cells in the sediment is not clear. Numerous tubular cells may appear in the urinary sediment after an intravenous pyelogram (IVP), and may be stained yellow by the dye. In other patients these cells may reflect a renal disorder. In patients with transplanted kidneys the presence of renal tubular cells in voided urine sediment may indicate rejection of the allograft (see p. 63).

Cells of Prostatic and Seminal Vesicle Origin

Occasionally cells of prostatic and seminal vesicle origin may be observed in the urinary sediment. Such cells, as a rule, accompany spermatozoa and their

precursor cells in specimens obtained after ejaculation or after prostatic massage. For description of these cells, see Chapter 7.

Macrophages

Macrophages or histiocytes belong to the family of cells with immune functions and are therefore most often observed in inflammatory reactions. The cells vary in sizes, may be mono- or multinucleated, and are characterized by the presence of fine cytoplasmic vacuoles that may contain phagocytised debris. Their appearance under various pathologic conditions will be discussed in the appropriate chapters.

Blood Cells

Erythrocytes

Erythrocytes are a frequent component of the urinary sediment. In the presence of clinical hematuria red blood cells dominate the sediment and may completely obscure the presence of other cells. However, small numbers of erythrocytes may occur, even in the absence of clinical hematuria. Thus, Freni and Freni-Titulaer (1977), using a careful urine collection technique, observed a few erythrocytes in all of 447 apparently healthy males; in 8.8% of this population, 10 or more erythrocytes per high-power field were ob-

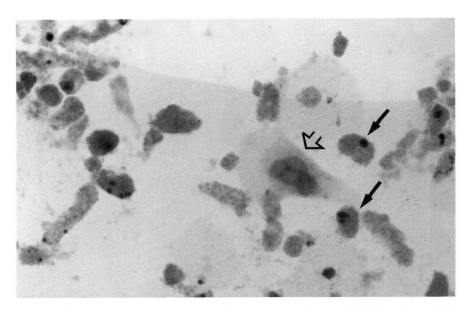

FIGURE 2-14.   Renal tubular cells—voided urine. Note the small cells with peripheral pyknotic nuclei and a granular cytoplasm (*arrows*). A multinucleated urothelial cell in the same field (*open arrow*) gives an idea of the size of the tubular cells (× 560).

served. Although it is customarily assumed that the presence of erythrocytes in the sediment indicates a pathological condition, this is frequently not the case, particularly if the sediment is well preserved, well stained, and carefully evaluated. In keeping with Freni's observations, in such material up to 10 erythrocytes per high-power field may be observed in the absence of documented disease.

MICROHEMATURIA

The significance of *microhematuria* has been extensively discussed in the literature. Microhematuria is usually defined as the presence of erythrocytes in the urinary sediment in the absence of gross hematuria. In voided urine sediments processed by Bales' method, which ensures optimal preservation of cells, the presence of scattered erythrocytes (from 1 to 10 per high-power field) is so common that little significance can be attributed to it. Most of the papers on this subject have relied on routine urinalysis, wherein unstained and unfixed urinary sediment was examined. Under these circumstances the preservation of the erythrocytes is far from optimal, and a substantial number of these cells must be present to be observed on microscopic examination. Even under these circumstances the follow-up of most patients is often completely negative and no lesions are found on extensive work-up. In a small proportion of these patients, stones, inflammatory events, or, rarely, tumors of the kidney or of the lower urinary tract will be observed.

The significance of microhematuria may depend on the patient's age and clinical symptoms. In earlier studies from the Mayo Clinic (Green et al., 1956; Carson et al., 1979), among elderly inpatients and patients specifically referred for urologic work–up, about 10% of the patients had bladder, renal, or prostatic tumors. In a study of a cohort of 1,000 young males (Froom et al., 1984) one tumor was observed. In 177 women followed for 10 years, Bard (1988) failed to observe any tumors. The summary of the key observations is shown in Table 2-1. Messing et al. (1987) pointed out that microhematuria is an event that may occur intermittently and may not occur at all in patients with significant disease.

How should one proceed with patients with microhematuria? As Carson et al. have shown, those patients with high-grade bladder tumors may have positive cytologic findings. Thus the first step in the work-up is cytologic examination of voided urine. A carefully performed cytologic examination will usually rule out a high-grade neoplastic lesion and may spare the patient tedious and costly invasive diagnostic procedures. If cytology is negative, further follow-up and work-up may depend on the clinical status of the patients. In older patients, tumors of the bladder (cystoscopy), kidney (intravenous pyelogram or ultrasound), and prostate (levels of prostate specific antigen [PSA] and ultrasound) should be ruled out. Otherwise, conservative follow-up is suggested (Mohr et al., 1986; Messing et al., 1987; Bard, 1988).

In the vast majority of patients, the source of eryth-

TABLE 2-1
Tumors in Patients With Microhematuria

Author	Patient Population	Neoplastic Disorders (Found)
Greene et al. (1955)	500 Mayo Clinic inpatients referred for urologic work-up	3 tumors of bladder (0.6%) 2 renal carcinomas (0.4%)
Carson et al. (1979)	200 Mayo Clinic patients referred for urologic work-up	22 tumors of bladder* (11%) 2 carcinomas of prostate (1%)
Froom et al. (1984)	1,000 young asymptomatic Air Force personnel, 387 with microhematuria	1 "transitional cell carcinoma" among patients with hematuria
Mohr et al. (1986)	2,312 general population with urinalysis; microhematuria in 13% of adult males and postmenopausal women	0.6% of patients with hematuria had bladder or renal tumors —all had other risk factors
Messing et al. (1987)	231 men over age 50 referred for urologic work-up; microhematuria intermittent during follow-up	3 bladder tumors (1.3%) 2 renal carcinomas (0.87%)
Bard (1988)	177 women with 10 years follow-up	None

*Urine cytology positive in 9 patients with flat carcinoma in situ

rocytes is never determined. The red blood cells are most likely derived from ruptured capillary vessels of various origins. Renal medical disorders are rarely asymptomatic. Blood chemistries and the determination of albumin in urine are the first step in the assessment of these patients.

RENAL VS. EXTRARENAL ORIGIN OF ERYTHROCYTES

The issue of differentiation of microhematuria due to parenchymal renal disease such as glomerulonephritis versus microhematuria of other origin has been extensively discussed, mainly in the European literature. Based on a review of the literature and their own experience, Rathert and Roth (1991) concluded that a morphologic examination of either very fresh or rapidly fixed voided urine sediment does allow the separation of the two cell types. Erythrocytes of renal origin were characterized by a dense periphery in the form of a double ring, and an "empty" center (see Fig. 4-20B in Chapter 4). Another manifestation of renal hematuria may be partial breakdown of erythrocytes with the appearance of small, irregular, oddly shaped cells. Erythrocytes of extrarenal origin may also form a double external ring but fail to show the empty center. Other extrarenal erythrocytes acquire features akin to poikilocytosis, with the periphery of the erythrocytes covered with spike-like excrescences.

A simpler approach was proposed by other authors (Mohammed et al., 1993; Van der Snoek et al., 1994). The presence of "dysmorphic" erythrocytes, *i.e.,* erythrocytes with abnormalities of shapes, was

considered as suggestive of a renal parenchymal disorder, whereas "isomorphic" erythrocytes (*i.e.,* red blood cells of normal shape) were considered to be representative of non-renal origin of hematuria. In Mohammed's work, using phase microscopy, the cut-off point of 20% of dysmorphic erythrocytes was shown to have a sensitivity of 90% and specificity of 100%. Van der Snoek used a cut-off point of 40%, achieving a sensitivity of 66.7%. It is evident from these data that "dysmorphic" erythrocytes are a common feature in the urinary sediment, regardless of the source of bleeding. An elaborate quantitative analysis of the proportion of such erythrocytes is necessary to identify the source of bleeding as either renal or extrarenal.

Leukocytes

Normal urine sediment contains very few leukocytes, usually lymphocytes, and, rarely, a few polymorphonuclear leukocytes. The presence of a large number of leukocytes may be suggestive of an important event.

NEUTROPHILIC POLYMORPHONUCLEAR LEUKOCYTES

A few neutrophils are fairly commonly seen in voided urine in the absence of significant clinical disease, particularly in women. Their origin is most likely in the genital tract. Larger numbers of these cells usually indicate an inflammatory process, discussed in Chapter 4, or a necrotic neoplastic event, discussed in Chapter 5.

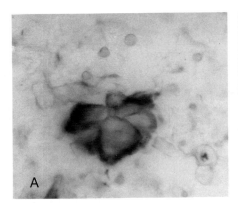 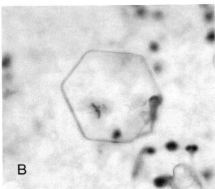

FIGURE 2-15.   (*A*) Uric acid crystal, voided urine (× 350). (*B*) Cystine crystal, voided urine (× 560).

LYMPHOCYTES

As a rule, lymphocytes are uncommonly seen in urinary sediment. Large numbers of lymphocytes may be observed in the presence of tumors, chronic inflammation, or in renal allograft rejection (see p. 63). If the lymphocytes are the dominant population in the sediment, the possibility of a tuberculosis, a leukemic process, or a malignant lymphoma must be raised (see Chaps. 4 and 5).

In a rare form of amaurotic familial idiocy, known as ceroid lipofuscinosis, Dolman et al. (1980) documented, by electron microscopy, the presence of the characteristic cytoplasmic inclusions in lymphocytes in spun urinary sediment. These authors proposed that the procedure can be used as a screening test for this disease.

Eosinophiluria

The presence of eosinophils, with their characteristic bilobate nuclei, is always indicative of a pathologic process. Such cells may be observed in allergic disorders, eosinophilic cystitis, which is usually seen as a consequence of prior bladder biopsies (Hellstrom et al., 1979), in the rare eosinophilic granulomas (Koss, 1975), or as a reaction to drugs (Nolan, 1986). Nolan suggested the use of Hansel's stain (methylene blue and eosin Y in methanol) for the diagnosis of drug-induced eosinophiluria.

NONCELLULAR COMPONENTS OF THE URINARY SEDIMENT

Crystals

Polygonal, transparent crystalline precipitations of *urates* are a common event in voided urine. Their presence is the result of a change in the pH of urine after collection and has no diagnostic significance. True *uric acid* crystals derived from urinary tract calculi are exceedingly rare (Fig. 2-15*A*). From time to time other crystals may be observed (Fig. 2-15*B*), but they are very rarely of diagnostic value. For a detailed description of crystals in the urinary sediment, see Naib (1985).

Contaminants

Voided urine, and sometimes specimens obtained by means of instrumentation, may contain crystals of surgical powder or cotton threads. Rarely other contaminants, such as the brown fungus *Alternaria,* derived from the water supply, may be observed (see Fig. 4-4*C*).

Renal Casts

Depending on the method of collection and processing of the urinary sediment, renal casts in variable numbers may be observed. They are best seen in unfixed urinary sediment but may also be seen in specimens fixed in 2% Carbowax in 70% ethanol and processed by the method of Bales (see p. 6).

The casts may be hyaline, granular, or cellular (Fig. 2-16). Hyaline casts are cylinders of variable length composed of a transparent, homogeneous protein precipitate (Fig. 2-16*B*). Granular casts are usually casts composed of the remnants of the granular cytoplasm of renal tubular cells that can no longer be identified. Cellular casts are usually composed of renal tubular cells (see Fig. 2-16*A;* compare to Fig. 2-14).

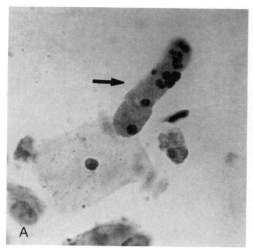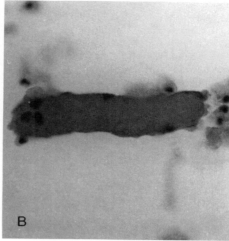

FIGURE 2-16. (*A*) Renal tubular cells forming a cast (*arrow*), voided urine. The small cells have a small, round, pyknotic nucleus and a granular cytoplasm. A mature, superficial squamous cell is adjacent. (*B*) Hyaline cast, voided urine (*A,B* × 560).

It is generally assumed in the medical literature that the presence of casts in the urinary sediment is an important indication of a serious disorder of the kidney or of organ rejection in renal transplant patients (see Chap. 4). However, using the Carbowax-alcohol fixative mentioned above, it became apparent that a small number of renal casts are commonly observed in healthy patients without any evidence of renal disease. It is likely that these casts represent a normal turnover of the renal epithelial tubular cells.

BIBLIOGRAPHY

General
Microhematuria
Eosinophiluria

General

Alm, P., and Colleen, S.: A histochemical and ultrastructural study of human urethral uroepithelium. Acta Path. Microbiol. Immunol. Scand., *90*, 103–111, 1982.
Alroy, J., Pauli, B. U., Weinstein, R. S., and Merk, F. B.: Association of asymmetric unit membrane plaque formation in the urinary bladder of adult humans with therapeutic radiation. Experientia, *33*, 1645–1647, 1977.
Bander, N. H.: Monoclonal antibodies: State of the art. J. Urol., *137*, 603–612, 1987.
Clark, B. G., and Gherardi, G. J.: Urethrotrigonitis or epidermidization of the trigone of the bladder. J. Urol. *87*, 545–548, 1962.
Cordon-Cardo, C., Bander, N. H., Fradet, Y., Finstad, C. L., Whitmore, W. F., Lloyd, K. O., Oettgen, H. F., Melamed, M. R., and Old, L. J.: Immunoanatomic dissection of the human urinary tract by monoclonal anti-

bodies. J. Histochem. Cytochem., *32*, 1035–1040, 1984.
Cordon-Cardo, C., Finstad, C. L., Bander, N., and Melamed, M. R.: Immunoanatomic distribution of cytostructural and tissue-associated antigens in the human urinary tract. Am. J. Path., *126*, 269–284, 1987.
Dolman, C. L., McLeod, P. M., and Chang, E. C.: Lymphocytes and urine in ceroid lipofuscinosis. Arch. Pathol. Lab. Med., *104*, 487–490, 1980.
Dorfman, H. D., and Monis, B.: Mucin-containing inclusions in multinucleated giant cells and transitional epithelial cells of urine: Cytochemical observations on exfoliated cells. Acta Cytol., *8*, 293–301, 1964.
Farsund, T.: Preparation of bladder mucosa for micro-flow fluorometry. Virch. Arch. B (Cell Path), *16*, 35–42, 1974.
Foot, N. C.: Glandular metaplasia of the epithelium of the urinary tract. South. Med., *37*, 137–142, 1944.
Herz, F., Gazivoda, P., Papenhausen, P. R., Katsuyama, J., and Koss, L. G.: Normal human urothelial cells in culture. Subculture procedure, flow cytometric and chromosomal analyses. Lab. Invest., *53*, 571–574, 1985.
Herz, F., Schermer, H. F., and Koss, L. G.: Short term culture of epithelial cells from urine of adults. Proc. Soc. Exp. Biol. Med., *161*, 153–157, 1979.
Hicks, R. M.: Fine structure of the transitional epithelium of rat ureter. J. Cell Biol., *26*, 25–48, 1966.
Hicks, R. M.: The function of the Golgi complex in transitional epithelium. Synthesis of the thick cell membrane. J. Cell Biol., *30*, 623–643, 1966.
Hicks, R. M.: The mammalian urinary bladder: An accommodating organ. Biol. Rev., *50*, 215–246, 1975.
Hicks, R. M.: The permeability of rat transitional epithelium. Keratinization and the barrier to water. J. Cell Biol., *28*, 21–31, 1966.
Hicks, R. M., and Newman, J.: Scanning electron micros-

copy of urinary sediment. *In*: Koss, L. G., and Coleman, D. V. (Eds.): Advances in Clinical Cytology. vol. 2. pp. 135–161. New York, Masson, 1984.

Hicks, R. M., Wakefield, J. S. J., and Chowaniec, J.: Evaluation of a new model to detect bladder carcinogens or co-carcinogens: Results obtained with saccharin, cyclamate and cyclophosphamide. Chem. Biol. Interact., *11*, 225–233, 1975.

Holmquist, N. D.: Diagnostic Cytology of Urinary Tract. Basel, S. Karger, 1977.

Ito, N., Hirose, M., Shirai, T., Tsuda, H., Nakanishi, K., and Fukushima, S.: Lesions of the urinary bladder epithelium in 125 autopsy cases. Acta Pathol. Jpn., *31*, 545–557, 1981.

Jacob, J., Ludgate, C. M., Forde, J., and Tulloch, W. S.: Recent observations on the ultrastructure of human urothelium. 1. Normal bladder of elderly subjects. Cell Tiss. Res., *543*, 543–560, 1978.

Kittredge, W. E., and Brannan, W.: Cystitis glandularis. J. Urol., *81*, 419–430, 1959.

Koss, L. G.: The asymmetric unit membrane of the epithelium of the urinary bladder of the rat. An electron microscopic study of a mechanism of epithelium maturation and function. Lab. Invest., *21*, 154–168, 1969.

Koss, L. G.: Tumors of the Urinary Bladder. Fascicle 11, 2nd Series, Atlas of Tumor Pathology. Washington, D.C. Armed Forces Institute of Pathology, 1975. Supplement, 1985.

Koss, L. G.: Diagnostic Cytology and Its Histopathologic Bases. 4th Ed. Philadelphia, J. B. Lippincott, 1992.

Koss, L. G.: Some ultrastructural aspects of experimental and human carcinoma of the bladder. Cancer Res., *37*, 2824–2835, 1977.

Lencioni, L.: L'Uro-cytogramme. *In* Diagnostic Cyto-Hormonal, à partir du sediment urinaire. 3rd Ed. Buenos Aires, Maloine, S. A. (Ed.): Editorial Medica Panamericana, 1972.

Lencioni, L. J., Amezaga, L. A. M., Alonso, C., Antonio, L., and DeCarmargo, H.: Urocytogram and pregnancy. II. Correlation with fetal condition at birth in high risk pregnancies. Acta Cytol., *17*, 125–127, 1973.

Lin, J. H., Wu, X. R., Krebich, G., and Sun, T. T.: Precursor sequences, processing, and urothelium-specific expression of a major 15-KD protein subunit of assymetric unit membrane. J. Biol. Chem., *269*, 1–10, 1994.

Martin, B. F.: Cell replacement and differentiation in transitional epithelium; a histological and autoradiographic study of the guinea-pig bladder and ureter. J. Anat., *112*, 433–455, 1972.

Morse, H. D.: The etiology and pathology of pyelitis cystica, ureteritis cystica, and cystitis cystica. Am. J. Pathol., *4*, 33–50, 1928.

Naib, Z. M.: Exfoliative Cytopathology. 3rd Ed. Boston, Little, Brown, 1985.

Newman, J., and Hicks, R. M.: Surface ultrastructure of the epithelia lining the normal human lower urinary tract. Br. J. Exp. Pathol., *62*, 232–251, 1981.

Pund, E. R., Yount, H. A., and Blumberg, J. M.: Variations in morphology of urinary bladder epithelium. Special reference to cystitis glandularis and carcinomas. J. Urol., *68*, 242–251, 1952.

Rathert, P., and Roth, S. E.: Urinzytologie. Praxis und Atlas. 2nd. Ed. Berlin, Springer Verlag, 1991.

Ro, J. Y., Ayala, A. G., and El Nagger, A.: Muscularis mucosae of urinary bladder: Importance for staging and treatment. Am. J. Surg. Path. *11*, 668–673, 1987.

Shokri-Tabibzadeh, S., Herz, F., and Koss, L. G.: Fine structure of cultured epithelial cells derived from voided urine of normal adults. Virchows Arch. [Cell Pathol], *39*, 41–48, 1982.

Streitz, J. M.: Squamous epithelium in the female trigone. J. Urol., *90*, 62–66, 1963.

Tyler, D. E.: Stratified squamous epithelium in the vesical trigone and urethra: Findings correlated with the menstrual cycle and age. Am. J. Anat., *111*, 319–325, 1962.

Walker, B. E.: Polyploidy and differentiation in the transitional epithelium of mouse urinary bladder. Chromosoma, *9*, 105–118, 1958.

Ward, G. K., Stewart, S. S., Price, G. B., and Mackillop, W. J.: Cellular heterogeneity in normal human urothelium: An analysis of optical properties and lectin binding. J. Histochem and Cytochem, *34*, 841–846, 1986.

Wiener, D. P., Koss, L. G., Sablay, B., and Freed, S. Z.: The prevalence and significance of Brunn's nests, cystitis cystica and squamous metaplasia in normal bladders. J. Urol., *122*, 317–321, 1979.

Wu, X. R., Manabe, M., Yu, J., and Sun, T. T.: Large scale purification and immunolocalisation of bovine uroplakins I, II, and III. J. Biol. Chem., *265*, 19170–19179, 1990.

Wu, X. R., and Sun, T. T.: Molecular cloning of a 47-KD tissue-specific and differentiation dependent urothelial cell surface glycoprotein. J. Cell Sci., *106*, 31–43, 1993.

Yu, J., Manabe, M., and Sun, T. T.: Identification of an 85–100-KD glycoprotein as a cell surface marker for an advanced stage of urothelial differentiation: Association with inter-plaque ('hinge') area. Epith. Cell Biol., *1*, 4–12, 1992.

Yu, J., Manabe, M., Wu, X. R., Xu, C., Surya, B., and Sun, T. T.: Uroplakin I: A 27-KD protein associated with the asymmetric unit membrane of mammalian urothelium. J. of Cell Biology, *111*, 1207–1216, 1990.

Microhematuria

Bard, R. H.: The significance of asymptomatic hematuria in women and its economic implications—A ten-year study. Arch. Int. Med., *148*, 2629–2632, 1988.

Carson, I. C. C., Segura, J. W., and Greene, L. F.: Clinical importance of microhematuria. J.A.M.A., *241*, 149–150, 1979.

Freni, S. C., and Freni-Titulaer, L. W. J.: Microhematuria found by mass screening of apparently healthy males. Acta Cytol., *21*, 421–423, 1977.

Froom, P., Ribak, J., and Benbassat, J.: Significance of microhaematuria in young adults. Br. Med. J., *288*, 20–22, 1984.

Golin, A. L., and Howard, R. S.: Asymptomatic microscopic hematuria. J. Urol., *124*, 389–391, 1980.

Greene, L. F., O'Shaughnessy, E. J., and Hendricks, E. D.:

Study of five hundred patients with asymptomatic microhematuria. J.A.M.A., *161*, 610–613, 1956.

Messing, E. M., Young, T. B., Hunt, V. B., Emoto, S. E., and Wehbie, J. M.: The significance of asymptomatic microhematuria in men 50 or more years old: Findings of a home screening study using urinary dipsticks. J. Urol., *137*, 919–922, 1987.

Mohammad, K. S., Bdesha, A. S., Snell, M. E., Witherow, R. O., and Coleman, D. V.: Phase contrast microscopic examination of urinary erythrocytes to localize source of bleeding: An overlooked technique? J. Clin. Path. *46*, 642–645, 1993.

Mohr, D. N., Offord, K. P., Owen, R. A., and Melton, I. L. J.: Asymptomatic microhematuria and urologic disease. J.A.M.A., *256*, 224–229, 1986.

Van der Snoek, B. F., Hoitsma, A. J., Van Weel, C., and Koene, R. A.: Dysmorphic erythrocytes in urinary sediment in differentiating urological from nephrological causes of hematuria (in Dutch). Nederlands Tijdschrift voor Geneeskunde, *138*, 721–726, 1994.

Eosinophiluria

Hellstrom, H. R., Davis, B. K., and Shonnard, J. W.: Eosinophilic cystitis. A study of 16 cases. Am. J. Clin. Pathol., *72*, 777–784, 1979.

Koss, L. G.: Diagnostic Cytology and Its Histopathologic Bases. 4th Ed. Philadelphia, J. B. Lippincott, 1992.

Madersbacher, H., and Bartsch, G.: Eosinophile Infiltrate der Harnblase. Urologia Internat., *27*, 149–159, 1972.

Nolan, I. C. R., Anger, M. S., and Kelleher, S. P.: Eosinophiluria—A new method of detection and definition of the clinical spectrum. N. Engl. J. Med., *315*, 1516–1519, 1986.

Wenzel, J. E., Greene, L. F., and Harris, L. E.: Eosinophilic cystitis. J. Pediatr., *64*, 746–749, 1964.

CHAPTER 3

The Makeup of the Urinary Sediment According to Collection Technique

The collection techniques described in Chapter 1 have a significant effect on the makeup of the urinary sediment. A thorough knowledge of the differences among the techniques used to obtain specimens is very important in the diagnostic interpretation.

VOIDED URINE

Cytologic Makeup of the Sediment of Normal Voided Urine

Spontaneously voided urine from normal patients contains relatively few urothelial cells (Color Plate 3-1*A*). These cells may occur singly or may desquamate in clusters. Smaller cells from the deeper layers of the epithelium are readily distinguished from the much larger umbrella cells (see Fig. 2-7 in Chapter 2). In voided urine, the nuclei of the small urothelial cells have a well-preserved nuclear membrane, are spherical in configuration, are pale and homogeneous or dark-staining, and may contain visible chromocenters (Fig. 3-1*A*). The cytoplasm is scanty, often frayed at the border, and faintly basophilic. Multinucleated umbrella cells are rare in spontaneously voided urine, except after diagnostic and therapeutic procedures (Fig. 3-1*B*).

Clusters of urothelial cells may be observed in voided urine in the absence of disease. The clusters are commonly observed after vigorous palpation of the bladder, catheterization, or diagnostic procedures.

They are composed of variable numbers of cells, from three or four to several hundred. Small clusters are usually flat, and the cells contained therein have the same characteristics as the isolated cells. Larger clusters may be three-dimensional and are often rounded (papillary) or oddly shaped, sometimes suggestive of fragments of papillary tumors (Fig. 3-2). In larger clusters the makeup of the individual cells may be difficult to determine. Nonetheless, the nuclei in such clusters are usually of monotonous size and show no hyperchromasia. *The presence of clusters should not be interpreted as indicating the presence of a pathological process in the bladder, particularly not the presence of a papillary tumor.* This issue will be discussed again in Chapter 4 in reference to lithiasis and in Chapter 5 in reference to papillary tumors.

Voided urine may contain a substantial number of squamous cells that often outnumber urothelial cells, particularly in female patients. Occasional macrophages, erythrocytes, and rare leukocytes complete the cytologic picture. (The issue of microhematuria was discussed in Chapter 2.) Voided urine may also contain cells showing a wide variety of benign abnormalities, discussed in Chapter 4.

Cell Preservation in Voided Urine

Because of low pH and high osmolarity, the preservation of epithelial cells in voided urine samples is usually satisfactory, particularly if the specimen is

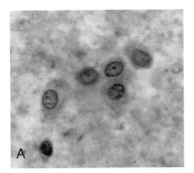

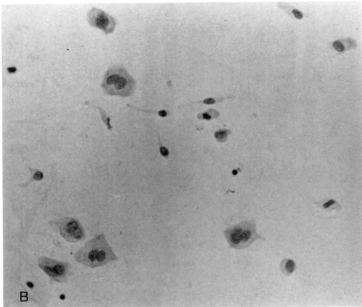

FIGURE 3-1. (*A*) Voided urine. Small urothelial cells with pale nuclei. (*B*) Voided urine sediment after catheterization. The sediment contains several binucleated superficial urothelial cells and a few scattered elongated small cells from the deeper layers of the urothelium. There was no evidence of any disorder of the lower urinary tract (*A* × 560; *B* × 350).

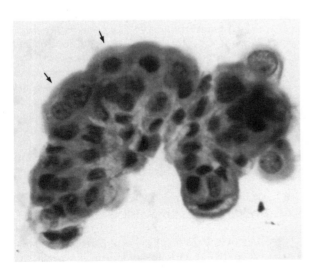

FIGURE 3-2. A detached papillary cluster of urothelial cells in voided urine after catheterization. The rounded umbrella cells are seen on the surface (*arrows*). There was no evidence of disease (× 560).

collected in a fixative (see p. 3). A common exception to this rule is the sediment obtained as a "first morning urine" which may contain a great many poorly preserved cells that may be difficult to interpret. It is for this reason that the optimal urine collection should be the second morning specimen (see p. 4). In the presence of inflammatory processes, described in Chapter 4, significant changes in the morphology of the cells may take place.

CYTOLOGIC MAKEUP OF BLADDER WASHINGS

Bladder washings display a full panorama of cells of urothelial origin. The superficial umbrella cells are usually well represented, as are cells from the deeper layers of the urothelium. Many of the cells form clusters, sometimes composed of several hundred cells. Of special significance is the excellent display of the nuclear features, described in Chapter 2. Specifically, the presence of multiple nuclei of variable sizes is common in the superficial cells, as is the presence of chromocenters and, occasionally, nucleoli (see Figs. 2-7 through 2-9). All of these features are normal. The cells from the deeper layers of the urothelium are often oddly shaped because of desmosomal attachments that tend to pull the cytoplasm (see Fig. 2-10). Cells of columnar shape, columnar cells with clear cytoplasm suggestive of mucus production, and sometimes ciliated cells may be observed. Specimens of bladder washings offer the best opportunity to study the makeup of urothelial cells.

The advantages of bladder washings are the clean population of epithelial cells, free of contaminants, that are suitable for microscopic examination. Although some observers claim that the cytologic diagnosis of bladder tumors is easier and more accurate than that of voided urine, I am not persuaded that this is the case. Further, bladder washings cannot be repeated in case of doubt as is the case with voided urine.

Cells secured by bladder washings can also be used in a number of experimental procedures such as image analysis, flow cytometry, molecular biology, and immunocytochemistry (see Chapters 9 through 11).

CYTOLOGIC MAKEUP OF NORMAL SPECIMENS OBTAINED BY RETROGRADE CATHETERIZATION (COLOR PLATE 3-1, *B THROUGH F*)

During retrograde catheterization the tip of the catheter passes through the narrow lumen of the ureter, scraping its lining epithelium. Consequently, retrograde catheterization specimens are characterized by a very rich population of urothelial cells occurring singly and in clusters of various sizes. The single cells are predominantly the mono- and multinucleated superficial umbrella cells, the latter containing from 2 to 50 or even more nuclei (see Chapter 2). The cell clusters may be of rounded or papillary configuration, or may be oddly shaped. The clusters are usually multilayered, hence the microscopic analysis of individual cells is often very difficult, except at the periphery, where the features of the normal urothelial cells may be recognized.

In my experience the clusters of normal cells and the multinucleated umbrella cells, obtained by retrograde catheterization, are the most common source of diagnostic errors. Such cell clusters are often interpreted as representing a papillary tumor.

CYTOLOGIC MAKEUP OF SMEARS OBTAINED BY BRUSHING

As is the case with retrograde catheterization, the brush forcibly removes large sheets of urothelial cells from the surface of the ureters on its way to and from the renal pelvis, often resulting in a complete denudation of the ureteral surface (see Color Plate 3-1*B* through *F*). Such large clusters display the enormous variety of urothelial cells and are often mistaken for fragments of papillary tumors (see Chap. 6). Many an unnecessary nephrectomy and ureterectomy has been performed as a result of such erroneous diagnoses. For the same reason brushings virtually never allow a differential diagnosis of stones. On rare occasions brushing may allow a *localization of a high-grade tumor* in the renal pelves or ureter (see Chap. 6).

EFFECTS OF INSTRUMENTATION

Catheterization of the bladder, retrograde catheterization of the ureter and renal pelves, and particularly brushings virtually always result in removal of urothelial cell clusters that may be mistaken for fragments of urothelial papillary tumors. This caveat is particularly important in the presence of spherical cell clusters. Another source of error is the multinucleated umbrella cells with large nuclei and nucleoli that are readily mistaken for cancer cells. As has been discussed in Chapter 2, a thorough knowledge of the great variability of normal urothelial cells is an essential prerequisite in the interpretation of cytologic specimens from the lower urinary tract, with special attention to cell clusters.

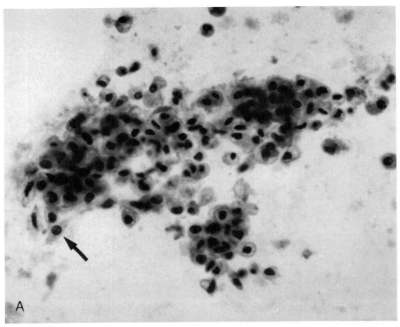

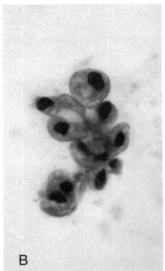

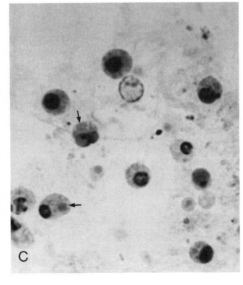

FIGURE 3-3. Ileal bladder urine. (*A*) There is a large cluster of small, predominantly spherical cells of intestinal origin with dark, hyperchromatic nuclei. The cytoplasm is generally clear. An occasional columnar cell may be noted (*arrow*). (*B*) Higher power view of a cluster of intestinal cells with vacuolated cytoplasm. In *C,* the common degenerative events are shown: the cytoplasm is granular or vacuolated and poorly preserved and often contains nonspecific eosinophilic inclusions (*small arrows*). The nuclei are spherical and pyknotic. A circular remnant of a dead cell is also seen (*A* × 350; *B,C* × 560).

CYTOLOGIC MAKEUP OF ILEAL BLADDER URINE

Ileal bladder urine is used in monitoring patients after cystectomy for cancer (see Chap. 5). The ileal urine normally contains a rich population of poorly preserved intestinal epithelial cells. Sometimes these cells preserve their columnar configuration and their mucus-producing, transparent cytoplasm. Such cells usually have a small, spherical, dark nucleus located toward the periphery. More often, however, the intestinal cells are rounded, have a vacuolated or granular

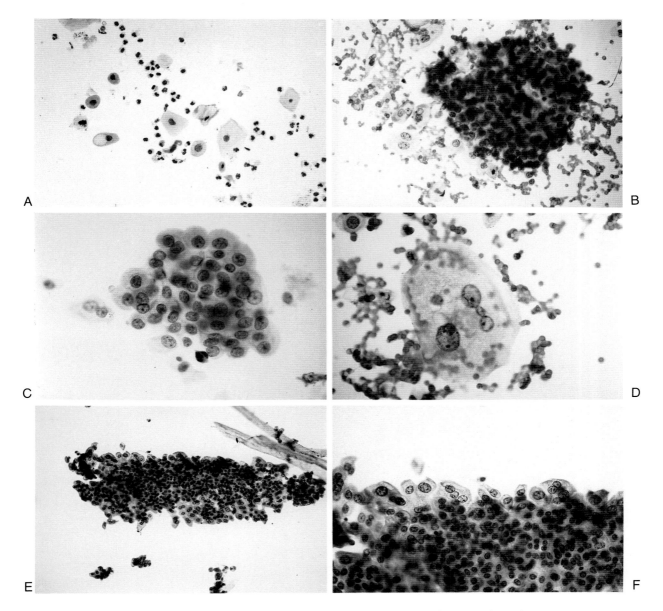

Color Plate 3-1. Normal cellular components of voided urine and retrograde washings or brushings. (*A*) Voided urine. The sediment contains scattered urothelial cells, squamous cells and leukocytes. The latter are suggestive of an inflammatory process. (*B–F*) Cells from retrograde washings or brushings in the absence of disease. (*B*) A large cluster of densely packed small urothelial cells. (*C*) Cluster of somewhat larger urothelial cells. (*D*) A very large, multinucleated umbrella cell. (*E* and *F*) Low- and high-power view of a densely packed sheet of small urothelial cells. The normal component cells may be seen at the periphery of the cluster (Original magnification: *A,B,F* × 100; *C,D* × 160; *E* × 40, enlarged about × 2.5).

TABLE 3-1
Principal Advantages and Disadvantages of Various Cytologic Methods of Investigation of the Lower Urinary Tract

Method	Advantages	Disadvantages	Remarks
Voided urine	Efficient method for diagnosis of high-grade tumors (including carcinoma in situ) of bladder, ureters, and renal pelves. The method is of value in monitoring patients with locally treated tumors and patients with renal transplant. Examination can be repeated without harming the patient.	The findings are not consistent, and three or more specimens should be examined for optimal results. Sources of error (see Chap. 1, 3, and 4) must be known.	All methods usually fail in the identification of low grade tumors. For exceptions, see Chapter 5.
Catheterized urine	Same as voided urine. Less contamination with cells of female genital tract.	Same as voided urine.	
Bladder washings	Same as voided urine, but results confined to bladder. The diagnosis of high-grade tumors is sometimes easier. Ideal medium for DNA measurements.	The method is poorly tolerated by ambulatory patients, particularly males. Optimal results may require cystoscopy.	Fragments of low-grade tumors may sometimes be recognized, but beware of errors.
Retrograde brushings	Occasionally useful in the identification and localization of high grade tumors of ureters and renal pelves.	A major source of diagnostic errors (see Chapter 2). The value of the procedure in the differential diagnosis of space-occupying lesions of ureters or renal pelves is very low.	
Drip urine collected from ureters	Efficient method of localization of high grade tumors of ureters and renal pelves.	A time-consuming procedure.	Separate catheters must be used for each side to avoid contamination.
Ileal bladder urine	Efficient in the diagnosis of metachronous high grade tumors of ureters and renal pelves after cystectomy for bladder cancer. Occasional primary lesions of ileal conduit may be observed.	Same as voided urine. Knowledge of cytologic presentation is essential.	A mandatory follow-up procedure after cystectomy for bladder cancer.

degenerating cytoplasm, often containing nonspecific eosinophilic cytoplasmic inclusions (see Chap. 4), and fragmented or pyknotic dark nuclei (Fig. 3-3). In such specimens cancer cells are readily recognized (see Chap. 6).

The advantages and disadvantages of the various collection techniques are summarized in Table 3-1.

BIBLIOGRAPHY

Harris, M. J., Schwinn, C. P., Morrow, J. W., Gray, R. L., and Brownell, B. M.: Exfoliative cytology of the urinary bladder irrigation specimen. Acta Cytol. *15*, 385–399, 1971.
Koss, L. G.: Diagnostic Cytology and Its Histopathologic Bases. 4th Ed. Philadelphia, J. B. Lippincott, 1992.

CHAPTER 4

Cytologic Manifestations of Benign Disorders Affecting Cells of the Lower Urinary Tract

A number of benign disorders described in this chapter may have a significant impact on the cytology of the urinary tract by causing cell changes that may either mimic or conceal the presence of malignant tumors. These disorders are described in this chapter, not necessarily in order of their importance but according to their etiology.

INFLAMMATORY DISORDERS

Bacterial Agents

A broad variety of bacterial agents may affect the epithelium of the urinary tract. The principal culprits are the colibacteria and other gram-negative rods. Bacterial infection may be either acute or chronic. The urinary tract may also be the portal of entry of Gram-negative organisms causing septicemia. Bacterial agents rarely cause significant abnormalities of cells in the urinary sediment.

Pyelonephritis

The clinical manifestations of the inflammatory disorders affecting the kidney and the renal pelves usually are high fever and flank pain. Sometimes the differential diagnosis of pyelonephritis includes renal pelvic calculi or tumors. Cytologic techniques are practically never used in the diagnosis of acute or chronic pyelonephritis.

The urinary sediment may contain a large number of polymorphonuclear leukocytes, necrotic material, and sometimes renal casts composed of leukocytes and renal tubular cells.

Cystitis

Acute cystitis is usually associated with high fever and major clinical symptoms that very rarely require confirmatory tissue biopsies or cytologic examination. The disruption of the mucus layer contributes to bacterial action (Cornish et al., 1988). Epithelial necrosis and ulcerations may occur. In the rare cases of cystitis when voided urine is studied, the urinary sediment may contain numerous desquamated urothelial cells, necrotic material and inflammatory cells, predominantly polymorphonuclear leukocytes (Fig. 4-1). It must be stressed that marked necrosis and inflammatory cells may also occur in the presence of necrotic tumors, particularly squamous carcinomas, as discussed in Chapter 5.

Chronic cystitis appears to affect women more often than men, usually as a consequence of childbearing or obstetrical trauma. In men chronic cystitis may be observed in outlet obstruction such as urethral stricture or prostatic enlargement.

Several histologic changes may be observed in chronic cystitis, caused by common bacterial pathogens: the wall of the bladder may be infiltrated with lymphocytes and macrophages; the epithelium may show a nonspecific hyperplasia; ulcerations of the epithelium may be observed and may lead to regenerative epithelial atypia.

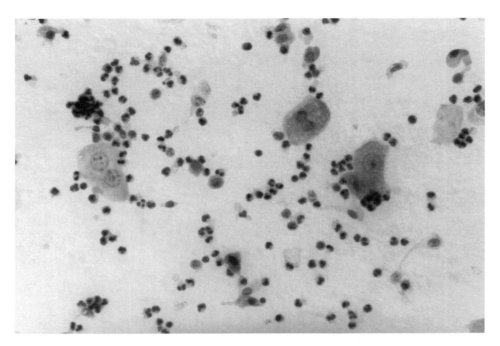

FIGURE 4-1. Voided urine sediment in acute cystitis. The background of the preparation contains numerous polymorphonuclear leukocytes and a scattering of benign urothelial cells, some of which are binucleated and some are necrotic (× 350).

The urinary sediment in such patients is usually characterized by a background composed of inflammatory cells and macrophages (Fig. 4-2). Erythrocytes are commonly seen. The urothelial cells may be abundant, albeit poorly preserved, occasionally forming small clusters. The cytoplasm may be granular and may contain vacuoles. The cytoplasm of such degenerated cells often shows spherical, eosinophilic inclusions that are of no diagnostic significance (see Fig. 4-2, *inset,* Color Plate 4-1*E,* and p. 55). Although some nuclear abnormalities may be observed in the form of slight nuclear enlargement and slight hyperchromasia, the contour of the nuclei is usually regular and the chromatin texture is usually finely granular and lacks the coarse granularity characteristic of urothelial cancer cells (see Chap. 5). Necrosis of urothelial cells in the form of nuclear pyknosis and marked cytoplasmic vacuolization is not uncommon. Very large sheets of urothelial cells may be observed in ulcerative cystitis.

Hunner's Ulcer

A form of chronic cystitis in women that is of unknown etiology and particularly unpleasant and difficult to treat is the *interstitial cystitis,* associated with chronic ulceration, known as Hunner's ulcer. I studied a number of voided urine sediments in women

with Hunner's ulcer. The findings were completely nonspecific and shed no light whatever on the etiology of this mysterious disease.

Inflammatory Pseudopolyp

Chronic cystitis of long duration may result in a protrusion of bladder epithelium around a core of inflamed stroma, resulting in a formation of an inflammatory pseudopolyp (Fig. 4-3*A*). The sediment in such cases shows atypical urothelial cells with vacuolated cytoplasm (Fig. 4-3*B,C*). Multinucleated cells, presumably degenerated umbrella cells, may also occur (Fig. 4-3*D*). The nuclei of urothelial cells, although somewhat enlarged, show a beaded nuclear membrane and a transparent center, most likely as evidence of impending cell death. The background of the preparations shows numerous inflammatory cells.

Eosinophilic Cystitis

Chronic cystitis with eosinophils as the dominant inflammatory cells may be sometimes observed in women and children with allergic disorders. In men, the disease has been observed after previous biopsies of the bladder; the eosinophilic reaction is thought to represent an autoimmune disorder (Hellstrom et al., 1979). Very rarely, an eosinophilic granuloma may occur. The latter is a space-occupying lesion that may

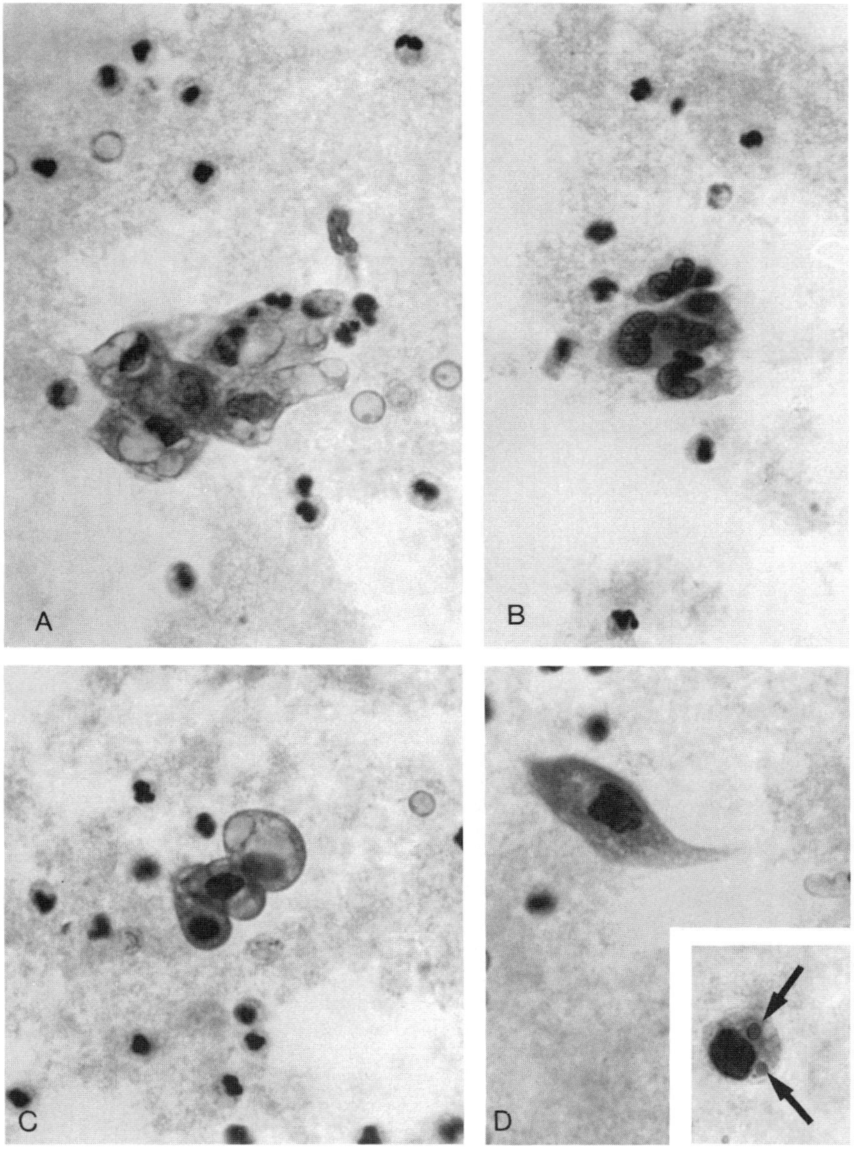

FIGURE 4-2. Voided urine sediment in severe chronic cystitis. (*A*) A cluster of urothelial cells with vacuolated cytoplasm in a background of leukocytes and erythrocytes. (*B*) A small cluster of urothelial cells with small, dark, hyperchromatic nuclei with a smooth nuclear membrane. (*C*) A small cluster of urothelial cells with vacuolated cytoplasm and spherical, hyperchromatic nuclei. (*D*) A poorly preserved umbrella cell, with multiple, small, spherical hyperchromatic nuclei mimicking a cancer cell. This is one of the rare events in inflammatory states that may be confused with cancer. (*Inset*) A small urothelial cell with nuclear changes consistent with a human polyomavirus infection (see text and Fig 4-8), containing two eosinophilic cytoplasmic inclusions (*arrows*) (*A–D* and *inset* × 560).

involve the bladder and the adjacent ureters and resembles identical lesions in more customary locations (Koss, 1975). Eosinophilic polymorphonuclear leukocytes with the characteristic bilobate nuclei may be observed in the urinary sediment in such cases. For further comments on eosinophiluria, see Chapter 2, p. 34.

Tuberculosis

Until recently, granulomatous inflammation of the lower urinary tract secondary to infection with *Mycobacterium tuberculosis* was exceedingly rare in the industrialized countries. Infrequent cases of cytologic findings in tuberculous cystitis were reported (Kapila and Verma, 1984; Piscioli et al., 1985). Two recent events have changed this situation. The spread of the acquired immunodeficiency syndrome (AIDS) has contributed significantly to revival of tuberculosis as a public health problem in the United States and in Western Europe. AIDS patients, with their low resistance to infection, may harbor not only the human variant of the organisms but also other, hitherto exceptional variants such as *Mycobacterium avium*. The second reason has to do with immunotherapy of cer-

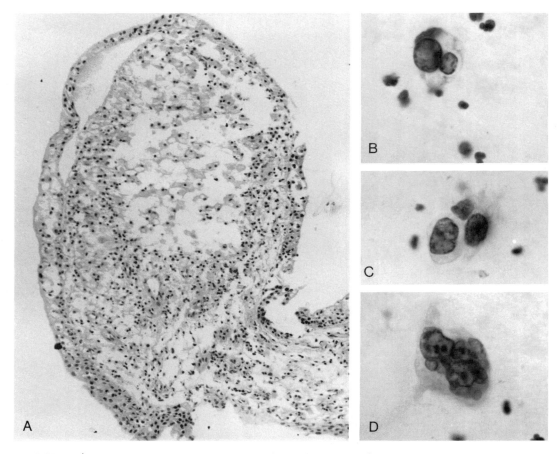

FIGURE 4-3. Inflammatory pseudopolyp in the bladder of an 86-year-old man with chronic cystitis of long duration. The histologic section (*A*) shows a polypoid lesion lined by a thin layer of urothelium surrounding a core of inflamed and edematous connective tissue. (*B,C,D*) Somewhat atypical urothelial cells from voided urine. Note the vacuolated cytoplasm and the nuclei with a "beaded" nuclear membrane and a transparent center. In *D* the multinucleated cell is most likely a macrophage (*A* × 80, *B,C,D* × 560).

tain forms of bladder cancer, notably flat carcinoma in situ, using the attenuated bovine mycobacterium known as bacille Calmette-Guérin (BCG) (see p. 59). In such patients the urinary sediment usually shows inflammatory cells and may contain fragments of tubercles in the form of clusters of elongated, carrot-shaped epithelioid cells, sometimes accompanied by multinucleated giant cells of Langhans' type. Similar findings have been reported by Piscioli et al. from patients with tuberculosis of the bladder (Color Plate 4-1*A*).

Piscioli et al. also pointed out that significant abnormalities of the urothelium may occur in such patients, resulting in significant atypias of urothelial cells in voided urine sediment. Although most atypias were transient and were attributed to reversible urothelial

hyperplasia, in some of the patients the level of urothelial cell atypia was sufficiently severe to warrant biopsies of bladder epithelium. In some of these patients, epithelial cell changes akin to carcinoma in situ were observed. In the absence of long-term follow-up, the significance of these changes is obscure. For further discussion of cell abnormalities in BCG treated patients, see Chapter 5, p. 126.

Actinomycosis

It is theoretically possible that *actinomycosis*, which may be observed in women wearing intrauterine contraceptive devices (IUDs), may occur in urinary sediment as the infection spreads from the uterus to the pelvic organs (Koss, 1992). The organism, which is now considered to be a bacterium rather

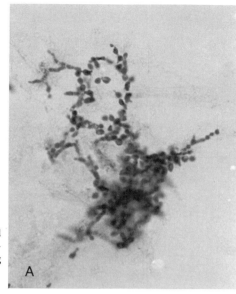
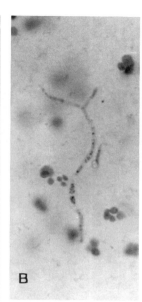

FIGURE 4-4. *Candida albicans* in voided urine sediment. (*A*) Yeast form of the fungus (conidia). (*B*) Filamentous, branching form of the fungus (pseudohyphae). (*B* × 560).

than a fungus, forms tightly bound balls of slender filaments with bulbous terminal swellings. The discovery of *Actinomyces* may be of clinical significance as it may indicate abscess formation in the pelvis.

Fungal Agents

Some fungal agents may affect the lower urinary tract, mainly the urinary bladder. Chief among these is *Candida albicans* (formerly *Monilia*). Although candidiasis of the lower urinary tract may occasionally be observed in the absence of any known disease state, it is most commonly observed in pregnant women, diabetics, and patients with impaired immunity. The latter group includes patients undergoing chemotherapy for cancer, bone marrow transplant recipients, and, perhaps most importantly, patients with AIDS. Moniliasis may be the first manifestation of infection with the human immunodeficiency virus. Unusual complications of candidiasis include the obstruction of ureters and septicemia.

The fungus is usually recognized in the urinary sediment in two forms: the yeast form, composed of small oval bodies, and the pseudohyphae form, characterized by oblong, often branching, non-encapsulated filaments (Fig. 4-4). The diagnosis of moniliasis in urine requires a rapid clinical evaluation of the patient.

Other fungi are uncommon. North American blastomycosis of the genitourinary tract has been observed, and the organism *Blastomyces dermatitidis* has been identified in the urinary sediment of the

infected patients as a part of the clinical syndrome. The yeast form of the fungi appears as spherical structures 8 to 15 μm in diameter, provided with a refractile, thick wall. A single spherical bud, attached to the mother organism by a flat surface, is characteristic of the fungus (Fig. 4-5*A*). Although the organisms can be recognized in any ordinary laboratory stain, special stains, such as Gomori's silver stain that stains the capsule of the fungus jet black, are sometimes helpful in identification.

Aspergillosis, a common opportunistic fungus infection in debilitated or immunosuppressed patients, has not been observed by me in urinary sediment. Because the infection may involve the female genital tract, the possibility that the organism will appear in the urinary sediment of such patients cannot be ruled out. The organism is usually recognized by its hyphae, which are long, encapsulated septated filaments, branching at an angle of 45 degrees (Fig. 4-5*B*). The fruiting head of the organism sometimes may be observed. A similar organism, *Mucormycosis,* has not been recognized in the urinary sediment so far.

A fungus of the species *Alternaria* is a common laboratory contaminant. Its oval, brown, septated spores are easy to recognize (see Fig. 4-5*C*).

Viral Agents (Table 4-1)

There are several important viral agents that cause significant morphologic abnormalities in urothelial cells, some of which may be confused with a malignant tumor. The dominant feature of viral infections is

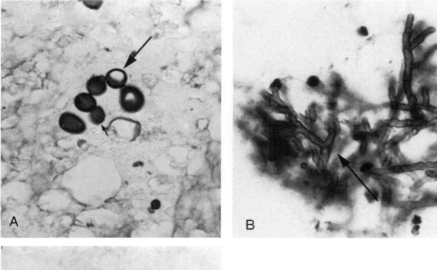

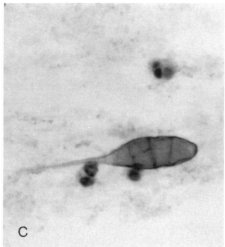

FIGURE 4-5. (*A*) North American blastomycosis. *Blastomyces dermatitidis* in sputum (Gomori's silver stain). The thick capsule is shown in one of the organisms (*large arrow*). A spherical budding organism with a flat surface is also shown (*small arrow*). (*B*) *Aspergillus fumigatus.* Fungus hyphae showing septa and branching at a 45° angle (*arrow*). (*C*) Brown spores of the fungus *Alternaria,* a common contaminant (*A,B,C* × 560).

TABLE 4-1
Viral Disorders Affecting the Urothelium

Virus	Nuclear Changes	Cytoplasmic Changes
Herpes simplex	*Early stages*: "ground-glass" appearance of nuclei. Multinucleation and "molding" are common. *Late stage*: eosinophilic central nuclear inclusions.	Giant cells (multinucleated)
Cytomegalovirus	Large, usually basophilic inclusions surrounded by a large clear zone (halo) and peripheral condensation of chromatin. Small satellite inclusions.	Cell enlargement; satellite inclusions
Polyomavirus (BK type)	*Early stage*: large basophilic nuclear inclusions filling the nucleus. *Later stage*: pale inclusions *Last stage*: coarse trabeculation of chromatin.	Cell enlargement
Human papillomavirus	Nuclear enlargement and homogeneous hyperchromasia	Perinuclear clear cytoplasmic zones (koilocytosis)

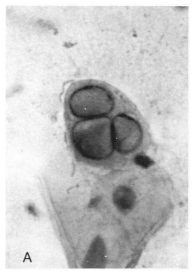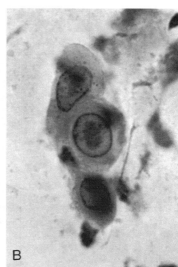

FIGURE 4-6. Herpesvirus infection in urine sediment. (*A*) Ground-glass appearance of the nuclei in early stage of infection. (*B*) The characteristic intranuclear eosinophilic inclusions reflect the second stage of infection (*A,B* × 1,000). (See also Plate 4-1*B*).

the formation of nuclear and cytoplasmic inclusions. Not all cytoplasmic inclusions, however, are of viral origin (see p. 55).

Herpes Simplex

Herpetic infection may occur in immunosuppressed patients, such as renal transplant recipients, in patients with tumors of the urinary bladder, in AIDS, and occasionally in the absence of any obvious disorder. Herpesvirus is an obligate cellular parasite, and florid infections with permissive replication of the virus, cause abnormalities in urothelial cells that are readily recognized. In the early stages of viral replication the nuclei of the infected cells become hazy, with a ground-glass appearance (Fig. 4-6*A*). Multinucleation is commonly observed in such cells, presumably the result of cell fusion in the presence of the virus. The multiple nuclei are often densely packed, with resulting nuclear "molding," recognized by tightly fitting contours of adjacent nuclei. In the second stage of the infection the viral particles are concentrated in the center of the nucleus, forming a brightly staining eosinophilic inclusion with a narrow clear zone or halo (Fig. 4-6*B*, Color Plate 4-1*B*). Inclusion-containing cells may contain single or multiple nuclei. Severe, acute inflammation may be present; consequently the infected cells in urinary sediment are often poorly preserved and the details of their nuclear structure cannot always be accurately observed. In such cases specific monoclonal antibody may be used to document the presence of the virus by immunocytochemistry. Molecular biologic techniques that will allow the recognition of the virus by South-

ern blot analysis or by polymerase chain reaction are currently being developed.

Cells with similar nuclear characteristics may also be observed in the urinary sediment in herpesvirus type 2 infection of the genital tract. This possibility must always be ruled out before considering the infection as primarily involving the urinary tract.

Cytomegalovirus

In years past, cytomegalovirus (CMV) infection was usually seen in newborn infants, usually with fatal consequences. The time-consuming and tedious search of the urinary sediment for the tell-tale abnormalities was the standard procedure until the 1970s, when rapid virologic diagnosis became possible. With the spread of AIDS, the infection has become fairly commonplace in adults. The virus causes very characteristic cellular changes that can be readily recognized in the urinary sediment. The principal abnormality is a large, usually basophilic but sometimes eosinophilic, nuclear inclusion surrounded by a large clear zone. There is a distinct outer belt of condensed nuclear chromatin. One or more small satellite inclusions may be observed in the nucleus and in the cytoplasm (Fig. 4-7). The cells bearing the inclusions are usually quite large and therefore readily recognized. Their origin is most likely in the renal tubules. Cytomegalovirus infection in the urinary sediment may be the first evidence of AIDS; the recognition of the virus-induced changes, therefore, may be of major clinical consequence. As in herpesvirus, a number of virologic and molecular biologic techniques that have recently been introduced are very specific for the recognition of this

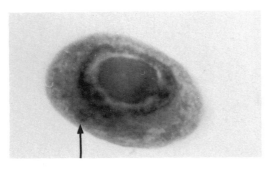

FIGURE 4-7. Cytomegalovirus infection—urinary sediment. The infected cell shows a large intranuclear inclusion, surrounded by a clear zone or halo. The nuclear chromatin is condensed at the periphery of the nucleus. A satellite inclusion is present in the cytoplasm (*arrow*). (× 1,600. Photograph courtesy of the late Dr. John K. Frost, Baltimore, MD.)

infection (Kimpton et al., 1990; Daiminger et al., 1994).

Human Polyomavirus (Decoy Cells)

Infection with human polyomavirus is widespread, and serologic studies have documented that nearly all adults show evidence of a past infection (Padget and Walker, 1976). The occult virus can become activated and recognized in voided urine sediment. There are two forms of the virus, both named after patients from whom they were isolated. The JC virus was first isolated from the brain of a patient with a rare disorder, progressive multifocal leukoencephalopathy (Padget et al., 1971). The BK virus was first isolated from the urinary tract of a patient with a renal transplant (Gardner et al., 1971).

The BK virus plays a major role in cytology of the urinary tract because it produces cell abnormalities that may be readily confused with cancer. The abnormalities were first recognized in the 1950s by Mr. Andrew Ricci, a cytotechnologist on the staff of my laboratory at the Memorial-Sloan Kettering Cancer Center, who named these cells "*decoy cells*." The changes were subsequently described in considerable detail by Coleman et al. in 1973 and ensuing years.

In permissive infections, the BK virus produces large, homogeneous, basophilic nuclear inclusions that occupy nearly the entire volume of the enlarged nucleus (Fig. 4-8, Color Plate 4-1C,D). Occasionally a very narrow rim of clearing separates the inclusion from the nuclear envelope. The infected cells are often enlarged and usually contain only a single nucleus, but bi- and sometimes large multinucleated cells are not uncommon (Fig. 4-8 *inset*, Color Plate 4-1C). With the passage of time the inclusions be-

come less basophilic and acquire a pale, homogeneous appearance (Fig. 4-8B, Color Plate 4-1D). The inclusions may also dissolve, presumably because the viral particles leach out, leaving behind a peculiar network of coarse nuclear chromatin that is as diagnostic of the infection as the classical inclusions (Fig. 4-8B). Such nuclei gave a positive immune reaction with an antibody prepared by Dr. Kertie Shah of the Johns Hopkins School of Public Health, Baltimore, MD, to a related papovavirus, SV40. In many infected cells, the nonspecific eosinophilic cytoplasmic inclusions may be simultaneously observed (Fig. 4-2D, *inset;* Color Plate 4-1D). In most cases of massive infection, the background of the cytologic preparation contains numerous cell debris and necrotic cells. Erythrocytes and leukocytes are commonly present. Viral inclusions may also be observed in the histologic sections of the urothelium (Fig. 4-9A).

Electron microscopic studies of the infected cells disclosed a crystalline network of viral particles, each measuring about 35 nm in diameter (Fig. 4-9B). Thus the ultrastructural appearance of the polyomavirus is similar to that of human papillomavirus, both viruses belonging to the family of papovaviridae. There is, however, a fundamental difference between the two viruses: while human papillomavirus is thought to have oncogenic properties in humans (see below and p. 114), there is no evidence whatever that the human polyomavirus is oncogenic in humans, although in experimental rodents induction of tumors with this viral species has been recorded. The cytopathic effects of the two viruses are also quite different, inasmuch as the papillomavirus does not produce conspicuous nuclear inclusions but produces nuclear and cytoplasmic alterations (koilocytosis) described on p. 114.

The activation of the BK type of human polyomavirus is most commonly observed in immunodeficient or immunosuppressed patients, such as those receiving organ transplants and patients on chemotherapy, particularly with cyclophosphamide (Cytoxan, Endoxan). The infection has also been observed in pregnant women (Coleman et al., 1980) and in diabetics. There is, however, a large group of people without any evidence of immunodeficiency or any other disorder in whom the permissive infection may occur. Such patients may experience nonspecific symptoms of urinary frequency that lead to examination of the urinary sediment. The cytologic picture in suitable cases may be quite dramatic and has often led to the erroneous diagnosis of carcinoma.

It has been proposed that in bone marrow transplant patients the infection with BK virus causes hemorrhagic cystitis (Arthur et al., 1986; Apperley et al., 1987). Subsequent study has documented that viral

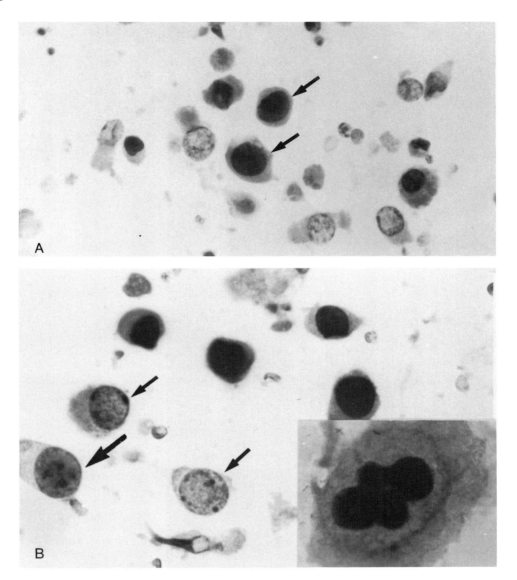

FIGURE 4-8. Polyomavirus infection, BK type (decoy cells), in urinary sediment. (*A*) Large, intranuclear, opaque basophilic inclusions (*arrows*) are characteristic of this infection. The background of the preparation contains cell debris and necrotic cells. (*B*) The classical, inclusion-containing cells are in the center of the figure. At the periphery, other changes, characteristic of polyomavirus infection, are shown: In two cells, the typical coarse chromatin network may be observed (*small arrows*). One cell (*large arrow*) shows a pale inclusion, probably an intermediate stage between the basophilic inclusions and the chromatin network (see Color Plate 4-1*D*). (*Inset*) A huge multinucleated cell, presumably an umbrella cell, with polyomavirus inclusions in all nuclei, observed in a 15-year-old woman after a bone marrow transplant (*A* × 560; *B* × 750; *inset* × 1,000; see also Color Plate 4-1*C* and *D*).

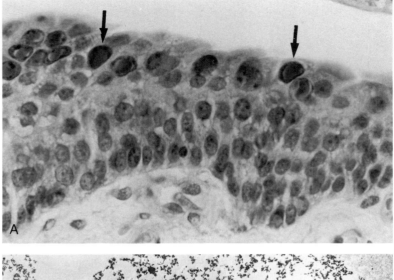

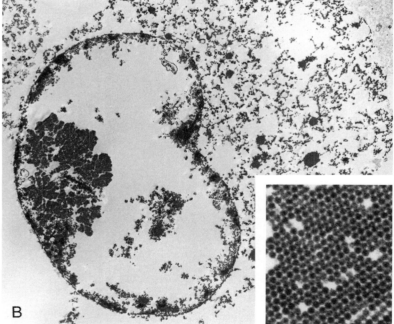

FIGURE 4-9. (*A*) Histologic section of ureter showing BK polyomavirus inclusion in the superficial cells (*arrows*). (*B*) Electronmicrograph of a urothelial cell, removed from a glass slide, with a nuclear inclusion due to BK virus. The cell was damaged during processing. (*Inset*) Crystalline array of viral particles measuring about 35 nm in diameter. (A × 560; B approx. × 10,000; *inset*, approx. × 80,000; Courtesy of Professor Dulcie Coleman, St. Mary's Hospital, London, U.K.)

activation and hemorrhagic cystitis in this group of patients are two independent phenomena: in most bone marrow transplant patients, the viral activation was unrelated to hemorrhagic cystitis (Cottler-Fox et al., 1991).

Progressive multifocal leukoencephalopathy, associated with the JC type of human polyomavirus, is now seen with increased frequency in patients with AIDS; hence the activation of this viral type is also related to immune deficiencies. As has been shown by Suhrland et al. (1987), the cytologic manifesta-

tions of this severe central nervous system disorder are very similar to those observed in the urinary tract: large basophilic inclusions occupy the nuclei of glial cells. The diagnosis can be established on aspiration biopsy of the brain of the affected patients. There are a few reports of a synchronous presence of leukoencephalopathy and malignant brain tumors (Sima et al., 1983).

Monoclonal antibodies to polyomaviruses and related viruses (SV40) have been produced and may be used for diagnostic purposes. However, the morphologic manifestations of this viral infection are so characteristic that it is very rarely necessary to resort to immunochemistry for diagnosis.

It has been documented by Koss et al. (1984) that cells with polyomavirus inclusions have an abnormal DNA content, and thus are an important source of aneuploid DNA histograms. I have repeatedly observed such events among patients monitored by DNA analysis after treatment of bladder tumors with resulting false alarms. For further discussion of DNA analysis in bladder tumors, see Chapter 9.

Human Papillomavirus

The current scientific and clinical interest in this group of viruses is due to their possible relationship to cancer of the uterine cervix. Over 70 types of this virus have been recognized. Most of the types are associated with skin disorders and some (types 6 and 11) with venereal warts (*Condylomata acuminata*). *Condylomata acuminata* may also occur within the lower urinary tract, mainly the urethra and the urinary bladder, and may cause significant cytologic abnormalities (koilocytosis), that will be discussed in Chapters 5 and 6, together with other benign tumors of the bladder and the urethra.

CELLULAR INCLUSIONS NOT DUE TO VIRAL AGENTS

Cytoplasmic and nuclear inclusions not due to viral agents may be observed in urothelial cells.

Nonspecific Cytoplasmic Eosinophilic Inclusions

Single or multiple spherical eosinophilic inclusions of various sizes frequently may be observed in degenerating urothelial cells, particularly in the presence of infection or inflammation. Although Bolande proposed in 1959 that the inclusions in childhood are due to a viral infection, subsequent studies failed to confirm the presence of the virus. The inclusions are usually observed in poorly preserved cells with a severely damaged, pyknotic, or karyorrhectic nucleus or in anucleated cell debris (see Fig. 4-2*D, inset;* Color Plate 4-1*E*). Such inclusions are also commonly observed in degenerating intestinal cells shed from ileal bladder (see p. 42 and Fig. 3-3*C*). The inclusions have no diagnostic significance and most likely represent condensed cytoplasmic filaments.

Inclusions Due to Lead Poisoning

As first reported in children with lead poisoning by Landing and Nakai in 1959, these are acid-fast homogeneous *nuclear* inclusions, occurring in renal tubular cells and found in the urinary sediment. In 1980 Schumann et al. reported the presence of such inclusions in the urinary sediment of industrial workers exposed to lead (Fig. 4-10). It is noteworthy that the cytologic examination of voided urine has not been used to identify children with high levels of exposure to lead-rich paint. This is a significant public health

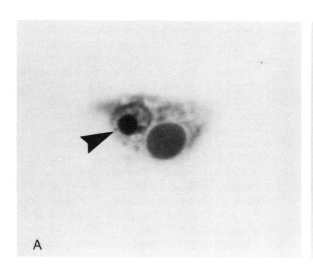
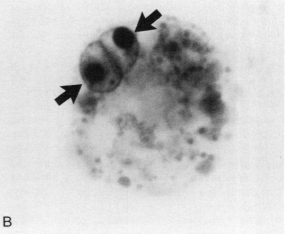

FIGURE 4-10. (*A and B*) Intranuclear inclusions (*arrowheads* in *A, arrows* in *B*) in lead poisoning, observed in exposed adult workers. The inclusions are of renal tubular origin and are acid-fast (× 1,000; Photographs courtesy of Dr. G. Berry Schumann, Dianon Systems, Stratford, CT).

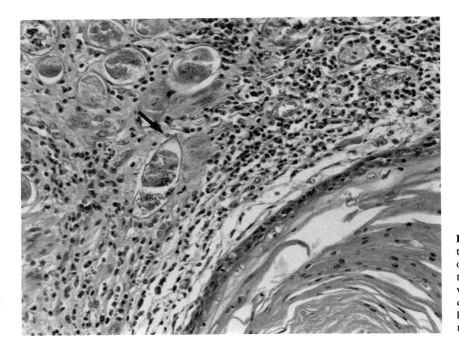

FIGURE 4-11. Histologic section of bladder with numerous ova of *S. haematobium,* adjacent to a focus of a deeply invasive, well-differentiated squamous carcinoma. The ovum indicated by an arrow shows the characteristic terminal spine (× 350).

dilemma because of the crippling effect of lead on childhood development.

Other Inclusions

Rouse *et al.* reported in 1986 the presence of eosinophilic nuclear inclusions in clusters of small epithelial cells in the urinary sediment of women. The nature and origin of these cells and their inclusions are not known in the absence of electron microscopic observations.

TREMATODES AND OTHER PARASITES

Trematodes or flukes are parasites commonly observed in tropical countries with a worldwide distribution. Most of the species require an intermediate host, usually a snail, to reproduce and infect humans. Of special interest in pathology of the urinary bladder is *Schistosoma haematobium* (Bilharzia), a parasite usually thought to be prevalent in Egypt, but widely distributed throughout the eastern littoral of Africa, including southern Africa (see also comments on p. 97). The infection is acquired by wading in shallow waters wherein the snails reside and release the mobile form of the parasite, the cercariae, that penetrate the exposed human skin. A reaction to the infection,

known as *swimmers' itch,* is commonly observed. The cercariae penetrate the lymphatics and the venules and migrate to the veins of their predilection, the pelvic plexus being the favored site for *S. haematobium.* The parasites mature in the venous plexus and deposit ova that are commonly observed in the bladder and the adjacent organs. The ova are excreted in urine and release a mobile form of the parasite known as the miracidium that penetrates the snail host, thus continuing the cycle. There is a known association of bladder cancer with heavy infestation with *S. haematobium.* In spite of many hypotheses, the mechanisms of this relationship remain completely unknown.

There are two important cytologic manifestations of the infection with *S. haematobium:* the recognition of the ova and of the malignant tumors that may be associated with it. The ova are oval structures with a thick transparent capsule, characterized by the presence of a sword-shaped protrusion, known as the terminal spine, located at the narrow end of the ova (Fig. 4-11). Whether fresh or calcified (as they often are) the ova are readily recognized in the urinary sediment. The embryonal form of the parasite, known as the miracidium, that is released in human stool and urine, also retains the shape of the ovum and its terminal spine. Because of movement of people across the continents, associated with air travel, sporadic cases of *S. haematobium* have been reported throughout the world, including a case report from the Massachusetts General Hospital (1994). The manifestations of bladder cancer associated with this infection will be discussed with other bladder tumors in Chapter 5.

Ova of other parasites may be occasionally recognized in the urinary sediment. Ova of common intestinal parasites such as *Ascaris lumbricoides* and *Enterobius vermicularis* (Oxyuris), may be occasionally observed. The reader is directed to other sources for description of these parasites and their ova (Koss, Diagnostic Cytology, 4th Ed., 1992, pp. 348–350). Filariasis may also be identified in voided urine (Webber and Eveland, 1982).

LITHIASIS

Pain, often radiating to the groin and gross hematuria, is the usual clinical symptom associated with lithiasis. Occasionally, however, a space-occupying lesion in the upper urinary tract, particularly if located in the renal pelvis, requires a diagnostic work-up. The customary differential diagnosis in such cases comprises lithiasis, urothelial tumors, and blood clots. Stones located in the renal pelves, the ureters, or the urinary bladder function as abrasive instruments. Therefore, the cytologic findings in voided urine may closely resemble the effects of instrumentation. In some patients, particularly if the stone is being expelled, numerous large rounded ("papillary") fragments of benign urothelium and an abundance of umbrella cells may be observed (Fig. 4-12). Highman and Wilson (1982) reported the presence of spherical ("papillary") clusters of urothelial cells in voided urine in the majority of patients with calculi, and claimed that this finding was much less common in control normal patients. This has not necessarily been my experience and, in my belief, the finding is nonspecific. Normal urothelium may desquamate in papillary clusters in the absence of disease, especially after instrumentation of any kind (see Chaps. 2 and 3). Further, such findings may also be observed in the presence of low grade papillary tumors (see Chap. 5), contributing still further to the complexity of the diagnostic decision. In my judgement, except under special circumstances described on p. 86, papillary clusters have minimal, if any, diagnostic value, particularly after vigorous palpation or instrumentation, and no diagnostic conclusion should be drawn from their presence in the voided urine sediment. As has been discussed on p. 41 the use of retrograde brushings or washings is rarely of value in attempting to differentiate a low-grade urothelial lesion from a stone because the cytologic presentation of these two entities is usually identical (see Fig. 4-2 and Fig. 3-2 in Chapter 3).

However, epidemiologic studies have documented that stones, particularly bladder stones, are a risk factor for urothelial carcinoma, particularly flat carcinoma in situ. The cytologic presentation of this important lesion will be discussed in Chapter 5. Suffice it to say that if suspicious or outright malignant cells are present in the urinary sediment in the presence of stones, a search for a malignant lesion must be instituted. Beyer-Boon et al. reported several patients with lithiasis with suspicious cells in the urinary sediment, but it is likely that in some of them a malignant lesion was present.

Significant noncancerous atypias of urothelial cells due to lithiasis are most uncommon. I have observed it in an occasional patient in the form of nuclear enlargement and hyperchromasia confined to a very few cells, some of them containing crystalline fragments in their cytoplasm (Koss, 1992).

LEUKOPLAKIA

Leukoplakia of the bladder is a condition of partial or complete keratinization of the squamous epithelium, replacing the urothelium, with resulting white appearance of the bladder mucosa on cystoscopy or gross inspection. Leukoplakia may be associated with lithiasis and is common in *S. haematobium* infestation, but quite often no known cause of this disorder can be identified. On microscopic examination the urothelium in leukoplakia is provided with a thick layer of surface keratin (Fig. 4-13). In the urinary sediment anucleated keratinized cells (so-called ghost cells) may be evident (Color Plate 4-1*F*). Leukoplakia per se is benign, but it may give rise to a squamous carcinoma. As will be discussed again in Chapter 5, the presence of anucleated squamous cells in a male patient calls for further investigation of the bladder. In women such cells may be derived from the genital tract and this source of origin must be first investigated.

EFFECT OF DRUGS

A number of drugs administered either locally or systemically may have a major impact on the make-up of the urothelium and cells derived therefrom. It is of interest that, in general, drugs administered locally for treatment of a disorder of the bladder have a much lesser effect on the urothelium than certain alkylating agents usually administered parenterally for the treatment of malignant diseases located outside of the lower urinary tract.

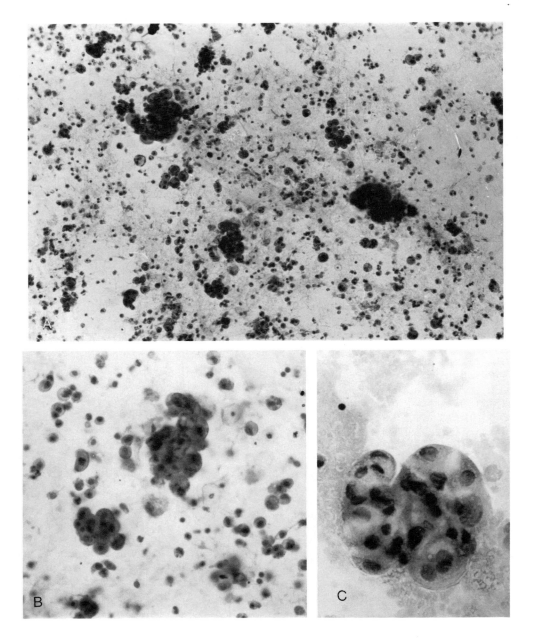

FIGURE 4-12.   Lithiasis of renal pelvis. Voided urine sediment after retrograde brushing. (*A*) Low-power view of the sediment with numerous large clusters and detached benign urothelial cells in the background. (*B*) Higher magnification of one field of *A*. Although the details of cell structure cannot be well seen, the overall presentation is typical of either a stone or instrumentation. In this case, an erroneous diagnosis of a papillary tumor was established that led to a nephrectomy. Only lithiasis of the renal pelvis was found. (*C*) Another "papillary" cluster of urothelial cells in voided urine sediment in a case of lithiasis (*A* × 140, *B* × 350, *C* × 560).

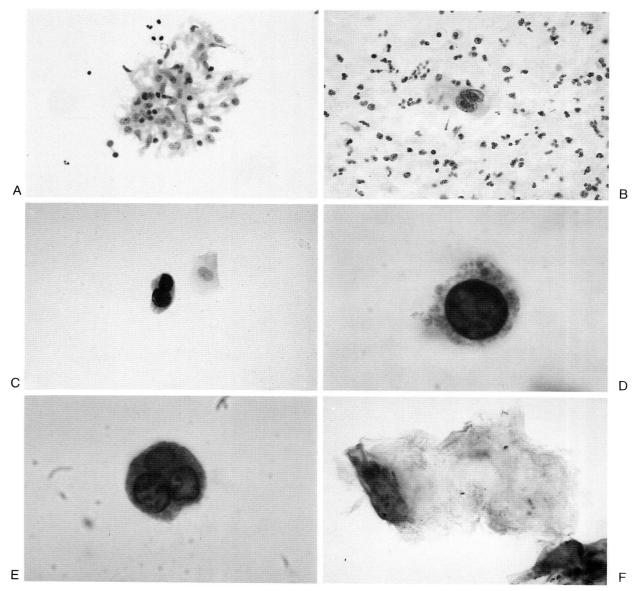

Color Plate 4-1.   (*A*) A granuloma found in urinary sediment of a patient treated with bacille Calmette-Guérin (BCG) for a carcinoma in situ of the bladder. Note that the spherical structure is made up of elongated epithelioid cells. (Photograph courtesy of Dr. Ruth Kreitzer, formerly of Mount Sinai Medical Center, New York, NY.) (*B*) Herpesvirus in sediment of voided urine in a 54-year-old male patient. In each nucleus of the binucleated cells there is a large, eosinophilic inclusion. The background of the smear shows evidence of marked inflammation. (*C,D*) Human polyomavirus infection in urinary sediment. (*C*) Binucleated umbrella cells. Both nuclei contain inclusions caused by human polyomavirus. (*D*) An oil immersion view of a urothelial cell with a classical, opaque inclusion due to human polyomavirus. The cytoplasm of the cell is degenerated and contains several small eosinophilic inclusions, not related to the virus. (*E*) Eosinophilic cytoplasmic inclusions, one large and several small, in a binucleated urothelial cell (voided urine). The pyknotic nuclei are at the periphery of the cells. The inclusions have no diagnostic significance. (*F*) Fully keratinized anucleated squamous cells ("ghost cells") in voided urine sediment in a case of leukoplakia of the bladder. Such cells may also occur in keratinizing squamous carcinoma. (Original magnification *A* × approx. 100; *B,C,F* × 160; *D,E* oil immersion × 400, enlarged about × 2.5.)

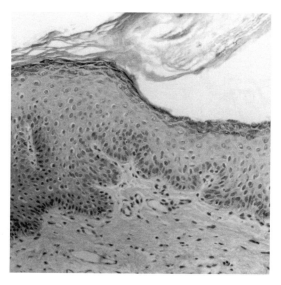

FIGURE 4-13. Leukoplakia of bladder epithelium. The epithelium is of squamous type with a heavy, partially detached layer of keratin on the surface. The cytologic presentation of leukoplakia is shown in Color Plate 4-1*F* (× 140). (From Koss, L. G.: Diagnostic Cytology and Its Histopathologic Bases, 4th Ed. Philadelphia, J. B. Lippincott, 1992.)

Intravesically Administered Drugs

Mitomycin C and Thiotepa are the two drugs commonly used for prevention of recurrence or for direct treatment of bladder tumors. The effects of these drugs on normal urothelium are relatively trivial. Occasionally cellular enlargement or vacuolization of the cytoplasm and the nucleus may be noted. There is occasionally a moderate enlargement of the cells, akin to the effect of radiotherapy (see below). In my experience, such changes virtually never mimic cell abnormalities associated with bladder cancer, to be described in Chapter 5, and very rarely cause a problem with differential diagnosis. Many of the cell changes described in the literature as allegedly specific effects of drugs were secondary to human polyomavirus activation, described in the preceding pages.

Bacille Calmette-Guérin (BCG) is used with increased frequency in the treatment of nonpapillary (flat) carcinoma in situ of the bladder. The drug may cause formation of granulomas in bladder wall and in the prostate. As was described on p. 48, the constituent cells of tubercules occasionally may be observed in the urinary sediment (see Color Plate 4-1*A*). The drug may also cause a major nonspecific inflammatory reaction, and the urinary sediment may contain a large number of leukocytes and macrophages. Again,

the use of this drug does not cause any cell changes that may be confused with cancer. *Regardless of the type of intravesical drug used, the presence of identifiable cancer cells strongly suggests that the tumor has not responded to the drug,* an issue that will be discussed again in reference to the monitoring of urothelial tumors (see Chap. 5, p. 126).

Systemically Administered Drugs

Alkylating agents, particularly cyclophosphamide and busulfan, may have a marked effect on the urothelium with resulting significant cell abnormalities.

Cyclophosphamide

Cyclophosphamide (Cytoxan, Endoxan), a widely used chemotherapeutic and immunosuppressive agent, has a remarkable effect on the urothelium. In humans, the drug administered in large doses causes hemorrhagic cystitis that may lead to death from exsanguination. In experimental animals, parenterally administered cyclophosphamide has been shown to cause a massive necrosis of the urothelium and of the underlying muscle, followed by an atypical epithelial regeneration and fibrosis of muscle (Koss, 1967; Bonikos and Koss, 1974). During the regenerative events bizarre epithelial cells may appear in the urine. It is likely that a similar mechanism of epithelial necrosis, followed by regeneration, accounts for major cytologic abnormalities in humans. As first described by Forni et al. (1964), in some cases the drug-induced changes result in oddly shaped, bizarre, abnormal urothelial cells with marked nuclear and nucleolar enlargement that mimic poorly differentiated cancer cells to perfection (Figs. 4-14 and 4-15).

In the past, hemorrhagic cystitis was principally observed in children and young adults treated with large doses of the drug for leukemia, lymphoma, or childhood malignant tumors. Since it was documented that massive hydration of the patient can prevent the effects of the drug on the bladder, such events have become rare. In more recent years, cytologic effects of cyclophosphamide have been observed in patients with leukemia and lymphoma under treatment, and mainly in recipients of bone marrow transplants. Prior to transplantation these patients receive a combination of chemotherapeutic agents that includes large doses of cyclophosphamide, and radiotherapy for the dual purpose of eradication of the tumor and immunosuppression. It is not known whether the cytotoxic effects of cyclophosphamide are enhanced by other modalities of therapy. Nonetheless, marked epithelial abnormalities, mimicking a malignant tumor, are common in such patients (Fig. 4-16). It is of incidental interest that

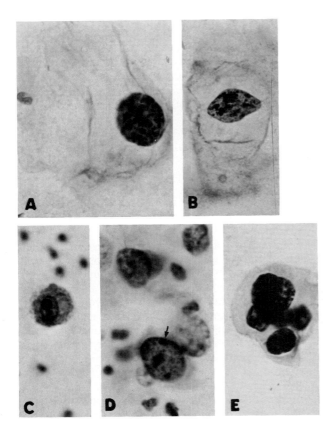

FIGURE 4-14. Voided urine sediment. Urothelial cell changes observed in patients treated with cyclophosphamide—there was no evidence of bladder tumor. (*A* and *B*) Note the coarse arrangement of nuclear chromatin, mimicking cancer. (*C* and *D*) Markedly enlarged nuclei. In *D*, a large sex chromatin body may be noted (*small arrow*). (*E*) A multinucleated cell with marked nuclear enlargement and hyperchromasia (A–E × 560). (Modified from Forni, A. M., Koss, L. G., and Geller, W.: Cytological study of the effect of cyclophosphamide on the epithelium of the urinary bladder in man. Cancer, *17,* 1348–1355, 1964.)

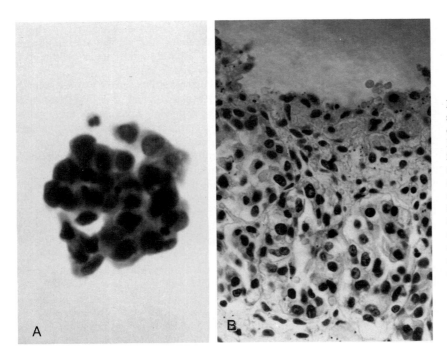

FIGURE 4-15. Voided urine sediment (*A*) and biopsy of bladder (*B*) in a patient, treated with large doses of cyclophosphamide for a lymphoma, who developed a hemorrhagic cystitis. (*A*) A cluster of urothelial cells with enlarged, hyperchromatic nuclei. (*B*) Bladder biopsy showing a marked atypia of the epithelium in the form of nuclear enlargement and hyperchromasia. The epithelium resembles somewhat a carcinoma in situ but there was no evidence of bladder disease after the acute reaction subsided. There was no long-term follow-up of this patient (*A* × 560, *B* × 250).

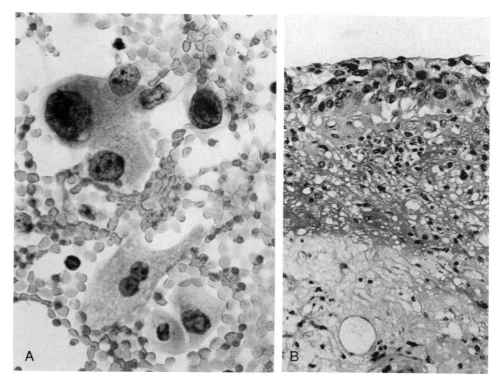

FIGURE 4-16. Cell changes mimicking cancer in voided urine (*A*) and bladder epithelium (*B*) of a 43-year-old man with a bone marrow transplant for leukemia. (*A*) The nuclear abnormalities in the form of granular hyperchromasia, irregular outline, and variability in size are identical to those seen in a high-grade carcinoma. (*B*) The abnormalities of the bladder epithelium at autopsy are similar to a flat carcinoma in situ. (*A* × 560, *B* × 200; Case courtesy of Dr. Denise Hidvegi, Northwestern University, Chicago, IL).

activation of the human polyomavirus infection may also occur in such patients, and the characteristic cell changes due to permissive viral infection may appear side-by-side with drug effects (see Fig. 4-8). The changes may be correctly identified with the knowledge of the patient's history.

As was mentioned on p. 52, it was suggested some years ago that human polyomavirus is responsible for hemorrhagic cystitis in bone marrow transplant patients (Arthur et al., 1986; Apperley et al., 1987). A study by Cottler-Fox et al., (1989) has shown that activation of the virus is independent of hemorrhagic cystitis which is most likely due to the effects of cyclophosphamide.

The cell changes induced by cyclophosphamide are not always innocuous. There are several reports (Wall et al., 1975; Fuchs et al., 1981; Pederson-Bjergaard et al., 1988; Travis et al., 1989) documenting that large doses of this drug may induce urothelial cancer, often of squamous type, in the urinary blad-

der, and sometimes in the renal pelvis (McDougal et al., 1981) and ureter (Schiff et al., 1982) (Fig. 4-17*A*). A few cases of leiomyosarcoma of the bladder have also been recorded (Thrasher et al., 1990), presumably as the result of drug effect on the smooth muscle of the bladder (Fig. 14-17*B*). In some of these reported cases, the malignant tumors occurred in patients treated for benign disorders.

Most of the recorded cases of cyclophosphamide-related cancers occurred in very young patients who would be very unlikely to develop spontaneous tumors of this type. Hence, the carcinogenic role of the drug must be assumed.

Busulfan

Several years ago, busulfan (Myleran), an alkylating agent, was the favored drug for the treatment of chronic myelogenous leukemia. The drug has since been replaced by other chemotherapeutic agents, but it is still being used in bone marrow transplant pa-

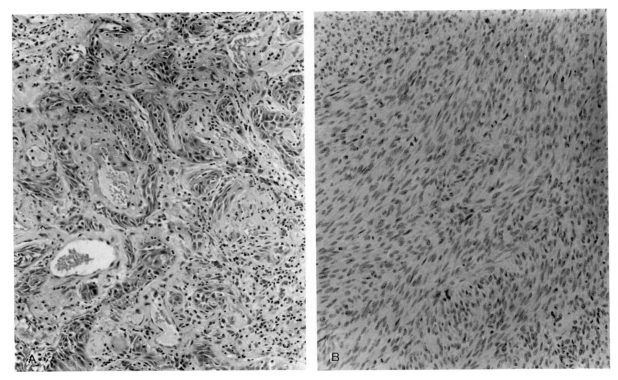

FIGURE 4-17. (*A*) Squamous carcinoma of bladder observed in a 19-year-old woman, treated for 24 months with cyclophosphamide for a malignant lymphoma (Case courtesy of Dr. K. P. Clausen, Ohio State University, Columbus, OH). (*B*) A huge leiomyosarcoma of bladder observed in a 17-year-old man after treatment with several hundred grams of cyclophosphamide for malignant lymphoma (× 150; Case courtesy of Dr. Lawrence Roth, Indianapolis, IN).

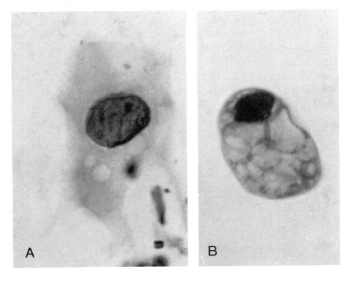

FIGURE 4-18. (*A,B*) Two examples of very large abnormal cells in the urinary sediment of a 68-year-old woman treated with large doses of busulfan for chronic myeologenous leukemia. The patient died of pulmonary fibrosis (busulfan lung) (× 560).

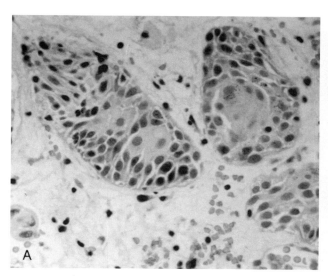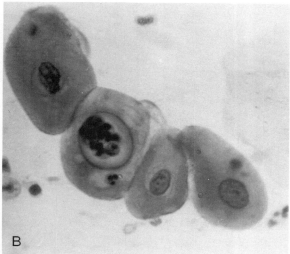

FIGURE 4-19. (*A*) Biopsy of bladder 2 years after administration of 60 cGy. Note the persisting marked nuclear enlargement in urothelial cells forming Brunn's nests. (*B*) Radiation effect on urothelial cells after 30 cGy (voided urine). Note cell enlargement and nuclear and cytoplasmic vacuole formation (*A* × 350, *B* × 560).

tients. When given in large doses over a long period of time it has a marked effect on the respiratory tract wherein it causes "busulfan lung." The disease consists of extensive pulmonary fibrosis and formation of bizarre giant cells in the bronchial and bronchiolar epithelium (for a detailed discussion of pulmonary changes, see Koss, L. G., Diagnostic Cytology, 4th Ed., 1992). The effect is not confined to the lungs, and bizarre cells with large, hyperchromatic nuclei may occur in epithelia of all other organs, including the urothelium. In the urinary sediment oddly-shaped cells with nuclear enlargement and hyperchromasia, mimicking cancer cells, may appear (Fig. 4-18). In the absence of clinical history it may be extremely difficult to identify such cells correctly.

EFFECTS OF RADIOTHERAPY

Radiotherapy, regardless of the target organ, has similar effects on epithelial cells. Marked cell enlargement, with a proportional enlargement of the nucleus, is the landmark of the effect of irradiation that may persist for several years after conclusion of treatment (Fig. 4-19A). Bizarre cell shapes and vacuolization of the nucleus and the cytoplasm are other stigmata of radiotherapy. Cells with these characteristics are usually fairly easy to recognize in the urinary

sediment (Fig. 4-19B). The effect may be observed not only in instances of direct irradiation of the target organ but also when the principal radiation beam is directed at an adjacent organ, and sometimes even when the target is anatomically distant. The term "abscopal radiation effect" has been applied to such events, which are extremely rare (Koss, 1992). It is of note that radiotherapy may be very effective in the eradication of invasive tumors of the bladder but that carcinoma in situ and related lesions may remain unaffected. Therefore, the finding of cancer cells in the urinary sediment of patients with bladder cancer may indicate persistence of carcinoma in situ. For further discussion of such events, see Chapter 5.

MONITORING OF RENAL TRANSPLANT PATIENTS

Urinary sediment has long been used to monitor renal transplant patients for evidence of rejection of the transplanted allograft. In a series of papers published from 1969 through 1979, Bossen et al. observed that the presence of renal tubular cells, fragments of tubules, tubular casts, lymphocytes, and cell necrosis correlated fairly well with impending rejection. Viruses, such as herpesvirus and cytomegalovirus, are often activated and may be recognized in urinary

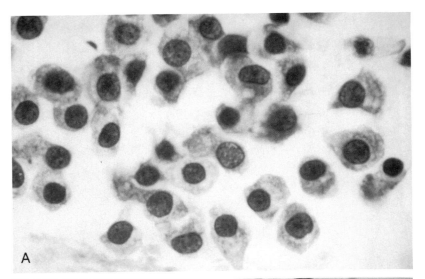

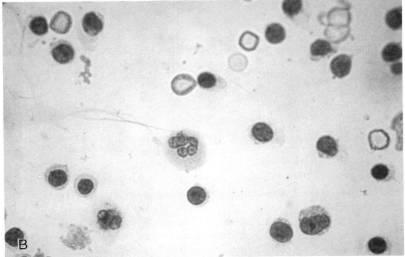

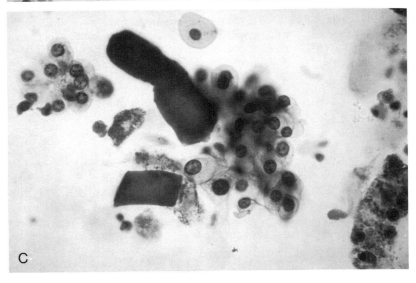

FIGURE 4-20. Urinary sediment in impending allograft rejection. (*A*) Well-preserved epithelial cells of renal collecting duct origin. A progressive increase in the number of such cells suggests impending rejection. (*B*) Lymphocytes (presumably T-cell type) and erythrocytes of renal origin, characterized by a thick outer border and transparent center, during acute allograft rejection. (*C*) Tissue fragments, presumably of renal tubular origin, and hyaline casts are suggestive of ischemic renal parenchymal necrosis (× 1,000; Photographs courtesy of Dr. G. Berry Schumann, Dianon Systems, Stratford, CT. From Schumann, G. B., Maxwell, G., Nelson, E., and De-Bells, C. C.: Predictive value of urinary cytodiagnosis in 60 consecutive renal allograft recipients [unpublished]).

sediment. The human polyomavirus, type BK, was first identified in the urinary sediment of a renal transplant recipient (Gardner et al., 1971). The activation of this virus is a very common event in all organ transplant patients. The identification of tubular cells is sometimes very difficult. Schumann et al. (1977) discussed at length the criteria leading to their recognition. In non-transplant patients, the renal tubular cells are generally poorly preserved and appear necrotic, whether occurring singly (see Fig. 2-14) or forming a part of a cast (see Fig. 2-16A). In renal transplant recipients, the epithelial cells of collecting tubules origin are much better preserved. The cells have a scanty but clearly visible, vacuolated cytoplasm and spherical, somewhat opaque nuclei (Fig. 4-20A). Another feature of impending rejection is the presence of numerous lymphocytes of T-cell type, accompanied by erythrocytes with a thick outer border and clear center, suggestive of renal origin (see p. 33 and Fig. 4-20B). Finally, tissue fragments, presumably necrotic renal tubules, and hyaline casts are also observed in impending allograft rejection (Fig. 4-20C). A recent study from our laboratory confirmed the predictive value of urinary sediment in allograft rejection (Cory et al., submitted for publication, 1995). Other techniques have recently been developed to monitor renal transplant recipients. Flow cytometry of samples directly aspirated from the transplanted kidney may disclose a dominance of T-lymphocytes that accumulate during the rejection process. Direct biopsies of the transplanted kidney are also used for this purpose.

Effect of Cyclosporine

Cyclosporine is an immunomodulatory drug extensively used in prevention of rejection of transplanted organs. The drug affects renal function in about 30% of the patients. Winkelmann et al. (1985) and Stella et al. (1987) described necrosis of epithelial cells derived from renal tubular epithelium and the presence of "tissue fragments" in the urine of bone marrow transplant patients as evidence of cyclosporine toxicity. So far as one could judge from the photographs, the changes were not specific for any drug effect. Similar conclusions were reached by Stilman et al. (1987). Most unfortunately, many observers knowledgeable about organ transplants are not familiar with the scope of urinary cytology. Thus, common findings are confused with transplant-specific findings.

As a notable exception, Kyo et al. (1992) attempted to differentiate the effects of cyclosporine toxicity from those of renal transplant rejection in voided urine by differential counts of mononuclear cells and tubular cells. In cases of transplant rejection, the counts of mononuclear cells (including several varieties of T lymphocytes) were higher than in cyclosporine toxicity. On the other hand, cyclosporine toxicity resulted in higher counts of tubular cells than rejection.

URINARY CYTOLOGY IN BONE MARROW TRANSPLANT RECIPIENTS

Total body irradiation and a battery of drugs, including cyclophosphamide and busulfan, are extensively used prior to bone marrow transplantation. Significant abnormalities of the urothelial cells, combining the features of radiation response and effects of cyclophosphamide, may be observed in the urinary sediment of such patients. Biopsies of the bladder may disclose lesions that are similar to a spontaneously occurring carcinoma in situ (see Fig. 4-14). Because of limited survival of many such patients the clinical significance of these abnormalities is unknown. A variety of viruses, besides human polyomavirus, may be activated in such patients, particularly cytomegalovirus and herpesvirus.

RARE BENIGN CONDITIONS

Malakoplakia

Malakoplakia was first identified in the urinary bladder in the form of soft, yellow plaques, hence the name of the disorder (from Greek, *malakos* = soft). It is now known that this disorder may occur in virtually any organ in the body. The disease reflects an enzymatic defect of macrophages that are unable to digest coliform bacteria. As a consequence of an infection with these organisms there is an accumulation of macrophages in tissues, accounting for the gross appearance of the lesion. The bacteria are absorbed by lysosomes, the disposal units of the cells, wherein they remain in an undigested state. The lysosomes become very large, visible under the microscope, resulting in the so-called *Michaelis-Guttmann bodies,* which often become calcified. The recognition of the cells characteristic of malakoplakia in urinary sediment has occurred in some instances, but usually after a biopsy, releasing the macrophages into the lumen of the bladder and thence in the urinary stream. The intracytoplasmic spherical, eosinophilic, or calcified Michaelis-Guttmann bodies in the cytoplasm of large macrophages are usually readily recognized (Fig. 4-21).

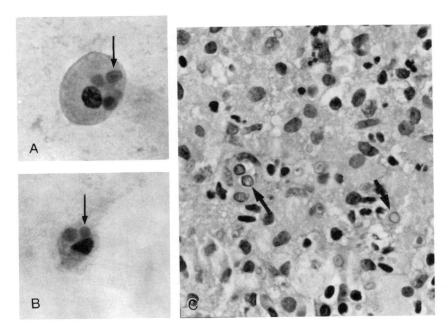

FIGURE 4-21. Urinary sediment and biopsy in a case of malakoplakia of the bladder. (*A,B*) Cells in voided urine after biopsy. The Michaelis-Guttmann bodies (*arrows*) are recognized as spherical cytoplasmic inclusions. (*C*) Biopsy of lesion composed of macrophages. Most of the Michaelis-Guttmann bodies are calcified (*arrows*). (*A,B* × 560, *C* × 350.)

Benign Giant Cells in Multiple Myeloma

One of the characteristic events in disseminated plasma cell myeloma is the formation of casts in distal convoluted and collecting renal tubules. The casts, composed of a variety of proteins, including the Bence-Jones protein, are surrounded by multinucleated giant cells, probably derived from macrophages.

Through the courtesy of Mr. Arthur Garutti, we studied a voided urine sediment in an elderly male with advanced multiple myeloma and Bence-Jones proteinuria. The sediment contained a moderate number of bizarre multinucleated giant cells with large, hyperchromatic nuclei (Fig. 4-22). The giant cells showed clear evidence of phagocytic activity, and hence most likely represented macrophages of renal origin.

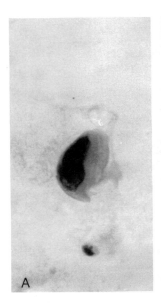
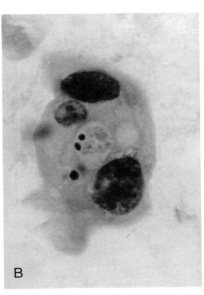

FIGURE 4-22. Multiple myeloma, urinary sediment. Two giant cells, probably originating in renal tubules are shown. Note the large, hyperchromatic nuclei. The larger cell contains phagocytized amorphous material and dense particles. The cells represent, most likely, renal tubular macrophages. (Case courtesy of Mr. Arthur Garutti, Port Jefferson, L.I., N.Y.; × 560.)

BIBLIOGRAPHY

Apperley, J. F., Rice, S. J., Bishop, J. A., et al.: Late-onset hemorrhagic cystitis associated with urinary excretion of polyomaviruses after bone marrow transplantation. Transplantation, 43, 108–112, 1987.

Arthur, R. R., Shah, K. V., Baust, S. T., Santos, G. W., and Saral, R.: Association of BK viruria with hemorrhagic cystis in recipients of bone marrow transplants. N. Engl. J. Med., 315, 230–234, 1986.

Ashton, P. R., and Lambird, P. A.: Cytodiagnosis of malakoplakia. Report of a case. Acta Cytol., 14, 92–94, 1970.

Bancroft, J., Seybolt, J. F., and Windhager, H. A.: Cytologic diagnosis of cytomegalic inclusion disease. Acta Cytol., 5, 182–186, 1961.

Bellin, H. J., Cherry, J. M., and Koss, L. G.: Effects of a single dose of cyclophosphamide. V. Protective effect of diversion of the urinary stream on dog bladder. Lab. Invest., 30, 43–47, 1974.

Berger, J. R., Kaszovitz, B., Post, M. J., and Dickinson, G.: Progressive multifocal leukoencephalopathy associated with human immunodeficiency virus infection: a review of the literature with a report of sixteen cases. Ann. Intern. Med., 107, 78–87, 1987.

Berkson, B. M., Lome, L. G., and Shapiro, I.: Severe cystitis induced by cyclophosphamide. Role of surgical management. J.A.M.A., 225, 605–606, 1973.

Beyer-Boon, M. E.: The efficacy of urinary cytology. Dissertation, Univ. of Leiden, the Netherlands, 1977.

Blanc, W. A.: Cytologic diagnosis of cytomegalic inclusion disease in gastric washings. Am. J. Clin. Pathol., 28, 46–49, 1957.

Bolande, R. P.: Inclusion-bearing cells in urine in certain viral infections. Pediatrics, 24, 7–12, 1959.

Bonikos, D. S., and Koss, L. G.: Acute effects of cyclophosphamide on rat urinary bladder muscle. Arch. Pathol., 97, 242–245, 1974.

Bossen, E. H., and Johnston, W. W.: Exfoliative cytopathologic studies in organ transplantation. IV. The cytologic diagnosis of Herpesvirus in the urine of renal allograft recipients. Acta Cytol., 19, 415–419, 1975.

Bossen, E. H., and Johnston, W. W.: Exfoliative cytopathologic studies in organ transplantation. V. The diagnosis of rejection in the immediate postoperative period. Acta Cytol., 21, 502–507, 1977.

Bossen, E. H., Johnston, W. W., Amatulli, J., and Rowlands, D. T.: Exfoliative cytopathologic studies in organ transplantation. I. The cytologic diagnosis of cytomegalic inclusions disease in the urine of renal allograft recipients. Am. J. Clin. Pathol., 52, 340–344, 1969.

Bossen, E. H., Johnston, W. W., Amatulli, J., and Rowlands, D. T.: Exfoliative cytopathologic studies in organ transplantation. III. The cytologic profile of urine during acute renal allograft rejection. Acta Cytol., 14, 176–181, 1970.

Brenner, D. W., and Schellhammer, P. F.: Upper tract urothelial malignancy after cyclophosphamide therapy. A case report and literature review. J. Urol., 137, 1226–1227, 1987.

Buckner, C. D., Rudolph, R. H., Fefer, A., Clift, R. A. and Epstein, R. B.: High dose cyclophosphamide therapy for malignant disease. Toxicity, tumor response, and the effects of stored autologous marrow. Cancer, 29, 357–365, 1972.

Chang, S. C.: Urinary cytologic diagnosis of cytomegalic inclusion disease in childhood leukemia. Acta Cytol., 14, 338–343, 1970.

Chappell, L. H., and Lundin, L.: A pitfall in urine cytology. A case report. Acta Cytol., 20, 162–163, 1976.

Clements, M. S., and Oko, T.: Cytologic diagnosis of schistosomiasis in routine urinary sediment. Acta Cytol., 27, 277–280, 1983.

Coleman, D. V.: The cytodiagnosis of human polyomavirus infection. Acta Cytol., 19, 93–96, 1975.

Coleman, D. V.: The cytological diagnosis of human polyomavirus infection and its value in clinical practice. In Koss, L. G., and Coleman, D. V. (eds.): Advances in Clinical Cytology, vol. 1. pp. 136–159. London, Butterworths, 1981.

Coleman, D. V., Field, A. M., Gardner, S. D., Porter, K. A., and Starzl, T. E.: Virus-induced obstruction of the ureteric and cystic duct in allograft recipients. Transplant. Proc., 5, 95–98, 1973.

Coleman, D. V., Gardner, S. D., and Field, A. M.: Human polyomavirus infection in renal allograft recipients. Br. Med. J., 3, 371–375, 1973.

Coleman, D. V., Wolfendale, M. R., Daniel, R. A., Dhanjal, N. K., Gardner, S. D., Gibson, P. E., and Field, A. M.: A prospective study of human polyomavirus infection in pregnancy. J. Infect. Dis., 142, 1–8, 1980.

Connery, D. B.: Leukoplakia of the urinary bladder and its association with carcinoma. J. Urol., 69, 121–127, 1953.

Cornish, J., Lecamwasam, J. P., Harrison, G., Vanderwee, M. A., and Miller, T. E.: Host defense mechanisms in the bladder. II. Disruption of the layer of mucus. Br. J. Exp. Path., 69, 759–770, 1988.

Cottler-Fox, M., Lynch, M., Deeg, H. J., and Koss, L. G.: Human polyomavirus: lack of relationship of viruria to prolonged or severe hemorrhagic cystitis after bone marrow transplant. Bone Marrow Trnspl., 4, 279–282, 1989.

Cowen, P. N.: False cytodiagnosis of bladder malignancy due to previous radiotherapy. Br. J. Urol., 47, 405–412, 1975.

Crabbe, J. G. S.: 'Comet' or 'decoy' cells found in urinary sediment smears. Acta Cytol., 15, 303–305, 1971.

Csapo, Z., Kuthy, E., Lantos, J., and Ormos, J.: Experimentally induced malakoplakia. Am. J. Pathol., 79, 453–462, 1975.

Daiminger, A., Schalasta, G., Betzl, D., and Enders, G.: Detection of human cytomegalovirus in urine samples by cell culture, early antigen assay and polymerase chain reaction. Infection 22, 24–28, 1994.

Dale, G. A., and Smith, R. B.: Transitional cell carcinoma of the bladder associated with cyclophosphamide. J. Urol., 112, 603–604, 1974.

deVoogt, H. J., Beyer-Boon, M. E., and Brussec, J. A. M.: The value of phase contrast microscopy for urinary cytology. Reliability and pitfalls. Acta Cytol., *19,* 542–546, 1975.

deVoogt, H. J., Rathert, P., and Beyer-Boon, M. E.: Urinary Cytology. New York, Springer-Verlag, 1977.

Dolman, C. L., McLeod, P. M., and Chang, E. C.: Lymphocytes and urine in ceroid lipofuscinosis. Arch. Pathol. Lab. Med., *104,* 487–490, 1980.

Dorfman, H. D., and Monis, B.: Mucin-containing inclusions in multinucleated giant cells and transitional epithelial cells of urine: cytochemical observations on exfoliated cells. Acta Cytol., *8,* 293–301, 1964.

Eggensperger, D. L., King, C., Gaudette, L. E., Robinson, W. M., and O'Dowd, G. J.: Cytodiagnostic urinalysis. Three years experience with a new laboratory test. Am. J. Clin. Pathol., *91,* 202–206, 1989.

Eickenberg, H. U., Amin, M., and Lich, R. J.: Blastomycosis of the genitourinary tract. J. Urol., *113,* 650–652, 1975.

Fetterman, G. H.: New laboratory aid in clinical diagnosis of inclusion disease of infancy. Am. J. Clin. Pathol., *22,* 424–425, 1952.

Fisher, E. R., and Davis, E.: Cytomegalic-inclusion disease in adult. N. Engl. J. Med., *258,* 1036–1040, 1958.

Forni, A. M., Koss, L. G., and Geller, W.: Cytological study of the effect of cyclophosphamide on the epithelium of the urinary bladder in man. Cancer, *17,* 1348–1355, 1964.

Frisque, R. J., Bream, G. L., and Cannella, M. T.: Human polyomavirus JC virus genome. J. Virol., *51,* 458–469, 1984.

Fuchs, E. F., Kay, R., Poole, R., Barry, J. M., and Pearse, H. D.: Uroepithelial carcinoma in association with cyclophosphamide ingestion. J. Urol., *126,* 544–545, 1981.

Gardner, S. D., Field, A. M., Coleman, D. V., and Hulme, B.: New human papovavirus (B.K.) isolated from urine after renal transplantation. Lancet, *1,* 1253–1257, 1971.

Gardner, S. D., MacKenzie, E. F. D., Smith, C., and Porter, A. A.: Prospective study of the human polyomaviruses BK and JC and cytomegalovirus in renal transplant recipients. J. Clin. Pathol., *37,* 578–586, 1984.

Glucksman, M. D.: Bladder cancer after cyclophosphamide therapy. Urology, *16,* 553, 1980.

Goudsmit, J., Wertheim-van Dillen, P., van Strein, A., and van der Noordaa, J.: The role of BK virus in acute respiratory tract disease and the presence of BKV DNA in tonsils. J. Med. Virol., *10,* 91–99, 1982.

Gupta, R. J., Schuster, R. A., and Christian, W. D.: Autopsy findings in a unique case of malakoplakia. Arch. Path., *93,* 42–48, 1972.

Harris, M. J., Schwinn, C. P., Morrow, J. W., Gray, R. L., and Brownell, B. M.: Exfoliative cytology of the urinary bladder irrigation specimen. Acta Cytol., *15,* 385–399, 1971.

Hellstrom, H. R., Davis, B. K., and Shonnard, J. W.: Eosinophilic cystitis. A study of 16 cases. Am. J. Clin. Pathol., *72,* 777–784, 1979.

Henry, L., and Fox, M.: Histological findings in pseudomembranous trigonitis. J. Clin. Pathol., *24,* 605–608, 1971.

Heritage, J., Chesters, P. M., and McCance, D. J.: The persistence of papovavirus BK DNA sequences in normal human renal tissue. J. Med. Virol., *81,* 143–150, 1981.

Highman, W., and Wilson, E.: Urine cytology in patients with calculi. J. Clin. Pathol., *35,* 350–356, 1982.

Hogan, T. F., Borden, E. C., McBain, J. A., Padgett, B. L., and Walker, D. L.: Human polyomavirus infection with JC and BK virus in renal transplant patients. Ann. Int. Med., *82,* 373–378, 1985.

Holmquist, N. D.: Diagnostic Cytology of Urinary Tract. Basel, S. Karger, 1977.

Houff, S. A., Major, E. O., Katz, D. A., Kufta, C. V., Sever, J. L., Pittaluga, S., Roberts, J. R., Gitt, J., Saini, N., and Lux, W.: Involvement of JC virus-infected mononuclear cells from the bone marrow and spleen in the pathogenesis of progressive multifocal leukoencephalopathy. N. Engl. J. Med., *318,* 301–305, 1988.

Hunner, G. L.: A rare type of bladder ulcer in women: Report of cases. Boston Med. Surg., *172,* 660–664, 1915.

Jayalakshmamma, B., and Pinkel, D.: Urinary-bladder toxicity following pelvic irradiation and simultaneous cyclophosphamide therapy. Cancer, *38,* 701–707, 1976.

Johnston, W. W., Bossen, E. H., Amatulli, J., and Rowlands, D. T.: Exfoliative cytopathologic studies in organ transplantation. II. Factors in the diagnosis of cytomegalic inclusion disease in urine of renal allograft recipients. Acta Cytol., *13,* 605–610, 1969.

Johnston, W. W., and Meadows, D. C.: Urinary bladder fibrosis and telangiectasia associated with long term cyclophosphamide therapy. N. Engl. J. Med., *284,* 290–294, 1971.

Kahan, A. V., Coleman, D. V., and Koss, L. G.: Activation of human polyomavirus infection—detection by cytologic technics. Am. J. Clin. Pathol., *74,* 326–332, 1980.

Kapila, K., and Verma, K.: Cytologic detection of tuberculosis of the urinary bladder. Acta Cytol., *28,* 90–91, 1984.

Kauffman, H. M., Clark, R. F., Magee, J. H., Ritenbury, M. S., Goldsmith, C. M., Prout, G. R., and Hume, D. M.: Lymphocytes in urine as an aid in the early detection of renal homograft rejection. Surg. Gynecol. Obstet., *119,* 25–36, 1964.

Kimpton, C. P., Corbitt, G., and Morris, D. J.: Comparison of polyethylene glycol precipitation and ultracentrifugation for recovery of cytomegalovirus from urine prior to detection of DNA by dot-blot hybridization. J. Virol. Meth. *28,* 141–145, 1990.

Klintmalm, G. B., Iwatsuki, S., and Starzl, T. E.: Nephrotoxicity of Cyclosporine A in liver and kidney transplant patients. Lancet, *1,* 470–471, 1981.

Koss, L. G.: Diagnostic Cytology and Its Histopathologic Bases, 4th Ed. Philadelphia, J. B. Lippincott, 1992.

Koss, L. G.: From koilocytosis to molecular biology: The impact of cytology on concepts of early human cancer. Modern Pathol., *2,* 526–535, 1989.

Koss, L. G.: A light and electron microscopic study of the effects of a single dose of cyclophosphamide on various organs in the rat. I. The urinary bladder. Lab. Invest., *16,* 44–65, 1967.

Koss, L. G.: Tumors of the Urinary Bladder. Atlas of Tumor Pathology, Second Series, Fascicle 11. Washington, D. C., Armed Forces Institute of Pathology, 1975.

Koss, L. G.: Tumors of the urinary bladder. Atlas of Tumor Pathology, Second Series, fascicle 11, Supplement. Washington, D.C., Armed Forces Institute of Pathology, 1985.

Koss, L. G.: Urinary tract cytology. *In* J. C. Connolly (ed.): Carcinoma of the Bladder. pp. 159–163. New York, Raven Press, 1981.

Koss, L. G., Melamed, M. R., and Mayer, K.: The effect of busulfan on human epithelia. Am. J. Clin. Pathol., *44*, 385–397, 1965.

Koss, L. G., Sherman, A. B., and Eppich, E.: Image analysis and DNA content of urothelial cells infected with human polyomavirus. Analyt. Quant. Cytol., *6*, 89–94, 1984.

Kyo, M., Gudat, F., Dalquen, P., Fujimoto, N., Ichikawa, Y., Fukuhishi, T., Najano, S., and Mihatsch, M. J.: Differential diagnosis of kidney transplant rejection and cyclosporine nephrotoxicity by urine cytology. Transp. Proceedings, *24*, 1388–1390, 1992.

Landing, B. H., and Nakai, H.: Histochemical properties of renal lead-inclusions and demonstration in urinary sediment. Am. J. Clin. Pathol., *31*, 499–503, 1959.

Lang, D. J., Kummer, J. F., and Hartley, D. P.: Cytomegalovirus in semen. Persistence and demonstration in extracellular fluids. N. Engl. J. Med., *291*, 121–123, 1974.

Lawrence, H. J., Simone, J., and Aur, R. J. A.: Cyclophosphamide-induced hemorrhagic cystitis in children with leukemia. Cancer, *36*, 1572–1576, 1975.

Lewin, K. J., Harell, G. S., Lee, A. S., and Crowley, L. G.: Malacoplakia. An electron-microscopic study: demonstration of bacilliform organisms in malacoplakic macrophages. Gastroenterology, *66*, 28–45, 1974.

Loveless, K. J.: The effects of radiation upon the cytology of benign and malignant bladder epithelia. Acta Cytol., *17*, 355–360, 1973.

Madersbacher, H., and Bartsch, G.: Eosinophile Infiltrate der Harnblase. Urologia Internat., *27*, 149–159, 1972.

Masukawa, T., Garancis, J. C., Rytel, M. W., and Mattingly, R. F.: Herpes genitalis virus isolation from human bladder urine. Acta Cytol., *16*, 416–428, 1972.

McDougal, W. S., Cramer, S. F., and Miller, R.: Invasive carcinoma of renal pelvis following cyclophosphamide therapy for nonmalignant disease. Cancer, *48*, 691–695, 1981.

Melamed, M. R.: The urinary sediment cytology in a case of malakoplakia. Acta Cytol., *6*, 471–474, 1962.

Melamed, M. R., and Wolinska, W. H.: On the significance of intracytoplasmic inclusions in the urinary sediment. Am. J. Pathol., *38*, 711–718, 1961.

Murphy, W. M.: Herpesvirus in bladder cancer. Acta Cytol., *20*, 207–210, 1976.

Myerson, D., Hackman, R. C., Nelson, J. A., Ward, D. C., and McDougall, J. K.: Widespread presence of histologically occult cytomegalovirus. Hum. Pathol., *15*, 430–439, 1984.

Naib, Z. M.: Exfoliative Cytopathology, 3rd Ed. Boston, Little Brown, 1985.

Norkin, L. C.: Papovaviral persistent infections. Microbiol. Rev., *46*, 384–425, 1982.

Nowels, K., Kent, E., Rinsho, K., and Oyasu, R.: Prostate specific antigen and acid phosphatase-reactive cells in cystitis cystica and glandularis. Arch. Pathol. Lab. Med., *112*, 734–737, 1988.

O'Flynn, J. D., and Mullaney, J.: Leukoplakia of the bladder. Br. J. Urol., *39*, 461–471, 1967.

O'Morchoe, P. J., Riad, W., Cowles, L. T., Dorsch, R. F., and Frost, J. K.: Urinary cytological changes after radiotherapy of renal transplants. Acta Cytol., *20*, 132–136, 1976.

Oravisto, K. J.: Epidemiology of interstitial cystitis. Ann. Chir. Gynaecol. Fenn., *64*, 75–77, 1975.

O'Reilly, R. J., Lee, F. K., Grossbard, E., et al.: Papovavirus excretion following marrow transplantation: incidence and association with hepatic dysfunction. Transplant Proc., *13*, 262–266, 1981.

Padgett, B. L., and Walker, D. L.: New human papillomaviruses. Prog. Med. Virol., *21*, 1–135, 1976.

Padgett, B. L., Walker, D. L., Zu Rhein, G. M., Eckroade, R. J., and Dessel, B. H.: Cultivation of papova-like virus from human brain with progressive multifocal encephalopathy. Lancet, *1*, 1257–1260, 1971.

Pedersen-Bjergaard, J., Ersboli, J., Hansen, V. L., Sorensen, B. L., Christoffersen, K., Hou-Jensen, K., Nissen, N. I., Knudsen, J. B., and Hansen, M. M.: Carcinoma of the urinary bladder after treatment with cyclophosphamide for non-Hodgkin's lymphoma. N. Engl. J. Med., *318*, 1028–1032, 1988.

Pinkert, T. C., Catlow, C. E., and Straus, R.: Endometriosis of the urinary bladder in a man with prostatic carcinoma. Cancer, *43*, 1562–1567, 1979.

Piscioli, F., Pusiol, T., Polla, E., Failoni, G., and Luciani, L.: Urinary cytology of [sic] tuberculosis of the bladder. Acta Cytol., *29*, 125–131, 1985.

Prescott, L. F.: Effects of acetylsalicylic acid, phenacetin, paracetamol, and caffeine on renal tubular epithelium. Lancet, *1*, 91–96, 1965.

Prescott, L. F., and Brodie, D. E.: A simple differential stain for urinary sediment. Lancet, *2*, 940, 1964.

Rasmussen, K., Petersen, B. L., Jacobo, E., Penick, G. D., and Sall, J.: Cytologic effects of Thiotepa and Adriamycin on normal canine urothelium. Acta Cytol., *24*, 237–243, 1980.

Rathert, P., and Roth, S. E.: Urinzytologie. Praxis und Atlas. 2nd Ed. Berlin, Springer Verlag, 1991.

Reeves, D. S., Thomas, A. L., Wise, R., Blacklock, N. J., and Soul, J. O.: Lack of homogeneity of bladder urine. Lancet, *1*, 1258–1259, 1974.

Rosen, S., Harmon, W., Krensky, A. M., and et al.: Tubulointerstitial nephritis associated with polyomavirus (BK type) infection. N. Engl. J. Med., *308*, 1192–1196, 1983.

Rouse, B. A., Donaldson, L. D., and Goellner, J. R.: Intranuclear inclusions in urinary cytology. Acta Cytol., *30*, 105–109, 1986.

Schiff, H. I., Finkel, M., and Schapira, H. E.: Transitional cell carcinoma of the ureter, associated with cyclophosphamide therapy for benign disease. A case report. J. Urol., *128*, 1023–1024, 1982.

Schistosomiasis of the urinary bladder. Case records of the Massachusetts General Hospital: N. Engl. J. Med., *330,* 51–57, 1994.

Schmid, G. H., Hornstein, O. P., Munstermann, M., and Potyka, J.: Periodical epithelial exfoliation of the urinary ducts in the male. Acta Cytol., *16,* 352–362, 1972.

Schneider, V., Smith, M. J. V., and Frable, W. J.: Urinary cytology in endometriosis of the bladder. Acta Cytol., *24,* 30–33, 1980.

Schumann, G. B., Berring, S., and Hill, R. B.: Use of the cytocentrifuge for the detection of cytomegalovirus inclusions in the urine of renal allograft patients. A case report. Acta Cytol., *21,* 167–172, 1977.

Schumann, G. G., Burleson, R. L., Henry, J. B., and Jones, D. B.: Urinary cytodiagnosis of acute renal allograft rejection using the cytocentrifuge. Am. J. Clin. Pathol., *67,* 134–140, 1977.

Schumann, G. B., Johnston, J. L., and Weiss, M. A.: Renal epithelial fragments in urine sediment. Acta Cytol., *25,* 147–153, 1981.

Schumann, G. B., Lerner, S. I., Weiss, M. A., Gawronski, L., and Lohia, G. K.: Inclusion bearing cells in industrial workers exposed to lead. Am. J. Clin. Path., *74,* 192–196, 1980.

Sima, A. A., Finkelstein, S. D., and McLachlan, D. R.: Multiple malignant astrocytomas in a patient with progressive multifocal leukoencephalopathy. Ann. Neurol., *14,* 183–188, 1983.

Sinclair-Smith, C., Kahn, L. B., and Cywes, S.: Malacoplakia in childhood. Case report with ultrastructural observations and review of the literature. Arch Pathol., *99,* 198–203, 1975.

Slavin, R. E., Millan, J. C., and Mullins, G. M.: Pathology of high dose intermittent cyclophosphamide therapy. Human Pathol., *6,* 693–709, 1975.

Smith, B. H., and Dehner, L. P.: Chronic ulcerating interstitial cystitis (Hunner's ulcer). A study of 28 cases. Arch. Pathol., *93,* 76–81, 1972.

Smith, M. G., and Vellios, F.: Inclusion disease or generalized salivary gland virus infection. Arch. Pathol., *50,* 862–884, 1950.

Spagnolo, D. V., and Waring, P. M.: Bladder granulomata after bladder surgery. Am. J. Clin. Pathol., *86,* 430–437, 1986.

Stella, F., Troccoli, R., Stella, C., Battistelli, S., Biagione, S., Giardini, C., Baroncoani, D., and Manenti, F.: Urinary cytologic abnormalities in bone marrow transplant recipients of Cyclosporin. Acta Cytol., *31,* 615–619, 1987.

Stilman, M. M., Freelund, M. C., and Schmitt, G. W.: Cytologic evaluation of urine after kidney transplantation. Acta Cytol., *31,* 625–630, 1987.

Suhrland, M. J., Koslow, M., Perchick, A., Weiner, S., Alba Greco, M., Colquhoun, F., Muller, W. D., and Burstein, D.: Cytologic findings in progressive multifocal leukoencephalopathy. Report of two cases. Acta Cytol., *31,* 505–511, 1987.

Taft, P. D., and Flax, M. H.: Urinary cytology in renal transplantation; association of renal tubular cells and graft rejection. Transpl., *4,* 194–204, 1966.

Thrasher, J. B., Miller, G. J., and Wettlaufer, J. N.: Bladder leiomyosarcoma following cyclophosphamide therapy for lupus nephritis. J. Urol., *143,* 119–121, 1990.

Travis, L. B., Curtis, R. E., Boice, J. D., Jr., and Fraumeni, J. F. Jr.: Bladder cancer after chemotherapy for non-Hodgkin's lymphoma. N. Engl. J. Med. *321,* 544–545, 1989.

Valente, P. T., Atkinson, B. F., and Guerry, D.: Melanuria. Acta Cytol., *29,* 1026–1028, 1985.

Wall, R. L., and Clausen, K. P.: Carcinoma of the urinary bladder in patients receiving cyclophosphamide. N. Engl. J. Med., *293,* 271–273, 1975.

Webber, C. A., and Eveland, L. K.: Cytologic detection of Wuchereria bancrofti microfilariae in urine collected during a routine workup for hematuria. Acta Cytol., *26,* 837–840, 1982.

Wenzel, J. E., Greene, L. F., and Harris, L. E.: Eosinophilic cystitis. J. Pediatr., *64,* 746–749, 1964.

White, F. A. I., Ishaq, M., Stoner, G. L., and Frisque, R. J.: JC virus DNA is present in many human brain samples from patients without progressive multifocal leukoencephalopathy. J. Virol., *66,* 5726–5734, 1992.

Winkelman, M., Burrig, K. F., Koldovsky, U., Witskowski, M., Grabensee, B., and Pfitzer, P.: Cyclosporin A altered renal tubular cells in urinary cytology. Lancet, *2,* 667, 1985.

Worth, P. H. L.: Cyclophosphamide and the bladder. Br. Med. J., *3,* 182, 1971.

CHAPTER 5

Tumors of the Bladder

UROTHELIAL (TRANSITIONAL CELL) TUMORS

Epidemiology

Tumors of the urinary bladder are the quintessential example of industrial neoplasms. They were first observed and reported by the German surgeon Rehn in 1895 and 1896 in workers employed in factories producing aniline dyes. It has since been shown that a number of aromatic amines such as benzidine, betanaphtylamine, para-aminodiphenyl, and related compounds produce bladder tumors in animals and in humans. The compound MBOCA, related to benzidine, recently has been shown to produce low-grade papillary tumors in exposed workers (Ward et al., 1988). As has been documented by Koss et al. in 1965, the risk factor with para-aminodiphenyl is not fully dose-related. Some workers with low exposure levels developed bladder cancers, whereas in the majority of the workers, bladder tumors did not occur in spite of massive exposure to the carcinogen (Koss et al., 1969). Clearly, powerful detoxification mechanisms protect most exposed people.

Besides exposure to carcinogenic chemicals, certain other occupations appear to put workers at high risk: rubber workers, leather workers, painters, and cooks have a high rate of bladder tumors (Cole et al., 1972). The first three groups are likely to be exposed to cancerogenic chemical compounds, but the reason for the high rate of bladder tumors in cooks remains unclear.

Paraplegic and quadraplegic patients surviving for many years after a spinal cord injury are prone to bladder cancer (Kaufman et al., 1977; Bejany et al., 1987; Bicket et al., 1991). In some of these patients occult invasive tumors were discovered by random bladder biopsies (Kaufman et al., 1977). Many of these patients develop squamous metaplasia and squamous carcinomas and hence show some similarities to patients with schistosomiasis (see p. 97). Whether the mechanism of disease is related to long-term catheterization or to urinary stasis is not known, pending further investigation.

Abuse of phenacetin, usually leading to tumors in the renal pelves and ureters, as discussed in Chapter 6, may also be associated with bladder cancer (Piper et al., 1985).

A number of drugs are associated with, or have been shown to cause bladder cancer. Thus, cyclophosphamide (Cytoxan, Endoxan), an alkylating agent widely used in the treatment of malignant lymphomas and other malignant tumors, may cause bladder carcinomas (and, very rarely, leiomyosarcomas) in patients receiving a large dose of the drug, as discussed in Chapter 4. Rarely, similar tumors may occur in renal pelves or ureters (see Chaps. 4 and 6). Chlornaphazin, a drug previously used in the treatment of lymphomas, has also been shown to be associated with bladder tumors, probably because its metabolites are aromatic amines (Videbaek, 1964; Laursen, 1970). Busulfan (Myelan) may also cause significant nuclear abnormalities in epithelial cells (see Chap. 4).

Another important association of bladder tumors is with *Schistosomia haematobium,* a parasite commonly present in Egypt and other parts of Eastern Africa (see p. 56). The mechanisms accounting for this association are unknown. Bladder tumors associated with schistosomiasis differ from spontaneously-occurring tumors inasmuch as the dominant histologic type is the keratin-producing squamous carcinoma that is comparatively uncommon in patients in other geographic locations. Cigarette smoking has been universally considered a carcinogenic event, but even this is not necessarily observed in patients with bladder tumors. In most patients with bladder tumors in the Western world there is no documented exposure to any known carcinogenic agents.

Histology and Natural History

Tumors of the urinary bladder may have diverse histologic patterns. By far the most common type of tumors are derived from and retain the configuration of the urothelium. In this chapter, the term "transitional cell tumors" has been replaced by "urothelial tumors." The unique structure of the epithelium of origin of these tumors, described in Chapter 2, is recognized by this terminology. The urothelial tumors are classified according to several features: configuration, grading, and staging.

The Concept of Two Pathways of Bladder Tumors: Papillary and Nonpapillary

For many years, neoplastic lesions of the urinary bladder have been considered as a single family of tumors, classified by grade and by stage. Even today, it is not uncommon to encounter published data wherein the bladder tumors are described as "superficial" or "invasive" without comments on their configuration, *i.e.,* papillary or nonpapillary, or grade (low-grade or high-grade). Yet there is ample evidence that the origin and behavior of the urothelial tumors of the bladder follow two separate, albeit overlapping, pathways. One pathway pertains to tumors originating in urothelium characterized by an increased number of epithelial layers without significant nuclear abnormalities (hyperplasia); such tumors are nearly always well-differentiated (low-grade) papillary tumors that have a very limited potential for invasion. The second pathway pertains to tumors derived from urothelial lesions characterized by marked

nuclear abnormalities such as flat carcinoma in situ and related lesions; such tumors may be either high-grade papillary or, more importantly, directly invading the wall of the bladder without a papillary component. Nearly all invasive bladder cancers are derived from the flat lesions (see below). This subdivision not only is of diagnostic and prognostic significance but also is supported by a number of observations, including DNA ploidy data, described in Chapter 9, blood group isoantigen distribution, described in Chapter 10, and by preliminary molecular genetic data, summarized in Chapter 11.

Papillary Tumors; Their Grading

Papillary tumors protrude into the lumen of the urinary bladder and are essentially composed of a richly vascularized core of connective tissue, supporting simple or complex epithelial folds (Fig. 5-1). The papillary tumors may have a single thin stalk or may be broad-based or sessile. The rich vascularity of these tumors accounts for one of the principal symptoms of this disease, hematuria. The papillary tumors may be classified into three grades, reflecting the degree of nuclear abnormality and the similarity of the epithelial component to the tissue of origin, or differentiation. Papillary tumors of Grade 1 closely resemble normal urothelium and show no significant nuclear abnormalities. Umbrella cells are commonly present on the epithelial surface of such tumors as evidence of normal maturation or differentiation (Fig. 5-2*A*). Papillary tumors of Grade 3 show marked nuclear abnormalities in the form of nuclear enlargement and hyperchromasia affecting all or nearly all component cells, and lack differentiating features, such as the presence of umbrella cells (Fig. 5-2*C,D*). Such tumors may be composed of large or small cancer cells or a mixture of cell sizes in different segments of the tumor. Grade 2 tumors are intermediate between grade 1 and grade 3 and show nuclear abnormalities of moderate grade, such as slight or moderate nuclear enlargement and hyperchromasia, in about half of the component cells. Grade 2 tumors retain many morphologic features of the epithelium of origin (Fig. 5-2*B*). Quite often different segments of a papillary tumor may show different grades of abnormality and are sometimes classified as grade 1 to 2, or 2 to 3.

Low-grade papillary tumors, including grade 1 papillary tumors and some grade 2 tumors are derived from areas of hyperplasia of the urothelium (see Fig. 5-8*A*). The early stages of tumor formation are characterized by increased vascularization of the hyper-

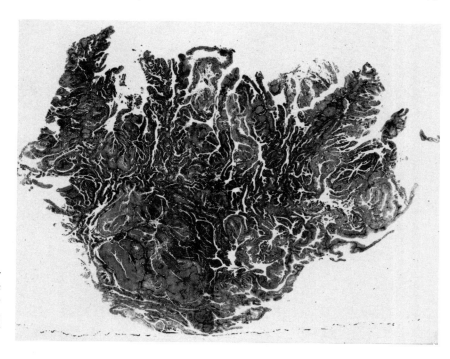

FIGURE 5-1. A low-power view of a papillary tumor of the urinary bladder. Note the complex pattern of delicate stalks, provided with a rich blood supply.

plastic epithelial segment. With the passage of time and continuing growth into the lumen of the bladder, the tumor acquires a stalk surrounded by epithelial folds. The roots of the tumor may extend into the lamina propria (stage T1) but such tumors *rarely progress to muscle-invading carcinoma. The extension into the lamina propria has no prognostic significance because it is not associated with metastases.* Low-grade papillary tumors may be accompanied by or followed by similar new tumors in the same, adjacent, or distant areas of the urothelium (Fig. 5-3). Nearly all grade 1 tumors and some grade 2 tumors with this behavior pattern have a diploid DNA content (see Chap. 9). *Because low-grade papillary tumors are usually lined by epithelium closely resembling normal urothelium, their cytologic recognition is poor.*

High-grade papillary tumors, comprising some grade 2 tumors and all grade 3 tumors, are usually derived from surface urothelium with various degrees of nuclear abnormality that may be classified either as carcinoma in situ or atypical hyperplasia (intraurothelial neoplasia), to be discussed below. These tumors are nearly always aneuploid and may progress to invasive cancer, sometimes directly but more often because of associated areas of carcinoma in situ. Such tumors *are composed of cells that are morphologically abnormal,* although the degree of abnormality depends on the grade and makeup of the tumor.

Nonpapillary Tumors; Their Grading

Nonpapillary tumors may be divided into noninvasive carcinomas, lining the surface of the bladder without evidence of invasion (*flat carcinomas in situ and related lesions, grouped as intraurothelial neoplasia*), and invasive tumors; the latter may again be graded as 2 or 3, depending on the level of nuclear abnormalities. Invasive grade 1 tumors, closely mimicking normal urothelium, are extremely uncommon. Invasive nonpapillary tumors may be composed of large or small cells, or a mixture of cells of different sizes. The invasive tumors may also show various patterns of differentiation: thus foci of squamous carcinoma or adenocarcinoma are frequently present in urothelial tumors. Such foci have no known prognostic significance. In many instances, the subsidiary patterns of differentiation may be dominant, resulting in an adenocarcinoma or squamous carcinoma (Fig. 5-4; see also pp. 97 and 99).

Invasive carcinomas are nearly always associated with significantly abnormal surface epithelium, are nearly always aneuploid, and are composed of morphologically highly abnormal cancer cells.

By far the most important high-grade neoplastic lesion of the urothelium is *nonpapillary or flat carcinoma in situ and related abnormalities, which are the source of most invasive urothelial cancers.* Such lesions are most commonly found in the urinary bladder

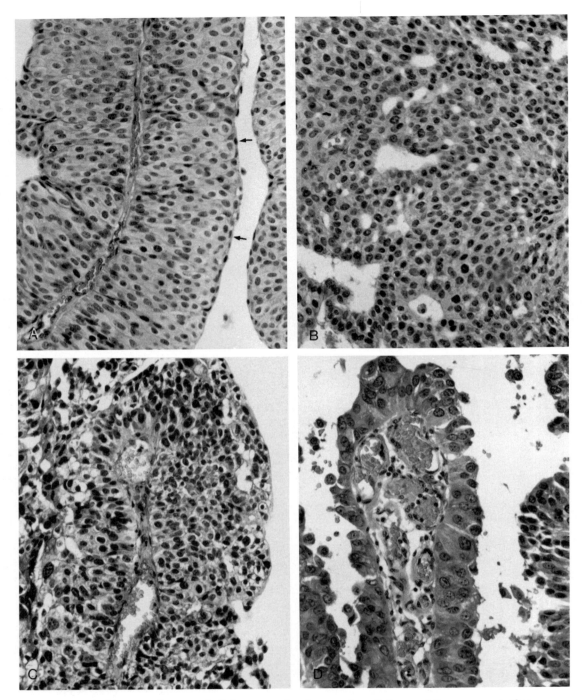

FIGURE 5-2. Papillary urothelial tumors of various grades, all shown at the same magnification. (*A*) Grade I papillary tumor. Note that the lining epithelium closely resembles normal urothelium with umbrella cells on the surface (*arrows*). (Compare with Fig. 2-1.) There are no nuclear abnormalities. (*B*) Grade II papillary tumor. Note that about half of the spherical nuclei in the epithelium are moderately enlarged and hyperchromatic. Compare the nuclei in *B* with those in *A* in the same panel. (*C,D*) Grade III papillary tumors with the epithelium composed of small (*C*) and large cancer cells (*D*). The enlarged nuclei are of variable sizes and configuration, and show marked hyperchromasia. (All figures × 250.)

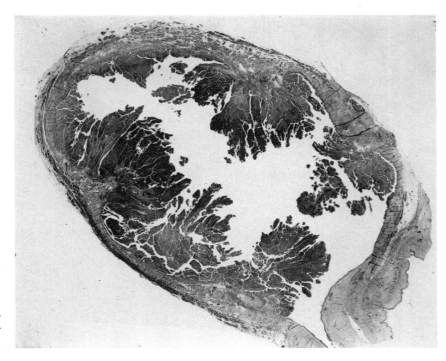

FIGURE 5-3. Whole human bladder mount showing multiple papillary tumors. Although the tunica muscularis is focally thinned, there was no evidence of invasion beyond the lamina propria. (Section courtesy of Dr. Rolph Schade, formerly of Newcastle-upon-Tyne, England.)

but are also known to occur in the ureters and renal pelves. Cytologic recognition of this group of tumors is excellent.

Precursor Lesions of Invasive Urothelial Carcinoma

Nonpapillary Carcinoma in Situ and Related Abnormalities (Intraurothelial Neoplasia or IUN)

Carcinoma in situ of the urinary bladder was first described by Melicow and Holloway in 1952, as "Bowen's disease or intraepithelial carcinoma." The lesion was initially observed as an incidental finding, adjacent to visible papillary tumors (Fig. 5-5). The full significance of this lesion has become evident within the last 30 years. A number of prospective studies on workers exposed to para-aminodiphenyl, a potent bladder carcinogen, have shown that invasive bladder cancer may develop in patients whose urinary sediment disclosed cancer cells in the absence of cystoscopically visible lesions (Melamed et al., 1960; Koss et al., 1965, 1969). Subsequent studies by mapping of bladders with papillary tumors also disclosed the presence of peripheral foci of carcinoma in situ and related lesions (Koss et al., 1974, 1977; Koss, 1985). Thus the lesion may be observed in two forms:

as an epithelial change accompanying papillary tumors, or as a primary lesion in the absence of prior neoplastic disease of the urothelium. *In either form, carcinoma in situ is the most important precursor lesion of invasive carcinoma.*

Primary Carcinoma in Situ

Primary carcinoma in situ does not form any visible tumors. Cystoscopy in such patients may disclose an area of redness of the bladder mucosa, mimicking inflammation, or other non-specific abnormalities, described as "cobblestone epithelium" or "interstitial cystitis." In many cases, there are hardly any visible abnormalities. The patients with this disease may complain of persisting "bladder irritation," nocturia, and sometimes dysuria, and may show microhematuria. Frank hematuria is uncommon. Thus the diagnosis of primary carcinoma in situ is based on either incidental biopsies of visible abnormalities or cytologic examination of voided urine. Many patients have no symptoms at all until invasive cancer develops. Short of a cytologic mass survey, such as we conducted on workers exposed to para-aminodiphenyl (see above), most carcinomas in situ remain occult.

Flat, nonpapillary carcinoma in situ is best defined as a lesion confined to the urothelium and composed of cancer cells. The morphologic configuration of carcinoma in situ may vary: the lesion may be composed

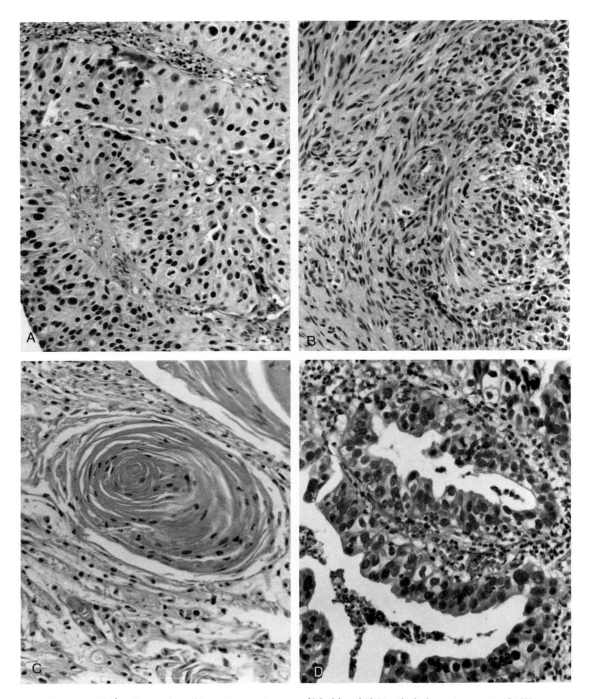

FIGURE 5-4. Examples of invasive carcinoma of bladder. (*A*) Urothelial carcinoma grade III mimicking a papillary tumor. (*B*) Urothelial carcinoma with a spindle cell component. (*C*) Well-differentiated squamous carcinoma with keratinization. (*D*) Adenocarcinoma. (A–D ×250).

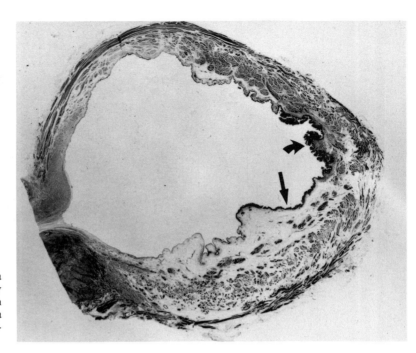

FIGURE 5-5. Cross section of a whole mount of a human urinary bladder showing a flat carcinoma in situ (*straight arrow*) adjacent to a papillary tumor (*curved arrow*). (Section courtesy of Dr. R. Schade.)

of small or large cancer cells forming from 4 to 20 or sometimes more layers of cells. The component cells usually show marked nuclear abnormalities in the form of large, often hyperchromatic, nuclei of odd shapes. In some lesions, prominent nucleoli may be noted. Occasionally, large clear cells akin to those observed in Paget's disease of the nipple may be present (Fig. 5-6D). It is of incidental interest that cancer of the bladder metastatic to the vagina or penis can also mimic Paget's disease (see p. 123 and Fig. 5-45).

Prospective studies of the behavior of primary carcinoma in situ were conducted in the 1960s. A number of observations have been reported that strongly suggested that biopsy-documented lesions, if untreated, are capable of producing invasive cancers of the urinary bladder in about 60% of patients (Koss, 1975 and 1985). At that time the only available effective treatment was cystectomy. With the advent of conservative chemo- and immunotherapy, the latter with an attenuated bovine tuberculosis bacterium known as bacille Calmette-Guérin (BCG), other important features of carcinoma in situ came to light. Because the treatment is effective only on direct contact with the diseased epithelium, it became apparent that an extension of the neoplasm into the prostatic ducts, where it was sheltered from the therapeutic agents, precluded effective therapy (Fig. 5-7). A study by Mahadevia et al. (1986) documented, by

mapping, that the extension of carcinoma in situ to prostatic ducts is fairly common. It occurred in nine of 16 patients with carcinoma in situ. In two patients, the involvement of the prostatic ducts was extensive, in seven focal. Clearly, an investigation of the anterior prostate by deep biopsies is an important step that should be undertaken in all male patients before conservative treatment is instituted.

Another important complication of carcinoma in situ of the bladder in both sexes is its extension into adjacent ureters (Fig. 5-7C) and urethra. Such involvement may occur with any high-grade advanced bladder tumor, whether or not the carcinoma in situ component has been identified. It has been recommended that the status of the ureters be checked by frozen section at the time of cystectomy. Stripping of the penile urethra epithelium is sometimes performed to prevent urethral recurrence (see also Chap. 6). Regardless of these considerations, in many patients the conservative therapy has only a transient effect or is not effective at all. Treatment by cystectomy still remains an option in such cases.

Flat carcinomas in situ virtually always have an aneuploid DNA content. Norming et al. (1992) observed that those carcinomas in situ that have or acquire two aneuploid populations of cells (multiploid tumors) lead to invasive carcinoma more often than tumors with a single aneuploid cell line. This obser-

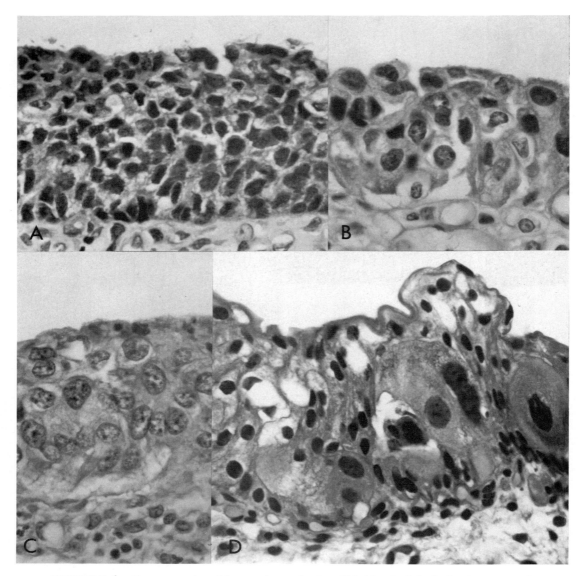

FIGURE 5-6.   Four examples of flat carcinoma in situ of bladder. In *A* the lesion is composed of small cells. In *B* and *C* the lesions are composed of larger cells—in *B* the nuclei show marked hyperchromasia, which is absent in *C.* In *D* the lesion contains a few giant cancer cells with vacuolated cytoplasm, surrounded by smaller cells. The pattern is similar to Paget's disease. (A–D × 560.)

vation suggests that increased instability of the genome of the cancer cells is an important factor in behavior, and hence in prognosis. It is also of interest that molecular genetic findings, discussed in Chapter 11, show major similarities between carcinoma in situ and invasive cancer.

The principal characteristics of nonpapillary carcinoma in situ are summarized in Table 5-1.

Lesser Degrees of Epithelial Abnormality ("Dysplasia," Intraurothelial Neoplasia)

Besides classical carcinomas in situ, composed of cancer cells of various sizes throughout its thickness, the epithelium of the bladder may show lesser degrees of abnormality. In such lesions, often designated as "dysplasia," there is usually some surface maturation,

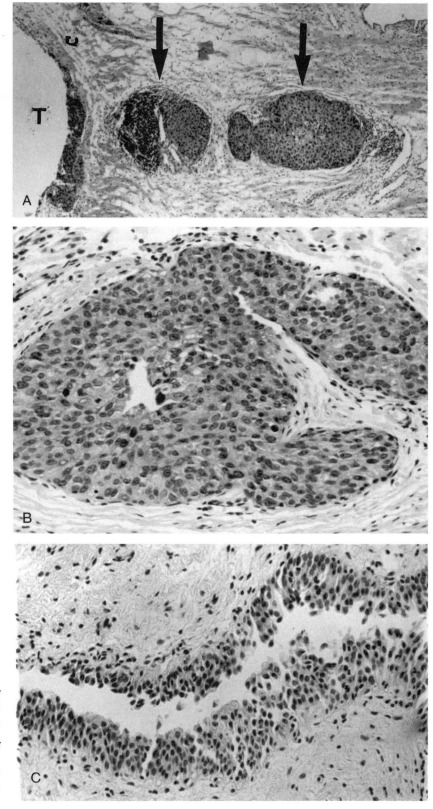

FIGURE 5-7. (*A*) Extension of a carcinoma in situ, lining the trigone of the bladder (T) to adjacent prostatic ducts (*arrows*). (*B*) Higher power view of one of the prostatic ducts with urothelial cancer. (*C*) Same patient: atypia of the epithelium of the distal ureter. (A × 90; *B,C* × 225).

TABLE 5-1
Characteristics of Nonpapillary Carcinoma in Situ of Bladder

1. The lesion, confined to the epithelium, is composed of cancer cells, replacing the normal urothelium.
2. The lesion cannot be recognized cystoscopically as a tumor. Cystoscopic abnormalities mimicking inflammation, "velvety redness," "cobblestone epithelium," or "interstitial cystitis" were recorded. In other cases there are no cystoscopic abnormalities whatever.
3. In males, the lesion often extends into the prostatic ducts. In both sexes, it may extend to the ureters and the urethra.
4. Because the lesion produces only nonspecific symptoms or may be asymptomatic, its diagnosis is based either on cytology of voided urine or on incidental biopsies of bladder epithelium.
5. If untreated, primary carcinomas in situ will progress to *invasive carcinoma in at least 60% of all patients within 5 years.*

for example formation of umbrella cells, even though the bulk of the epithelium is composed of cells with significant nuclear abnormalities. I proposed that all intraepithelial neoplastic abnormalities should be designated as *intraurothelial neoplasia (IUN)* (Koss, 1992).

The term is similar to those used to describe precancerous lesions in the female genital tract. The lesions may be graded, with IUN grade 1 corresponding to epithelial hyperplasia, grade 2 lesions to atypical hyperplasia (moderate dysplasia), and grade 3 lesions to severe dysplasia or classical carcinoma in situ (Fig. 5-8). As has been described above, epithelial hyperplasia is the source of origin of low-grade papillary tumors. Admittedly, epithelial hyperplasia may also be reactive, for example, as a response to a subepithelial tumor, such as a leiomyoma, but these two forms of hyperplasia cannot be separated from one another by microscopic examination.

Moderate degrees of epithelial abnormalities (IUN grade 2) play a less well-defined role as precursor lesions of invasive carcinoma than classical carcinoma in situ. IUN grade 2 may give rise to papillary tumors and to invasive cancer and must be considered to be high-risk lesions. In mapping studies of the bladder, progression of such lesions to invasive cancer has been observed (Koss, 1979). Several prospective studies have also documented that patients with

such lesions are at a substantial risk for invasive cancer, although the percentage of progressive lesions is probably somewhat below the classical carcinoma in situ or IUN grade 3 (Eisenberg et al., 1960; Schade and Swinney, 1968; Althausen et al., 1976; Wolf et al., 1983, 1987).

More recently, Mufti and Singh (1992) documented that abnormal "random" mucosal biopsies ("dysplasia" or carcinoma in situ) in patients with superficial (papillary) tumors, grade I to II, accurately predicted tumor recurrence. The incidence of freedom from new tumors was 66% of 88 patients without peripheral abnormalities and only 33% in 27 patients with abnormal biopsies (p = 0.002).

In support of the neoplastic nature of "dysplasia" are the observations of Hofstädter et al. (1986) who measured by image analysis the DNA ploidy in Feulgen-stained nuclei isolated from "dysplasia." Most of the cases of "dysplasia" were tetraploid, whereas nuclei from carcinomas in situ were aneuploid. Thus "dysplasia" or IUN grade 2 may represent an intermediate stage between normal epithelium and classical carcinoma in situ.

Secondary Carcinoma in Situ

There is some controversy about the significance of carcinomas in situ accompanying papillary tumors. Such lesions are usually discovered in "random"

FIGURE 5-8. Various grades of intraurothelial neoplasia (IUN) in urinary bladder. (*A*) IUN grade I—epithelial hyperplasia. There is an increase in the number of epithelial layers with trivial nuclear atypia. Such lesions are the source of low-grade papillary tumors. (*B*) IUN grade II—urothelium with moderate nuclear atypia. Note the structural similarity to normal urothelium. Such lesions, sometimes classified as "dysplasia," may give rise to papillary tumors of grade II or higher grade and sometimes to invasive carcinoma. (*C*) IUN grade III—"severe dysplasia" or carcinoma in situ. Compare with the classical carcinomas in situ shown in Fig. 5-5. This lesion is dangerous inasmuch as it may lead directly to invasive carcinoma. (A–C × 350).

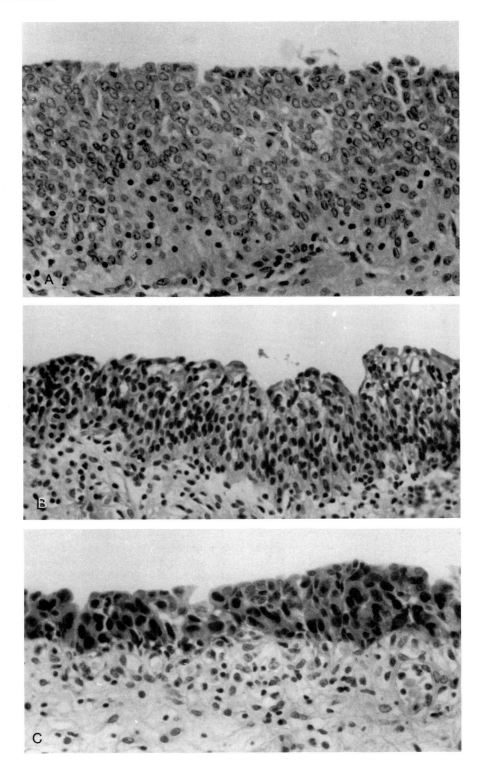

"cold cup" epithelial biopsies of patients with papillary tumors, a practice that was suggested as a consequence of mapping of entire bladders with papillary tumors (summary in Koss, 1985). Positive urine cytology in the presence of a low-grade papillary tumor is strongly suggestive of the presence of a carcinoma in situ and should lead to cystoscopic biopsies of seemingly normal or inflamed bladder mucosa or a search for such tumors in the ureters or renal pelves (Schwalb et al., 1993).

The likelihood of finding a peripheral carcinoma in situ (or related lesions) increases with the grade of the primary papillary tumor. Carcinomas in situ are very uncommon in patients with low-grade papillary tumors but are found in many cases of high grade papillary tumors. In most such instances, the carcinoma in situ is immediately adjacent to the papillary tumors, suggesting a relationship of the two lesions, as discussed above. Carcinomas in situ that are peripheral to the papillary tumor can be uncovered by mucosal biopsies guided by cytology. Also of significance in this regard are flow cytometric DNA ploidy studies of peripheral biopsies in patients with bladder tumors (Norming et al., 1989). As discussed at length in Chapter 9 (p. 263), aneuploidy in peripheral biopsies was observed mainly in the presence of aneuploid tumors, usually grade III, sometimes grade II. There was also considerable concordance of DNA ploidy patterns between primary tumors and their peripheral biopsies, suggesting a link between the visible and invisible lesions. Melamed et al. (1964) noted that about 50% of such lesions can progress to invasive carcinoma. Prout (1983, 1987), on the other hand, proposed that such lesions are less likely to progress to invasion than primary carcinomas in situ. Significant follow-up studies of untreated patients can no longer be conducted, and treatment of one type or another is likely to be applied to all these patients, with a significant modification of their natural history. Therefore, the full significance of these lesions may never become known. In my judgment, for all practical intents and purposes, these lesions should be considered as potentially threatening to the patient and should be treated.

Needless to say, carcinoma in situ or a related lesion is nearly always present adjacent to invasive cancers, although documentation may be difficult because of destruction of the in situ lesion by the invasive tumor or because of necrosis.

The Derivation of Invasive Urothelial Cancer

Studies of the natural history of invasive cancer of the bladder, notably those by Brawn (1982) and by Kaye and Lange (1982), pointed out that in about 80% of such patients there has been no prior history

or clinical evidence of papillary disease. Hence the conclusion that most of these invasive lesions originated in occult flat carcinoma in situ and related epithelial abnormalities. There is also excellent evidence that the status of the peripheral epithelium of the bladder in patients with papillary tumors is of prognostic significance: those patients whose peripheral epithelium shows varying degrees of abnormality are at greater risk for recurrent or invasive cancer than patients whose peripheral epithelium is normal (see above). In a study by Althausen et al. (1976), 80% of a small group of patients with carcinoma in situ of the bladder, peripheral to papillary tumors of low grade, progressed to invasive carcinoma.

The origin of invasive carcinoma in bladders of patients with papillary tumors has also been studied by mapping of bladders removed by cystectomy for recurrent papillary tumors (Koss et al., 1974, 1977; Koss, 1979). It could be documented that in such cases invasive cancer develops in areas of carcinoma in situ and related lesions that may be remote from the papillary tumors (Fig. 5-9). At the time of the cystectomies, the existence of the occult invasive foci was not suspected. These observations have led to the adoption of multiple biopsies of bladder epithelium as a routine procedure in the evaluation of patients with papillary tumors (see p. 126). In another study it could also be shown that flat carcinoma in situ of the ureter or renal pelvis is an unfavorable prognostic sign in these tumors (Mahadevia et al., 1983; also see Chap. 6).

Characteristics of Two Groups of Urothelial Tumors

It is evident from the preceding discussion that the subdivision of urothelial tumors into two groups has considerable bearing on their behavior, and hence on their treatment and prognosis. Besides the basic morphologic differences described above, the two groups of tumors vary in several other respects. The DNA ploidy patterns are different (Tribukait, 1984, 1987; Koss et al., 1989; Norming et al., 1992): the low-grade tumors are predominantly diploid, whereas the high-grade tumors, whether in situ or invasive, are predominantly aneuploid. For further discussion of this issue, see Chapter 9.

The two groups of tumors also differ in their density of nuclear pores, which is lower in the low-grade diploid tumors than in high-grade aneuploid tumors (Czerniak et al., 1984). In addition, the reactivity of the cells with a monoclonal antibody known as Ca1 (epitectin) is higher in aneuploid than diploid tumors (Czerniak and Koss, 1985). The expression of blood group isoantigens is common in diploid tumors but variable in aneuploid tumors (summary in Malmstrom, 1988). Early evidence suggests that the two

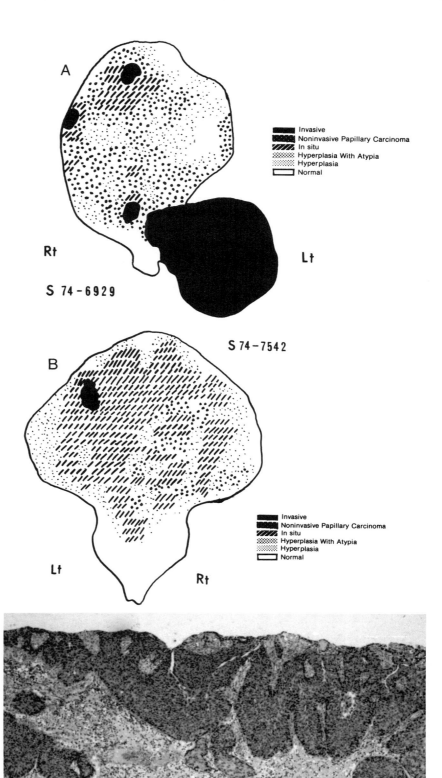

FIGURE 5-9. (*A,B*) Two examples of mapping of the urinary bladder with occult invasive carcinoma derived from carcinoma in situ. (*A*) Bladder removed because of a bulky papillary tumor of low grade with extension to the lamina propria. Three foci of invasive carcinoma derived from carcinoma in situ were observed in areas of the bladder remote from the papillary tumor. (*B*) Bladder removed for an extensive carcinoma in situ. A focus of occult invasive carcinoma was observed in an area of the bladder with a relatively normal surface. (*C*) An example of occult invasive carcinoma derived from a carcinoma in situ of the bladder. (× 80); *A* and *B* modified from Koss, L. G., Nakanishi, I., and Freed, S. Z.: Nonpapillary carcinoma in situ and atypical hyperplasia in cancerous bladders. Further studies of surgically removed bladders by mapping. Urology *9,* 442–455, 1977.

TABLE 5-2
Characteristics of Two Groups of Urothelial Tumors

	Low-Grade Papillary Tumors	High-Grade Papillary Tumors, Nonpapillary Tumors and Invasive Carcinomas
Epithelial abnormality of origin	Epithelial hyperplasia	Carcinoma in situ and related abnormalities (intraurothelial neoplasia or dysplasia)
Invasive potential	Low	High
DNA ploidy pattern*	Predominantly diploid	Predominantly aneuploid
Density of nuclear pores[†]	Normal	Increased
Expression of Ca antigen (Epitectin)[‡]	As in normal urothelium	Increased
Blood group isoantigen expression[§]	Usually present	Variable
Molecular genetic differences	See Chapter 11	
Cytologic recognition	Very poor	Good to outstanding, depending on grade and DNA ploidy

*Tribukait, 1984, 1987; Koss et al., 1989; Norming, et al., 1992.
[†]Czerniak et al., 1984.
[‡]Czerniak and Koss, 1985.
[§]Summary in Malmstrom, 1988.

families of bladder tumors may also show molecular genetic differences (see Chap. 11). Most importantly in the context of this work is the recognition of cancer cells in the cytologic samples, which is high for high-grade aneuploid tumors and low for low-grade diploid tumors. Table 5-2 and Fig. 5-10*A* summarize the differences between the two groups of urothelial tumors.

STAGING OF TUMORS OF THE BLADDER

Jewett and Strong (1946) laid down the foundations for staging of bladder tumors with significant prognostic implications based on extensive studies of bladder cancers at the autopsy table. Jewett's system of staging disclosed that the depth of invasion of bladder wall was directly related to prognosis. Tumors invading the muscularis (stages B or C) fared less well than more superficial tumors (stages 0 or A), whereas for tumors with metastases either to regional lymph nodes or to more distant organ sites (stage D), the prognosis was nearly hopeless (Fig. 5-10*B*).

With the introduction of the international TNM protocols, three factors are considered in staging: T (tumor—extent of invasion in the organ of origin), N (lymph node metastases), and M (distant metastases). From the point of view of this narrative, the most important changes occurred in separation of the non-invasive tumors into two categories: T_{is}, indicating a flat carcinoma in situ, and T_a, indicating a papillary non-invasive tumor. This is an important recognition that these two tumor types have vastly different behav-

ior patterns and prognosis. Clearly, T_{is} is the source of most invasive cancers (see above).

Another comment pertains to tumors stage T_1, *i.e.*, tumors extending into the lamina propria. In my experience, low-grade papillary tumors often extend to the lamina propria, but this finding is of no prognostic significance. I consider this to be the equivalent of "roots of a tree", necessary for the tumor to survive. On the other hand, invasion of the lamina propria by cells derived from a high-grade tumor such as a carcinoma in situ, particularly if there are numerous foci of invasion, is a form of *microinvasive carcinoma,* of major clinical significance because it usually heralds an invasive bladder cancer.

Higher grade tumors (T_2 and T_3, tumor invading the muscularis; T_4 tumor spreading beyond the bladder) represent a clinical dilemma as to the most effective form of treatment by surgery, radiotherapy, and chemotherapy.

The TNM nomenclature is reflected in Fig. 5-10*B*, superimposed on the Jewett nomenclature.

TARGETS OF CYTOLOGIC EXAMINATION OF THE LOWER URINARY TRACT

Nonpapillary (flat) carcinoma in situ and related epithelial lesions constitute the most important group of epithelial abnormalities in the lower urinary tract. *A timely diagnosis, treatment, and monitoring of these precancerous changes is the best means of prevention of invasive cancer* with its high mortality rate.

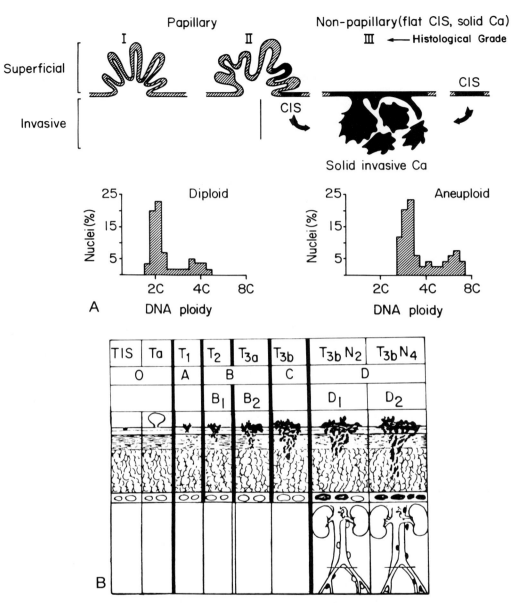

FIGURE 5-10. (*A*) Schematic representation of data presented in Table 5-2, reflecting the morphology, grading, behavior pattern, and DNA ploidy of the two families of urothelial tumors. (Diagram by Dr. Bogdan Czerniak.) (*B*) Schematic representation of staging of bladder tumors. The prognosis depends significantly on the depth of invasion of bladder wall and the presence or absence of metastases. Note in stage 0 the separation of carcinoma in situ (TIS) from non-invasive papillary tumors (Ta), two lesions with very different behavior pattern and prognosis.

Fortunately, cytologic techniques are exquisitely sensitive in the identification of these lesions. **Hence, the principal target of cytologic evaluation of the lower urinary tract is the detection, diagnosis and monitoring of flat cancerous abnormalities of the urothelium.** High-grade papillary lesions and nearly all invasive carcinomas can also be identified cytologically but, in such cases, the cytologic verdict merely confirms clinical and histologic data. *The method generally fails,* however, *in the identification of low-grade papillary lesions and epithelial hyperplasia without nuclear abnormalities.*

Cytologic Diagnosis of Urothelial Tumors

The fundamental issue in understanding the performance of cytology in the diagnosis of tumors of the lower urinary tract is the separation of the neoplastic events into two principal categories: tumors lined by normal or nearly normal urothelium (low-grade tumors) and tumors lined by or composed of identifiable malignant cells (high-grade tumors). This division corresponds closely to the separation of urothelial tumors into two groups, as discussed above (Table 5-2 and Fig. 5-10A). In the context of this summary, certain cytologic characteristics of these tumors must be emphasized.

Tumors Composed of Cells That Resemble Normal Urothelium

Tumors that are lined by cells that resemble very closely normal urothelium shed cells that generally cannot be identified as abnormal.

This group of tumors comprises the low-grade, well-differentiated papillary tumors, customarily classified as "papillomas," papillary tumors grade 1, and about one half of papillary carcinomas grade 2, particularly those with normal (diploid) DNA distribution patterns. Such tumors may shed clusters of urothelial cells, sometimes of spherical (papillary) configuration.

The morphologic characteristics of such clusters are generally identical with those shed from normal urothelium after palpation or instrumentation or in the presence of inflammation or stones (Fig. 5-11; see also pp. 41 and 57). Even if the urine is obtained prior to clinical examination, the margin of error in linking clusters of urothelial cells to the presence of a low-grade tumor is very high.

There are a few exceptions to this rule: *in voided urine, spontaneously shed complex clusters* of morphologically benign urothelial cells with loosely structured periphery may be consistent with (but are *not diagnostic* of) a papillary tumor, provided that a trauma, such as palpation or instrumentation, can be ruled out (Fig. 5-11C). A secure diagnosis of a low-grade tumor can also be established *when tumor fragments with a clearly identified connective tissue stalk or a central capillary vessel are present in the sediment.*

Another exception to this rule occurs in the uncommon low-grade papillary tumor with a squamoid configuration, *i.e.,* features resembling squamous epithelium. In such cases, the urine sediment may contain urothelial cells, arranged in concentric fashion ("epithelial pearls"), without any evidence of significant nuclear abnormalities (Fig. 5-12). Such "pearls" must be differentiated from a similar cell arrangement observed in squamous cancers, wherein marked nuclear abnormalities and heavy cytoplasmic keratinization are usually observed (see Color Plate 5-1F).

Many attempts have been made to define the morphologic microscopic characteristics of tumor fragments to differentiate them from normal urothelial cell clusters but, except for the circumstances described above, no significant objective criteria have emerged. If one considers that lithiasis may contribute to the shedding of clusters of urothelial cells and that one of the main points of differential diagnosis of space-occupying lesions of the urinary tract is between low-grade papillary tumors and lithiasis, the limitations of cytology become very clear: **the method is not suitable for differentiation between effects of instrumentation, lithiasis and low-grade papillary tumors.**

These conclusions are at a considerable variance with published writing, wherein several authors claimed that grade 1 tumors shed recognizable cells in the urinary sediment. Thus, Murphy et al. (1984) claimed that cells with increased nucleocytoplasmic (NC) ratio, enlarged and eccentric nuclei (but no nucleoli) are characteristic and can be recognized in 70% of these tumors. Wiener et al. (1993) reported 33% of correct cytologic diagnoses in grade 1 tumors without describing her criteria. Kannan and Bose (1993) specifically addressed the issue of differentiation between artifacts of instrumentation and low-grade tumors. They concluded that "cell clusters with ragged borders" characterize the tumors, whereas normal urothelial cells "form clusters with smooth borders, lined with denser staining of cytoplasmic collar." In my experience, however, none of the described criteria are fully reliable, and I have seen many errors of diagnosis based on what I consider flimsy cytology evidence.

It is for these reasons that numerous attempts have been made to identify cells from low-grade tumors by additional techniques. For example, Bonner et al. (1993) used as a tumor marker the M344 antibody in combination with DNA ploidy, with Hoechst 33258 dye as a DNA fluorochrome (see Chapters 9 and 10). The sensitivity of the system was claimed to be 88% for low-grade tumors (combining grade 1 and grade 2 tumors) and 95% for high-grade tumors. Sagerman et al. (1994) used three glycoprotein antigens, Lewis X, M344, and 19A211 (see Chapter 10), combined with cytology. In 14 of 15 low-grade tumors the cytochemical reaction was positive, whereas cytologic abnormalities were observed in only 6 of the 15 patients. Non-specific staining was observed in 2 negative control patients. Baars et al. (1994) searched for immunologic expression of keratin 7 (see Chapter

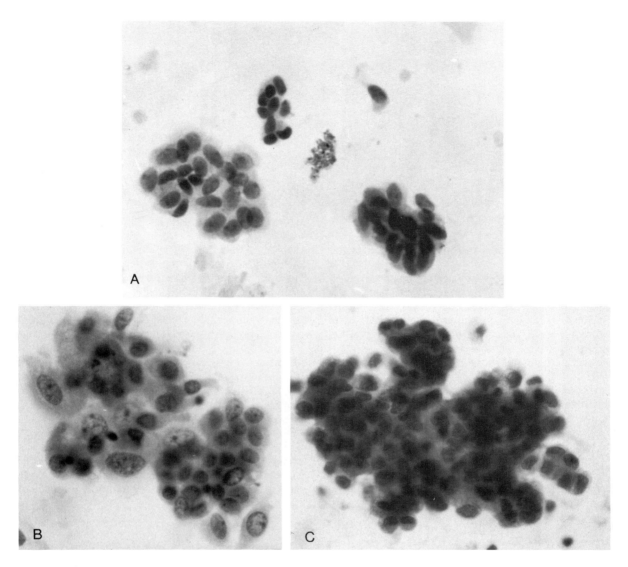

FIGURE 5-11. (*A*) Urine sediment in patients with histologically documented low-grade papillary tumors. Several clusters of morphologically benign urothelial cells are seen. Such findings are *not* of diagnostic value and do not allow the differentiation of a low-grade papillary tumor from effects of trauma, palpation, instrumentation, or stones. (*B*) A higher power view of a cluster of urothelial cells in another case of a grade I tumor. The loose structure and ragged edges of the cluster may suggest a papillary tumor but, in my judgment, the findings are not specific. (*C*) A complex cluster of morphologically benign urothelial cells in spontaneously voided urine. Note the loosely structured surface of the cluster. Under appropriate clinical circumstances such clusters may be consistent with but are *not diagnostic* of a low-grade papillary tumor. Compare with Figs. 2-11A and 4-2C. (*A,C* × 350; B × 560).

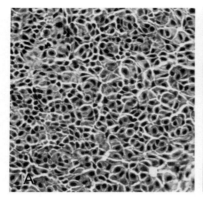 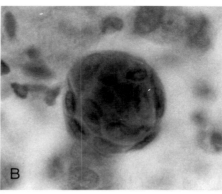

FIGURE 5-12. Low-grade papillary tumor with squamoid features. (*A*) Tissue section. (*B*) Urinary sediment showing a benign "pearl" of urothelial derivation (*A* × 250; *B* × 1000).

10) with positive results in 6 papillary urothelial tumors, grades 2–3.

Perhaps the most sophisticated approach was taken by Cajulis et al. (1994) using fluorescence in situ hybridization (FISH) technique in bladder washing specimens, searching for numerical abnormalities of chromosomes 8 and 12. One of the three grade 1 tumors showed aneuploidy by FISH and by DNA measurements by flow cytometry. The chromosomal FISH signals were abnormal in 83% of 26 bladder tumors of all grades. Amberson and Laino (1993) supplemented conventional urine cytology with DNA ploidy analysis of Feulgen stained smears by image analysis. The recognition of low-grade tumors, using the combination of the two techniques and a ranking algorithm, rose from 15.2% to 47.8%.

For further comments on the use of these and other techniques in the search for diagnostic and prognostic parameters in urothelial tumors, see Chapters 9, 10, and 11.

Tumors Composed of Cells That Differ Morphologically From Normal Urothelium

Tumors composed of cells that differ from normal urothelium can be identified under the microscope as cancer cells. This group of tumors comprises some papillary carcinomas grade 2, all papillary carcinomas grade 3, and most importantly, **flat carcinomas in situ and nearly all invasive carcinomas and the relatively rare other types of primary and metastatic cancers. The cells shed from such tumors differ markedly from benign urothelial cells by virtue of cytoplasmic and nuclear abnormalities.**

It is this latter group of tumors that are the target of cytologic study. The clinical value of cytologic diagnosis of cystoscopically visible high-grade papillary tumors is debatable. In most such instances the lesion is either biopsied or removed. The principal value of cytology is therefore in the diagnosis and monitoring of high-grade tumors that are not clearly evident on cystoscopic examination: carcinomas in situ and related lesions and occult invasive cancers. Carcinomas in situ may be primary or may accompany or follow papillary tumors, thus changing completely the prognostic outlook for the patient.

Voided urine is an excellent diagnostic medium for identifying high-grade tumors, notably nonpapillary carcinoma in situ of the bladder, ureters, and renal pelvis. The method is also very efficient in the identification of invasive tumors. As reported under Results (see p. 124), three sequential voided urine morning samples, appropriately processed and interpreted, will identify virtually all flat carcinomas in situ and nearly all other high-grade tumors, including invasive cancers. The tumors that will not be identified usually shed necrotic debris that will obscure the presence of cancer cells.

Urothelial Cancer Cells in Voided Urine

Recognition of urothelial cancer cells *in voided urine* is based on cytoplasmic and nuclear abnormalities and changes in the nucleocytoplasmic ratios. The urothelial cancer cells vary in size, depending on the composition of the tumor, and may be either small or large. Most cancer cells are of irregular shape. The principal *nuclear features* of cancer cells are nuclear enlargement (with a change in the nucleocytoplasmic ratio in favor of the nucleus), coarse granulation of nuclear chromatin, hyperchromasia, and abnormal nuclear contours. Multinucleated cancer cells and mitoses may occur (Figs. 5-13, 5-14; Color Plate 5-1*A*–*C*). In very-high-grade tumors, poorly differentiated cancer cells with scanty, often poorly preserved, cytoplasm and vesicular (open) nuclei with irregular, very large nucleoli, may be ob-

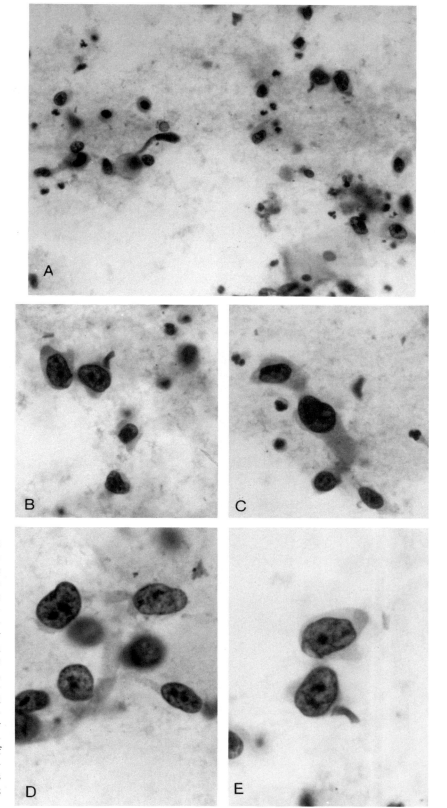

FIGURE 5-13. Voided urine sediment in a patient with invasive urothelial carcinoma, grade 3. (*A*) Overview: numerous cancer cells may be observed. The background contains some necrotic debris. (*B,C*) A higher power view of cancer cells to show the bizarre cell configuration with a high nucleocytoplasmic ratio, irregular nuclear contour, and coarse granulation of chromatin, rendering the nuclei hyperchromatic but *not* homogeneous. (*D*) High-power view of cancer cell nuclei to demonstrate the coarse granulation of chromatin and the irregular nuclear contour. (*E*) Cancer cells with large nucleoli. (*A* × 350; *B,C* × 560; *D,E* × 900.)

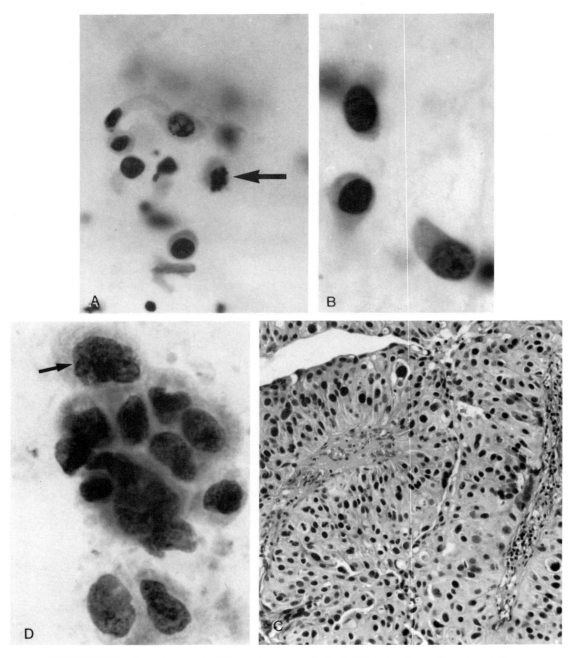

FIGURE 5-14.   Invasive urothelial carcinoma grade 2–3. Voided urine sediment and tissue section. (*A*) Overview of the sediment. A mitosis can be observed (*arrow*). (*B*) Urothelial cancer cells. Note the bizarre shapes and coarse granulation of chromatin. (*C*) Histologic section of the invasive tumor. (*D*) A cluster of cancer cells from another case with a papillary carcinoma grade III accompanied by invasive carcinoma. Note a multinucleated cancer cell (*arrow*). (*A* × 200; *B,D* × 900; *C* × 200.)

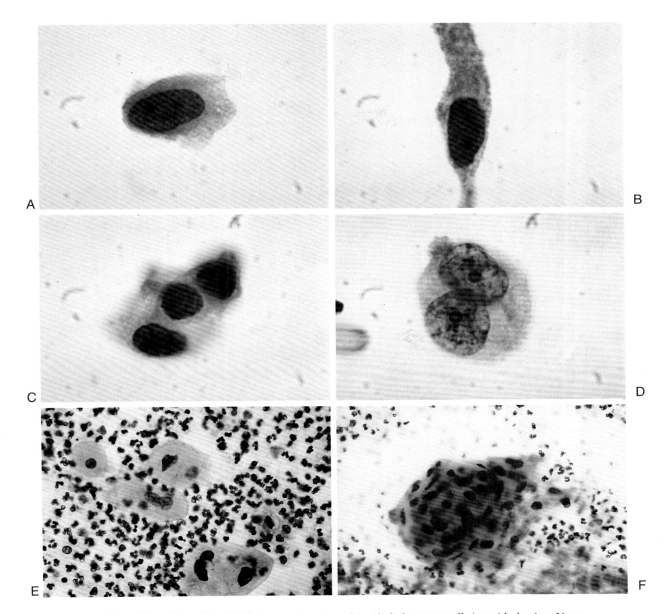

Color Plate 5-1. (*A–C*) Oil immersion view of urothelial cancer cells in voided urine. Note the bizarre cell shapes, altered nucleocytoplasmic ratio, irregular nuclear outline, and coarse granulation of chromatin. (*D*) Urothelial cancer cell with two nuclei, each provided with a large nucleolus. Such cells are seen mainly in poorly differentiated tumor. (*E,F*) Squamous carcinoma of bladder. In *E* there are several squamous cancer cells with orange-colored thick cytoplasm and pyknotic nuclei. The smear background shows marked inflammation and necrosis. In *F* there is a squamous "pearl," characteristic of this tumor type. (Original magnification *A–D* oil immersion × 400; *E,F* × 160, enlarged about × 2.5.)

served (Fig. 5-13*E,* Color Plate 5-1*D*). Such cells sometimes desquamate in clusters. Cytologic findings in rare variants of urothelial cancer are described on pp. 107–113.

Cancer Cells in Bladder Washings (Barbotage) or Brushings

As a general rule, the preservation of cancer cells in washings is superior to those observed in voided urine. Still, the general characteristics of urothelial cancer cells remain generally the same. One exception to this rule is a *lesser degree of nuclear hyperchromasia* with resulting better visualization of nuclear features. *Large nucleoli,* occurring in high-grade tumors, are more often observed with these techniques than in voided urine. Because brushing specimens often contain a large component of benign urothelial cells with their enormous morphologic variability, the interpretation of the cytologic findings is sometimes much more difficult in such samples than it is in voided urine or washings. (For a discussion of general characteristics of specimens obtained by washings and brushings, see Chapter 2.)

Cytologic Recognition of High-Grade Urothelial Carcinoma

CARCINOMA IN SITU

Flat carcinomas in situ are characterized by the presence of cancer cells that are often fairly uniform in size. In most lesions, the dominant cancer cells are small (Figs. 5-15 through 5-17). There are, however, carcinomas in situ with larger cancer cells (Fig. 5-18). The background of the smears in untreated carcinoma in situ is often "clean," *i.e.,* free of necrotic debris and inflammatory cells. There are, however, some instances wherein the cancer cells are accompanied by an inflammatory component. Occasionally, particularly after biopsies, the cancer cell population may become more heterogeneous, and may contain very large cancer cells.

The question whether a diagnosis of carcinoma in situ may be rendered on the basis of cytologic material alone is difficult to answer unequivocally. In some cases, such a diagnosis may be strongly suggested if the cancer cells are numerous, of approximately equal sizes, and the background of the preparation is clean. In the presence of an inflammatory component, it is wiser not to establish this diagnosis because invasive cancer cannot be ruled out.

INTRAUROTHELIAL NEOPLASIA GRADE 2 (DYSPLASIA)

A specific recognition of cell changes corresponding to this level of epithelial abnormality is rarely possible. In some such cases, the cytologic presentation is similar to classical carcinoma in situ, thus providing yet another link between these lesions. In other instances, only atypical urothelial cells, described below, may be observed.

INVASIVE CARCINOMA

In instances of very-high-grade invasive tumors, the recognition of advanced cell changes does not usually cause any significant difficulty. Bizarre cancer cells are quite common (see Figs. 5-13, 5-14; Color Plate 5-1*A–D*). To be sure, cells in the sediment of voided urine may be poorly preserved, particularly in the presence of inflammation and necrosis, and may show a variety of degenerative changes such as frayed or vacuolated cytoplasm, pyknotic or distorted nuclei, and nonspecific cytoplasmic eosinophilic inclusions. Such smears may also contain cells with inclusions and nuclear changes created by the polyomavirus infection that must be differentiated from cancer cells by their regular nuclear contour and nuclear features, described on p. 52.

In less advanced or better differentiated invasive carcinomas, the cancer cells resemble those seen in carcinoma in situ, although the variability of cell sizes and configuration is often greater and the background often shows evidence of inflammation and necrosis. As discussed above, superficially invasive carcinomas, derived from carcinoma in situ and related abnormalities, cannot be specifically recognized as invasive tumors in cytologic samples.

HIGH-GRADE PAPILLARY TUMORS

Papillary tumors of grade 3 shed cancer cells identical to those observed in invasive urothelial cancer. Clusters of cancer cells, such as those shown in Figure 5-14*D,* are somewhat more common than in invasive cancer, but isolated cancer cells, either singly or in groups of two or three, are the dominant cytologic feature. To be sure, a positive urinary sediment in the case of a high-grade papillary tumor does not allow the distinction between a non-invasive and invasive tumor and sheds no light on the presence of a peripheral carcinoma in situ. However, if the cytology remains positive after surgical removal of the visible tumor, the implication of residual high grade neoplastic disorder is clear.

Papillary tumors grade 2 often present a diagnostic challenge: in many of them, no abnormal cells are observed beyond those described for low-grade tumors. In a small proportion of these cases (perhaps 10–15%) clear-cut cancer cells may be noted. In about 30–40% of such tumors, atypical urothelial cells may be observed.

Atypical Urothelial Cells

In a significant proportion of cases of urothelial tumors grade 2, the urinary sediment contains cells

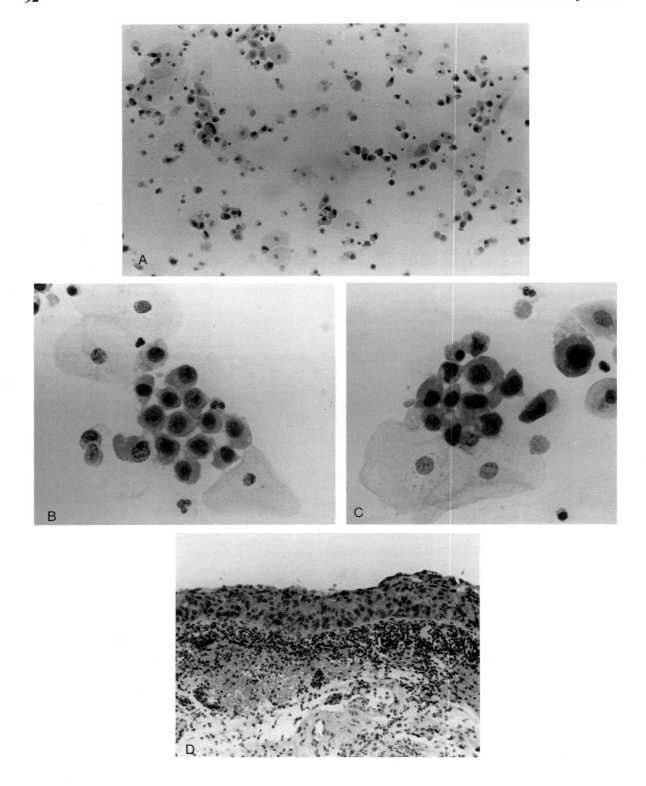

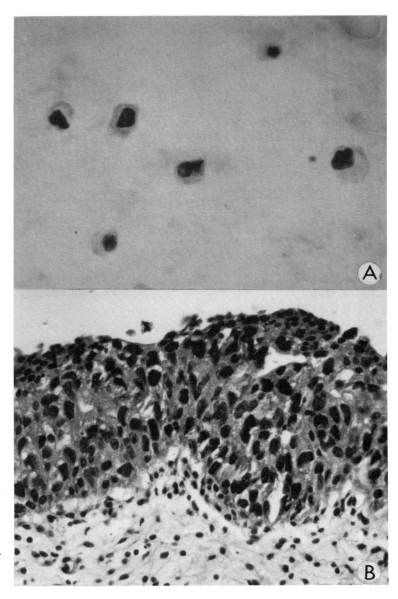

FIGURE 5-16. Flat urothelial carcinoma in situ. Voided urine sediment and tissue section. (*A*) Note the relatively uniform size of the small cancer cells against the clean background. Also note the irregular nuclear contours and hyperchromasia. (*B*) Histologic section of the corresponding biopsy. (*A* × 560; *B* × 350.)

FIGURE 5-15. Flat urothelial carcinoma in situ. Voided urine sediment and a tissue section. (*A*) Overview of the voided urine sediment. There are numerous cancer cells next to benign urothelial and squamous cells. (*B,C*) Cancer cells, singly and in clusters. Note the relatively uniform size of the small cancer cells and the clean background of the smear. The nuclear sizes of the small cancer cells may be compared with the nuclei of benign squamous cells in the same field. (*D*) Biopsy of carcinoma in situ. Note that an inflammatory infiltrate is present beneath the cancerous epithelium. (*A,D* × 150; *B,C* × 560.)

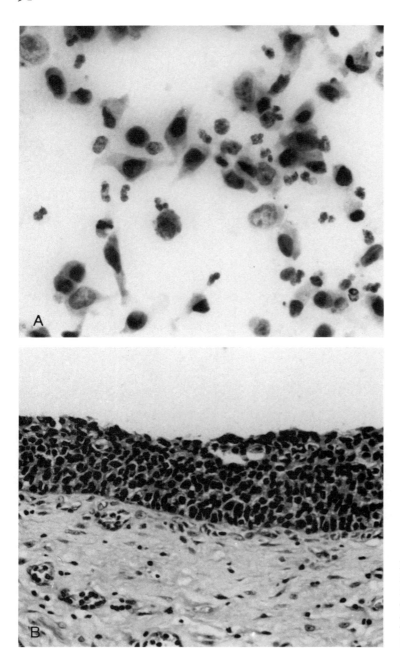

FIGURE 5-17. Nonpapillary carcinoma in situ. (*A*) Voided urine sediment. There is a rich population of small cancer cells of bizarre shapes. Note the abnormal nuclear contour and hyperchromasia. (*B*) The corresponding tissue section. (*A* × 560; *B* × 250.)

that differ from normal urothelial cells but do not fulfill the criteria of malignant cells, outlined above. Such cells resemble normal urothelial cells from deeper layers, but are characterized by slight to moderate nuclear enlargement and some hyperchromasia, without, however, the coarse granularity of chromatin, abnormalities of the nuclear contour, or large nucleoli characteristic of cancer cells. Such cells may be

identified as atypical (Fig. 5-19). In a study of such cells conducted several years ago (Koss et al., 1977), it could be demonstrated by computer algorithms that the atypical cells belong to two categories: those corresponding to benign conditions, and those reflecting urothelial tumors. Unfortunately, in daily microscopic work these fine points of differentiation cannot be recognized. Therefore, for all practical intents and

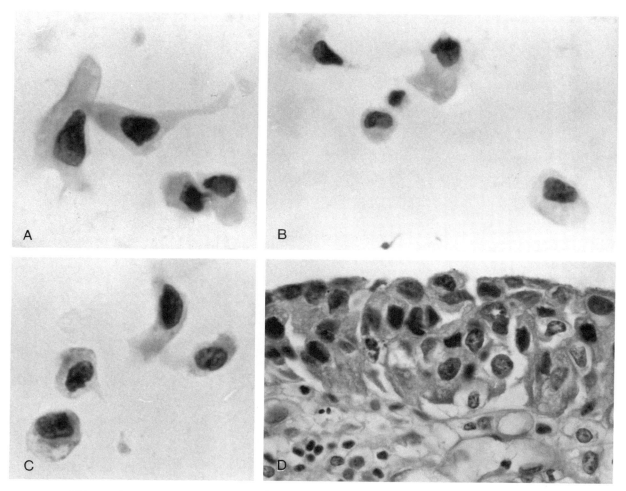

FIGURE 5-18.   Nonpapillary carcinoma in situ composed of large cells. (*A,B,C*) Voided urine sediment. Note the bizarre shape of the cancer cells and the distorted configuration of the nuclei that also display a coarse chromatin pattern. Note the clean background of the smear. (*D*) Histologic appearance of the tumor. (*A,B,C* × 900; *D* × 560.)

purposes, the diagnosis of atypical cells should be avoided whenever possible. The consequences of the diagnosis of cytologic atypia are unpredictable. In some patients, a biopsy may confirm the presence of a carcinoma, grade 2 or an intraurothelial neoplasia, grade 2 (dysplasia). In the absence of a visible tumor the cytologic examination should be repeated until a clear diagnosis of either cancer or no cancer can be established. In some cases of atypia, measuring the DNA ploidy in bladder washings sometimes may be of value as suggested by Amberson and Laino (1993). A normal DNA pattern suggests that there is no occult high-grade cancer. An abnormal DNA pattern should lead to further search for an occult cancer. *Polyomavirus infection is an important source of error as*

such cells usually give an aneuploid DNA pattern. For further details on the methods of DNA analysis, see Chapter 9.

Cytologic Grading of Bladder Tumors

In 1972, Esposti and Zajicek from Stockholm proposed that bladder tumors could be graded based on the appearance of cancer cells in the sediment of bladder washings. Grade 1 tumors could not be distinguished from normal urothelium. However, some grade 2 tumors shed cancer cells with a somewhat more abundant cytoplasm and a somewhat lesser degree of nuclear abnormality than grade 3 and 4 tumors (in this work combined as grade 3). This grading system has been used by other Scandinavian invest-

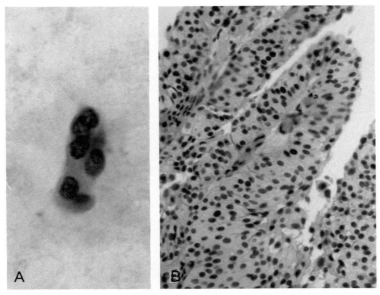

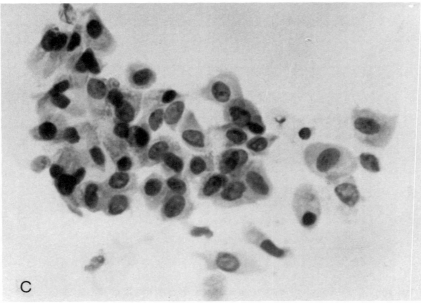

FIGURE 5-19. (*A,B*) Grade 2 papillary tumor of bladder with atypical urothelial cells in voided urine sediment. (*A*) A cluster of urothelial cells with nuclear hyperchromasia and slight nuclear enlargement but no other nuclear abnormalities characteristic of fully developed cancer cells. (*B*) Histologic section of the corresponding papillary tumor. (*C*) Another example of atypical urothelial cells in a grade 2 papillary tumor in bladder washings. Note the slight nuclear enlargement and hyperchromasia. (*A,C* × 560; *B* × 150.)

igators but very rarely elsewhere. The value of the cytologic grading system is limited and has been superseded by DNA ploidy analysis.

Principal Sources of Diagnostic Errors in Cytologic Diagnosis of Urothelial Tumors

Most of the important sources of diagnostic errors have been discussed in Chapters 3 and 4; hence only a brief summary is provided here. The errors pertain mainly to benign cell changes that may be mistaken for cancer cells. Their knowledge is fundamental in the practice of cytology of the urinary tract.

Effects of Trauma or Instrumentation

An important feature of normal urothelium is its tendency to desquamate in the form of tissue fragments which often contract, thus forming round or oval structures that are commonly designated as "papillary clusters" (see Figs. 2-7, 3-2, and Color Plate 3-1). Almost any diagnostic procedure such as vigorous palpation, catheterization, or any other form of instrumentation, particularly brushing, may thus result in the formation of such epithelial clusters. Such clusters, particularly when present in large numbers, are often misinterpreted as representing papillary tumors, more so if the observer is not familiar with the cytologic complexity of normal urothelium, described in Chapter 2. Another important source of error is the presence of numerous superficial urothelial cells (umbrella cells) that may be mistaken by an inexperienced observer for cancer cells because of their unusual nuclear features (See p. 21, Figs. 2-8 and 2-9 and Color Plate 3-1*D*).

Cell Preservation

Cells in the sediment of voided urine, particularly the first morning voiding, are often poorly preserved, and this feature may add to the difficulties of interpretation. It is a sound principle of cytologic diagnosis not to make the diagnosis of cancer in the absence of persuasive evidence.

Human Polyomavirus

Infection with human polyomavirus is a fairly frequent event, as discussed on p. 52. Polyomavirus infection may also occur in the presence of cancer. As described on p. 52, the virus forms large intranuclear inclusions that may mimic cancer cell nuclei, except for their homogeneous configuration and the absence of coarse granularity of the chromatin (see Fig. 4-8). To the best of our current knowledge, the infection has no clinical significance in the urinary tract, but it is an important source of diagnostic errors that may lead to a costly and entirely unnecessary cancer work-up of the patient.

Lithiasis

A further common cause of diagnostic errors is lithiasis. Stones, located anywhere in the lower urinary tract may act as abrasive instruments and dislodge epithelial fragments that sometimes may be quite large and have the "papillary" morphologic appearance and may mimic fragments of papillary tumors (see Fig. 4-12). The presence of numerous umbrella cells, common in such specimens, may add to the diagnostic confusion.

Drugs and Other Therapeutic Procedures

Certain drugs, mainly cyclophosphamide but occasionally other alkylating agents, radiotherapy, and other interventions may also cause cell changes that may be difficult to differentiate from cancer (see p. 57). A further source of diagnostic difficulty may be the synchronous infection with human polyomavirus that may occur in these patients, who are often immunosuppressed. It must also be noted that urothelial cancers and even sarcomas may develop in

patients receiving large doses of cyclophosphamide for the treatment of malignant lymphomas (see p. 61).

OTHER VARIANTS OF MALIGNANT TUMORS OF THE BLADDER

Squamous Carcinoma

Keratin-forming invasive squamous carcinomas are common in Africa in patients infected with *Schistosoma haematobium,* but are relatively uncommon in Western countries, where they constitute no more than 2% to 3% of bladder tumors (see Fig. 4-11). Squamous carcinomas have been observed with increasing frequency in long-term survivors with severe spinal injury (see p. 71). Squamous carcinomas usually develop in the background of a markedly keratinized squamous epithelium, replacing the urothelium. Because of a thick surface layer of keratin such epithelium has the cystoscopic appearance of a white patch, and hence is known as leukoplakia (see p. 57 and Fig. 4-13). A classical squamous carcinoma in situ is uncommon, but the presence of slight to moderate nuclear abnormalities in the form of nuclear enlargement or hyperchromasia within the keratinized epithelium may occur, and is the lesion at origin of squamous cancer. It is sometimes very surprising how inconspicuous the nuclear abnormalities may be in the histologic sections of such precancerous lesions (Fig. 5-20*E*). The experience with *cytologic presentation of squamous carcinoma in situ* of the bladder is very limited. Figure 5-20 shows the cells found in the urinary sediment of one such patient. It may be noted that the cells are large, closely resembling mature squamous cells, and have a conspicuous, eosinophilic, sharply demarcated cytoplasm. The nuclei are enlarged and some of them are hyperchromatic (Fig. 5-20, *C* and *D*). In other, heavily keratinized cells, the nuclei were pale, as is often the case with keratin-forming cancers. Of special note was the presence of perinuclear cytoplasmic clear zones (Fig. 5-20, *A* and *D*), similar to the findings in koilocytes, cells infected with human papillomaviruses, also observed in bladder condylomas (see p. 114 and Figs. 5-35 and 5-36). The possibility that some of the squamous carcinomas may be derived from flat condylomas of the bladder is discussed on p. 114.

Invasive squamous carcinomas may display varying degrees of differentiation. Highly keratinized, hence well-differentiated, squamous carcinomas show mainly local growth and may occlude the bladder. Distant metastases derived from such tumors are infrequent and the patients usually die of uremia. Less well-differentiated squamous cancers may form me-

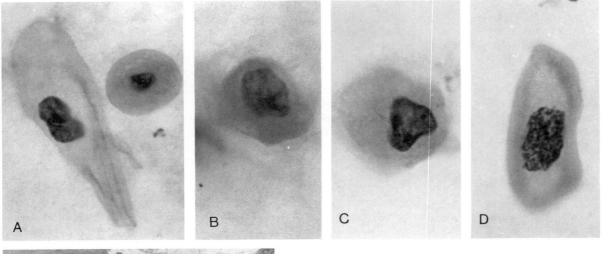

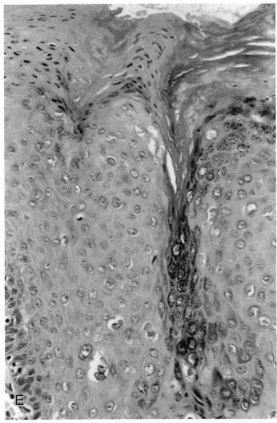

FIGURE 5-20. Squamous carcinoma in situ developing in leukoplakia. (*A–D*) Squamous cancer cells in the urinary sediment. Note the sharply demarcated cell border, characteristic of squamous cancer and the large, irregular hyperchromatic nuclei. The perinuclear clear zones are similar to those observed in squamous cells infected with human papillomavirus (Compare to Fig. 5-36), the so-called koilocytes. (*E*) Tissue section of the lesion showing a markedly keratinized squamous epithelium with relatively inconspicuous nuclear abnormalities. (*A–D,* × 900; *E* × 250.)

tastases, sometimes to the abdominal wall. DNA ploidy studies of squamous cancer are discussed in Chapter 9 (p. 267).

The *cytologic presentation* of well-differentiated invasive squamous carcinoma in voided urine is fairly characteristic. In Papanicolaou stain such tumors shed markedly keratinized cells with thick, yellow or orange-colored cytoplasm and large, irregular, often dark and pyknotic nuclei (Color Plate 5-1*E*). The so-called "squamous pearls," cell aggregates concentrically arranged around a core of keratin, may be observed (Color Plate 5-1*F*). The smear background often shows evidence of marked inflammation and necrosis. Anucleated keratin fragments, also known as ghost cells, are not uncommon (see Color Plate 4-1E). Although such ghost cells occur in benign leukoplakia, they should always be investigated further to rule out squamous carcinoma that may be masquerading as leukoplakia. Of special interest in the differential diagnosis of well-differentiated squamous carcinomas are the relatively rare condylomata acuminata of the urethra or bladder that may mimic cytologically squamous cancers (see below, p. 114).

Poorly differentiated squamous carcinomas shed, in urine, a mixture of cancer cells. Some of them show a sharply demarcated, eosinophilic cytoplasm and large pyknotic nuclei, characteristic of squamous cancer (Fig. 5-21). Other cancer cells are poorly differentiated, with scanty cytoplasm and very large nuclei of uneven size with coarsely granular chromatin and prominent, large nucleoli (Fig. 5-21E).

Metastatic squamous carcinomas of various primary origins may also occur in the bladder. *In women,* squamous carcinoma of the uterine cervix or vagina that may invade the bladder is of particular importance in this regard. *Squamous cancer cells in the sediment of voided urine may also be derived from precancerous lesions or cancer of the cervix, vagina, or vulva.* In fact, in my experience, in women such contaminants are more common than primary or metastatic squamous carcinoma. If the squamous cancer cells cannot be traced to a bladder lesion, investigation of the genital tract is mandatory.

Adenocarcinoma of the Bladder and its Variants

Primary adenocarcinomas of the urinary bladder often closely resemble intestinal carcinomas, reflecting the origin of the bladder in the cloaca, the terminal portion of the embryonal intestinal tract. Similar tumors derived from the urachus, the vestigial omphaloenteric duct, usually involve the dome of the bladder. Adenocarcinomas of intestinal type are also known to occur in children with exstrophy, a congenital abnormality in which the bladder is located outside the abdominal wall.

Precursor Lesions of Primary Adenocarcinoma

Most pure adenocarcinomas of the bladder can be traced to benign precursor lesions. The most common of these lesions is cystitis cystica (see Fig. 2-4C), followed by intestinal metaplasia (Fig. 5-22A). This latter variant of bladder epithelium is rare, and it usually comes to light as a result of an incidental biopsy

for symptoms of cystitis. I have seen it mainly in young people with otherwise normal bladders and in exstrophy. The epithelium resembles colonic mucosa and may also contain Paneth cells and argentaffine cells. In two examples described by Gordon (1963), the intestinal type of epithelium completely replaced the urothelium of the renal pelves, ureters, and the bladder. In most instances, however, the change is focal. The frequency of conversion of the intestinal type of epithelium to adenocarcinoma is unknown in adults, although in children with untreated exstrophy it occurs with a fair frequency. Petersen (1992) summarized 80 such cases culled from the world literature: 85% were adenocarcinomas and the remainder squamous cancers.

It is not clear why the intestinal type of epithelium within the urinary tract has a higher potential for malignant transformation than normal urothelium (Willén, 1992). It must be noted, however, that colonic polyps and carcinomas of the colon are a known complication of implantation of the ureters into sigmoid colon (ureterosigmoidostomy) (Brekkan et al., 1972; Sooriyaarachchi et al., 1976; Berg et al., 1987). Primary carcinomas of the ileal conduit are also known to occur (see p. 157). It appears that the contact of urine with intestinal type epithelium may have a carcinogenic effect. Frieri et al. (1984) and Jannoni et al. (1986) observed abnormal patterns of colonic mucins following urinary diversion and hypothesized that this may account for some of the neoplastic events.

Another potential precursor of adenocarcinoma is the extremely rare villous adenoma of the bladder that resembles very closely a similar lesion of the colon (Fig. 5-22B).

A third lesion that has shown transition to adenocarcinoma is the so-called *nephrogenic adenoma,* which I prefer to call *adenosis* of the bladder (Koss, 1985). This uncommon and complex lesion of the wall of the bladder is composed of glandular and tubular spaces lined by flat or cuboidal cells (Fig. 5-22C). Many papers have been published on the frequency and significance of this lesion (Bhagavan et al., 1981; Molland et al., 1976; Young et al., 1986; Gonzales et al., 1988) but none have provided proof that the lesion is acquired. There are, however, several documented cases of adenocarcinoma developing in this, presumably congenital, abnormality (Koss, 1985).

CYTOLOGY OF PRECURSOR LESIONS OF ADENOCARCINOMA

Except for the presence of mucus-containing columnar cells, commonly observed in the urinary sediment, that reflect the presence of areas of colonic epithelium, there are no cytologic abnormalities that would reflect the presence of the precursor lesions.

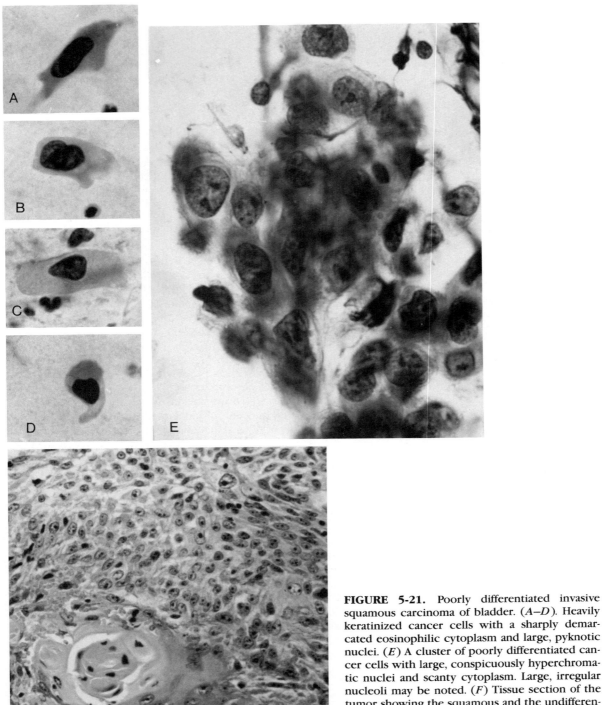

FIGURE 5-21. Poorly differentiated invasive squamous carcinoma of bladder. (*A–D*). Heavily keratinized cancer cells with a sharply demarcated eosinophilic cytoplasm and large, pyknotic nuclei. (*E*) A cluster of poorly differentiated cancer cells with large, conspicuously hyperchromatic nuclei and scanty cytoplasm. Large, irregular nucleoli may be noted. (*F*) Tissue section of the tumor showing the squamous and the undifferentiated components of the tumor. (*A–E* × 900; *F* × 250.)

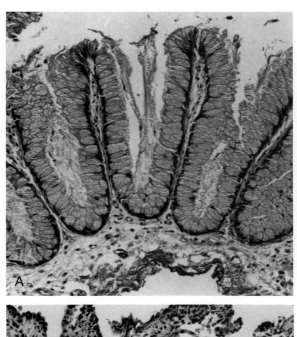

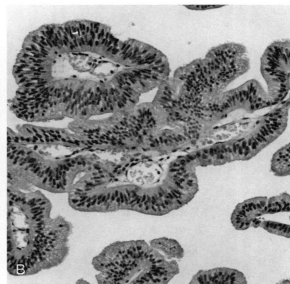

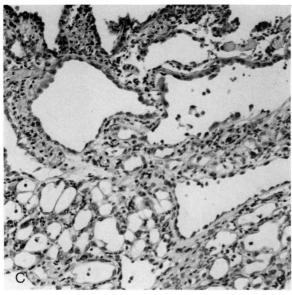

FIGURE 5-22. Precursor lesion of adenocarcinoma of the bladder. (*A*) Area of colonic epithelium with large goblet cells, observed in the bladder of a 31-year-old man. The lesion was a "red patch" in the bladder. (*B*) Villous adenoma of colonic type observed in the trigone of a 43-year-old man. (*C*) The so-called nephrogenic adenoma (adenosis) of bladder—an incidental finding at the autopsy of an 82-year-old man. The gland-like spaces of variable sizes are lined by flat or cuboidal cells, giving the epithelium a "hobnail" appearance. (*A,B,C* × 150.)

Although it was proposed that nephrogenic adenomas shed recognizable cells (Stilman et al., 1986; Troster et al., 1986) the two reports are contradictory and not well documented. I have personally not observed any cell changes that could be considered characteristic of this lesion.

Types of Adenocarcinoma

Adenocarcinoma in situ lining the surface of the bladder has been observed (Fig. 5-23*A,B*). Mor-

phologic variants of adenocarcinoma include carcinomas mimicking colonic cancers of varying degrees of differentiation. Less common are mucus-producing signet-ring cell carcinomas, infiltrating the bladder wall and causing a "leather-bottle" bladder, similar to the "leather bottle" stomach (Fig. 5-23*C,D*). Other variants of adenocarcinomas include clear cell carcinomas (Fig. 5-23*E*) and poorly differentiated adenocarcinomas that may be difficult to classify further. Mixed forms of cancer are discussed below.

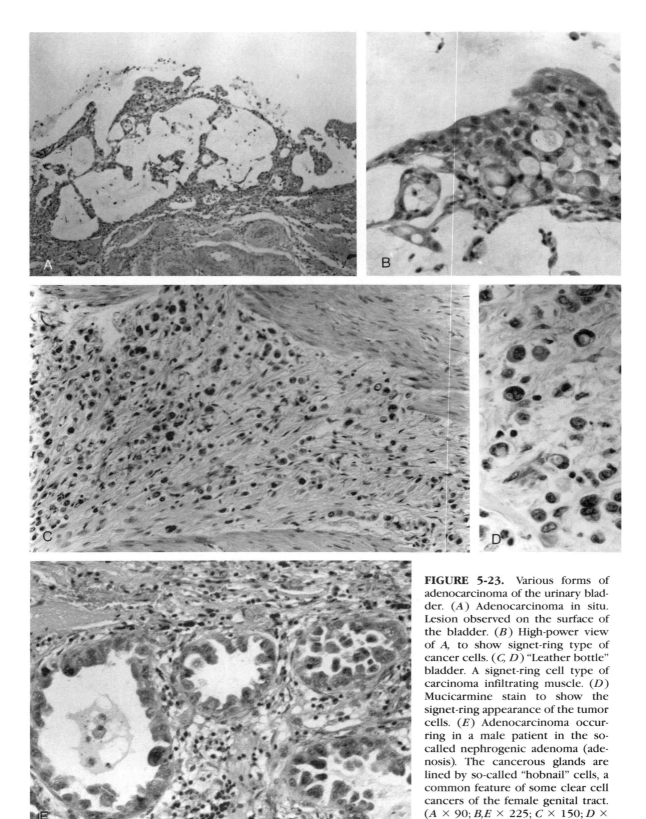

FIGURE 5-23. Various forms of adenocarcinoma of the urinary bladder. (*A*) Adenocarcinoma in situ. Lesion observed on the surface of the bladder. (*B*) High-power view of *A,* to show signet-ring type of cancer cells. (*C, D*) "Leather bottle" bladder. A signet-ring cell type of carcinoma infiltrating muscle. (*D*) Mucicarmine stain to show the signet-ring appearance of the tumor cells. (*E*) Adenocarcinoma occurring in a male patient in the so-called nephrogenic adenoma (adenosis). The cancerous glands are lined by so-called "hobnail" cells, a common feature of some clear cell cancers of the female genital tract. (*A* × 90; *B,E* × 225; *C* × 150; *D* × 350.)

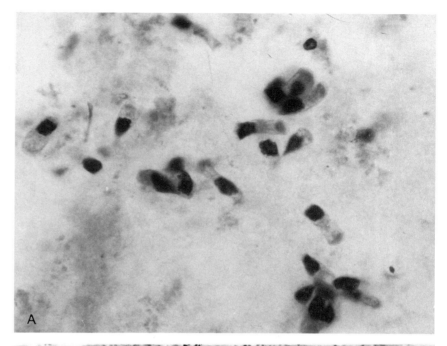

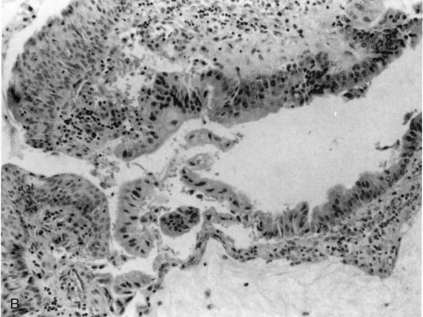

FIGURE 5-24. Adenocarcinoma of enteric type, urinary bladder. (*A*) Urinary sediment with columnar cancer cells. (*B*) A field from the histologic section in the same case. Adenocarcinoma, presumably originating in cystitis cystica. The surface urothelium shows only hyperplasia. (*A* × 560; *B* × 150.)

CYTOLOGIC PRESENTATION

In classical cases of adenocarcinoma of colonic type the urinary sediment often contains columnar cancer cells with large, often hyperchromatic nuclei and large nucleoli, sometimes forming clusters (Fig. 5-24). In less classical cases, such as the poorly differentiated, mucus-producing carcinomas, the cancer cells are smaller, more spherical or cuboidal in shape, and are provided with fairly large, hyperchromatic nuclei. Prominent nucleoli may be present. The cytoplasm is usually basophilic, often scanty, sometimes

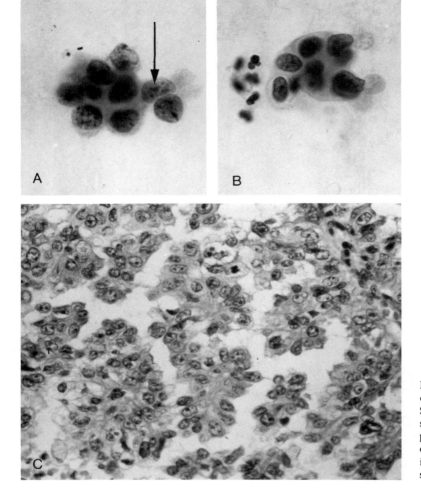

FIGURE 5-25. Clear cell adenocarcinoma of the urinary bladder. (*A,B*) Small, rounded "papillary" clusters of small cancer cells with scanty, transparent cytoplasm. Note the granularity of the nuclei and prominent nucleoli in *A* (*arrow*). (*C*) Tissue section of the same tumor. (*A,B* × 560; *C* × 350.)

poorly preserved. In very poorly differentiated tumors, the type of tumor cannot be established on cytologic grounds. In the presence of large cytoplasmic vacuoles, usually containing mucus, the nuclei may be pushed to the periphery of the cell (signet-ring cells). In clear cell adenocarcinoma the cancer cells are usually quite large, have an abundant, faintly granular or finely vacuolated cytoplasm and open, vesicular nuclei with prominent nucleoli (Fig. 5-25). Such cells usually form rounded ("papillary") clusters.

The differential diagnosis of primary adenocarcinoma of the bladder comprises metastatic adenocarcinomas of various origins, particularly of the rectum or colon, that may have a very similar histologic and cytologic makeup (see p. 118).

Mixed Type Carcinomas

It is not uncommon for bladder cancers to display more than one pattern of morphologic differentiation. For example, urothelial carcinomas may contain foci of squamous carcinoma or adenocarcinoma. Occasionally such diverse cancer types may occur in different anatomic locations within the bladder and grow as separate tumors. In such cases the intervening epithelium of the bladder often shows a flat carcinoma in situ. The cytologic presentation of such tumors rarely allows the diagnosis of the complex carcinomas. Usually one cytologic pattern is dominant, and the complexity of the tumor in biopsies is usually a surprise. However, there are exceptions to this rule, and mixed populations of cancer cells are sometimes observed

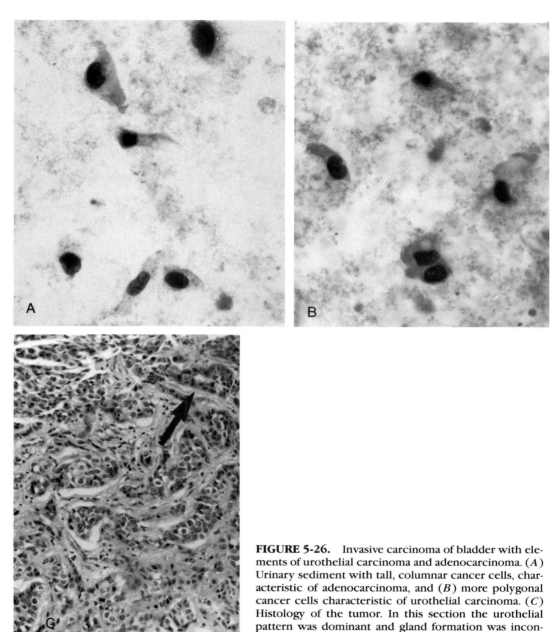

FIGURE 5-26. Invasive carcinoma of bladder with elements of urothelial carcinoma and adenocarcinoma. (*A*) Urinary sediment with tall, columnar cancer cells, characteristic of adenocarcinoma, and (*B*) more polygonal cancer cells characteristic of urothelial carcinoma. (*C*) Histology of the tumor. In this section the urothelial pattern was dominant and gland formation was inconspicuous (*arrow*). (*A,B* × 560; *C* × 150.)

(Fig. 5-26). If flat carcinoma in situ is present, the cytologic presentation often reflects its presence (see above, p. 91).

Bladder Tumors in Diverticula

Bladder diverticula are fairly common and may sometimes harbor urothelial or squamous carcinomas, although the number of such reported tumors is small (Petersen, 1992). Because most diverticula are discovered incidentally and may be resected, the examination of the urinary sediment may lead to the diagnosis of an occult carcinoma (Fig. 5-27). The simple procedure is desirable because it offers a better therapeutic outcome, whereas advanced and symptomatic diverticular carcinomas have a poor prognosis (Knappenberger, 1960). Exceptionally, tumors of other

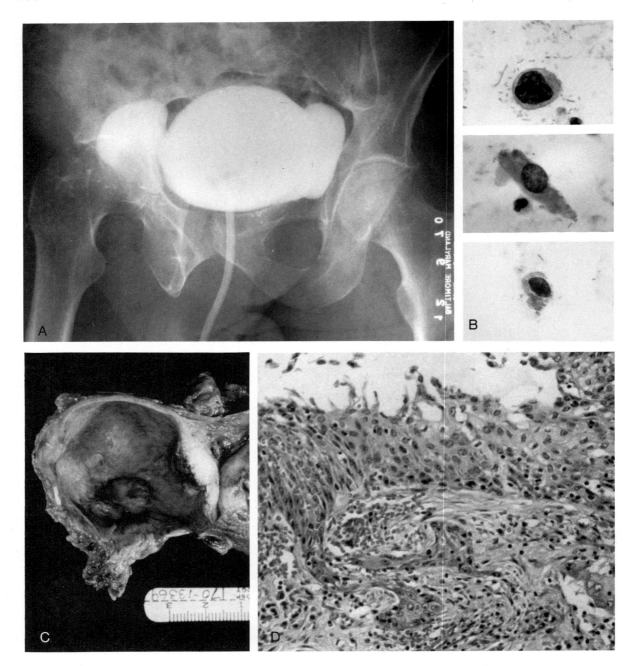

FIGURE 5-27. Invasive urothelial carcinoma in bladder diverticulum discovered incidentally in voided urine cytology. (*A*) Cystogram showing two diverticuli of the bladder. (*B*) Composite picture of cancer cells in voided urine. (*C*) Gross appearance of the resected right diverticulum. A flat tumor is present. (*D*) Histology of the surface of the carcinoma that was deeply invasive elsewhere. (*B* × 1,000; *D* × 250.)

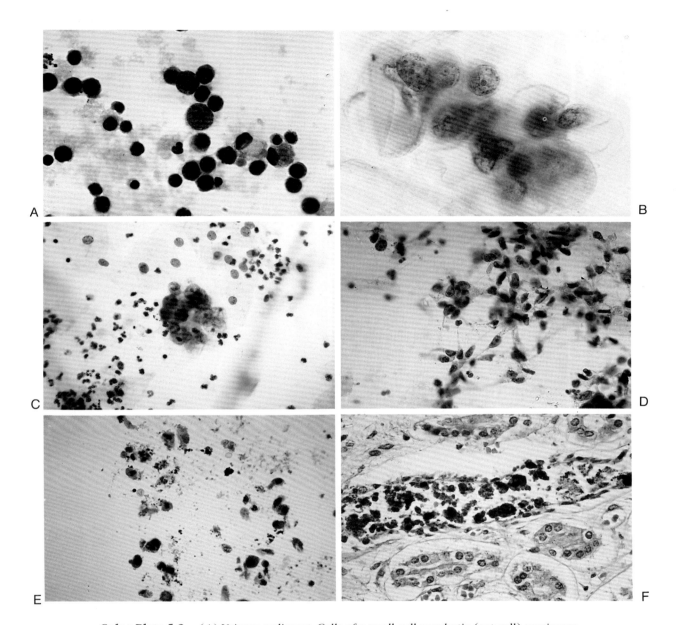

Color Plate 5-2. (*A*) Urinary sediment. Cells of a small cell anaplastic (oat cell) carcinoma under high magnification. The histology is shown in Fig. 5-28. Note the short string or rouleaux of cancer cells. (*B*) Urinary sediment. Metastatic ovarian carcinoma. Note the huge size of the cancer cells. (*C*) Urinary sediment. Adenocarcinoma of the urethra. Note the papillary cluster of cancer cells with scanty cytoplasm, large, open, somewhat hyperchromatic nuclei, and prominent nucleoli. (*D*) Urinary sediment. Metastatic colonic carcinoma to bladder. Note the large number of columnar cancer cells. (*E*) Melanuria in the urinary sediment and (*F*) the renal tubules with melanin pigment in a patient who died with disseminated malignant melanoma. (Original magnification: *A* × 256; *B,C,E* × 160; *D,F* × 100, enlarged about × 2.5.)

types may also occur in diverticuli (summary in Petersen, 1992).

Bladder Cancer and Lithiasis

Bladder stones are a risk factor in bladder cancer (Wynder, 1963, 1977). Although lithiasis per se may result in atypia of urothelial cells (see p. 57), these changes are rarely severe enough to mimic cancer cells. Beyer-Boon (1977) observed 11 cases of lithiasis with significant cellular abnormalities, suggestive of carcinoma in 5 cases. In the absence of follow-up information the significance of this observation remains unknown. Therefore, the presence of cancer cells calls for an investigation of the bladder that may harbor a carcinoma in situ.

Bladder Cancer and Prostatic Enlargement

Prostatic enlargement, whether caused by a benign hypertrophy or a carcinoma, is a risk factor for tumors of the bladder. In a review of our files from 1974 to 1977, there were 60 patients with bladder cancer associated with prostatic enlargement, 47 with benign hypertrophy, and 13 with prostatic carcinoma. In 19 of these patients, bladder cancer was occult and was discovered by cytology of urine. In many such cases, the bladder disease was a carcinoma in situ with extension to prostatic ducts (see p. 77). In 1986, Mahadevia et al. presented mapping studies of 20 cystoprostatectomy specimens from male patients treated for invasive bladder cancer or for extensive carcinoma in situ. In nine of these patients, there was extension of the urothelial carcinoma into the adjacent prostatic ducts. In 14 of these 20 patients, prostatic carcinoma was also found; it was occult in 13 of these patients.

It is evident from the above that cytologic examination of voided urine in patients with prostatic enlargement is mandatory, as it may lead to the discovery of occult carcinoma in situ of the bladder. This observation received strong support from de la Rosette et al. (1993) who examined the urinary sediments in 206 patients with symptoms of prostatic dysfunction. Six high-grade carcinomas of the bladder, one of them a carcinoma in situ and five grade 2 or 3 papillary tumors, four of them with carcinoma in situ, were observed in patients with "severe cytologic atypia." In my experience, the common site of such lesions is the trigone. A careful examination of the epithelium of the trigone is mandatory in any specimen of transurethral prostatic resection (TUR).

UNCOMMON MALIGNANT TUMORS OF THE BLADDER

Rare types of carcinomas, sarcomas, and other malignant tumors may be observed in the urinary bladder. Some of them can be identified on cytologic examination of the urinary sediment, although specific tumor patterns are rarely recognized.

Uncommon Types of Carcinomas

Endocrine Tumors

This group of tumors with divergent histologic presentation have in common the presence of dense core cytoplasmic endocrine granules that may produce a wide variety of polypeptide hormones, such as calcitonin, gastrin, and even insulin. The presence of the granules may be documented by electron microscopy, whereas their products may be documented by immunostaining. It is uncommon for these tumors to produce clinical syndromes associated with hormone production. The one exception is *pheochromocytoma* (paraganglioma), which is capable of producing neuropeptide hormones capable of inducing paroxysmal hypertension. Pheochromocytomas, however, are intramural within the bladder and cannot be detected by cytologic examination of the urinary sediment. For comments on diagnosis of adrenal or retroperitoneal pheochromocytomas by aspiration biopsy, see Chapter 8.

SMALL CELL CARCINOMAS

Small cell carcinomas (oat cell carcinomas) of the bladder are highly malignant and very aggressive tumors, identical in appearance and behavior to similar tumors of the lung and other organs. The endocrine nature of these tumors may require the finding of dense core cytoplasmic granules by electron microscopy. The cancer cells are small, about four times the size of lymphocytes, and are characterized by compact, often pyknotic nuclei and very scanty, usually basophilic cytoplasm. There are no visible nucleoli within the nuclei (Fig. 5-28). Of diagnostic significance in the cytologic presentation of oat cell carcinoma is the presence of small clusters or rouleaux of tightly packed tumor cells with nuclear molding (Color Plate 5-2A). The absence of nucleoli and the presence of cell clusters are very helpful in differentiating the cells of oat cell carcinoma from a malignant lymphoma wherein cells, as a rule, do not cluster and are usually provided with nucleoli (see below). The cytologic diagnosis of oat cell carcinoma of the lung is fairly commonplace either in sputum or by aspiration

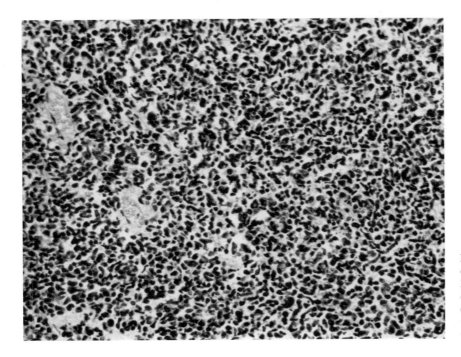

FIGURE 5-28. Small cell (oat cell) carcinoma of bladder. Note the small, spindly cancer cells resembling grains of oats (× 150). (Cytologic presentation of this tumor is shown in Color Plate 5-2*A*.)

biopsy. In urinary sediment, I have seen this tumor only once, as shown in Color Plate 5-2*A*.

CARCINOID TUMORS

Carcinoid tumors are extremely uncommon in the urinary bladder. Their customary appearance is in sheets and ribbons of small, uniform tumor cells with an intimate relationship to the capillaries (Fig. 5-29).

I have observed carcinoid tumor structure as a part of highly malignant urothelial carcinomas and adenocarcinomas. In urinary sediment, under such circumstances, the presence of the carcinoid component was concealed by malignant cells of the dominant tumor types (already described). I have not observed a pure carcinoid tumor in the urinary sediment. In other organs, such as the lung or liver metastases from other

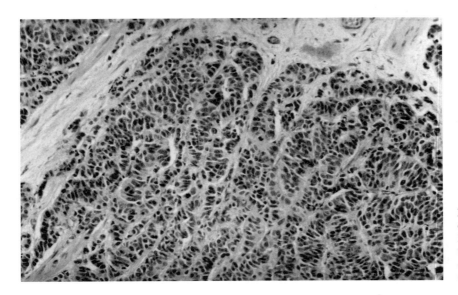

FIGURE 5-29. Carcinoid tumor of bladder. Note the ribbon-like arrangement of cells. The urinary sediment in this case did not contain any tumor cells (× 150).

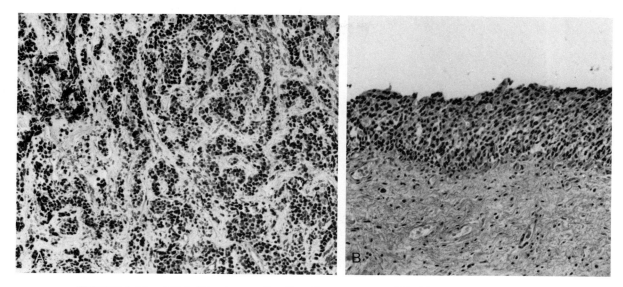

FIGURE 5-30. (*A*) Infiltrating small cell malignant tumor of bladder, composed of ribbons of small cells, akin to a carcinoid. The Grimelius silver stain reaction was positive in the cytoplasm of the tumor cells. (*B*) In the adjacent epithelium there was a flat carcinoma in situ, composed of small cells, the likely source of the invasive tumor. (*A,B* × 150.)

sites, uniform, small tumor cells with basophilic cytoplasm and enlarged, often peripherally placed nuclei have been observed. Within the nuclei tiny nucleoli could be seen. The tumor cells may show a remarkable similarity to plasma cells, except for their much larger size (Koss et al., 1992). Exceptionally, *endocrine tumors of mixed type,* composed of small and larger cells, have been observed. There are no documented instances of their cytologic identification in the urinary tract.

Very rarely, invasive small cell malignant tumors with some features of carcinoids, such as formation of ribbons and the presence of endocrine granules, may be observed. In the example shown in Figure 5-30, the adjacent epithelium showed a flat carcinoma in situ, undoubtedly the precursor lesion of the invasive cancer.

Spindle Cell Carcinomas (Spindle and Giant Cell Carcinomas, Carcinosarcomas).

Spindle cell carcinomas are highly malignant epithelial tumors in which the customary epithelial component is accompanied or replaced by malignant spindle cells, sometimes resembling a sarcoma. Giant tumor cells with multiple, highly abnormal nuclei, are sometimes present. In such tumors the epithelial deri-

vation of the spindle cells can be easily documented by immunostaining with antikeratin antibodies (Fig. 5-31). We have not observed this tumor type in the urinary sediment.

Malignant Mesodermal Mixed Tumors

Malignant mesodermal mixed tumors are highly malignant tumors composed of malignant epithelial and sarcomatous components. The epithelial components may have variable appearance and areas of urothelial carcinoma, squamous carcinoma, and adenocarcinoma may be observed in the same tumor. The sarcomatous component may be undifferentiated and composed of small cells resembling primitive mesenchyme, or may be differentiated in the form of chondrosarcoma, rhabdomyosarcoma, angiosarcoma, or osteosarcoma. We studied one malignant mixed tumor over a period of its evolution and observed that the initial lesion was a flat urothelial carcinoma in situ, from which the malignant mixed tumor developed (Fromowitz et al., 1984). The urinary sediment was dominated by small cancer cells, presumably derived from the elements of carcinoma. A few cells may have represented the component of chondrosarcoma that was also present in the tumor. The final diagnosis was based on histologic examination (Fig. 5-32).

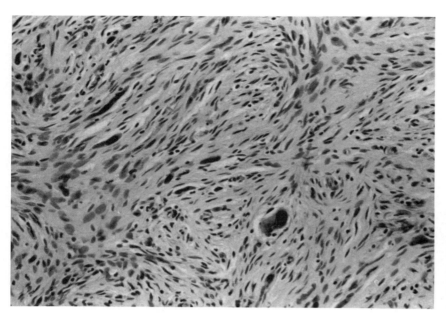

FIGURE 5-31. Spindle cell carcinoma with giant cells in the urinary bladder. Such tumors may be mistaken for sarcomas but the cytoplasm stains strongly with antikeratin antibodies, identifying the tumor as of epithelial origin (× 150).

Sarcomas

Sarcomas of muscle are by far the most common form of sarcomas in the urinary bladder. *Rhabdomyosarcoma* may occur in two forms: the juvenile or embryonal form, occurring mainly in pediatric patients, known as *botryoid sarcoma* (grape-like sarcoma), and the rare *adult forms* in which the tumor cells may be well-differentiated and form cytoplasmic cross-striations. Several configurations or subtypes of the adult form of tumor are known to occur. The clinical presentation of botryoid sarcoma is characteristic, inasmuch as the tumor forms grape-like, opaque, moist protrusions into the lumen of the bladder. Histologically the tumor is composed of undifferentiated small cancer cells with a few cells showing accumulation of myoglobin in the cytoplasm (strap cells), and some cells showing cytoplasmic cross-striations. In the urine sediment of a child with a botryoid sarcoma, I observed a few small cancer cells, insufficient for the diagnosis of tumor type, which was determined from the clinical presentation (Fig. 5-33). Adult rhabdomyosarcomas are usually intramural and cannot be recognized in the urinary sediment, unless the tumor breaks through into the lumen of the bladder. A case report of rhabdomyosarcoma cells in the urinary sediment was published by Krumerman and Katatikarn (1976).

Malignant Lymphoma

Primary malignant lymphomas may occur in the urinary bladder. In most such instances the tumor develops in the wall of the bladder and is covered by a hyperplastic urothelium, hence cannot be detected in the urinary sediment. As will be discussed below, *metastatic malignant lymphomas and leukemias* may be identified in the urinary sediment, and it is likely that the cytologic presentation of primary malignant lymphomas would be identical (see p. 119). Such a case has been reported by Mincione (1982).

Other Sarcomas

Leiomyosarcomas are uncommonly observed in the urinary bladder. The tumors, which are composed

FIGURE 5-32. Mesodermal mixed tumor of urinary bladder. (*A*) A composite of six small malignant cells observed in the urinary sediment. A precise classification of these cells was not possible, although epithelial origin was favored. (*B,C*) Two histologic aspects of the same tumor: in *B* the dominant lesion is a carcinoma, in *C* an area of cartilage surrounded by undifferentiated small cell sarcoma. Elsewhere there was a flat carcinoma in situ (*not shown*), the site of origin of this tumor. (*A* × 560; *B,C* × 150) (see Fromowitz, F. B., Bard, R. H., and Koss, L. G.: The epithelial origin of a malignant mesodermal mixed tumor of the bladder: report of a case with long-term survival. J. Urol. *132*, 2385–2389, 1984).

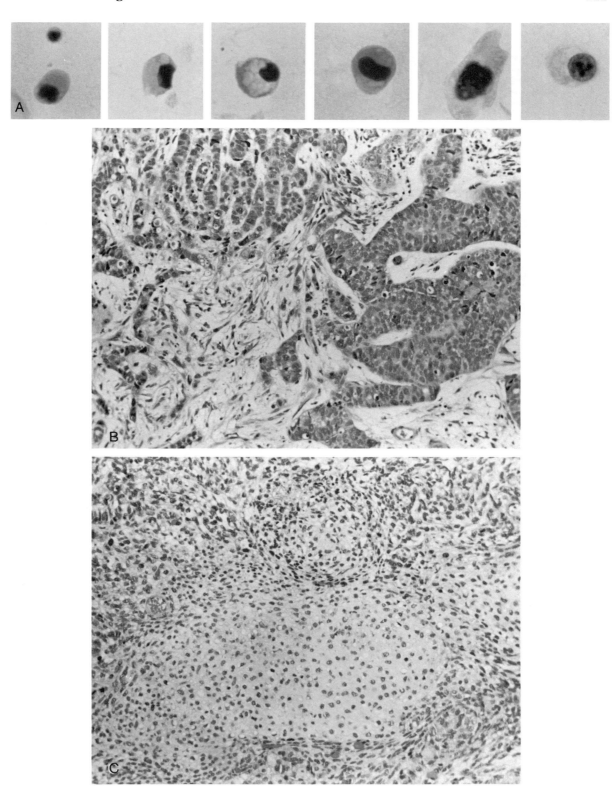

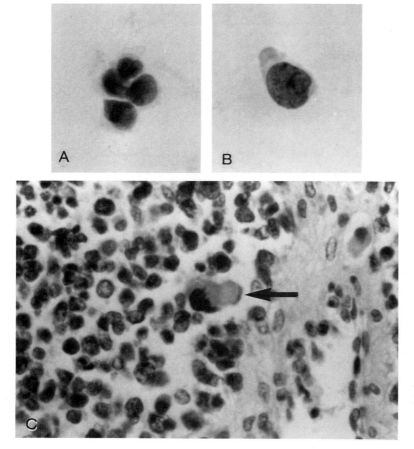

FIGURE 5-33. Embryonal rhabdomyosarcoma of the bladder in a child. Urinary sediment and tissue section. (*A*) Small cancer cells forming a small cluster. (*B*) A single cancer cell with whispy cytoplasm. (*C*) Section of tumor composed mainly of small cancer cells. One cell (*arrow*) had an abundant strongly eosinophilic cytoplasm (a so-called "strap cell"). (*A,B* × 1,000; *C* × 560.)

of abnormal smooth muscle cells, usually have a slow evolution and are subepithelial and therefore cannot be identified in the urinary sediment. An example of this tumor is shown in Figure 4-17*B*.

Other Malignant Tumors

Choriocarcinoma

A case of primary *choriocarcinoma* of the urinary bladder in an 82-year-old man, confirmed by immunocytochemical analysis of the tumor, was studied by us (Obe et al., 1983). Histologically the tumor was composed of cytotrophoblasts and multinucleated syncytiotrophoblasts, invading bladder wall. The tumor, which expressed high levels of human chorionic gonadotropin (hCG), metastasized widely. In the urinary sediment small cancer cells and a few multinucleated cancer cells were observed (Fig. 5-34). The tumor was preceded by a carcinoma in situ, and it was proposed that it represented a modification of a urothelial carcinoma (also see above: mesodermal mixed tumors). There is increasing evidence to support this concept, first expressed in 1983. In recent years, several documented cases of a transformation of a urothelial cancer into a choriocarcinoma have been reported in male patients (summary in Yokoyama et al., 1992). It was also documented that high-grade urothelial tumors may produce hCG and even cause gynecomastia (Wurzel et al., 1987).

Two cases of primary choriocarcinoma of bladder with cytologic findings were described by Yokoyama et al. (1992). Both patients were elderly males. In one of them, the tumor was associated with urothelial carcinoma, and in the other it was a pure choriocarcinoma. As in our case, the urinary sediment contained mono- and multinucleated cancer cells, the latter interpreted as syncytiotrophoblasts.

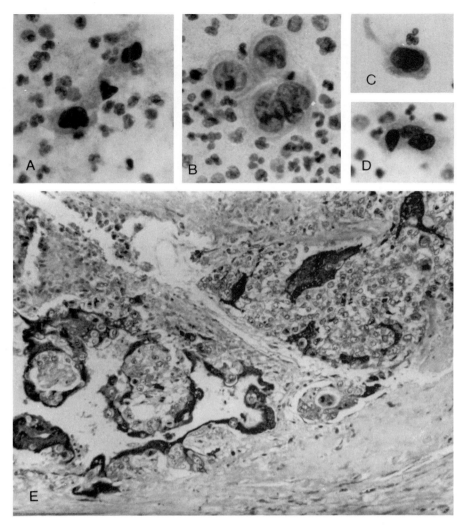

FIGURE 5-34. Choriocarcinoma of the urinary bladder in an elderly man. (*A–D*) Cancer cells in the urinary sediment, reminiscent of a carcinoma. (*E*) Tumor at autopsy, immunostained for human chorionic gonadotropin (*black*). The tumor was structurally reminiscent of placental chorionic villi, composed of small cytotrophoblasts in the center and large syncytiotrophoblasts at the periphery. The initial biopsy on this patient disclosed a carcinoma in situ (*not shown*); hence, it was proposed that the tumor represented a modification of a carcinoma. (*A–D* × 560; *E* × 150.) (see Obe, J. A., Rosen, N., and Koss, L. G.: Primary choriocarcinoma of the urinary bladder. Report of a case with probable epithelial origin. Cancer *52*, 1405–1409, 1983).

Malignant Melanomas

Primary malignant melanomas of the bladder are exceptional (Ainsworth and Clark, 1976), and I have no knowledge of a case with cytologic presentation. For cytologic presentation of *metastatic melanoma* see p. 122.

BENIGN TUMORS AND TUMOROUS CONDITIONS

There are benign neoplasms of the bladder urothelium that may have some impact on the cytology of the urinary sediment.

Inverted Papilloma

Inverted papilloma is an uncommon benign tumor of the urinary bladder that usually affects the trigone. The tumors may be bulky and pedunculated, and may obstruct bladder neck. The surface of the tumors is usually smooth, because the lining is composed of an uninterrupted layer of urothelium. The tumor itself is composed of anastomosing strands of urothelium, usually without nuclear abnormalities but occasionally with focal nuclear enlargement. It has been claimed that inverted papilloma may produce specific abnormalities of urothelial cells in urinary sediment. This has not been the case in my experience, and I do not believe that this tumor can be identified cytologically. A case of bladder carcinoma derived from an inverted papilloma has been reported (Koss, 1985).

Nephrogenic Adenoma

This entity was discussed in conjunction with adenocarcinoma of bladder on p. 99.

Condylomas of the Bladder

Condylomas (condylomata acuminata) of the urinary bladder are uncommon tumors sometimes associated with condylomas of the external genitalia or the urethra. The tumors are similar in configuration to condylomas of the skin or to common warts, and are composed of anastomosing strands of squamous epithelium that may have a papillary surface. The epithelium of the condylomas is often atypical (see Fig. 5-36*F* and *G*). Toward the epithelial surface the large squamous cells usually display perinuclear clear zones and nuclear abnormalities in the form of nuclear enlargement and hyperchromasia. Such abnormalities of the squamous cells are known as *koilocytosis* (Koss and Durfee, 1956), a characteristic cell change occurring in lesions associated with permissive proliferation of the *human papillomavirus* (Fig. 5-35). In fact, the presence of types 6 and 11 of this virus has been documented in bladder condylomas by in situ hybridization by Del Mistro et al. (1988). These and other types of human papillomavirus have also been implicated in precancerous and cancerous lesions of the genital tract, mainly the cervix, vulva, and vagina. Thus, although the presence of koilocytes in the voided urine sediment in males may indicate a lesion in the bladder or the urethra, in women the possibility of a lesion of the lower genital tract with an incidental pick-up of such cells by the urinary stream must be considered. The interested reader is referred to Koss (1992) for a de-

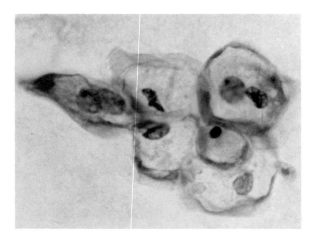

FIGURE 5-35. Koilocytes in voided urine sediment. The squamous cells are characterized by enlarged, moderately hyperchromatic single or double nuclei, surrounded by a clear cytoplasmic zone or halo. The halo is sharply demarcated toward its periphery. Such cells are pathognomonic of a permissive human papillomavirus infection. In males they suggest the presence of condylomata acuminata in the penile urethra or the bladder. In women they may also represent a lesion of the lower genital tract with the cells incidentally picked up in the urinary stream ($\times$ 560).

tailed discussion of the relationship of human papillomavirus to neoplastic events in the female genital tract (for further comments on condylomata acuminata of the urethra and their significance, see Chapter 6).

Condylomas of the urinary bladder may shed abnormal cells in the urinary sediment. These cells are usually squamous in nature and have large, hyperchromatic nuclei (Fig. 5-36). Some cells may display large perinuclear clear zones or halos, identifying them as koilocytes. Such abnormal cells may mimic to perfection cells of squamous carcinoma, a lesion with which they may be confused (see p. 97 and Figs. 5-20 and 5-21). In fact, there is some evidence that condylomas of the bladder may become malignant and produce squamous carcinomas capable of metastases. We observed this sequence of events in one of our patients.

Endometriosis

Endometriosis may involve the urinary bladder and may form a space-occupying lesion. The lesions are usually observed during childbearing age and are often associated with endometriosis of other organs.

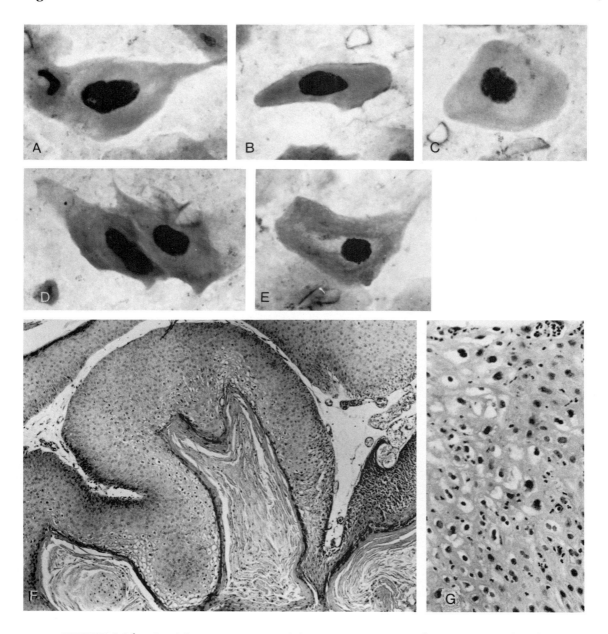

FIGURE 5-36. Condyloma acuminatum of the urinary bladder in a 43-year-old man. (*A–E*) Abnormal cells in the urinary sediment. Note nuclear hyperchromasia and thick, keratin-bearing cytoplasm accounting for the similarity of such cells with squamous cancer cells (see also Fig. 5-20). In *E* there is a perinuclear clear zone suggestive of koilocytosis (see also Fig. 5-35). (*F*) A low-power view of the bladder tumor shows the folds of squamous epithelium with surface keratinization. (*G*) A high-power view of an epithelial segment documents nuclear abnormalities and koilocytosis. (*A–G* × 1,000; *F* × 80; *G* × 350.)

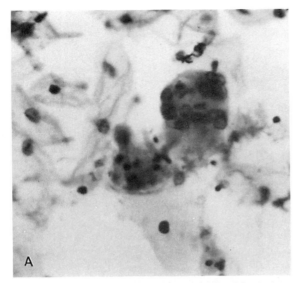

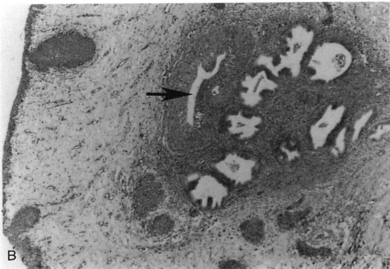

FIGURE 5-37. Endometriosis of the bladder in a 27-year-old woman with voiding discomfort, particularly severe during menstruation. The patient had previously documented endometriosis of the umbilicus and, on cystoscopy, showed characteristic "blue dome" cysts in the wall of the bladder. (*A*) A cluster of endometrial glandular cells in bladder washings. In the absence of clinical history, the exact identification of such cells would be very difficult. (*B*) Section of urinary bladder showing endometrial glands and stroma in the bladder wall. An inclusion of normal urothelium is shown (*arrow*). Elsewhere a focus of endometriosis was ulcerated, accounting for the presence of endometrial cells in urine and bladder washings. (*A* × 500; *B* × 120. Photographs courtesy of Dr. Volker Schneider, Freiburg i/B, Germany. From Schneider, V., Smith, M. J. V., and Frable, W. J.: Urinary cytology in endometriosis of the bladder. Acta Cytol. *24,* 30–33, 1980 with permission.)

The characteristic clinical complaint is painful voiding, mainly at the time of menstrual bleeding. One such lesion was reported in an elderly male receiving estrogen treatment for prostate cancer (Pinkert et al., 1979). On cystoscopy, the lesions are usually seen as "blue dome" cysts in the wall of the bladder. Histologically, endometrial glands and stroma are observed in the wall of the bladder. Schneider et al. (1980) reported the presence of glandular cells of endometrial type in urine sediment of a woman with endometriosis. The case is shown in Fig. 5-37.

Pseudotumors of the Bladder and Pseudosarcomatous Stromal Reaction

Exuberant proliferation of connective tissue may occur in the urinary bladder as a result of a surgical trauma and sometimes as a spontaneous event. The patterns of proliferation of large fibroblasts, often showing mitotic activity and large nucleoli, may mimic a sarcoma (Fig. 5-38). There is no documented cytologic counterpart of these uncommon lesions. Pseudotumors of the bladder must be dif-

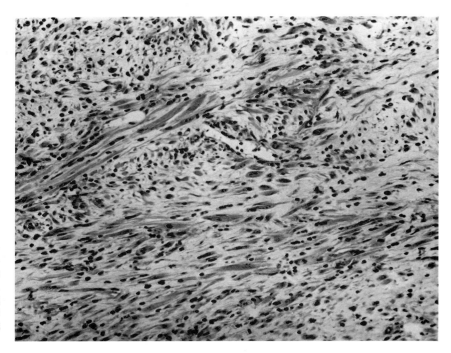

FIGURE 5-38. Pseudosarcomatous proliferation of connective tissue in the wall of the bladder after a surgical trauma. Sheets of actively proliferating fibroblasts mimic a sarcoma. The lesion is benign and self-limiting (× 150).

ferentiated from a similar reaction accompanying primary or metastatic urothelial tumors (Mahadevia et al., 1989). The spindly cells, some of which are cancer cells recognizable by staining with antikeratin antibodies, may lead to an erroneous diagnosis of a benign lesion, particularly in a small biopsy specimen (Fig. 5-39). In such cases, the urinary sediment may disclose the presence of urothelial cancer cells.

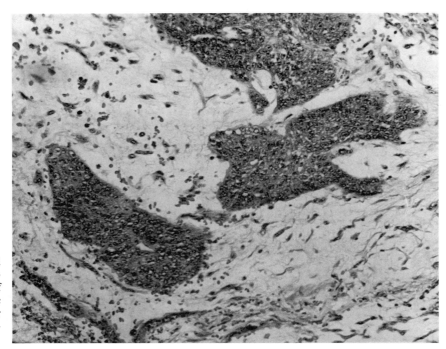

FIGURE 5-39. A spindle cell reaction accompanying invasive squamous carcinoma of bladder. Some of the spindle cells were shown to be cancer cells by staining with antikeratin antibodies (× 150).

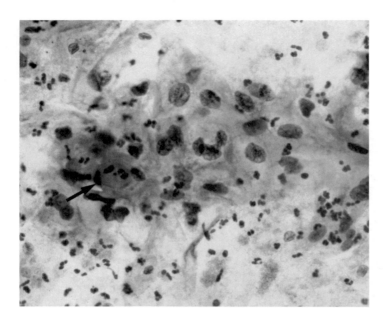

FIGURE 5-40. An example of cancer cells derived from an epidermoid carcinoma in situ of the uterine cervix in urinary sediment (× 350).

METASTATIC TUMORS

A broad spectrum of metastatic malignant tumors may be observed in the urinary sediment. By far the most common metastatic tumors are derived from adjacent organs: the uterine cervix and sometimes the endometrium or the ovary in women, the prostate in men, and the colon and the rectum in both sexes.

Carcinoma and Precancerous States of the Uterine Cervix, Vagina and Vulva

This is an important source of abnormal cells in the urinary sediment. In cancers invading the bladder wall, cancer cells may desquamate directly into the lumen of the urinary bladder. In precancerous states the cells desquamating from the surface of the cervix or adjacent organs may be picked up by the urinary stream. In both situations, the cells usually have the characteristics of a squamous or epidermoid carcinoma, to wit, orange- or yellow-stained cytoplasm (in Papanicolaou stain), and large, hyperchromatic nuclei (Fig. 5-40). If such cells are found in the urinary sediment of women in the absence of a documented primary bladder carcinoma, it is advisable to have these patients undergo a gynecologic examination, including a cervical smear and, if necessary, a colposcopic examination of the uterine cervix and the vagina.

Other Carcinomas of the Female Genital Tract

Endometrial and ovarian adenocarcinomas may invade the wall of the urinary bladder and may display in the urinary sediment single cancer cells or, more commonly, cell clusters, characteristic of these diseases. Cells derived from endometrial carcinoma are usually quite small, with variable amounts of basophilic, sometimes vacuolated cytoplasm. The nuclei are usually provided with prominent nucleoli. On the other hand, cells of ovarian cancer may be large, or even very large, depending on tumor type, and are characterized by a basophilic, often vacuolated cytoplasm and open, vesicular, large nuclei, provided with large nucleoli (Color Plate 5-2*B*). Such cells rarely, if ever, occur in primary adenocarcinoma of the bladder.

Adenocarcinomas of the female urethra may also shed cells into the urinary stream. They cannot be specifically identified as to the site of origin but often show a classical cytologic presentation of an adenocarcinoma (Color Plate 5-2*C*). The cell clusters are approximately spherical ("papillary"). The cells composing such clusters are often arranged in a multilayered structure. The cytoplasm is variable, sometimes vacuolated. The nuclei are open, minimally hyperchromatic and provided with prominent nucleoli of moderate sizes. For further comments on urethral carcinoma, see Chapter 6.

Prostatic Carcinomas

Prostatic adenocarcinomas, usually in advanced stages of the disease, may invade the urinary bladder or metastasize to it. The cancer cells in the urinary sediment are usually quite small, often spherical, but sometimes columnar in configuration. Small cell clusters may be observed. The cytoplasm of the cancer cells is usually basophilic; the nuclei are open, vesicular, and usually are provided with conspicuous nucleoli (see Fig. 7-4 in Chapter 7). The cells have few morphologic characteristics that allow their differentiation from other forms of adenocarcinomas. Immunostaining for specific prostatic antigen or for prostatic acid phosphatase allows their identification. Still, it must be stressed that *some bladder tumors originating in the trigone may share the immune characteristics with prostatic cells.* Therefore, the knowledge of clinical history is helpful.

Another important point in the differential diagnosis of prostatic carcinoma is the *synchronous presence of prostatic and bladder tumors,* as extensively documented by mapping studies (Mahadevia et al., 1986). As discussed above (see p. 107), it is not uncommon to observe *urothelial carcinomas,* sometimes *as flat carcinomas in situ, accompanying prostatic disease.* We have observed repeatedly the presence of *urothelial cancer cells* in the urinary sediment *as the first evidence of prostatic carcinoma,* particularly in younger men with aggressive prostatic cancers. It must be stressed, once again, that carcinomas in situ of the bladder may extend into the prostatic ducts (see p. 77 and Fig. 5-7).

Carcinomas of the Colon and Rectum

As discussed in reference to primary adenocarcinoma of the urinary bladder, the cancer cells of large bowel origin cannot be differentiated from cells of primary bladder adenocarcinoma of the intestinal type (see p. 103). The columnar configuration of these cancer cells, whether observed singly or in clusters, is common to both types of tumors. Tumor identification is based on clinical and histologic examination (Fig. 5-41 and Color Plate 5-2*D*).

Metastatic Carcinomas From Distant Sites

Although uncommon, such events may happen and sometimes cancer cells from remote origin may be observed in the urinary sediment. *In women,* by far the most common such cancers are of mammary origin. Sometimes the origin of such cells may be suggested, if they display the characteristic features of a lobular carcinoma: such cells are small signet-ring type cells, with a peripheral nucleus and a cytoplasmic vacuole, with a condensation of mucus within the vacuole, appearing as a central dot. Staining with mucicarmine is usually positive and identifies such cells with certainty. For further discussion of such cells the reader is referred to other sources (Koss, 1992).

In men, the most common source of metastatic carcinoma is lung cancer. As a rule, the cancer cells do not display any specific characteristics but may be readily recognized as malignant (Fig. 5-42). *In both sexes,* metastatic carcinomas from a variety of other distant sites may be observed, for example, of renal and pancreatic origin. Undoubtedly from time to time cancer cells from other primary sites will be observed.

Malignant Lymphomas and Leukemia

These disorders are one of the important sources of metastatic disease.

Non-Hodgkin's Lymphomas

Non-Hodgkin's lymphomas, particularly of the large cell type, may be identified in the sediment of voided urine. The tumor cells usually appear singly and *do not form clusters,* have scanty cytoplasm, and show significant nuclear abnormalities of various types. Thus the nuclei may be of bizarre shapes or show the characteristic nuclear protrusions or "nipples" (Fig. 5-43). In other cells the nuclei may be indented or cleaved. Prominent nucleoli, sometimes multiple, are commonly observed. Non-Hodgkin's lymphomas have a variety of cytologic presentations, depending on tumor type. A case of K1–positive, large cell lymphoma diagnosed in urine sediment was reported by Tanaka et al. (1993). For further discussion of malignant lymphomas, see Chapter 8.

Hodgkin's Disease

I have not observed persuasive evidence of metastatic Hodgkin's disease in the urinary sediment. Theoretically one should be able to recognize Reed-Sternberg cells, but this event must be extraordinarily rare. The cytologic presentation of Hodgkin's disease is discussed in Chapter 8.

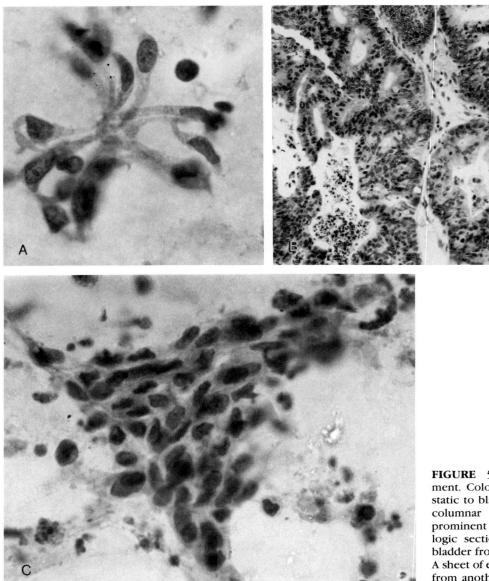

FIGURE 5-41. Urinary sediment. Colonic carcinoma metastatic to bladder. (*A*) Elongated, columnar cancer cells with prominent nucleoli. (*B*) Histologic section of biopsy of the bladder from the same case. (*C*) A sheet of elongated cancer cells from another case. (*A,C* × 900; *B* × 225.)

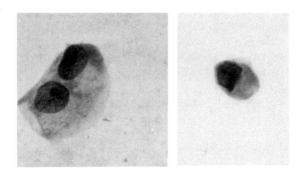

FIGURE 5-42. Urinary sediment. Cells of metastatic bronchogenic adenocarcinoma. The specific organ of origin cannot be established on cytology alone (× 560).

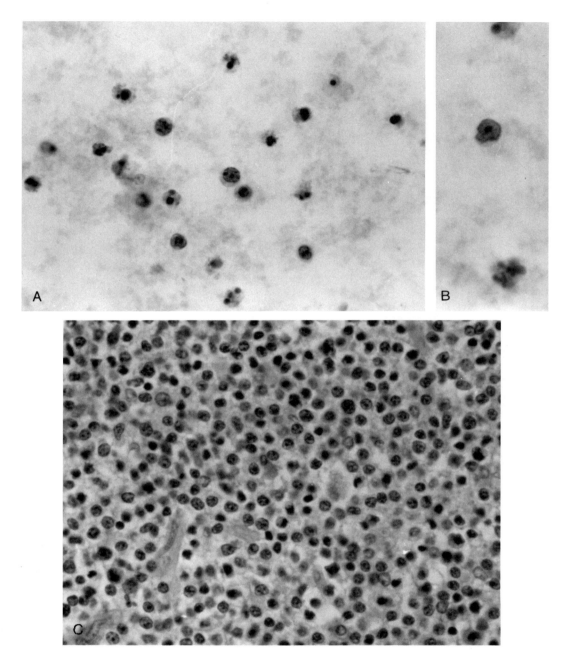

FIGURE 5-43. Metastatic high-grade non-Hodgkin's lymphoma in urinary sediment. (*A*) Numerous isolated lymphoid cells are present. (*B*) High-power view of one of the cells shows a nucleus with protrusion and a large nucleolus. (*C*) Histologic section of primary tumor. (*A,C* × 350; *B* × 560.)

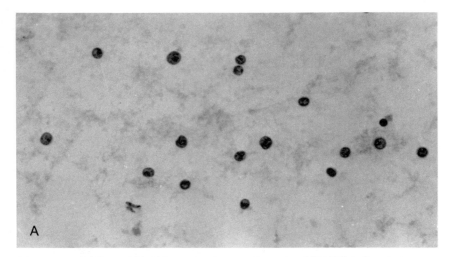

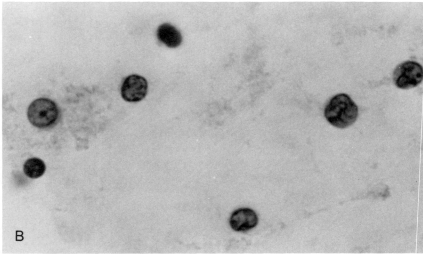

FIGURE 5-44. Lymphoblastic leukemia, with hematuria as its first manifestation. Urinary sediment. (*A*) A large number of blast cells was present in the urinary sediment. (*B*) A high-power view of the blasts shows the large nucleoli (*A* × 350; *B* × 900).

Leukemia

Leukemias sometimes may be identified in the urinary sediment *as a primary diagnostic medium.* The patients usually give a history of hematuria that may be the first manifestation of leukemia. Leukemic blast cells may be first identified in the urinary sediment. They are usually very numerous, spherical cells the size of very large lymphocytes, with scanty cytoplasm, large, open nuclei, and central large nucleoli (Fig. 5-44).

Malignant Melanomas

Metastatic malignant melanomas may involve the urinary tract directly or by producing melanuria. In melanuria the cytoplasm of the cells in the urinary sediment, some derived from renal tubules, may contain abundant brown melanin pigment (Color Plate 5-2*E,F*). Thus the recognition of the malignant characteristics of cancer cells is important in making the diagnosis. The presence of melanin pigment per se is not diagnostic of metastatic melanoma to the urinary tract. Cells of malignant melanoma are characterized by significant abnormalities in cell size, configuration, and nuclear structure. In most instances the cancer cells are large, sometimes very large, and contain one, two, or sometimes more nuclei, often located at the periphery of the cell. Melanin pigment may obscure the nucleus. When visible, the nuclei are large, and are provided with very large nucleoli (Fig. 5-45). Another common feature of cells of malignant

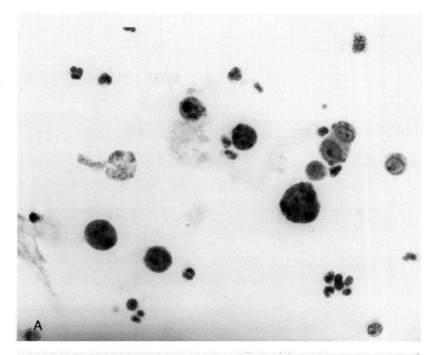

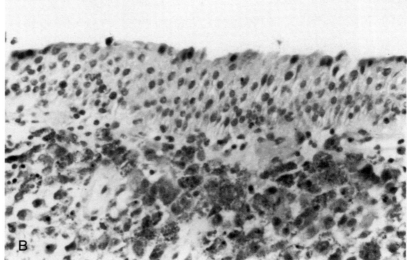

FIGURE 5-45. Metastatic heavily pigmented malignant melanoma of skin in the wall of the urinary bladder. (*A*) Sediment of voided urine contains numerous large cells carrying brown pigment, obscuring the nuclei. In cells relatively free of pigment large nuclei and prominent nucleoli can be seen. (*B*) Biopsy of bladder showing a subepithelial metastatic deposit of heavily pigmented metastatic melanoma (*A* × 560; *B* × 150).

melanoma is the presence of intranuclear clear zones or nuclear cytoplasmic inclusions, representing cytoplasmic infolding into the nucleus. It is not possible to determine from the positive urinary sediment which part of the urinary tract is involved by tumor, which may affect the kidneys, the ureters, the bladder, or sometimes all sites at once.

Metastatic Urothelial Carcinoma to Other Organs

It is of note that metastatic urothelial cancer to the vagina or to the penis may produce changes identical to extramammary Paget's disease (Fig. 5-46). Metastatic urothelial carcinoma to distant organs can

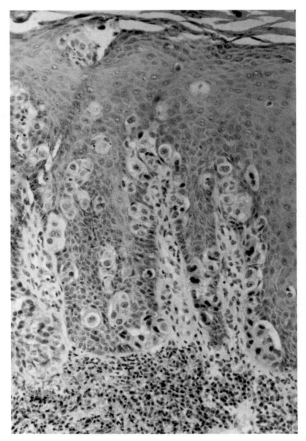

FIGURE 5-46. Metastatic bladder carcinoma to the skin of glans penis. The histologic presentation is typical of Paget's disease with numerous large, clear Paget's cells in the epidermis (× 150).

sometimes be recognized in cytologic preparations because of the formation of fairly typical umbrella cells.

RESULTS OF CYTOLOGIC EXAMINATION OF URINARY SEDIMENT

Voided Urine

Without understanding of the two pathways of bladder tumors and the pitfalls in their diagnosis, the early published results of urine cytology reflect a poor performance of the method. For example, Foot et al. (1958) reported accurate cytologic diagnosis (suspicious or positive) in 78.9% of 212 patients with bladder tumors and a "false positive" rate in 9.2% of 423 patients without tumors. With better understanding of the accomplishments and pitfalls of the method, it can be stated that voided urine is an accurate medium of diagnosis of high-grade urothelial tumors, particularly nonpapillary carcinoma in situ and related lesions. In a study of performance of voided urine cytology based on 3 sequential specimens of voided urine (processed by the method of Bales, described on pp. 6–9) in 203 cases, summarized in Table 5-3, it may be noted that failures to establish a cytologic diagnosis are mainly with well-differentiated tumors (grade 1), and to some extent with grade 2 tumors. The diagnostic performance was generally excellent with high-grade tumors, particularly carcinoma in situ and invasive cancers (Koss et al., 1985), as also reported by other observers (Johnson, 1964; Esposti and Zajicek, 1972). As discussed on p. 86, the claims of high

TABLE 5-3
Highest Cytologic Diagnosis Based on Three Sequential Specimens of Voided Urine in 203 Instances of Bladder Tumors

Highest Histologic Diagnosis of Tumor	*No. of Cases*	*Highest Cytologic Diagnosis*	
		NEGATIVE/ATYPICAL	SUSPICIOUS/POSITIVE
Noninvasive papillary tumors (all)	136	29 (22%)	107 (78%)
Grade 1	6	5 (83%)	1* (17%)
Grade 2	68	20 (29%)	48 (71%)
Grade 3	62	4 (6%)	58 (94%)
Nonpapillary carcinoma in situ	14	0	14 (100%)
Invasive carcinoma (all grades)	27	2 (7%)	25 (93%)
Carcinoma of the ureter	4	0	4
Other cancers	2	1	1
No evidence of cancer	20	20 (100%)	0

(From Koss, L. G., et al. Diagnostic value of cytology of voided urine. Acta Cytol. *29*, 810–816, 1985.)
*This patient was subsequently shown to have a high-grade tumor.

TABLE 5-4
Clinical Interpretation of Cytologic Findings

Clinical Finding	Cytologic Diagnosis	Significance
Visible papillary tumor	Negative (no abnormal cells)	Low-grade papillary tumor
Visible papillary tumor	Suspicious or positive (cancer cells present)	a. High-grade tumor with or without carcinoma in situ b. Low-grade tumor with carcinoma in situ
No visible tumor	Suspicious or positive	Carcinoma in situ or tumor in upper urinary tract.

accuracy in the cytologic diagnosis of low-grade bladder tumors are not based on reproducible criteria.

There is a remarkable similarity in the performance of diagnostic cytology on voided urine with the distribution of DNA ploidy values in urothelial tumors, as will be discussed in Chapter 9.

Washings and Brushings

There are no reliable data on the efficacy of bladder washings when compared with other modes of diagnosis, except in reference to flow cytometry (see below). In reference to washings and brushings of other components of the lower urinary tract, such as the ureters, renal pelves, or penile urethra, only anecdotal information is available (see Chap. 6).

Clinical Interpretation of Cytologic Findings

There is considerable confusion among urologists and pathologists alike as to the correlation of cytologic findings with clinical disease. Nothing is more frustrating to a urologist than a "negative" (no tumor identified) diagnosis in the presence of a visible, sometimes large lesion, unless it is clearly understood that such lesions, when of low grade and lined by normal or nearly normal urothelium do not shed identifiable abnormal cells. On the other end of the diagnostic spectrum, the diagnosis of cancer in the absence of visible disease is a source of bewilderment and sometimes anger, because it is not understood that carcinoma in situ may not be visible and yet shed cancer cells. A brief correlation of the cytologic findings is given in Table 5-4.

It must be clearly understood that the diagnosis of cancer rendered by a competent observer on multiple urine samples must be taken with utmost seriousness. This usually indicates the presence of a life-threatening disease. It must be remembered that invasive cancer is in most instances not associated with visible, papillary disease but with the invisible carcinoma in situ and that ignoring a positive cytologic report may lead to a disaster for the patient. It is of additional significance that patients undergoing local chemotherapy, whether by thiotepa, mitomycin C, or bacille Calmette-Guérin (BCG) are not exempt from this rule. In such cases the presence of cancer cells in the sediment indicates treatment failure. It is rare for the drug effect to be confused with cancer.

Biopsy Documentation of Carcinoma in Situ

The biopsy proof of carcinoma in situ, diagnosed by cytology, in the absence of significant cystostopic abnormalities, is sometimes quite difficult. Multiple cystoscopic biopsies of the bladder must be obtained, starting with areas of visible abnormality (i.e., redness) but also encompassing apparently normal urothelium. The cancerous epithelium may be very fragile and, therefore, the material must be handled with great care by the clinician and by the laboratory. DeBellis and Schumann (1986) proposed that in such cases the fixative used for small bladder biopsies should be centrifuged and the sediment carefully examined for detached fragments of cancerous epithelium.

It is suggested that, at a minimum, biopsies should be obtained from the trigone (which should encompass the anterior prostatic ducts—see p. 77), the posterior wall, the lateral walls, and the dome of the bladder. It is advisable to have separate containers filled with buffered formalin prepared and labeled in advance for each biopsy site.

After removal of the biopsy from the fixative, it is advisable to filter the fixative and embed all residual tissue fragments as they may contain diagnostically valuable material.

A protocol for handling the patients is shown below.

PROTOCOL FOR HANDLING NEOPLASTIC LESIONS OF THE BLADDER

1. *Asymptomatic patients* exposed to known carcinogens
Check for hematuria
Urinary cytology × 3 q 6 months
Cystoscopy and multiple biopsies of bladder if indicated
2. *Symptomatic patients* (hematuria, frequency, nocturia, pain, mucous discharge)
Urinary cytology × 3
Cystoscopy
Multiple biopsies if cytology positive
    Lesion (if visible)
    Lateral walls
    Posterior wall
    Trigone, including prostatic ducts
    Dome
    Upper urinary tract, if bladder is negative
3. *Follow-up after removal of localized lesions*
Cytology × 3 q 3 months
Cystoscopy and multiple biopsies if cytologic or cystoscopic abnormalities are present.
Investigation of the upper urinary tract, if necessary

Schwalb et al. (1993) proposed a series of management algorithms for patients with positive urinary cytology in the absence of visible lesions. The algorithms for previously untreated patients, patients after complete transurethral resection, and after complete clinical response to intravesical therapy, differ little from the protocol outlined above. These authors stressed once again the importance of occult disease in the prostatic ducts and the upper urinary tract (ureters and renal pelves).

CYTOLOGIC TECHNIQUES IN MONITORING BLADDER TUMORS

Cytology of voided urine is perhaps the most useful and least expensive modality of follow-up of bladder tumors, particularly in patients with either primary or secondary carcinoma in situ, but also in patients with other tumor types. The method is especially valuable in patients treated with immuno- or chemotherapy for flat cancerous lesions. *The presence of malignant cells, even in the absence of a visible lesion, must lead to further investigation of the patient, particularly of the prostatic ducts, wherein foci of occult high-grade carcinoma may be hiding.* I have seen several documented instances of treated patients whose positive urinary sediments were not investigated further because "there was nothing to see" in the bladder, and who subsequently developed metastatic carcinoma and died of it. Voided urine may be supplemented with bladder washings and DNA ploidy determination by either flow cytometry or image analysis (see Chap. 9). Abnormalities of DNA patterns are sometimes an indication of a recurrent tumor, although the margin of error of such measurements is substantial. For further discussion of this topic, see Chapter 9.

Schwalb et al. (1994) presented pattern of disease recurrence in 75 patients, 69 with carcinoma in situ, with full clinical response to BCG and positive cytology 1 or more years after treatment. In 62 patients, cystoscopically visible and/or biopsy confirmed recurrences were observed within a median of 6 months (range 2 to 60 months) after positive cytology. In 39 of these patients the recurrent disease occurred in the bladder, with carcinoma in situ the most commonly observed lesion. In 11 patients the disease occurred in the upper urinary tract, in 7 in prostatic ducts, and in 9 patients in a combination of these sites. In 13 patients with positive cytology the source of cancer cells could not be found at the time of writing of the paper.

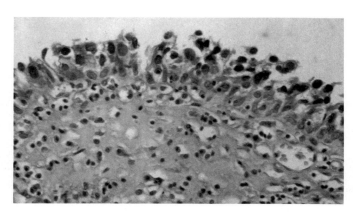

FIGURE 5-47. Carcinoma in situ of the urinary bladder after eradication of invasive cancer by radiotherapy. This is a source of treatment failure (× 150).

Schwalb et al. stress the need for aggressive evaluation of such patients, leading to the diagnosis of recurrent disease at a treatable stage.

Radiotherapy of bladder tumors also warrants monitoring with voided urine sediment. In some patients so treated, the invasive tumor may be eradicated but a carcinoma in situ may remain (Fig. 5-47). Undoubtedly, this is the source of radiation failure.

Laser Treatment of Bladder Tumors

Fanning et al. (1993) described a treatment artifact in patients whose bladder tumors were treated by Nd-YAG laser. Spindly cells in bundles, presumably tumor cells, were described and illustrated. Fanning noted that this artifact precluded the evaluation of the sediment for the presence or absence of residual tumor.

RESEARCH ON BLADDER TUMORS

Tumors of the urinary bladder have been the subject of an extensive research effort pertaining to the cytogenetics, immunology, DNA content, and molecular biology. Specific aspects of research will be discussed in Chapters 9, 10, and 11.

BIBLIOGRAPHY

Urothelial (Transitional Cell) Tumors
Rare Bladder Tumors
Bladder Tumors-Monitoring

Urothelial (Transitional Cell) Tumors

Allegra, S. R., Broderick, P. A., and Corvese, N. L.: Cytologic and histogenetic observations in well differentiated transitional cell carcinoma of bladder. J. Urol., *107*, 777–782, 1972.

Alroy, J., Pauli, B. U., and Weinstein, R. S.: Correlation between numbers of desmosomes and the aggressiveness of transitional cell carcinomas in human urinary bladder. Cancer, *47*, 104–112, 1981.

Althausen, A. F., Prout, G. R., Jr., and Daly, J. J.: Noninvasive papillary carcinoma of bladder associated with carcinoma in situ. J. Urol., *116*, 575–580, 1976.

Alvaro, A. S., Dalbagni, G., Cordon-Cardo, C., Zhang, Z. F., Sheinfeld, J., Fair, W. R., Herr, H. W., and Reuter, V. E.: Nuclear overexpression of p53 protein in transitional cell bladder carcinoma: A marker for disease progression. J. Natl. Cancer Inst., *85*, 53–59, 1993.

Amberson, J. B., and Laino, J.: Image cytometric deoxyribonucleic acid analysis of urine specimens as an adjunct to visual cytology in the detection of urothelial cell carcinoma. J. Urol., *149*, 42–45, 1993.

Anderstrom, C., Johansson, S., and Nilson, S.: The significance of lamina propria invasion on the prognosis of patients with bladder tumors. J. Urol., *124*, 23–26, 1980.

Ashall, F., Bramwell, M. E., and Harris, H.: A new marker for human cancer cells: The Ca antigen and the Ca1 antibody. Lancet, *2*, 1–7, 1982.

Austen, G. J., and Friedell, G. H.: Observations of local growth patterns of bladder cancer. Trans. Am. Assoc. Genitourin. Surg., *56*, 38–43, 1964.

Baars, J. H., De Ruijter, J. L. M., Smedts, F., Van Niekerk, C. C., Poels, L. G., Seldenrijk, C. A., and Ramaekers, F. C. S.: The applicability of a keratin 7 monoclonal antibody in routinely Papanicolaou-stained cytologic specimens for the differential diagnosis of carcinomas. Am. J. Clin. Pathol., *101*, 257–261, 1994.

Baird, S. S., Bush, L., and Livingstone, A. G.: Urethrectomy subsequent to total cystectomy for papillary carcinoma of the bladder. Case reports. J. Urol., *74*, 621–625, 1955.

Bales, C. E.: A semi-automated method for preparation of urine sediment for cytologic evaluation. Acta Cytol., *25*, 323–326, 1981.

Banigo, O. G., Waisman, J., and Kaufman, J. J.: Papillary (transitional) carcinoma in an ileal conduit. J. Urol., *114*, 626–627, 1975.

Barlebo, H., Sorensen, B. L., and Soeberg Ohlsen, A.: Carcinoma in situ of the urinary bladder. Flat intraepithelial neoplasia. Scand. J. Urol. Nephrol., *6*, 213–223, 1972.

Barlebo, H., and Sorensen, B. L.: Flat epithelial changes in the urinary bladder in patients with prostatic hypertrophy. Scand. J. Urol. Nephrol., *6 (Suppl 15)*, 121–128, 1972.

Bejany, D. E., Lockhart, J. L., and Rhamy, R. K.: Malignant vesical tumors following spinal cord injury. J. Urol., *138*, 1390–1392, 1987.

Bergkvist, A., Ljunggvist, A., and Moberger, G.: Classification of bladder tumors based on the cellular pattern. Preliminary report of a clinical-pathological study of 300 cases with a minimum follow-up of eight years. Acta Chir. Scand., *130*, 371–378, 1965.

Beyer-Boon, M. E.: The efficacy of urinary cytology. Dissertation, Univ. of Leiden, the Netherlands, 1977.

Bhagavan, B. S., Tiamson, E. M., Wenk, R. E., Berger, B. W., Hamamoto, G., and Eggelstone, J. C.: Nephrogenic adenoma of the urinary bladder and urethra. Human Path., *12*, 907–916, 1981.

Bickel, A., Culkin, D. J., Wheeler, J. S., Jr.: Bladder cancer in spinal cord injury patients. J. Urol., *146*, 1240–1242, 1991.

Bonner, R. B., Hemstreet, G. P., Fradet, Y., Rao, J. Y., Min, K. W., and Hurst, R. E.: Bladder cancer risk assessment with quantitative fluorescence image analysis of tumor markers in exfoliated bladder cells. Cancer, *72*, 2461–2469, 1993.

Bonser, G. M., Clayson, D. B., Jull, J. W., and Pyrah, L. N.: Carcinogenic properties of 2-amino-1-naphthol hydrochloride and its parent amine 2-naphthylamine. Br. J. Cancer, *6*, 412–424, 1952.

Boon, M. E., Blomjous, C. E., Zwartendijk, J., Heinhuis, R. J., and Ooms, E. C. M.: Carcinoma in situ of the urinary bladder. Clinical presentation, cytologic pattern, and stromal changes. Acta Cytol., *30,* 360–366, 1986.

Borland, R. N., Partin, A. W., Epstein, J. I., and Brendler, C. B.: The use of nuclear morphometry in predicting recurrence of transitional cell carcinoma. J. Urol., *149,* 272–275, 1993.

Bracken, R. B., and Grabstald, H.: Bladder carcinoma involving the lower abdominal wall. J. Urol., *114,* 715–721, 1975.

Brawn, P. N.: The origin of invasive carcinoma of the bladder. Cancer, *50,* 515–519, 1982.

Brekkan, E., Colleen, S., Myrvold, B., Schnurer, L. B., and Fritjofsson, A.: Colonic neoplasia: A late complication of ureterosigmoidostomy. Scand. J. Urol. Nephrol., *6,* 197–202, 1972.

Cajulis, R. S., Haines, G. K., Frias-Hidvegi, D., and McVary, K.: Interphase cytogenetics as an adjunct in the cytodiagnosis of urinary bladder carcinoma. A comparative study of cytology, flow cytometry and interphase cytogenetics in bladder washes. Anal. Quant. Cytol. Histol., *16,* 1–10, 1994.

Chin, J. L., Huben, R. P., Nava, E., Rustum, Y. M., Greco, J. M., Pontes, E., and Frankfurt, O. S.: Flow cytometric analysis of DNA content in human bladder tumors and irrigation specimens. Cancer, *56,* 1677–1681, 1985.

Cifuentes Delatte, L., Oliva, H., and Navarro, V.: Intraepithelial carcinoma of the bladder. Urol. Int., *25,* 169–186, 1970.

Cole, P., Hoover, R., and Friedell, G. H.: Occupation and cancer of the lower urinary tract. Cancer, *29,* 1250–1260, 1972.

Cole, P., Monson, R., Haning, H., and Friedell, G. H.: Smoking and cancer of the lower urinary tract. N. Engl. J. Med., *284,* 129–134, 1971.

Coon, J. S., McCall, A., Miller, A. W., Farrow, G. M., and Weinstein, R. S.: Expression of blood-group-related antigens in carcinoma in situ of the urinary bladder. Cancer, *56,* 797–804, 1985.

Cooper, P. H., Waisman, J., Johnston, W. H., and Skinner, D. G.: Severe atypia of transitional epithelium and carcinoma of the urinary bladder. Cancer, *31,* 1055–1060, 1973.

Crabbe, J. G. S.: Cytology of voided urine and special reference to 'benign' papilloma and some of the problems encountered in the preparation of the smears. Acta Cytol., *5,* 233–240, 1961.

Culp, O. S., Utz, D. C., and Harrison, E. G. J.: Experience with ureteral carcinoma in situ detected during operations for vesical problems. J. Urol., *97,* 679–682, 1967.

Cutler, S. J., Heney, N. M., and Friedell, G. H.: Longitudinal study of patients with bladder cancer: factors associated with disease recurrence and progression. *In* Bonney, W. W., and Prout, G. R., Jr. (Eds.): Bladder Cancer. AUA Monographs. vol. 1, p. 35. Baltimore, Williams & Wilkins, 1982.

Czerniak, B., Cohen, G. L., Etkin, P., Deitch, D., Sim-

mons, H., Herz, F., and Koss, L. G.: Concurrent mutations of coding and regulatory sequences of the Ha-ras gene in urinary bladder carcinoma. Hum. Path., *23,* 1199–1204, 1992.

Czerniak, B., Deitch, D., Simmons, H., Etkind, P., Herz, F., and Koss, L. G.: Ha-ras gene codon 12 mutation and ploidy in urinary bladder cancer. Brit. J. Cancer, *62,* 762–763, 1990.

Czerniak, B., and Koss, L. G.: Expression of Ca antigen on human urinary bladder tumors. Cancer, *55,* 2380–2383, 1985.

Czerniak, B., Koss, L. G., and Sherman, A.: Nuclear pores and DNA ploidy in human bladder carcinomas. Cancer Res., *44,* 3752–3756, 1984.

De Jager, R., Guinan, P., Lamm, D., Khanna, O., Brosman, S., De Kernion, J., Williams, R., Richardson, C., Muenz, L., Reitsma, D., et al.: Long-term complete remission in bladder carcinoma in situ with intravesical bacillus Calmette Guérin. Overview analysis of six phase II clinical trials. Urology, *38,* 507–513, 1991.

De la Rosette, J. J. M., Hubregtse, M. R., Wiersma, A. M., and Debruyne, F. M. J.: Value of urine cytology in screening patients with prostatitis syndrome. Acta Cytol., *37,* 710–712, 1993.

Dean, P. J., and Murphy, W. M.: Carcinoma in situ and dysplasia of the bladder urothelium. World J. Urol., *5,* 103–107, 1987.

Dean, P. J., and Murphy, W. M.: Importance of urinary cytology and future role of flow cytometry. Urology, *26* (Suppl.), 11–15, 1985.

DeBellis, C. C., and Schumann, G. B.: Cystoscopic biopsy supernate. A new cytologic approach for diagnosing urothelial carcinoma in situ. Acta Cytol., *30,* 356–359, 1986.

Deden, C.: Cancer cells in urinary sediment. Acta Radiol. (Suppl.), *115,* 1–75, Figs. 1–36, 1954.

Del Mistro, A., Koss, L. G., Braunstein, J., Bennett, B., Saccomano, G., and Simons, K. M.: Condylomata acuminata of the urinary bladder. Am. J. Surg. Pathol., *12,* 205–215, 1988.

DeMay, R. M., and Grathwohl, M. A.: Signet-ring-cell (colloid) carcinoma of the urinary bladder. Acta Cytol., *29,* 132–136, 1985.

deVoogt, H. J., Beyer-Boon, M. E., and Brussec, J. A. M.: The value of phase contrast microscopy for urinary cytology. Reliability and pitfalls. Acta Cytol., *19,* 542–546, 1975.

deVoogt, H. J., Rathert, P., and Beyer-Boon, M. E.: Urinary Cytology. Springer-Verlag, New York, 1977.

DiBonito, L., Musse, M. M., Dudine, S., and Falconieri, G.: Cytology of transitional-cell carcinoma of the urinary bladder: Diagnostic yield and histologic basis. Diagn. Cytopathol., *8,* 124–127, 1992.

Dimmette, R. M., Sproat, H. F., and Klimt, C. R.: Examination of smears of urinary sediment for detection of neoplasms of bladder: survey of an Egyptian village infested with Schistosoma hematobium. Am. J. Clin. Pathol., *25,* 1032–1042, 1955.

Domagala, W., Kahan, A. V., and Koss, L. G.: The ultrastructure of surfaces of positively identified cells in the human urinary sediment: A correlative light and scanning electron microscopic study. Acta Cytol., 23, 147–155, 1979.

Droller, M. J.: A rose is a rose is a rose, or is it? (Editorial). J. Urol., 136, 1057–1058, 1986.

Eisenberg, R. B., Roth, R. B., and Schweisberg, M. H.: Bladder tumors and associated proliferative mucosal lesions. J. Urol., 84, 544–550, 1960.

El-Bolkainy, M., and Chu, E. W.: Detection of bladder cancer associated with schistosomiasis. Cairo, Egypt, National Cancer Institute, Cairo University, Al Ahram Press, 1981.

Elliot, G. B., Moloney, P. L., and Anderson, G. H.: 'Denuding cystitis' and in situ urothelial carcinoma. Arch. Pathol., 96, 91–94, 1973.

Esposti, P. L., Moberger, G., and Zajicek, J.: The cytologic diagnosis of transitional cell tumors of the urinary bladder and its histologic basis. A study of 567 cases of urinary-tract disorder including 170 untreated and 182 irradiated bladder tumors. Acta Cytol., 14, 145–155, 1970.

Esposti, P. L., and Zajicek, J.: Grading of transitional cell neoplasms of the urinary bladder from smears of bladder washings. A critical review of 326 tumors. Acta Cytol., 16, 529–537, 1972.

Falor, W. H.: Chromosomes in noninvasive papillary carcinoma of the bladder. J.A.M.A., 216, 791–794, 1971.

Falor, W. H., and Ward, R. M.: Cytogenetic analysis: A potential index for recurrence of early carcinoma of the bladder. J. Urol., 115, 49–52, 1976.

Falor, W. H., and Ward, R. M.: Fifty-three month persistence of ring chromosome in noninvasive bladder carcinoma. Acta Cytol., 20, 271–274, 1976.

Fanning, C. V., Staerkel, G. A., Sneige, N., Thomsen, S., Myhre, M. J., and Von Eschenbach, A. C.: Spindling artifact of urothelial cells in post-laser treatment urinary cytology. Diagn. Cytopathol., 9, 279–281, 1993.

Farrow, G. M., Barlebo, H., Enjoji, M., Chisholm, G., Friedell, G. H., Jackse, G., Kakizoe, T., Koss, L. G., Kotake, T., and Vahlensieck, W.: Transitional cell carcinoma in situ. In Denis, L., Nijima, T., Prout, G., and Schröder, F. H. (eds.): Developments in Bladder Cancer. New York, Alan R. Liss, 1986, pp. 85–96.

Farrow, G. M., Utz, D. C., Rife, C. C., and Greene, L. F.: Clinical observations on 69 cases of in situ carcinoma of the urinary bladder. Cancer Res., 37, 2794–2798, 1977.

Farrow, G. M., Utz, D. C., and Rife, C. C.: Morphological and clinical observations of patients with early bladder cancer treated with total cystectomy. Cancer Res., 36, 2495–2501, 1976.

Foot, N. C., and Papanicolaou, G. N.: Early renal carcinoma in situ detected by means of smears of fixed urinary sediment. J.A.M.A., 139, 356–358, 1949.

Foot, N. C., Papanicolaou, G. N., Holmquist, N. D., and Seybolt, J. F.: Exfoliative cytology of urinary sediments: review of 2,829 cases. Cancer, 11, 127–137, 1958.

Forni, A., Ghetti, G., and Armell, G.: Urinary cytology in workers exposed to carcinogenic aromatic amines: A six-year study. Acta Cytol., 16, 142–145, 1972.

Fossa, S. D.: Feulgen-DNA-values in transitional cell carcinoma of the human urinary bladder. Beitr. Pathol., 155, 44–55, 1975.

Fossa, S. D., and Kaalhus, O.: Nuclear size and chromatin concentration in transitional cell carcinoma of the human urinary bladder. Beitr. Pathol., 157, 109–125, 1976.

Fox, A. J., and White, G. C.: Bladder cancer in rubber workers. Do screening and doctors' awareness distort the statistics? Lancet, 1, 1009–1011, 1976.

Friedell, G. H., Soloway, M. S., Hilgar, A. G., and Farrow, G. M.: Summary of workshop on carcinoma in situ of the bladder. J. Urol., 136, 1047–1048, 1986.

Garner, J. W., Goldstein, A. M. B., and Cosgrove, M. D.: Histologic appearance of the intestinal urinary conduit. J. Urol., 114, 854–857, 1975.

Gonzales, J. A., Watts, J. C., and Alderson, T. P.: Nephrogenic adenoma of bladder: report of 10 cases. J. Urol., 139, 45–47, 1988.

Gonzales-Zulueta, M., Ruppert, J. M., Tokino, K., Tsai, Y. C., Spruck, C. H. I., Miyao, N., Nichols, P. W., Hermann, G. G., Horn, T., Steven, K., Summerhayes, I. C., Sidransky, D., and Jones, P. A.: Microsatellite instability in bladder cancer. Cancer Res., 53, 5620–5623, 1993.

Gordon, A.: Intestinal metaplasia of urinary tract epithelium. J. Path. Bact., 85, 441–444, 1963.

Granberg-Ohman, I., Tribukait, B., and Wijkstrom, H.: Cytogenetic analysis of 62 transitional cell bladder carcinomas. Cancer Genet. Cytogenet., 11, 69–85, 1984.

Grogono, J. L., and Shepheard, B. G. F.: Carcinoma of the urachus. Br. J. Urol., 41, 222–227, 1969.

Gustafson, H., Tribukait, B., and Esposti, L.: DNA profile and tumor progression in patients with superficial bladder tumors. Urol. Res., 10, 13–18, 1982.

Harris, M. J., Schwinn, C. P., Morrow, J. W., Gray, R. L., and Browell, B. M.: Exfoliative cytology of the urinary bladder irrigation specimen. Acta Cytol., 15, 385–399, 1971.

Harrison, J. H., Bostford, T. W., and Tucker, M. R.: The use of urinary sediment in the diagnosis and management of neoplasms of the kidney and bladder. Surg. Gyn. Obst., 92, 129–139, 1951.

Harving, N., Wolf, H., and Melsen, F.: Positive urinary cytology after tumor resection: An indicator for concomitant carcinoma in situ. J. Urol., 140, 495–497, 1988.

Helpap, B., Bodekar, J., and Pfitzenmaier, N.: Histologische und zytologische Aspekta der urotherlialen Atypie (Dysplasie). Pathologe, 6, 292–297, 1985.

Herz, F., Barlebo, H., and Koss, L. G.: Modulation of alkaline phosphatase activity in cell cultures derived from human urinary bladder carcinoma. Cancer, 34, 1934–1943, 1974.

Hicks, R. M., and Newman, J.: Scanning electron microscopy of urinary sediment. In Koss, L. G., and Coleman, D. V. (Eds.): Advances in Clinical Cytology, Vol. 2, pp. 135–161. New York, Masson, 1984.

Hofstädter, F., Delgado, R., Jakse, G., and Judmaier, W.: Urothelial dysplasia and carcinoma in situ of the bladder. Cancer, 57, 356–361, 1986.

Holmquist, N. D.: Diagnostic Cytology of the Urinary Tract. Basel, S. Karger, 1977.

Houston, W., Koss, L. G., and Melamed, M. R.: Bladder cancer and schistosomiasis: A preliminary cytological study. Trans. Roy. Soc. Trop. Med. Hyg., *60*, 89–91, 1966.

Hueper, W. C.: Occupational and environmental cancers of the urinary system. Yale University Press, New Haven, 1969.

Jacobs, J. B., Arai, M., Cohen, S. M., and Friedell, G. H.: Early lesions in experimental bladder cancer: Scanning electron microscopy of cell surface markers. Cancer Res., *36*, 2512–2517, 1976.

Jannoni, C., Marcheggiono, A., Pallone, F., Gallucci, M., Di Silvero, O., and Caprilli, R.: Abnormal patterns of colorectal mucin secretion after urinary diversion of different types. Human Path., *17*, 834–840, 1986.

Jewett, H. J., Lowell, R. K., and Shelley, W. M.: A study of 364 cases of infiltrating bladder cancer: Relation of certain pathological characteristics to prognosis after extirpation. J. Urol., *92*, 668–678, 1964.

Jewett, H. J., and Strong, G. H.: Infiltrating carcinoma of bladder: Relation of depth of penetration of bladder wall to incidence of local extension and metastases. J. Urol., *35*, 366–372, 1946.

Johnston, W. D.: Cytopathologic correlations in tumors of the urinary bladder. Cancer, *17*, 867–880, 1964.

Jordan, A. M., Weingarten, J., and Murphy, W. M.: Transitional cell neoplasms of the urinary bladder. Can biologic potential be predicted from histologic grading? Cancer, *60*, 2766–2774, 1987.

Kakudo, K., Itatani, H., and Uematsu, K.: Non-papillary carcinoma in situ of the urinary bladder. An electron microscopic study. Acta Pathol. Jpn., *34*, 345–353, 1984.

Kalnins, Z. A., Rhyne, A. L., Morehead, R. P., and Carter, B. J.: Comparison of cytologic findings in patients with transitional cell carcinoma and benign urologic diseases. Acta Cytol., *14*, 743–749, 1970.

Kannan, V., and Bose, S.: Low grade transitional cell carcinoma and instrument artifact. A challenge in urinary cytology. Acta Cytol., *37*, 899–902, 1993.

Kaufman, J. M., Fam, B., Jacobs, S. C., Gabilondo, F., Yalla, S., Kane, J. P., and Rossier, A. B.: Bladder cancer and squamous metaplasia in spinal cord injury patients. J. Urol., *118*, 967–970, 1977.

Kaye, K. W., and Lange, P. H.: Mode of presentation of invasive bladder cancer: Reassessment of the problem. J. Urol., *128*, 31–33, 1982.

Kern, W. H.: The cytology of transitional cell carcinoma of the urinary bladder. Acta Cytol., *19*, 420–428, 1975.

Kern, W. H., Bales, C. E., and Webster, W. W.: Cytologic evaluation of transitional cell carcinoma of the bladder. J. Urol., *100*, 616–622, 1968.

Knappenberger, S. T., Uson, A. C., and Melicow, M. M.: Primary neoplasms occurring in vesical diverticula: A report of 18 cases. J. Urol., *83*, 153–159, 1960.

Koss, L. G.: Tumors of the Urinary Bladder. Atlas of Tumor Pathology, Second Series, Fascicle 11. Washington, D.C. Armed Forces Institute of Pathology, 1975.

Koss, L. G.: Tumors of the urinary bladder. Atlas of Tumor Pathology, Second Series, Fascicle 11, Supplement. Washington, D.C., Armed Forces Institute of Pathology, 1985.

Koss, L. G.: Formal discussion of 'clinical observations on 69 cases of in situ carcinoma of the urinary bladder.' Cancer Res., *37*, 2799, 1977.

Koss, L. G.: Some ultrastructural aspects of experimental and human carcinoma of the bladder. Cancer Res., *37*, 2824–2835, 1977.

Koss, L. G.: Mapping of the urinary bladder: Its impact on the concepts of bladder cancer. Hum. Pathol., *10*, 533–548, 1979.

Koss, L. G.: Environmental carcinogenesis and cytology (Editorial). Acta Cytol., *24*, 281–282, 1980.

Koss, L. G.: Urinary tract cytology. In Connolly, J. C. (Ed.): Carcinoma of the Bladder. New York, Raven Press, 1981, pp. 159–163.

Koss, L. G.: Evaluation of patients with carcinoma in situ of the bladder. In Sommers, S. C., and Rosen, P. P. (Eds.): Pathology Annual, Part II, Vol. 17, pp. 353–359. Appleton-Century-Crofts, 1982.

Koss, L. G.: The role of cytology in the diagnosis, detection and follow-up bladder cancer. In Denis, L., et al. (Eds.): Developments in Bladder Cancer. New York, Alan R. Liss, pp. 97–108, 1986.

Koss, L. G.: Precursor lesions of invasive bladder cancer. Eur. Urol., *14*, (Suppl. 1), 4–6, 1988.

Koss, L. G.: From koilocytosis to molecular biology: The impact of cytology on concepts of early human cancer. Modern Pathol., *2*, 526–535, 1989.

Koss, L. G.: Bladder cancer from a perspective of 40 years. J. Cell Biochem., *Sup. 161*, 23–29, 1992.

Koss, L. G.: Diagnostic Cytology and Its Histopathologic Bases, 4th Ed. Philadelphia, J. B. Lippincott, 1992.

Koss, L. G., Bartels, P. H., Bibbo, M., Freed, S. Z., Taylor, J., and Wied, G. L.: Computer discrimination between benign and malignant urothelial cells. Acta Cytol., *19*, 378–391, 1975.

Koss, L. G., Bartels, P. H., Bibbo, M., Freed, S. Z., Sychra, J. J., Taylor, J., and Wied, G. L.: Computer analysis of atypical urothelial cells. I. Classification by supervised learning algorithms. Acta Cytol., *21*, 247–260, 1977.

Koss, L. G., Bartels, P. H., Sychra, J. J., and Wied, G. L.: Computer analysis of atypical urothelial cells. II. Classification by unsupervised learning algorithms. Acta Cytol., *21*, 261–265, 1977.

Koss, L. G., and Czerniak, B.: Image analysis and flow cytometry of tumors of prostate and bladder. With a comment on molecular biology of urothelial tumors. In Weinstein, R., and Gardner, W. A., Jr. (Eds.): Pathology and Pathobiology of the Urinary Bladder and Prostate. Baltimore, Williams & Wilkins, 1992.

Koss, L. G., Deitch, D., Ramanathan, R., and Sherman, A. B.: Diagnostic value of cytology of voided urine. Acta Cytol., *29*, 810–816, 1985.

Koss, L. G., Eppich, E. M., Medler, K. H., and Wersto, R. P.: DNA cytophotometry of voided urine sediment: Comparison with results of cytologic diagnosis and image analysis. Anal. Quant. Cytol. Hist., 9, 398–404, 1987.

Koss, L. G., Esposti, L., Nagayama, T., De Voogt, H., Farsund, T., et al.: The role of cytology in the diagnosis, detection, and follow-up of bladder cancer. In Denis, L., Nijima, T., Prout, G., and Schröder, F. H. (eds.): Developments in Bladder Cancer. pp. 97–108. New York, Alan R. Liss, 1986.

Koss, L. G., and Lavin, P.: Studies of experimental bladder carcinoma in Fischer 344 female rats. I. Induction of tumors with diet low in vitamin B6 containing N-2 fluorenylacetamide after single dose of cyclophosphamide. J. Nat. Cancer Inst., 46, 585–595, 1971.

Koss, L. G., Melamed, M. R., and Kelly, R. E.: Further cytologic and histologic studies of bladder lesions in workers exposed to para-aminodiphenyl: Progress report. J.N.C.I., 43, 233–243, 1969.

Koss, L. G., Melamed, M. R., and Mayer, K.: The effect of busulfan on human epithelia. Am. J. Clin. Pathol., 44, 385–397, 1965.

Koss, L. G., Melamed, M. R., Ricci, A., Melick, W. F., and Kelly, R. E.: Carcinogenesis in the human urinary bladder. Observations after exposure to para-aminodiphenyl. N. Engl. J. Med., 272, 767–770, 1965.

Koss, L. G., Nakanishi, I., and Freed, S. Z.: Nonpapillary carcinoma in situ and atypical hyperplasia in cancerous bladders. Further studies of surgically removed bladders by mapping. Urology, 9, 442–455, 1977.

Koss, L. G., Tiamson, E. M., and Robbins, M. A.: Mapping cancerous and precancerous bladder changes. A study of the urothelium in ten surgically removed bladders. J.A.M.A., 227, 281–286, 1974.

Koss, L. G., Wersto, R. P., Simmons, D. A., Deitch, D., Herz, F., and Freed, S. Z.: Predictive value of DNA measurements in bladder washings. Comparison of flow cytometry, image cytophotometry, and cytology in patients with a past history of urothelial tumors. Cancer, 64, 916–924, 1989.

Koss, L. G., Woyke, S., and Olszewski, W.: Aspiration biopsy. Cytologic Interpretation and Histologic Bases. 2nd Ed. New York, Igaku Shoin, 1992.

Lamm, D. L.: Carcinoma in situ. Urol. Clin. North Am., 19, 499–508, 1992.

Lange, P. H., and Limas, C.: Molecular markers in the diagnosis and prognosis of bladder cancer. J. Urol., 23S, 46–49, 1984.

Laursen, B.: Cancer of the bladder in patients treated with chlornaphazine. Br. Med. J., 3, 684–685, 1970.

Lederer, B., Mikuz, G., Gutter, W., and zur Neiden, G.: Zytophotometrische Untersuchungen von Tumoren des Ubergangsepithels der Harnblase. Vergleich zytophotometrischer Untersuchungsergebnisse mit dem histologischen Grading. Beitr. Pathol., 147, 379–389, 1972.

Lerman, R. I., Hutter, R. V., and Whitmore, W. F., Jr.: Papilloma of the urinary bladder. Cancer, 25, 333–342, 1970.

Levi, P. E., Cooper, E. H., Anderson, C. K., and Williams, R. E.: Analysis of DNA content, nuclear size and

cell proliferation of transitional cell carcinoma in man. Cancer, 23, 1074–1085, 1969.

Limas, C., and Lange, P.: A, B, H Antigen detectability in normal and neoplastic urothelium. Influence of methodologic factors. Cancer, 49, 2476–2484, 1982.

Limas, C., and Lange, P. H.: Lewis antigens in normal and neoplastic urothelium. Am. J. Path., 121, 176–183, 1985.

Limas, C., and Lange, P.: T-antigen in normal and neoplastic urothelium. Cancer, 58, 1236–1245, 1986.

Linker, D. G., and Whitmore, W. F.: Ureteral carcinoma in situ. J. Urol., 113, 777–780, 1975.

Lönn, U., Lönn, S., Nylen, U., Friberg, S., and Stenkvist, B.: Gene amplification detected in carcinoma cells from human urinary bladder washings by the polymerase chain reaction method. Cancer, 71, 3605–3610, 1993.

Mahadevia, P. S., Alexander, J. E., Rojas-Corona, R., and Koss, L. G.: Pseudosarcomatous stromal reaction in primary and metastatic urothelial carcinoma. Am. J. Surg. Path., 13, 782–790, 1989.

Mahadevia, P. S., Karwa, G. L., and Koss, L. G.: Mapping of urothelium in carcinomas of the renal pelvis and ureter. A report of nine cases. Cancer, 51, 890–897, 1983.

Mahadevia, P. S., Koss, L. G., and Tar, I. J.: Prostatic involvement in bladder cancer: Prostate mapping in 20 cystoprostatectomy specimens. Cancer, 58, 2096–2102, 1986.

Malmström, P. U.: Prognosis of transitional cell bladder carcinoma. With special reference to ABH blood group isoantigen expression and DNA analysis. Scand. J. Urol. Nephrol. Suppl., 112, 1–55, 1988.

Marcheggiono, A., Jannoni, C., Pallone, F., Frieri, G., Gallucci, M., and Caprilli, R.: Abnormal patterns of colonic mucin secretion after ureterosigmoidostomy. Human Path., 15, 630–647, 1984.

Marshall, V. F.: Current clinical problems regarding bladder tumors. Cancer, 9, 543–550, 1956.

McDougal, W. S., Cramer, S. F., and Miller, R.: Invasive carcinoma of renal pelvis following cyclophosphamide therapy for nonmalignant disease. Cancer, 48, 691–695, 1981.

Melamed, M. R., Grabstald, H., Whitmore, W. F., Jr.: Carcinoma in situ of bladder: Clinico-pathologic study of case with suggested approach to detection. J. Urol., 96, 466–471, 1966.

Melamed, M. R., Koss, L. G., Ricci, A., Whitmore, W. F., Jr.: Cytohistological observations on developing carcinoma of urinary bladder in man. Cancer, 13, 67–74, 1960.

Melamed, M. R., Traganos, F., Sharpless, T., and Darzynkiewicz, Z.: Urinary cytology automation. Preliminary studies with acridine orange stain and flow-through cytofluorometry. Invest. Urol., 13, 331–338, 1976.

Melamed, M. R., Voutsa, N. G., and Grabstald, H.: Natural history and clinical behavior of in situ carcinoma of the human urinary bladder. Cancer, 17, 1533–1545, 1964.

Melick, W. F., Escue, H. M., Naryka, J. J., Mezera, R. A., and Wheeler, E. P.: First reported cases of human bladder tumors due to new carcinogen xenylamine. J. Urol., *74*, 760–766, 1955.

Melicow, M. M.: Carcinoma in situ: An historical perspective. Urologic Clinics of North America, *3*, 5–11, 1976.

Melicow, M. M.: Histological study of vesical urothelium intervening between gross neoplasms in total cystectomy. J. Urol., *68*, 261–278, 1952.

Melicow, M. M.: Tumors of the bladder: A multifaceted problem. J. Urol., *112*, 467–478, 1974.

Melicow, M. M., and Hollowell, J. W.: Intraurothelial cancer: carcinoma in situ, Bowen's disease of the urinary system: discussion of thirty cases. J. Urol., *68*, 763–772, 1952.

Molland, E. A., Trott, P. A., Parris, A. M. I., and Blandy, J. P.: Nephrogenic adenoma: a form of adenomatous metaplasia of the bladder. A clinical and electromicroscopical study. Brit. J. Urol., *48*, 453–462, 1976.

Morse, N., and Melamed, M. R.: Differential counts of cell populations in urinary sediment smears from patients with primary epidermoid carcinoma of bladder. Acta Cytol., *18*, 312–315, 1974.

Mostofi, F. K.: Pathological aspects and spread of carcinoma of the bladder. J.A.M.A., *206*, 1764–1769, 1968.

Mostofi, F. K.: Pathology and spread of carcinoma of the urinary bladder. *In* Johnson, D. E., and Samuels, M. L. (Eds.): Cancer of the Gentourinary Tract. New York, Raven Press, 1979, p. 303.

Mostofi, F. K., Thomson, R. V., and Dean, A. L., Jr.: Mucous adenocarcinoma of urinary bladder. Cancer, *8*, 741–758, 1955.

Mufti, G. R., and Singh, M.: Value of random mucosal biopsies in the management of superficial bladder cancer. Eur. Urol., *22*, 288–293, 1992.

Murphy, W. M., Crabtree, W. N., Jukkola, A. F., and Soloway, M. S.: The diagnostic value of urine versus bladder washings in patients with bladder cancer. J. Urol., *126*, 320–322, 1981.

Murphy, W. M., Emerson, L. D., Chandler, R. W., Moinuddin, S. M., and Soloway, M. S.: Flow cytometry versus urinary cytology in the evaluation of patients with bladder cancer. J. Urol., *136*, 815–819, 1986.

Murphy, W. M., and Soloway, M. S.: Developing carcinoma (dysplasia) of the urinary bladder. Pathol. Annu., *17*, 197–217, 1982.

Murphy, W. M., Soloway, M. S., Jukkola, A. F., Grabtree, W. N., and Ford, K. S.: Urinary cytology and bladder cancer. The cellular features of transitional cell neoplasms. Cancer, *53*, 1555–1565, 1984.

Nielsen, K., Colstrup, H., Nilsson, T., and Gundersen, H. J. G.: Stereological estimates of nuclear volume correlated with histopathological grading and prognosis of bladder tumor. Virchows Arch. B (Cell Pathol.), *52*, 41–54, 1986.

Norming, U., Nyman, C. R., and Tribukait, B.: Comparative flow cytometric deoxyribonucleic acid studies on exophytic tumors and random mucosal biopsies in un-treated carcinoma of the bladder. J. Urol., *142*, 1442–1447, 1989.

Norming, U., Tribukait, B., Gustafson, H., Nyman, C. R., Wang, N., and Wijkstrom, H.: Deoxyribonucleic acid profile and tumor progression in primary carcinoma in situ of the bladder: A study of 63 patients with grade 3 lesions. J. Urol., *147*, 11–15, 1992.

Olsen, P. R., Wolf, H., Schroeder, T., Fischer, A., and Hojgaard, K.: Urothelial atypia and survival rate of 500 unselected patients with primary transitional cell tumor of the urinary bladder. Scand. J. Urol. Nephrol., *22*, 257–263, 1988.

Ooi, A., Herz, F., Ii, S., Cordon-Cardo, C., Fradet, Y., Mayall, B. H., et al.: Ha-ras codon 12 mutation in papillary tumors of the urinary bladder. A retrospective study. Int. J. Onc., *4*, 85–90, 1994.

Pamukcu, A. M., Gorsoy, S. K., and Price, J. M.: Urinary bladder neoplasms induced by feeding bracken fern (Pteris aquilina) to cows. Cancer Res., *27*, 917–924, 1964.

Papanicolaou, G. N., and Marshall, V. F.: Urine sediment smears as diagnostic procedure in cancers of urinary tract. Science, *101*, 519–520, 1945.

Pedersen-Bjergaard, J., Ersboli, J., Hansen, V. L., Sorensen, B. L., Christoffersen, K., Hou-Jensen, K., Nissen, N. I., Knudsen, J. B., and Hansen, M. M.: Carcinoma of the urinary bladder after treatment with cyclophosphamide for non-Hodgkin's lymphoma. N. Engl. J. Med., *318*, 1028–1032, 1988.

Petersen, R. O.: Urologic Pathology, 2nd Ed. Philadelphia, J. B. Lippincott, 1992.

Pettersson, S., Hansson, G., and Blohme, I.: Condyloma acuminatum of the bladder. J. Urol., *115*, 535–536, 1976.

Piper, J. M., Tonascia, J., and Matanoski, G. M.: Heavy phenacetin use and bladder cancer in women aged 20 to 49 years. N. Engl. J. Med., *313*, 292–295, 1985.

Prout, G. K. J.: Current concepts: Bladder carcinoma. N. Engl. J. Med., *287*, 86–90, 1972.

Prout, G. R., Barton, B. A., Griffin, P. P., and Friedell, G. H.: Treated history of noninvasive grade 1 transitional cell carcinoma. J. Urol., *148*, 1413–1419, 1992.

Prout, G. R., Griffin, P. P., Daly, J. J., and Heney, N. M.: Carcinoma in situ of the urinary bladder with and without associated neoplasms. Cancer, *52*, 524–532, 1983.

Prout, G. R., Griffin, P. P., and Daly, J. J.: The outcome of conservative treatment of carcinoma in situ of the bladder. J. Urol., *138*, 766–770, 1987.

Pugh, R. C. B.: The pathology of bladder tumours. *In* Wallace, D. M. (Ed.): Neoplastic Disease at Various Sites: Tumours of the Bladder. Vol. 2, pp. 116–156. Edinburgh, E. & S. Livingstone, 1959.

Pugh, R. C. B.: The pathology of cancer of the bladder. An editorial overview. Cancer, *32*, 1267–1274, 1973.

Rehn, L.: Blasengeschwuelste bei Anilinarbeitern. Arch. Klin. Chir., *50*, 588–600, 1895.

Rehn, L.: Blasengeschwuelste bei Fuchsinarbeitern. Arch. Klin. Chir., *53*, 383–392, 1896.

Reichborn-Kjennerud, S., and Hoeg, K.: The value of urine

cytology in the diagnosis of recurrent bladder tumors. A preliminary report. Acta Cytol., *16,* 269–272, 1972.

Richards, B., Parmer, M. K. B., Anderson, C. K., Ansell, I. D., Grigor, K., Hall, R. R., et al.: Interpretation of biopsies of 'normal' urothelium in patients with superficial bladder cancer. Br. J. Urol., *67,* 369–375, 1991.

Rife, C. C., Farrow, G. M., and Utz, D. C.: Urine cytology of transitional cell neoplasms. Urol. Clin. North Am., *6,* 599–612, 1979.

Ro, J. Y., Ayala, A. G., and El Nagger, A.: Muscularis mucosae of urinary bladder: importance for staging and treatment. Am. J. Surg. Path., *11,* 668–673, 1987.

Roland, S. I., and Marshall, V. F.: Reliability of Papanicolaou technique when cancer cells are found in urine. Surg. Gynecol. Obstet., *104,* 41–44, 1957.

Rosa, B., Cazin, M., and Dalian, G.: Urinary cytology for carcinoma in situ of the urinary bladder. Acta Cytol., *29,* 117–124, 1985.

Rosenkilde, O. P., Wolf, H., Schroeder, T., Fischer, A., and Hjgaard, K.: Urothelial atypia and survival rate of 500 unselected patients with primary transitional-cell tumor of the urinary bladder. Scand. J. Urol. Nephrol., *22,* 257–263, 1988.

Sagerman, P. M., Saigo, P. E., Sheinfeld, J., Charitonowics, E., and Cordon-Cardo, C.: Enhanced detection of bladder cancer in urine cytology with Lewis X, M344 and 19A211 antigens. Acta Cytol., *38,* 517–523, 1994.

Sarnacki, C. T., McCormack, L. J., Kiser, W. S., Hazard, J. R., McLaughlin, T. C., and Belovich, D. M.: Urinary cytology and clinical diagnosis of urinary tract malignancy: A clinicopathologic study of 1,400 patients. J. Urol., *106,* 761–764, 1971.

Schade, R. O. K., Serck-Hanssen, A., and Swinney, J.: Morphological changes in the ureter in cases of bladder carcinoma. Cancer, *27,* 1267–1272, 1971.

Schade, R. O. K., and Swinney, J.: Precancerous changes in bladder epithelium. Lancet, *2,* 943–946, 1968.

Schade, R. O. K., and Swinney, J.: The association of urothelial atypism with neoplasia: Its importance in treatment and prognosis. J. Urol., *109,* 619–622, 1973.

Schistosomiasis of the urinary bladder. Case records of the Massachusetts General Hospital (case 1-1994).: N. Engl. J. Med., *330,* 51–57, 1994.

Schneider, V., Smith, M. J. V., and Frable, W. J.: Urinary cytology in endometriosis of the bladder. Acta Cytol., *24,* 30–33, 1980.

Schulte, P. A., Ringen, K. N., Hemstreet, G. P., et al.: Risk assessment of a cohort exposed to aromatic amines. Initial results. J. Occupat. Med., *27,* 115–121, 1985.

Schulte, P. A., Ringen, K., Hemstreet, G. P., et al.: Risk factors of bladder cancer in a cohort exposed to aromatic amines. Cancer, *58,* 2156–2162, 1986.

Seemayer, T. A., Knaack, J., Thelmo, W. L., Wang, N. S., and Ahmed, M. N.: Further observations on carcinoma in situ of the urinary bladder: Silent but extensive intraprostatic involvement. Cancer, *36,* 514–520, 1975.

Shaaban, A. A., Tribukait, B., Abdel-Fattah, A. E-B., and Ghoneim, M. A.: Characterisation of squamous cell

bladder tumors by flow cytometric deoxyribonucleic acid analysis: a report of 100 cases. J. Urol., *144,* 879–883, 1990.

Shaaban, A. A., Tribukait, B., El-Bedeiwy, A. F. A., and Ghoneim, M. A.: Prediction of lymph node metastases in bladder carcinoma with deoxyribonucleic acid flow cytometry. J. Urol., *144,* 884–887, 1990.

Sherman, A. B., Koss, L. G., Wyschogrod, D., Melder, K. H., Eppich, E. M., and Bales, C. E.: Bladder cancer diagnosis by computer image analysis of cells in the sediment of voided urine using a video scanning system. Analyt. Quant. Cytol., *8,* 177–186, 1986.

Shibutani, Y. F., Schoenberg, M. P., Carpiniello, V. L., and Malloy, T. R.: Human papillomavirus associated with bladder cancer. Urology, *40,* 15–17, 1992.

Sidransky, D., Von Eschenbach, A., Tsai, Y. C., Jones, P., Summerhayes, I., Marshall, F., Paul, M., Green, P., Hamilton, S. R., Frost, P., and Vogelstein, B.: Identification of p53 gene mutations in bladder cancers and urine samples. Science, *252,* 706–709, 1991.

Simon, W., Cordonnier, J. J., and Snordgrass, W. T.: The pathogenesis of bladder carcinoma. J. Urol., *88,* 797–802, 1962.

Skinner, D. G., Richie, J. P., Cooper, P. H., Waisman, J., and Kaufman, J. J.: The clinical significance of carcinoma in situ of the bladder and its association with overt carcinoma. J. Urol., *112,* 68–71, 1974.

Smeets, A. W. G., Pauwels, R. P. E., Beck, J. P. M., Geraedts, J. P. M., Debruyne, F. M. J., Laarakers, L., Feitz, W. F. J., Vooijs, G. P., and Ramaekers, F. C. S.: Tissue specific markers in flow cytometry of urological cancers. III. Comparing chromosomal and flow cytometric DNA analysis of bladder tumors. Int. J. Cancer, *39,* 304–310, 1987.

Smith, A. F.: An ultrastructural and morphometric study of bladder tumours. Virchows Arch. [Pathol. Anat.], *406,* 7–16, 1985.

Sooriyaarachchi, G. S., Johnson, R. O., and Cartone, P. P.: Neoplasms of the large bowel following ureterosigmoidostomy. Arch. Surg., *112,* 1174–1177, 1977.

Starklint, H., Jensen, N. K., and Thybo, E.: The extent of carcinoma in situ in urinary bladders with primary carcinoma. Acta Pathol. Microbiol. Scand., *Sect. A, 84,* 130–136, 1976.

Starklint, H., Kjaergaard, J., and Jensen, N. K.: Types of metaplasia in forty urothelial bladder carcinomas. A systematic histological investigation. Acta Pathol. Microbiol. Scand., *84,* 137–142, 1976.

Stilman, M., Murphy, J. L., and Merriam, J. C.: Cytology of nephrogenic adenoma. Acta Cytol., *30,* 35–40, 1986.

Suprun, H., and Bitterman, W.: A correlative cytohistologic study on the interrelationship between exfoliated urinary bladder carcinoma cell types and the staging and grading of these tumors. Acta Cytol., *19,* 265–273, 1975.

Temkin, I. S.: Industrial Bladder Carcinogenesis. New York, Pergamon Press, 1963.

Thelmo, W. L., Seemayer, T. A., Madarnas, P., Mount, B. M. M., and Mackinnon, K. J.: Carcinoma in situ of the bladder with associated prostatic involvement. J. Urol., *111*, 491–494, 1974.

Travis, L. B., Curtis, R. E., Boice, J. D., Jr., Fraumeni, J. F., Jr.: Bladder cancer after chemotherapy for non-Hodgkin's lymphoma. N. Engl. J. Med., *321*, 544–545, 1989.

Tribukait, B.: Flow cytometry in assessing the clinical aggressiveness of genito-urinary neoplasms. World J. Urol., *5*, 108–122, 1987.

Troster, M., Wyatt, J. K., and Alen-Halagah, J.: Nephrogenic adenoma of the urinary bladder. Histologic and cytologic observations in a case. Acta Cytol., *30*, 41–44, 1986.

Trott, P. A., and Edwards, L.: Comparison of bladder washings and urine cytology in the diagnosis of bladder cancer. J. Urol., *110*, 664–666, 1973.

Tyrkus, M., Powell, I., and Fakr, W.: Cytogenetic studies of carcinoma in situ of the bladder: Prognostic implications. J. Urol., *148*, 44–46, 1992.

Umiker, W.: Accuracy of cytologic diagnosis of cancer of the urinary tract. Acta Cytol., *8*, 186–193, 1964.

Umiker, W., Lapides, J., and Soureene, R.: Exfoliative cytology of papillomas and intraepithelial carcinomas of the urinary bladder. Acta Cytol., *6*, 255–266, 1962.

Utz, D. C., Hanash, K. A., and Farrow, G. M.: The plight of the patient with carcinoma in situ of the bladder. J. Urol., *103*, 160–164, 1970.

Utz, D. C., Schmitz, S. E., Fugelso, P. D., and Farrow, G. M.: A clinicopathologic evaluation of partial cystectomy for carcinoma of the urinary bladder. Cancer, *32*, 1075–1077, 1973.

Utz, D. C., and Zincke, H.: The masquerade of bladder cancer in situ as interstitial cystitis. Trans. Amer. Assoc. Genitourin. Surg., *75*, 64–65, 1973.

Videbaek, A.: Chlornaphazin (Erysan) may induce cancer of the urinary bladder. Acta Med. Scand., *176*, 45–50, 1964.

Voutsa, N. G., and Melamed, M. R.: Cytology of in situ carcinoma of the human urinary bladder. Cancer, *16*, 1307–1316, 1963.

Wallace, D.: Cancer of the bladder. Am. J. Roentgenol. Rad. Ther. Nucl. Med., *102*, 581–586, 1968.

Ward, E., Halperin, W., Thun, M., Grossman, H. B., Fink, B., Koss, L. G., Osorio, A. M., and Schulte, P.: Bladder tumors in two young males occupationally exposed to MBOCA. Am. J. Indus. Med., *14*, 267–272, 1988.

Webber, M. M.: A study of malignant bladder mucosa using autoradiography of exfoliated epithelial cells. Acta Cytol., *13*, 128–132, 1969.

Weinstein, R. S.: Changes in plasma membrane structure associated with malignant transformation in human urinary bladder epithelium. Cancer Res., *36*, 2518–2524, 1976.

Weinstein, R. S., Alroy, J., Farrow, G. M., Miller, A. W., and Davidsohn, I.: Blood group isoantigen detection in carcinoma in situ of the urinary bladder. Cancer, *43*, 661, 1979.

Weinstein, R. S., Coon, J. S., Schwartz, D., Miller, A. W., and Pauli, B. U.: Pathology of superficial bladder cancer

with emphasis on carcinoma in situ. Urology, (*26 Suppl.*), 2–10, 1985.

Wheeler, J. D., and Hill, W. T.: Adenocarcinoma involving urinary bladder. Cancer, *7*, 119–135, 1954.

Whitmore, W. F., Jr.: Bladder cancer: An overview. Ca—A Cancer Journal for Clinicians, *38*, 213–223, 1988.

Widran, J., Sanchez, R., and Gruhn, J.: Squamous metaplasia of the bladder: A study of 450 patients. J. Urol., *112*, 479–482, 1974.

Wiener, H. G., Vooijs, G. P., and van't Hof-Grootenboer, B.: Accuracy of urinary cytology in the diagnosis of primary and recurrent bladder cancer. Acta Cytol., *37*, 163–169, 1993.

Wiggishoff, C. C., and McDonald, J. H.: Urinary exfoliative cytology in the diagnosis of bladder tumors. Acta Cytol., *16*, 139–141, 1972.

Wijkstrom, H., Lundh, B., and Tribukait, B.: Urine or bladder washings in the cytologic evaluation of transitional cell carcinoma of the urinary tract. Scand. J. Urol. Nephrol., *21*, 119–123, 1987.

Willen, R.: Morphologic changes of intestinal mucosa in contact with urine. Scand. J. Urol. Nephrol., *Suppl. 142*, 26–30, 1992.

Wolf, H., and Hjøgaard, K.: Urothelial dysplasia concomitant with bladder tumours as a determinant factor for future new occurrences. Lancet, *2*, 134–136, 1983.

Wolf, H., Olsen, P. R., Fischer, A., and Hjøgaard, K.: Urothelial atypia concomitant with primary bladder tumor. Scand. J. Urol. Nephrol., *21*, 33–38, 1987.

Wolinska, W. H., Melamed, M. R., and Klein, F. A.: Cytology of bladder papilloma. Acta Cytol., *29*, 817–822, 1985.

Wurzel, R. S., Yamase, H. T., and Nieh, P. T.: Ectopic production of human chorionic gonadotrophin by poorly differentiated transitional cell tumors of the urinary tract. J. Urol., *137*, 502–504, 1987.

Wynder, E. L., and Goldsmith, R.: The epidemiology of bladder cancer. A second look. Cancer, *40*, 1246–1268, 1977.

Wynder, E. L., Onderdonk, J., and Mantel, N.: An epidemiologic investigation of cancer of the bladder. Cancer, *16*, 1388–1407, 1963.

Yamada, T., Masawa, N., Honma, K., Yokogawa, M., Fukui, I., and Mitani, G.: Nonpapillary intraepithelial and/or early invasive cancer arising in the urinary bladder—their developmental and advancing courses. Dokkyo J. Med. Sci., *11*, 51–69, 1984.

Yamada, T., Yokogawa, M., Mitani, G., Inada, T., Ohwada, F., and Fukui, I.: Two different types of cancer development in the urothelium of the human urinary bladder with different prognosis. Jap. J. Clin. Oncol., *5*, 77–90, 1975.

Yates-Bell, A. J.: Carcinoma in situ of the bladder. Br. J. Surg., *58*, 359–364, 1971.

Young, R. H., and Scully, R. E.: Nephrogenic adenoma: A report of 15 cases, review of the literature, and comparison with clear cell carcinoma. Am. J. Surg. Path., *10*, 286–275, 1986.

Zincke, H., Utz, D. C., and Farrow, G. M.: Review of

Mayo Clinic experience with carcinoma in situ. Urology, *26, (Suppl. 4)*, 39–46, 1985.

Rare Bladder Tumors

Ainsworth, A. M., Clark, W. H., Jr., Mastrangelo, M., and Conger, K. B.: Primary malignant melanoma of the urinary bladder. Cancer, *37*, 1928–1936, 1976.

Andrion, A., Gaglio, A., and Zai, G.: Bladder involvement in disseminated malignant lymphoma diagnosed by voided urine cytology. Cytopathology, *4*, 115–117, 1993.

Auvert, J., Boureau, M., and Weisberger, G.: Embryonal sarcoma of the lower urinary tract in children: 5-year survival in two cases after radical treatment. J. Urol., *112*, 396–401, 1974.

Auvigne, R., Auvigne, J., and Kerneis, J.: Un cas de plasmocytome de la vessie. J. d'Urol., *62*, 85–90, 1956.

Berenson, R. J., Flynn, S., Freiha, F. S., Kempson, R. L., and Torti, F. M.: Primary osteogenic sarcoma of the bladder: Report of a case and review of the literature. Cancer, *57*, 350–355, 1987.

Bhansali, S. K., and Cameron, K. M.: Primary malignant lymphoma of the bladder. Br. J. Urol., *32*, 440–454, 1960.

Brinton, J. A., Ito, Y., and Olsen, B. S.: Carcinosarcoma of the urinary bladder. Cancer, *25*, 1183–1186, 1970.

Cheson, B. D., Schumann, G. B., and Johnston, J. L.: Urinary cytodiagnosis of renal involvement in disseminated histiocytic lymphoma. Acta Cytol., *28*, 148–152, 1984.

Cheson, B. D., Schumann, J. L., and Schumann, G. B.: Urinary cytodiagnostic abnormalities in 50 patients with non-Hodgkin's lymphomas. Cancer, *54*, 1914–1919, 1984.

Crane, A. R., and Tremblay, R. G.: Primary osteogenic sarcoma of the bladder. Ann. Surg., *118*, 887–908, 1943.

Das Gupta, T., and Grabstald, H.: Melanoma of the genitourinary tract. J. Urol., *93*, 607–614, 1965.

Davis, B. H., Ludwig, M. E., Cole, S. R., and Patuszak, W. T.: Small cell neuroendocrine carcinoma of the urinary bladder: Report of three cases with ultrastructural analysis. Ultrastr. Path., *4*, 197–204, 1983.

Del Mistro, A., Koss, L. G., Braunstein, J., Bennett, B., Saccomano, G., and Simons, K. M.: Condylomata acuminata of the urinary bladder. Am. J. Surg. Pathol., *12*, 205–215, 1988.

Fletcher, M. S., Aker, M., Hill, J. T., Pryor, J. P., and Whimster, W. F.: Granular cell myoblastoma of the bladder. Brit. J. Urol., *57*, 109–110, 1985.

Foote, J. W., Seemayer, T. A., and Duignan, J. P.: Desmoid tumor involving the bladder: Case report. J. Urol., *114*, 147–149, 1975.

Fromowitz, F. B., Bard, R. H., and Koss, L. G.: The epithelial origin of a malignant mesodermal mixed tumor of the bladder: Report of case with long-term survival. J. Urol., *132*, 2385–2389, 1984.

Ganem, E. J., and Batal, J. T.: Secondary malignant tumors of the urinary bladder metastatic from primary foci in distant organs. J. Urol., *75*, 965–972, 1956.

Holtz, F., Fox, J. E., and Abell, M. R.: Carcinosarcoma of the urinary bladder. Cancer, *29*, 294–304, 1972.

Jao, W., Soto, J. M., and Gould, V. E.: Squamous carcinoma of bladder with pseudosarcomatous stroma. Arch. Pathol., *100*, 461–466, 1975.

Javaheri, P., and Raafat, J.: Malignant pheochromocytoma of the urinary bladder: report of two cases. Brit. J. Urol., *47*, 401–404, 1975.

Klinger, M. E.: Secondary tumors of the genitourinary tract. J. Urol., *65*, 144–153, 1951.

Koss, L. G.: Tumors of the Urinary Bladder. Atlas of Tumor Pathology, Second Series, Fascicle 11. Washington, D.C., Armed Forces Institute of Pathology, 1975.

Koss, L. G.: Tumors of the urinary bladder. Atlas of Tumor Pathology, Second Series, Fascicle 11, Supplement. Washington, D.C., Armed Forces Institute of Pathology, 1985.

Koss, L. G., and Durfee, G. R.: Unusual patterns of squamous epithelium of uterine cervix; cytologic and pathologic study of koilocytotic atypia. Ann. N.Y. Acad. Sci., *63*, 1245–1261, 1956.

Kotani, H., Sugihara, S., Yamada, K., and Matsuda, M.: Cytologic detection of malignant lymphoma cells in urine and hydrocele fluid. Acta Cytol., *31*, 362–364, 1987.

Krumerman, M. S., and Katatikarn, V.: Rhabdomyosarcoma of the urinary bladder with intraepithelial spread in an adult. Arch. Pathol. Lab. Med., *100*, 395–397, 1976.

MacKenzie, A. R., Sharma, T. C., Whitmore, W. F., Jr., and Melamed, M. R.: Non-extirpative treatment of myosarcomas of the bladder and prostate. Cancer, *28*, 329–334, 1971.

MacKenzie, A. R., Whitmore, W. F., Jr., and Melamed, M. R.: Myosarcomas of the bladder and prostate. Cancer, *22*, 833–843, 1968.

Mills, S. E., Wolfe, J. T., III, Weiss, M. R., Swanson, P. E., Wick, M. R., Fowler, J. E., and Young, R. H.: Small cell undifferentiated carcinoma of the urinary bladder. Am. J. Surg. Path., *11*, 606–617, 1987.

Mincione, G. P.: Primary malignant lymphoma of the urinary bladder with positive cytologic report. Acta Cytol., *26*, 69–72, 1982.

Narayana, A. S., Loening, S., Weimer, G. W., and Culp, D. A.: Sarcoma of the bladder and prostate. J. Urol., *119*, 72–76, 1978.

Obe, J. A., Rosen, N., and Koss, L. G.: Primary choriocarcinoma of the urinary bladder. Report of a case with probable epithelial origin. Cancer, *52*, 1405–1409, 1983.

Ordonez, N. G., Khorsand, J., Ayala, A. G., and Sneige, N.: Oat cell carcinoma of the urinary tract. An immunohistochemical and electron microscopic study. Cancer, *58*, 2519–2530, 1986.

Pang, S. C.: Bony and cartilaginous tumours of the urinary bladder. J. Pathol. Bact., *76*, 357–377, 1958.

Parton, I.: Primary lymphosarcoma of the bladder. Br. J. Urol., *34*, 221–223, 1962.

Pettersson, S., Hansson, G., and Blohme, I.: Condyloma

acuminatum of the bladder. J. Urol., *115,* 535–536, 1976.

Peven, D. R., and Hidvegi, D. F.: Clear-cell adenocarcinoma of the female urethra. Acta Cytol., *29,* 142–146, 1985.

Pinkert, T. C., Catlow, C. E., and Straus, R.: Endometriosis of the urinary bladder in a man with prostatic carcinoma. Cancer, *43,* 1562–1567, 1979.

Piva, A., and Koss, L. G.: Cytologic diagnosis of metastatic malignant melanoma in urinary sediment. Acta Cytol., *8,* 398–402, 1964.

Pringle, J. P., Graham, R. C., and Bernier, G. M.: Detection of myeloma cells in the urine sediment. Blood, *43,* 137–143, 1974.

Samaan, N. A., Hickey, R. C., and Shutts, P. E.: Diagnosis, localisation, and management of pheochromocytoma: Pitfalls and follow-up in 41 patients. Cancer, *62,* 2451–2460, 1988.

Sano, M. E., and Koprowska, I.: Primary cytologic diagnosis of a malignant renal lymphoma. Acta Cytol., *9,* 194–196, 1965.

Santino, A. M., Shumaker, E. J., and Garces, J.: Primary malignant lymphoma of the bladder. J. Urol., *103,* 310–313, 1970.

Stitt, R. B., and Colapinto, V.: Multiple simultaneous bladder malignancies: primary lymphosarcoma and adenocarcinoma. J. Urol., *96,* 733–736, 1966.

Su, C., and Prince, C. L.: Melanoma of the bladder. J. Urol., *87,* 365–367, 1962.

Tanaka, T., Yoshimi, N., Sawada, K., Takami, T., Sugie, S., Etori, F., Kachi, H., and Mori, H.: Ki-1-positive large cell anaplastic lymphoma diagnosed by urinary cytology. A case report. Acta Cytol., *37,* 520–524, 1993.

Valente, P. T., Atkinson, B. F., and Guerry, D.: Melanuria. Acta Cytol., *29,* 1026–1028, 1985.

Wang, C. C., Scully, R. E., and Leadbetter, W. F.: Primary malignant lymphoma of the urinary bladder. Cancer, *24,* 772–776, 1969.

Weinberg, T.: Primary chorionepithelioma of the urinary bladder in a male. Report of a case. Am. J. Pathol., *15,* 783–795, 1939.

Yam, L. T., and Janckila, A. J.: Immunocytochemical diagnosis of lymphoma from urine sediment. Acta. Cytol., *29,* 827–832, 1985.

Yokoyama, S., Hayashida, Y., Nagahama, J., Nakayama, I., Kashima, K., and Ogata, J.: Primary and metaplastic choriocarcinoma of the bladder. A report of two cases. Acta Cytol., *36,* 176–182, 1992.

Young, R. H., and Scully, R. E.: Clear cell adenocarcinoma of the bladder and urethra: a report of three cases and review of the literature. Am. J. Surg. Path., *9,* 816–826, 1985.

Bladder Tumors-Monitoring

Aamodt, R. L., Coon, J. S., Deitch, A., deVere White, R. W., Koss, L. G., Melamed, M. R., Weinstein, R. S., and Wheeless, L. L.: Flow cytometric evaluation of bladder cancer: recommendations of the NCI flow cyto-

metry network for bladder cancer. World J. Urol., *10,* 63–67, 1992.

Alvaro, A. S., Dalbagni, G., Cordon-Cardo, C., Zhang, Z. F., Sheinfeld, J., Fair, W. R., Herr, H. W., and Reuter, V. E.: Nuclear overexpression of p53 protein in transitional cell bladder carcinoma: A marker for disease progression. J. Natl. Cancer Inst., *85,* 53–59, 1993.

Amberson, J. B., and Laino, J.: Image cytometric deoxyribonucleic acid analysis of urine specimens as an adjunct to visual cytology in the detection of urothelial cell carcinoma. J. Urol., *149,* 42–45, 1993.

Badalament, R. A., Fair, W. R., Whitmore, W. F., Jr., and Melamed, M. R.: The relative value of cytometry and cytology in the management of bladder cancer: The Memorial Sloan-Kettering Cancer Center experience. Semin. Urol., *6,* 22–30, 1988.

Badalament, R. A., Gary, H., Whitmore, W. F., Jr., et al.: Monitoring intravesical bacillus Calmette-Guerin treatment of superficial bladder carcinoma by serial flow cytometry. Cancer, *58,* 2751–2757, 1986.

Badalament, R. A., Hermansen, D. K., Kimmel, M., et al.: The sensitivity of bladder wash flow cytometry, bladder wash cytology, and voided cytology in the detection of bladder carcinoma. Cancer, *60,* 1423–1427, 1987.

Blomjous, C. E., Schipper, N. W., Baak, J. P., van Galen, E. M., de Voogt, H. J., and Meyer, C. J.: Retrospective study of prognostic importance of DNA flow cytometry of urinary bladder carcinoma. J. Clin. Pathol., *41,* 21–25, 1988.

Blomjous, E. C., Schipper, N. W., Baak, J. P., Vos, W., De Voogt, H. J., and Meijer, C. J.: The value of morphometry and DNA flow cytometry in addition to classic prognosticators in superficial urinary bladder carcinoma. Am. J. Clin. Pathol., *91,* 243–248, 1989.

Borgstrom, E., and Wahren, B.: Clinical significance of A, B, H isoantigen deletion of urothelial cells in bladder carcinoma. Cancer, *58,* 2428–2434, 1986.

Borgstrom, E., Wahren, B., and Gustafson, H.: Fluorescence methods for measuring the A, B, and H isoantigens on cytological material from bladder carcinoma. Urol. Res., *13,* 43–45, 1985.

Borland, R. N., Partin, A. W., Epstein, J. I., and Brendler, C. B.: The use of nuclear morphometry in predicting recurrence of transitional cell carcinoma. J. Urol., *149,* 272–275, 1993.

Chin, J. L., Huben, R. P., Nava, E., Rustum, Y. M., Greco, J. M., Pontes, E., and Frankfurt, O. S.: Flow cytometric analysis of DNA content in human bladder tumors and irrigation specimens. Cancer, *56,* 1677–1681, 1985.

Collste, L. G., Devonec, M., Darzynkiewicz, Z., Traganos, F., Sharpless, T. K., Whitmore, W. F., Jr., and Melamed, M. R.: Bladder cancer diagnosis by flow cytometry. Correlation between cell samples from biopsy and bladder irrigation fluid. Cancer, *45,* 2389–2394, 1980.

Coon, J. S., McCall, A., Miller, A. W., Farrow, G. M.,

and Weinstein, R. S.: Expression of blood-group-rel antigens in carcinoma in situ of the urinary bladc Cancer, *56,* 797–804, 1985.

Coon, J. S., and Weinstein, R. S.: Detection of A, B, H tissue isoantigens by immunoperoxidase methods in normal and neoplastic urothelium. Comparison with the erythorocyte adherence method. Am. J. Clin. Pathol., *76,* 163–171, 1981.

Cordon-Cardo, C., Reuter, V. E., Lloyd, K. O., Sheinfeld, J., Fair, W. R., Old, L. J., and Melamed, M. R.: Blood group-related antigens in human urothelium: Enhanced expression of precursor, lex, and ley determinants in urothelial carcinoma. Cancer Res., *48,* 4113–4120, 1988.

Czerniak, B., Cohen, G. L., Etkin, P., Deitch, D., Simmons, H., Herz, F., and Koss, L. G.: Concurrent mutations of coding and regulatory sequences of the Ha-ras gene in urinary bladder carcinoma. Hum. Path., *23,* 1199–1204, 1992.

Czerniak, B., Deitch, D., Simmons, H., Etkind, P., Herz, F., and Koss, L. G.: Ha-ras gene codon 12 mutation and ploidy in urinary bladder cancer. Brit. J. Cancer, *62,* 762–763, 1990.

Dean, P. J., and Murphy, W. M.: Importance of urinary cytology and future role of flow cytometry. Urology, *26(Suppl.),* 11–15, 1985.

DeHarven, E., He, S., Hanna, W., Bootsma, G., and Connolly, J. G.: Phenotypically heterogeneous deletion of the A,B,H antigen from the transformed bladder urothelium. A scanning electron microscope study. J. Submicrosc. Cytol., *19,* 639–649, 1987.

deVere White, R. W., Deitch, A. D., Baker, W. C., Jr., and Strand, M. A.: Urine: A suitable sample for deoxyribonucleic acid flow cytometry studies in patients with bladder cancer. J. Urol., *139,* 926–928, 1988.

Devonec, M., Darzynkiewicz, Z., Whitmore, W. F., and Melamed, M. R.: Flow cytometry for followup examinations of conservatively treated low stage bladder tumors. J. Urol., *126,* 166–170, 1981.

Falor, W. H., and Ward, R. M.: Cytogenetic analysis: A potential index for recurrence of early carcinoma of the bladder. J. Urol., *115,* 49–52, 1976.

Falor, W. H., and Ward, R. M.: DNA banding patterns in carcinoma of the bladder. J.A.M.A., *226,* 1322–1327, 1973.

Farsund, T.: Selective sampling of cells for morphological and quantitative cytology of bladder epithelium. J. Urol., *128,* 267–271, 1982.

Flanigan, R. C., King, C. T., Clark, T. D., Cash, J. B., Greenfield, B. J., Sniecinski, I. J., and Primus, F. J.: Immunohistochemical demonstration of blood group antigens in neoplastic and normal human urothelium: A comparison with standard red cell adherence. J. Urol., *130,* 499–503, 1983.

Fossa, S. D.: Feulgen-DNA-values in transitional cell carcinoma of the human urinary bladder. Beitr. Pathol., *155,* 44–55, 1975.

Fradet, Y., Cordon-Cardo, C., Thomson, T., Daly, M. E., Whitmore, W. F., Jr., Lloyd, K. O., Melamed, M. R.,

Old, L. J.: Cell surface antigens of human bladder ıcer defined by mouse monoclonal antibodies. Proc. atl. Acad. Sci. USA, *81,* 224–228, 1984.

ıdet, Y., Cordon-Cardo, C., Whitmore, W. F., Melamed, M. R., and Old, L.: Cell surface antigens of human bladder tumors: Definition of tumor subsets by monoclonal antibodies and correlation with growth characteristics. Cancer Res., *46,* 5183–5188, 1986.

Fradet, Y., Islam, N., Boucher, L., Parent-Vaugeois, C., and Tardif, M.: Polymorphic expression of a human superficial bladder tumor antigen defined by mouse monoclonal antibodies. Proc. Natl. Acad. Sci. USA, *84,* 7227–7231, 1987.

Gustafson, H., Tribukait, B., and Esposti, L.: DNA profile and tumor progression in patients with superficial bladder tumors. Urol. Res., *10,* 13–18, 1982.

Harving, N., Wolf, H., and Melsen, F.: Positive urinary cytology after tumor resection: An indicator for concomitant carcinoma in situ. J. Urol., *140,* 495–497, 1988.

Hopkins, S., Ford, K. S., and Soloway, M. S.: Invasive bladder cancer: Support for screening. J. Urol., *130,* 61–64, 1983.

Jacobsen, A. B., Fossa, S. D., Thorud, E., Lunde, S., Melvik, J. E., and Pettersen, E. O.: DNA flow cytometric values in bladder carcinoma biopsies obtained from fresh and paraffin-embedded material. A.P.M.I.S., *96,* 25–29, 1988.

Klein, F. A., Herr, H. W., Sogani, P. C., Whitmore, W. F., and Melamed, M. R.: Detection and follow-up of carcinoma of the urinary bladder by flow cytometry. Cancer, *50,* 389–395, 1982.

Klein, F. A., Herr, H. W., Whitmore, W. F., Sogani, P. C., and Melamed, M. R.: An evaluation of automated flow cytometry (FCM) in detection of carcinoma in situ of the urinary bladder. Cancer, *50,* 1003–1008, 1982.

Koss, L. G.: Diagnostic Cytology and Its Histopathologic Bases. 4th Ed. Philadelphia, J. B. Lippincott, 1992.

Koss, L. G.: The role of cytology in the diagnosis, detection and follow-up bladder cancer. *In* Denis, L., et al. (Eds.): Developments in Bladder Cancer. New York, Alan R. Liss, 1986, pp. 97–108.

Koss, L. G.: Urinary tract cytology. *In* Connolly, J. C. (Ed.): Carcinoma of the Bladder. pp. 159–163. New York, Raven Press, 1981.

Koss, L. G., Bartels, P., and Wied, G. L.: Computer-based diagnostic analysis of cells in the urinary sediment. J. Urol., *123,* 846–849, 1980.

Koss, L. G., Deitch, D., Ramanathan, R., and Sherman, A. B.: Diagnostic value of cytology of voided urine. Acta Cytol., *29,* 810–816, 1985.

Koss, L. G., Esposti, L., Nagayama, T., De Voogt, H., Farsund, T., et al.: The role of cytology in the diagnosis, detection, and follow-up of bladder cancer. *In* Denis, L., et al. (Eds.): Developments in Bladder Cancer. New York, Alan R. Liss, 1986, pp. 97–108.

Koss, L. G., Wersto, R. P., Simmons, D. A., Deitch, D., Herz, F., and Freed, S. Z.: Predictive value of DNA measurements in bladder washings. Comparison of flow cytometry, image cytophotometry, and cytology in patients with a past history of urothelial tumors. Cancer, *64*, 916–924, 1989.

Kovarik, S., Davidsohn, I., and Stejkal, R.: ABO antigen in cancer: detection with the mixed cell agglutination reaction. Arch. Pathol., *86*, 12–21, 1968.

Lederer, B., Mikuz, G., Gutter, W., and zur Neiden, G.: Zytophotometrische Untersuchungen von Tumoren des Ubergangsepithels der Harnblase. Vergleich zytophotometrischer Untersuchungsergebnisse mit dem histologischen Grading. Beitr. Pathol., *147*, 379–389, 1972.

Levi, P. E., Cooper, E. H., Anderson, C. K., and Williams, R. E.: Analysis of DNA content, nuclear size and cell proliferation of transitional cell carcinoma in man. Cancer, *23*, 1074–1085, 1969.

Limas, C., and Lange, P.: A, B, H Antigen detectability in normal and neoplastic urothelium. Influence of methodologic factors. Cancer, *49*, 2476–2484, 1982.

Limas, C., and Lange, P.: Lewis antigens in normal and neoplastic urothelium. Am. J. Pathol., *121*, 176–183, 1985.

Limas, C., and Lange, P.: T-antigen in normal and neoplastic urothelium. Cancer, *58*, 1236–1245, 1986.

Malmstrøm, P. U.: Prognosis of transitional cell bladder carcinoma. With special reference to ABH blood group isoantigen expression and DNA analysis. Scand. J. Urol. Nephrol. Suppl., *112*, 1–55, 1988.

Melamed, M. R., and Klein, F. A.: Flow cytometry of urinary bladder irrigation specimens. Hum. Pathol., *15*, 302–305, 1984.

Melamed, M. R., Traganos, F., Sharpless, T., and Darzynkiewicz, Z.: Urinary cytology automation. Preliminary studies with Acridine Orange stain and flow-through cytofluorometry. Invest. Urol., *13*, 331–338, 1976.

Melder, K. K., and Koss, L. G.: Automated image analysis in the diagnosis of bladder cancer. Applied Optics, *26*, 3367–3372, 1987.

Murphy, W. M., Crabtree, W. N., Jukkola, A. F., and Soloway, M. S.: The diagnostic value of urine versus bladder washings in patients with bladder cancer. J. Urol., *126*, 320–322, 1981.

Murphy, W. M., Emerson, L. D., Chandler, R. W., Moinuddin, S. M., and Soloway, M. S.: Flow cytometry versus urinary cytology in the evaluation of patients with bladder cancer. J. Urol., *136*, 815–819, 1986.

Orihuela, E., Varadachay, S., Herr, H. W., Melamed, M. R., and Whitmore, W. F.: The practical use of tumor marker determination in bladder washing specimens. Assessing the urothelium of patients with superficial bladder cancer. Cancer, *60*, 1009–1016, 1987.

Rife, C. C., Farrow, G. M., and Utz, D. C.: Urine cytology of transitional cell neoplasms. Urol. Clin. North Am., *6*, 599–612, 1979.

Schwalb, D. M., Herr, H. W., and Fair, W. R.: The management of clinically unconfirmed positive urinary cytology. J. Urol., *150*, 1751–1756, 1993.

Schwalb, M. D., Herr, H. W., Sogani, P. C., Russo, P., Sheinfeld, J., and Fair, W. R.: Positive urinary cytology

following a complete response to intravesical bacillus Calmette-Guerin therapy: pattern of recurrence. J. Urol., *152*, 382–387, 1994.

Shaaban, A. A., Tribukait, B., El-Bedeiwy, A. F. A., and Ghoneim, M. A.: Prediction of lymph node metastases in bladder carcinoma with deoxyribonucleic acid flow cytometry. J. Urol., *144*, 884–887, 1990.

Sherman, A., Koss, L. G., Adams, S., Schreiber, K., Moussouris, H. F., Fred, S. Z., Bartels, P. H., and Wied, G. L.: Bladder cancer diagnosis by image analysis of cells in voided urine using a small computer. Anal. Quant. Cytol., *3*, 239–249, 1981.

Sherman, A. B., Koss, L. G., Wyschogrod, D., Melder, K. H., Eppich, E. M., and Bales, C. E.: Bladder cancer diagnosis by computer image analysis of cells in the sediment of voided urine using a video scanning system. Anal. Quant. Cytol. Histol., *8*, 177–186, 1986.

Sherman, A. B., Koss, L. G., and Adams, S. E.: Interobserver and intraobserver differences in the diagnosis of urothelial cells. Comparison with classification by computer. Anal. Quant. Cytol., *6*, 112–120, 1984.

Spooner, M. E., and Cooper, E. H.: Chromosome constitution of transitional cell carcinoma of the urinary bladder. Cancer, *29*, 1401–1412, 1972.

Tribukait, B.: Flow Cytometry in Surgical Pathology and Cytology of Tumors of the Genito-Urinary Tract. *In* Koss, L. G., and Coleman, D. V. (Eds.): Advances in Clinical Cytology, Vol. 2, pp. 163–189. New York, Masson, 1984.

Tribukait, B.: Flow cytometry in assessing the clinical aggressiveness of genito-urinary neoplasms. World J. Urol., *5*, 108–122, 1987.

Tribukait, B., Gustafson, H., and Esposti, M. D.: Ploidy and proliferation of human bladder tumors as measured by flow-cytofluorometric DNA-analysis and its relations to histopathology and cytology. Cancer, *43*, 1742–1751, 1979.

Weinstein, R. S., Alroy, J., Farrow, G. M., Miller, A. W., and Davidsohn, I.: Blood group isoantigen detection in carcinoma in situ of the urinary bladder. Cancer, *43*, 661, 1979.

Weinstein, R. S., Coon, J., Alroy, J., and Davidsohn, I.: Tissue-associated blood group antigens in human tumors. *In* DeLellis, R. A. (Ed.): Diagnostic Immunohistochemistry. New York, Masson, 1981, pp. 239–261.

Wheeless, L. L., Coon, J. S., Deitch, A. D., et al.: Comparison of automated and manual techniques for analysis of DNA frequency distributions in bladder washings. Cytometry, *9*, 600–604, 1988.

Wied, G. L., Bartels, P. H., Bahr, G. F., and Oldfield, D. G.: Taxonomic intracellular analytic system (TICAS) for cell identification. Acta Cytol., *12*, 180–204, 1968.

Wijkstrom, H., Granberg-Ohman, I., and Tribukait, B.: Chromosomal and DNA patterns in transitional cell bladder carcinoma. A comparative cytogenetic and flow-cytofluorometric DNA study. Cancer, *53*, 1718–1723, 1984.

Wijkstrom, H., Lundh, B., and Tribukait, B.: Urine or bladder washings in the cytologic evaluation of transitional cell carcinoma of the urinary tract. Scand. J. Urol. Nephrol., *21,* 119–123, 1987.

Yamase, H. T., Powell, G. T., and Koss, L. G.: A simplified method of preparing permanent tissue sections for the erythrocyte adherence test. Am. J. Clin. Pathol., *75,* 178–181, 1981.

CHAPTER 6

The Urethra, Ureters, Renal Pelves, and Ileal Conduit

THE URETHRA

Histologic Recall

Male

In males, the urethra extends from the bladder to the tip (meatus) of the penis. The urethra may be divided into the proximal (posterior) urethra, lined by the urothelium (see Chap. 2), and the distal (anterior) part, lined by squamous epithelium. A transitional zone between the two epithelial types is lined by a stratified columnar epithelium. The epithelial lining of the urethra is not necessarily uniform: patches of different epithelial types may occur in various locations. The posterior urethra contains an elevated area, the verumontanum, wherein open the ejaculatory ducts. In between the ejaculatory ducts there opens a short sinus, the prostatic utricle, a remnant of the fused Müllerian ducts. The utricle is lined by cuboidal or columnar epithelium and may be the site of carcinomas of endometrial type (see p. 146). Numerous prostatic ducts also open into the posterior urethra. The mucus-secreting bulbourethral or Cowper's glands open into the anterior urethra.

Female

In females, the urethra is only about 3 cm long, stretching from the bladder to its opening just posterior to the clitoris. The urethra is lined by urothelium, except for its most anterior part, which is lined by squamous epithelium. The glands of Skene open into the urethra. Diverticula may occur.

Methods of Investigation

In the male, the status of the epithelium of the urethra may be investigated in voided urine, in washings of the urethra, or by direct removal of cytologic samples by an applicator or a small brush. *In the female,* the tumors are usually visible to the naked eye and are diagnosed by a direct biopsy. Occasionally these tumors may be diagnosed in voided urine or by direct brushings.

Inflammatory Diseases

Acute or chronic urethritis is most often caused by *Neisseria gonorrhoeae* or *Chlamydia trachomatis.* Neither disease calls for a cytologic examination. Urethral strictures, usually seen in the male as a consequence of urethritis, do not shed cells of diagnostic value.

Giacomini et al. (1989) used a small, especially constructed sampling instrument to study urethral cytology in males. In a number of patients, they reported characteristic cytologic findings consistent with a number of infectious processes. In gonorrhea, gram-negative diplococci were observed. In *Chlamydia* infection, degenerative cell changes were noted. This

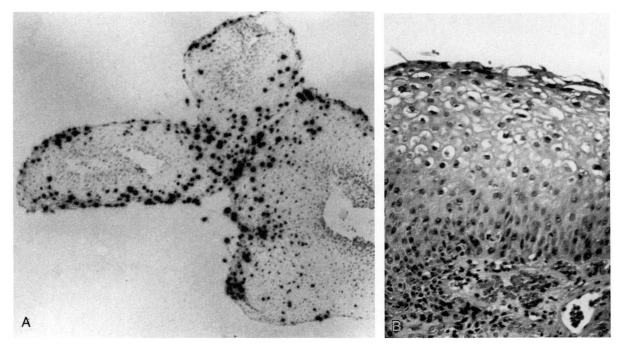

FIGURE 6-1. (*A*) Condyloma acuminatum of the urethral meatus of the penis. Results of in situ hybridization with a probe to human papillomavirus type 6 (*black nuclei*). It may be noted that the upper epithelial layers show a stronger hybridization signal than deeper layers, corresponding to the distribution of viral DNA. (*B*) Histologic appearance of the epithelial lining in the same tumor. Toward the surface note the presence of cells with enlarged, hyperchromatic nuclei and perinuclear halos, the so-called koilocytes. (*A* × 60; *B* × 150.)

infection must be confirmed by culture (Koss, 1992). The presence of *Trichomonas vaginalis* was also noted in urethral smears, as were changes related to human papillomavirus infection (see below).

Benign Tumors

Condylomata Acuminata (Venereal Warts)

The wart-type lesions affecting the skin and the mucosal membranes of external genitalia of both sexes are a sexually transmitted disease caused by human papillomavirus (HPV) types 6 or 11. Histologically the tumors are composed of folds of squamous epithelium, often showing significant nuclear abnormalities in the form of nuclear hyperchromasia and abnormal mitotic figures (Fig. 6-1). If located within the male urethra, the condylomas are usually flattened and may be mistaken for squamous carcinoma (Fig. 6-2*A,B*). Even though condylomata acuminata must be classified as benign tumors, the mucosal lesions, whether located in the penile urethra or

in the bladder, are very difficult to treat and may recur. The possibility that some of these tumors could transform into a squamous carcinoma was previously discussed (see p. 114).

Until the early 1980s, the venereal warts were thought of as a nuisance rather than a serious disorder. With progress in the understanding of a possible carcinogenic role of the human papillomavirus in carcinomas of the female genital tract, particularly of the uterine cervix (summary in Koss, 1992), and carcinoma of the penis (Malek et al., 1993), condylomata acuminata acquired a new significance. Today the presence of condylomata acuminata must be considered a risk factor for other disorders associated with human papillomavirus (HPV), and such patients and their sexual partners require a careful and thorough examination which, in the female, must include a cervical (Papanicolaou) smear and a colposcopic examination (Levine et al., 1984).

It is still far from certain whether the penises and penile urethras of all male partners of women with precancerous lesions or cancer of the cervix, vagina, or vulva should be examined for HPV related lesions.

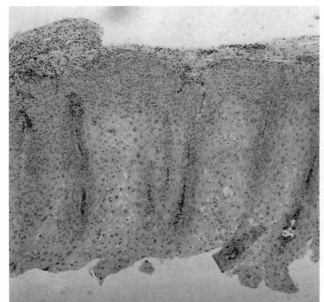

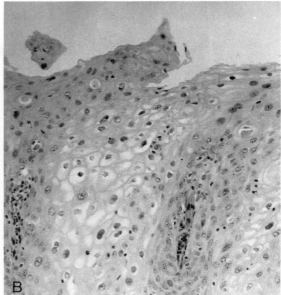

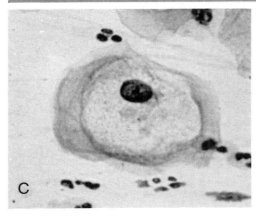

FIGURE 6-2. (*A*) Flattened condyloma acuminatum located within penile urethra. Note the deep invagination of the rete pegs and the nuclear abnormalities, better shown in *B*. (*B*) Koilocytes are present within the epithelium. The lesion was initially thought to be a squamous carcinoma in situ. The presence of human papillomavirus was demonstrated by immunochemistry. (*C*) A koilocyte in a urethral brush specimen. Note the large, opaque nucleus and the perinuclear clear zone, sharply demarcated towards the periphery of the cell (compare to Figs. 5-35 and 5-36). (*A* × 60; *B* × 150; *C* × 800.)

Although in some of them visible and treatable condylomas may be present (Levine et al., 1984; Fralick et al., 1994), most of them have no visible lesions. Sedlacek et al. (1986) and Barrasso et al. (1987) proposed the use of "penoscopy," *i.e.*, the application of colposcopy to the skin of the penis after application of 3% acetic acid solution to recognize the aceto-white lesions. This still does not rule out the possibility of an intraurethral lesion. Fralick et al. (1994) advocated the use of urethroscopy with a small pediatric cystoscope. It was proposed by Ceccini et al. (1988) and Giacomini et al. (1989) that a male equivalent of the cervical smears in the form of direct sampling of the urethra with a small brush or a small sampling instrument serves to uncover occult condylomas in the male.

A discussion of the possible role of human papillomavirus infection as a putative carcinogenic agent is beyond the scope of this book, and the reader is referred to other sources for a detailed analysis of the evidence (see Syrjänen et al., 1987; Koss, 1992). Suffice it to say that carcinoma of the uterine cervix and its precursor stages (cervical intraepithelial neoplasia), carcinomas of the vagina, and, to a lesser extent, of the vulva and penis, have been linked to infection with human papillomavirus types 16, 18, 31, 35, 42, and a few other recently identified types. A distinct disorder of the shaft of the penis, the giant condyloma of Buschke-Löwenstein, has also been shown to be associated with HPV type 11. These tumors, very difficult to treat, may show invasive behavior but, as a rule, do not form metastases. A reversible disorder of the skin of the genital region in both sexes, Bowenoid papulosis, has been shown to be associated with human papillomavirus type 16. The precise sequence of events characterizing the role of the virus in cancer is far from clear. Still, it is known that some of the proteins produced by the virus may interact with proteins of cancer inhibitory genes, known as Rb gene and p53 gene.

CYTOLOGIC FINDINGS

In both sexes, the characteristic cytologic finding in condylomata acuminata is the identification of *koilocytes* (Fig. 6-2C; see also Fig. 5-35). These are squamous cells of intermediate type, sometimes significantly larger than normal, characterized by large, sometimes multiple, hyperchromatic opaque nuclei, surrounded by a clear cytoplasmic zone or cavity. At its periphery the cavity is usually sharply demarcated. The term was derived by Koss and Durfee in 1956 from the Greek word *koilos,* meaning a hollow or a cavity. Ultrastructural studies disclosed that the nuclei of koilocytes often contain crystalline arrays of human papillomavirus particles, whereas the peripheral clear zone reflects cytoplasmic necrosis, demarcated by a condensation of cytoplasmic filaments. Thus the koilocytes are dead cells with evidence of a *permissive viral infection* caused by proliferation and accumulation of mature viral particles. A direct scraping of the surface of a condyloma acuminatum may also yield other abnormal cells that may mimic to perfection cells of a squamous carcinoma. Such cells have keratinized cytoplasm and large, irregularly configured hyperchromatic or pyknotic nuclei (see Color Plate 6-1A and Fig. 5-36). Without knowing the source of such cells, an erroneous diagnosis of squamous carcinoma can be readily established.

The efficacy of cytology of voided urine in discovering urethral changes associated with HPV infection in men was compared with urethroscopy and biopsies of lesions by Fralick et al. (1994). Cytology was positive in 5 of 135 patients but only 1 of the 5 had a documented lesion. In 14 patients with biopsy-documented urethral disease only one had abnormal cytology. Unfortunately, the description of histology of the HPV induced lesions of the urethra was inadequate and not illustrated. Thus the results of this study must be considered questionable. On the other hand the cytologic findings in urethral brush specimens reported by Ceccini et al. (1988) and Giaccomini et al. (1989) were not verified by biopsies, and thus the entire issue of cytologic diagnosis of HPV related urethral disease in males is worthy of a thorough reexamination. The issue is complicated still further because no effective treatment of intraurethral lesions is available.

Other Benign Tumors of the Urethra

Except for condylomata acuminata, other benign tumors of the urethra are rare. A painful inflammatory polypoid lesion of the female urethra, a caruncle, may be sometimes observed. Other benign polypoid lesions are essentially the same as found in the urinary bladder (see Chap. 5). None of these lesions can be recognized by cytologic techniques.

Primary Malignant Tumors of the Urethra

Primary cancers of the urethra are uncommon. They differ significantly according to sex, and, in the male, are usually related to the tumors of the urinary bladder.

Primary Malignant Tumors of the Female Urethra

Malignant tumors of the female urethra are most commonly epidermoid or squamous carcinomas, followed by urothelial type carcinomas and adenocarcinomas. Some of the adenocarcinomas are of the clear cell type (Young and Scully, 1985; Meis et al., 1987). Carcinomas of mixed type (adenosquamous or mucoepidermoid carcinomas) are uncommon. Because these tumors are usually discovered late in the course of the disease, their prognosis is often poor. Very rare malignant tumors are malignant melanomas, rhabdomyosarcomas and leiomyosarcomas. We have not observed any metastatic tumors to the female urethra.

CYTOLOGIC FINDINGS

Malignant cells of squamous or urothelial type may be observed in the sediment of voided urine or in direct scrape samples of the tumor. For descriptions of the characteristic cells, see pp. 88 and 97. If tumor cells are found in the sediment of voided urine, tumors of the bladder and tumors of the genital tract must be ruled out before the urethra can be considered as a primary source of the cancer cells.

We observed several examples of urethral adenocarcinoma, some originating in urethral diverticula, in the sediment of voided urine. The tumor cells formed round (papillary) clusters wherein the cells were superimposed. The large cancer cells had an abundant, basophilic cytoplasm and large, vesicular nuclei with prominent large nucleoli (Fig. 6-3 and Color Plate 6-1B,C; see also p. 118 and Color Plate 5-2C). Peven and Hidvegi (1985) described the cytologic findings in a case of a clear cell adenocarcinoma in a female patient. The findings were identical to

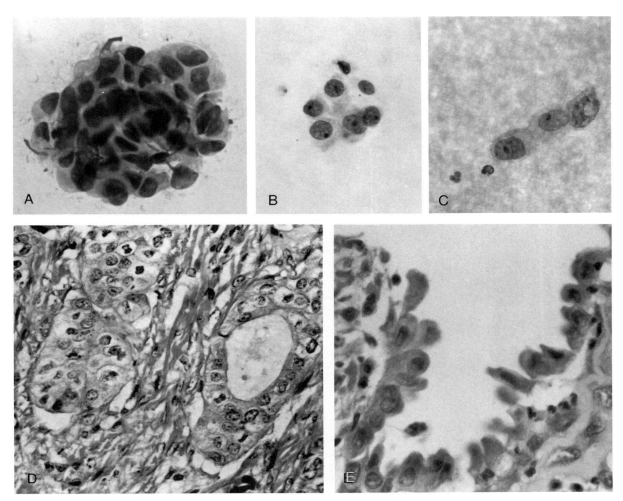

FIGURE 6-3. Adenocarcinoma of urethral diverticulum in a 54-year-old woman. (*A–C*) Cells and cell clusters in voided urine sediment. (*A*) A somewhat air-dried cluster of spherical (papillary) configuration, composed of cancer cells with large, irregular hyperchromatic nuclei. The fine details of nuclear structure cannot be seen in this cluster. (*B* and *C*) Better preserved clusters of cancer cells, showing a finely granular chromatin, prominent nucleoli, and scanty, faintly stained cytoplasm. (*D*) Histologic section of the tumor. (*E*) Lining of an adjacent area of the diverticulum with a carcinoma in situ. The same case is shown in Color Plate 6-1, *B, C*. (*A,B,C* × 560; *D,E* × 350.)

those described and illustrated in clear cell adenocarcinoma of the bladder (see p. 104 and Fig. 5-25).

Primary Malignant Tumors of the Male Urethra

Most malignant tumors of the male urethra are related to high-grade carcinomas of the urinary bladder. The urethral involvement may be in the form of a urothelial carcinoma in situ or invasive carcinoma. Both types of lesions are morphologically identical to the corresponding tumors of the urinary bladder. Be-

cause of the high frequency of urethral involvement in bladder cancer, stripping of the penile urethra is often performed at the time of cystectomy for advanced bladder disease. A rare form of urethral involvement in bladder cancer is Paget's disease, characterized by the presence of large cells with clear cytoplasm in the cancerous epithelium (see Fig. 5-46). Such cells usually stain positively for mucus, in a fashion similar to Paget's cells in the nipple or in the vulva. The mechanism of this event is unknown.

Primary cancers of the penile urethra, not related

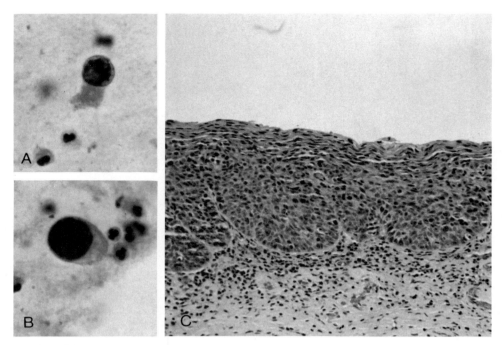

FIGURE 6-4. Urothelial carcinoma in situ of penile urethra, following several cystoscopic resections of high-grade urothelial carcinomas of bladder. (*A,B*) Cancer cells in voided urine. (*C*) Histologic section of urethral biopsy. (*A,B* × 560; *C* × 150.)

to carcinoma of the bladder, are uncommon. Adeno-carcinomas derived from the prostatic utricle and mimicking endometrial adenocarcinomas are sometimes observed (Melicow and Tannenbaum, 1971). The derivation of these tumors is still questionable (Petersen, 1992). The meatus of the urethra may become involved in cancers of the skin of the penis. As mentioned above, intraurethral condylomata acuminata may be mistaken for squamous carcinomas of the urethra.

CYTOLOGIC FINDINGS

Although voided urine may contain cells of urothelial carcinoma originating in the urethra, the origin of such cells cannot be ascertained (Fig. 6-4). Urethral washings, on the other hand, have been, in our hands, an efficient means of following patients with bladder tumors for evidence of urethral involvement. Several cases of carcinoma in situ, characterized by small urothelial cancer cells, have been diagnosed in this way (Fig. 6-5). In a case of an adenocarcinoma of the prostatic utricle, voided urine disclosed clusters of large malignant cells with columnar configuration suggestive of an adenocarcinoma (Fig. 6-6).

Other Malignant Tumors

Malignant melanoma of the urethra has been observed in both sexes, with a slight preponderance in females (summary in Petersen, 1992). We observed a carcinoma of the sweat glands of the penis with a component of Paget's disease of the skin of the penis that was initially thought to represent a urothelial carcinoma (Mitsudo et al., 1981). A few other exceedingly rare tumors have been reported, including a carcinoid (Sylsora et al., 1975), but none with cytologic correlation.

Metastatic Tumors

The only example of metastatic carcinoma encountered by us was a case of prostatic carcinoma that most likely extended from the bladder trigone to the urethra. Small cancer cells consistent with prostatic origin were observed in that case. For a description of prostatic cancer cells in the urinary sediment, see Chapter 8. As was discussed on p. 123, metastatic urothelial carcinoma may cause Paget's disease of the skin of the penis (see Fig. 5-46).

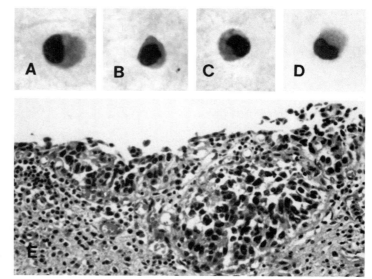

FIGURE 6-5. Urothelial carcinoma in situ of penile urethra observed in a 57-year-old man after several episodes of high-grade bladder carcinomas. (*A–D*) Small cancer cells observed in washings of the urethra. (*E*) Histologic section of lesion. (*A–D* × 560; *E* × 150.)

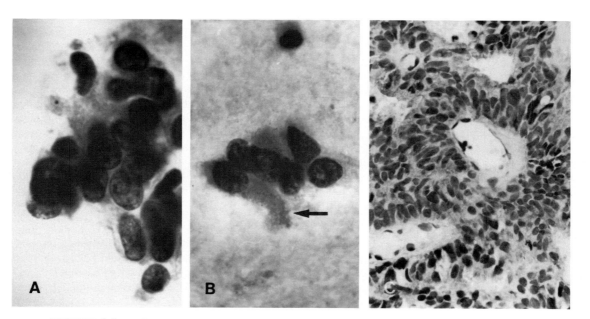

FIGURE 6-6. Adenocarcinoma of prostatic utricle in a 57-year-old man. (*A,B*) Clusters of cancer cells in voided urine. Note the columnar configuration of some cells (*arrow*), which is strongly suggestive of an adenocarcinoma. (*C*) Histologic section of the tumor. (*A,B* × 1,000; *C* × 350). Modified from Koss, L. G.: Diagnostic Cytology and Its Histopathologic Bases. 4th Ed. Philadelphia, J. B. Lippincott, 1992.

THE URETERS AND THE RENAL PELVES

Histologic Recall

The ureters and the renal pelves are lined by urothelium, with occasional patches of columnar, mucus-secreting epithelium. Nests of Brunn and cyst formation, identical to those observed in the bladder, are commonly observed (see Chap. 2).

Space-Occupying Lesions

The investigation of space-occupying lesions of the ureters and the renal pelves is usually triggered either by hematuria or by an episode of flank pain. The lesions are usually discovered by roentgenologic methods, such as an intravenous or retrograde pyelogram, or by computed tomography. The differential diagnosis usually comprises a tumor, a stone, a vascular malformation, or, infrequently, an inflammatory lesion. The urologist seeking an answer to his questions often expects too much of the cytologic examination, which has strict limitations, as will be set forth below.

Methods of Investigation

By far the best universal method of examination of the ureters and renal pelves is voided urine. As discussed in reference to the urinary bladder (see Chap. 5), urine sediment is an excellent and sensitive method of diagnosis of high-grade urothelial tumors, whether in situ or invasive. *The method fails in the identification of well-differentiated, low-grade tumors and is of very limited value in the identification of lithiasis or inflammatory lesions.* To be sure, the presence of cancer cells in voided urine does not indicate the origin of such cells, which may be derived from the urinary bladder, either one of the ureters, or the renal pelves. Therefore a positive specimen still calls for localizing procedures. The methods commonly used for this purpose are retrograde washings, brushings, or careful collection of urine from each ureter. As discussed in Chapter 3, the three methods present different degrees of difficulty of interpretation. Recently fiberoptic instruments allowing for a visual inspection and biopsies of the ureters and renal pelves have been introduced.

Retrograde brushings or washings usually result in removal of large fragments of the urothelium from the lining of the ureter. Such clusters, as discussed and illustrated in Chapter 3, are frequently mistaken for fragments of low-grade papillary tumors, a common source of diagnostic error in urinary cytology. *It must be repeated that clusters of urothelial cells are a common denominator of instrumentation, low-grade papillary tumors, and lithiasis.*

Occasionally, in the presence of a *high-grade tumor,* a retrograde procedure may lead to a confirmatory diagnosis and a localization of the lesion. In performing the procedures, care must be exercised to avoid cross contamination, by using separate instruments for each side. A much better procedure is collection of urine from each ureter by inserting the catheter for only a short distance and letting the urine drip into a container with a fixative (see Chap. 1). The procedure is time-consuming, but this type of material is usually free of the massive presence of normal urothelial cells, it is easier to interpret, and therefore allows for a better localization of the lesion. The retrograde fiberoptic instruments have not been fully evaluated at the time of this writing (1994).

Benign Lesions

Inflammatory Lesions Mimicking Tumors

These are comparatively infrequent in the Western world, where *tuberculosis* involving the kidney and the excretory portions of the urinary tract has become an uncommon disease. Even with the recently reported recrudescence of tuberculosis as a consequence of AIDS, renal involvement is still very rare. The diagnosis of tuberculosis of the upper urinary tract must be confirmed by bacteriologic evidence. Although tuberculosis sometimes may be suspected on the analysis of the urinary sediment because of the presence of a marked inflammation, necrosis, and sometimes carrot-shaped epithelioid cells and multinucleated Langhans' cells, this finding is distinctly uncommon in lesions of the ureters and renal pelves. *Malakoplakia,* a disorder of macrophages incapable of digestion of coliform baccilli, may form a space-occupying lesion, but it is uncommon in the ureters or renal pelves. As discussed in Chapter 4, the cytologic diagnosis of malakoplakia is unlikely in the absence of an ulceration of the underlying epithelium. For further comments on cytologic diagnosis of malakoplakia, see p. 65.

Benign Tumors

Excluding papillomas of the urothelium, which will be discussed with urothelial tumors, other benign tumors of the ureters and the renal pelves are very uncommon. *Inverted papilloma* has been described in both locations, but some of the lesions of the ureter, on further scrutiny and follow-up, turned out to be low-grade urothelial tumors, capable of recurrence. This proved to be the case with one such ureteral tumor described by Fromowitz, et al. (1981) from our laboratories. The error is usually due to a flattening of the surface of the tumor within the narrow lumen of the organ, mimicking the uninterrupted surface of the inverted papilloma. *Fibrous polyps* and hamartomatous polyps have also been described. In women, *endometriosis* may involve both the renal pelves and the ureter, sometimes forming a constrictive lesion of the latter. None of these lesions has been identified in cytologic samples to date. For cytologic presentation of endometriosis in the urinary bladder, see p. 114 and Fig. 5-45.

A case of a tumor-forming pyelitis cystica, the equivalent of cystitis cystica in a renal pelvis, was described by Dabbs (1992). The cytologic finding in retrograde washings were those of normal urothelium and, regrettably, not diagnostic of this disorder.

Malignant Tumors

Malignant tumors are most often of urothelial derivation and configuration. However, adenocarcinomas and squamous carcinomas may also occur.

Urothelial Tumors

RISK FACTORS

Although urothelial tumors of the ureters and the renal pelves may occur as single, independent events, they are commonly intimately associated with similar tumors occurring elsewhere in the lower urinary tract, mainly in the urinary bladder. The sequence of events cannot be predicted. In most patients tumors of the bladder are followed by tumors of the renal pelves or ureters, but the sequence may be reversed, with bladder tumors following tumors occurring in the upper urinary tract. A synchronous involvement of all these organs may also occur. Distal ureters may also be involved in high-grade bladder cancers, particularly carcinoma in situ, perhaps by direct extension of the cancerous process (see p. 77). The epithelium of distal ureters may show either an atypical hyperplasia or carcinoma in situ (Fig. 6-7). For this reason the performance of frozen sections on ureteral margins is advocated at the time of cystectomy for bladder cancer. These well-known observations have always been interpreted as showing the "field effect" of the urothelium in its response to carcinogenic agents, although in many instances the exact nature of such agents has not been identified, except in industrial

workers exposed to known carcinogens. Cigarette smoking is the customary villain.

Carcinomas of the ureters and renal pelves are known to occur in analgesic abusers, mainly women, who consume large doses of phenacetin (Bengtsson et al., 1968; Johansson et al., 1974). It is of interest that in this group of patients vascular abnormalities in the form of capillary sclerosis of the lower urinary tract are commonly observed (Mihatsch et al., 1979; Palvio et al., 1987). In patients with Balkan nephropathy, an endemic familial disease of unknown etiology observed along the Danube in Yugoslavia, carcinomas of the renal pelves and ureters were also reported (review in Petkowic, 1978). Tumors of the renal pelves and ureters were also observed in patients treated with large doses of cyclophosphamide (McDougal et al., 1981; Schiff et al., 1982; Brenner and Shellhammer, 1987), as were tumors of the urinary bladder (see p. 61).

HISTOLOGY

The similarities among urothelial tumors of various component organs of the lower urinary tract are also evident in their morphologic presentation. Tumors of the ureters and of the renal pelves are either well-differentiated papillary tumors of low grade, sometimes identified as papillomas or low-grade urothelial tumors, or high-grade tumors associated with carcinoma in situ and related abnormalities (intraurothelial neoplasia, see p. 75). Mahadevia et al. (1983) have documented by mapping that high-grade tumors of the renal pelves and ureters are always associated with peripheral epithelial abnormalities. In four of the nine cases, there was a classic carcinoma in situ in the adjacent urothelium (Fig. 6-8). This latter finding was of prognostic significance, inasmuch as patients with this disorder may succumb to their tumor rapidly or may develop metachronous tumors in the bladder more often than patients in whom carcinoma in situ cannot be observed. Renal pelvic tumors are also capable of extension into the renal collecting ducts. Similar observations on the association of grossly visible lesions with peripheral flat epithelial abnormalities were presented by Lomax-Smith and Seymour (1980) in a case of a carcinoma of the ureter developing in analgesic nephropathy, and by Chasko et al. (1981) in 30 mapped cases of tumors of the renal pelves and ureters.

Also in keeping with tumors of the urinary bladder, DNA ploidy studies performed on 11 patients with urothelial tumors of the renal pelves and ureters disclosed aneuploid DNA pattern in all grade III tumors, two carcinomas in situ, and in two of five grade II tumors (Oldbring et al., 1989). Aneuploidy correlated well with invasiveness of the tumors, whereas the

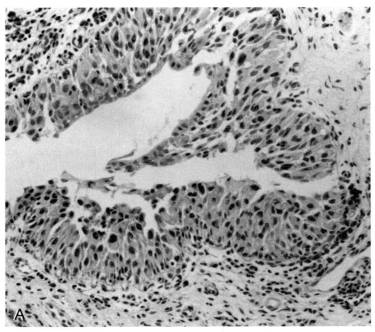

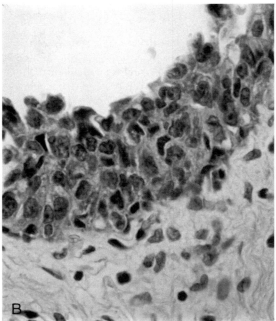

FIGURE 6-7. Abnormalities of distal ureters at the time of cystectomy for high-grade bladder cancer with a major component of carcinoma in situ. (*A*) Markedly atypical hyperplasia of urothelium. (*B*) Carcinoma in situ. (*A* × 225; *B* × 560.)

FIGURE 6-8. Results of mapping of seven carcinomas of the renal pelvis and two of the ureter. The distribution of the various levels of epithelial abnormalities is shown. It may be noted that areas of carcinoma in situ and epithelial atypia (UIN II; see Chapter 5) accompany every tumor. Tumor extension into the renal collecting tubules was observed in six of the seven carcinomas of renal pelves. (From Mahadevia, P. S., Karwa, G. L., and Koss, L. G.: Mapping of urothelium in carcinomas of the renal pelvis and ureter. A report of nine cases. Cancer *51,* 890–897, 1983, with permission.)

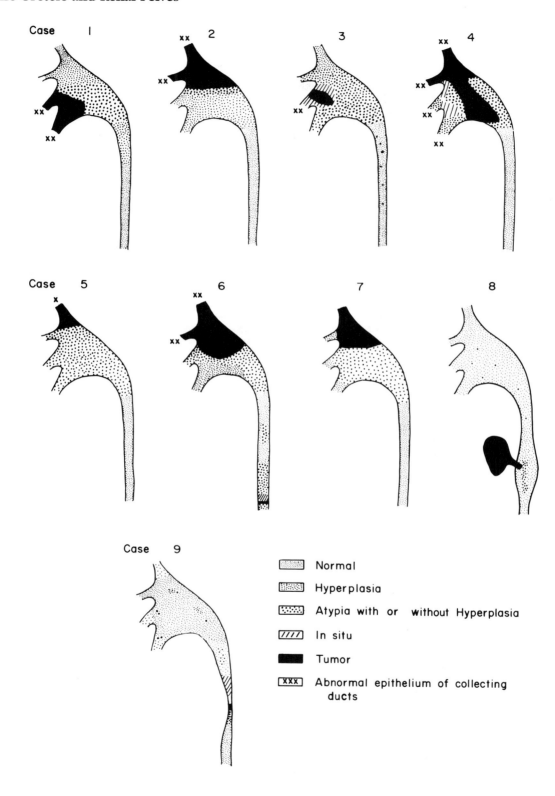

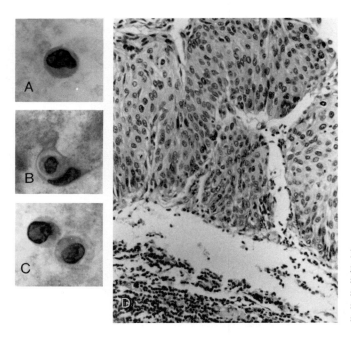

FIGURE 6-9. Urothelial papillary carcinoma, grade 2, of the ureter. Voided urine and histologic section. (*A–C*) Cancer cells found in the urinary sediment. In *B* a "cell in cell" image, common in squamous carcinoma, may be observed. (*D*) Tissue section of the tumor. (*A–C* × 560; *D* × 150.)

three diploid grade 2 tumors were non-invasive. For further discussion of DNA analysis in urothelial tumors, see Chapter 9.

CYTOLOGIC PRESENTATION

As is the case with urothelial tumors of the urinary bladder, the cytologic presentation of the urothelial tumors of the ureters and the renal pelves depends greatly on their histologic makeup. Grade I papillary tumors cannot be recognized either in voided urine or in washings or brushings of the ureters or renal pelves because the component tumor cells and cell clusters cannot be differentiated from normal urothelium (see p. 86). Aneuploid grade 2 papillary tumors may shed recognizable cancer cells (Fig. 6-9), whereas diploid grade 2 tumors shed, at best, atypical cells. High-grade tumors have the same cytologic characteristics as the corresponding tumors of the urinary bladder (see p. 88). Their recognition as malignant tumors in voided urine is sometimes surprisingly easy because of numerous, easily recognizable cancer cells (Fig. 6-10 and Color Plate 6-1*D*).

Localization of Occult Urothelial Carcinomas and Carcinomas In Situ

The finding of cancer cells in urine in the presence of a clinically and radiologically obvious space-occupying lesion usually offers sufficient guidance for treatment. There are, however, situations in which the positive urine cytology is not supported by clinical findings. The customary procedure in such cases is to rule out a lesion of the bladder by cystoscopy, bladder washings, and biopsies (see p. 125). In the absence of a lesion in the bladder, further efforts at localization of the tumor must be made. In the case illustrated in Figure 6-11, the localization of the high-grade tumor to a renal pelvis could be secured by retrograde brushings. In my experience, however, drip-urine from the ureters usually offers better morphologic evidence of tumor.

Foot and Papanicolaou reported in 1949 on a case of a carcinoma in situ of the renal pelvis, first diagnosed in voided urine. Such cases are rare, and very few additional cases, some located in the ureter, have been reported (summary in Khan et al., 1979). In the case illustrated in Figure 6-12, an occult carcinoma in situ was first diagnosed in voided urine and subsequently localized to the left renal pelvis by retrograde catheterization. Another case with high-grade urothelial cancer cells observed in renal pelvic washings is shown in Color Plate 6-1*E,F*. In most cases some symptoms, usually hematuria, trigger the search for the occult carcinoma. Cytologic presentation of renal pelvic carcinomas in renal aspiration biopsy is discussed in Chapter 7 on p. 125.

TREATMENT

The customary therapy for urothelial tumors of the upper urinary tract is surgical removal, usually a nephroureterectomy. Unfortunately, in patients either with bilateral tumors or who are very poor surgical risks, this therapy may cause significant problems.

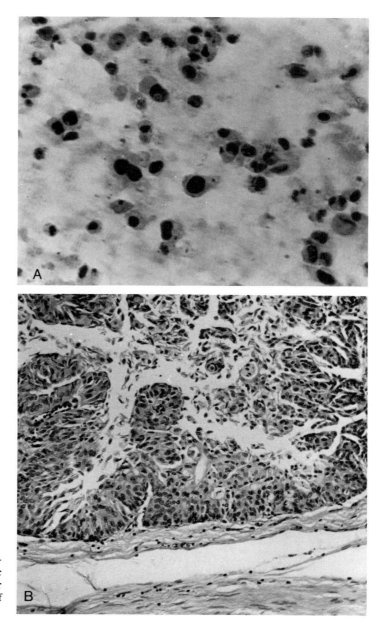

FIGURE 6-10. Urothelial papillary carcinoma, grade 3, of renal pelvis. Voided urine and histologic section. (*A*) Numerous cancer cells in voided urine. (*B*) Tissue section of the tumor. (*A* × 360; *B* × 150.)

Recently, bacille Calmette-Guérin (BCG) has been used for treatment of urothelial lesions of the upper urinary tract. The therapeutic agent was administered by retrograde catheterization in patients who were poor surgical risks, or who had prior nephroureterectomy, or who had bilateral disease (Sharpe et al., 1993). The indications for this therapy were based on positive cytology. Seven of 11 patients reverted to normal cytology with a median follow-up of 36 months. Longer-term follow-up is required to ascertain the long-term efficacy of this therapy.

Other Primary Malignant Tumors

Squamous carcinomas are known to occur in renal pelves but are very rare. More common are *adenocarcinomas,* which may have a variety of presentations, usually resembling carcinomas of the gastrointestinal tract. We have observed a clear cell carcinoma and a

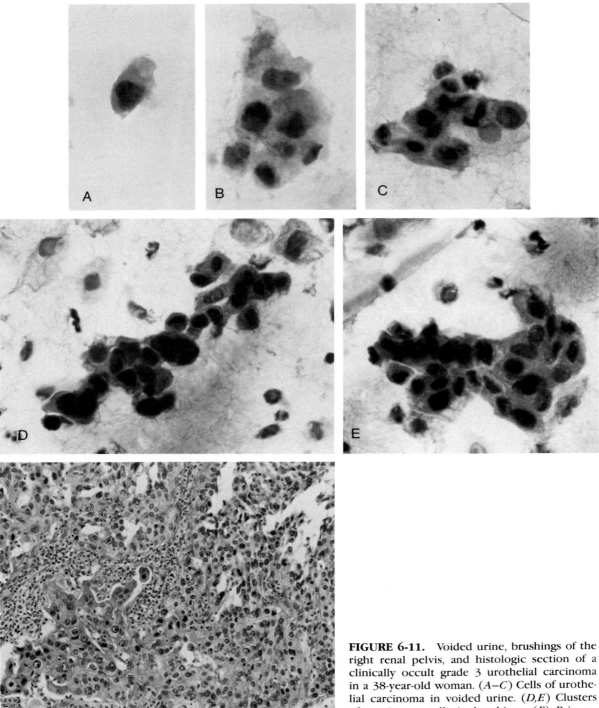

FIGURE 6-11. Voided urine, brushings of the right renal pelvis, and histologic section of a clinically occult grade 3 urothelial carcinoma in a 38-year-old woman. (*A–C*) Cells of urothelial carcinoma in voided urine. (*D,E*) Clusters of carcinoma cells in brushings. (*F*) Primary urothelial carcinoma, grade 3, of the right renal pelvis. The tumor invaded the kidney. (*A–E* × 560; *F* × 150.)

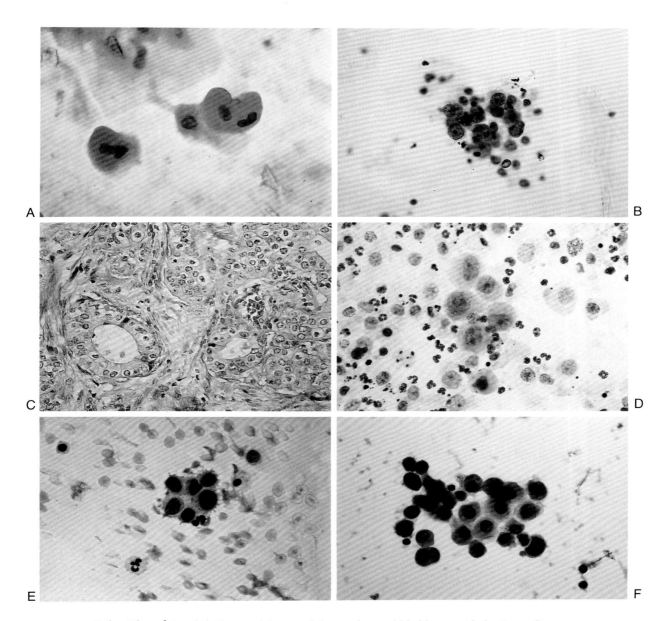

Color Plate 6-1. (*A*) Flat condylomas of the urethra and bladder—voided urine sediment. Very atypical squamous cells are reminiscent of cells of squamous carcinoma. (*B,C*) Adenocarcinoma of the urethral diverticulum in a 49-year-old woman (same case as Fig. 6-3). (*B*) A cluster of cancer cells in voided urine sediment. Note the papillary configuration of the cluster and the prominent nucleoli. (*C*) Histologic appearance of tumor. (*D–F*) Examples of cytologic findings in urothelial carcinomas of the renal pelves. (*D*) Voided urine sediment—cells of a poorly differentiated tumor in a 39-year-old male. Note the prominent nucleoli in the cancer cells. (*E,F*) Renal pelvic washings—cells of a high-grade urothelial carcinoma. (Original magnification *A,B* × 160; *C* × 100; *D–F* × 560, enlarged about × 2.5.)

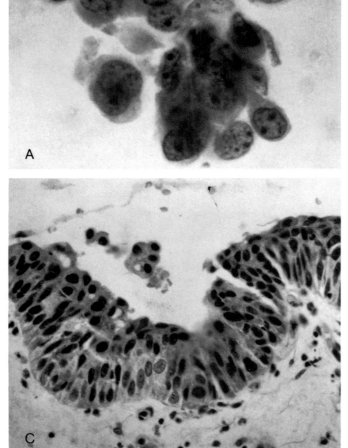

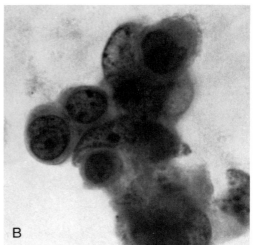

FIGURE 6-12. Radiologically occult carcinoma in situ of the right renal pelvis in a woman age 80, diagnosed in renal washings. (*A,B*) Cancer cells in washings of right renal pelvis. Note in *A* large irregular nucleoli characteristic of high-grade lesions. (*C*) Section of pelvic epithelium with carcinoma in situ. (*A,B* × 1,000; *C* × 650. Case courtesy of Dr. Harold Bloch, El Paso, Texas.)

mucus-producing carcinoma with signet ring cells, the latter occurring in the renal pelvis of young female patients with a congenital anomaly of the bladder treated with ureteral implantation into the sigmoid colon.

CYTOLOGIC PRESENTATION

Squamous carcinomas of the renal pelves and ureters are so rare that we have not observed any examples of them. It may be safely assumed that the cytologic presentation would be identical to that of corresponding tumors of the urinary bladder (see p. 97). This is also true of adenocarcinomas (see p. 99). To my knowledge, there are no reported

examples of cytologic findings in such tumors of the renal pelves.

Rare Primary Malignant Tumors

The repertory of malignant tumors other than those described above is limited (summary in Petersen, 1992). We observed a case of a spindle and giant cell carcinoma of the renal pelvis, characterized by highly abnormal spindly cells and numerous giant tumor cells resembling osteoclasts. Unfortunately no cytologic examination was conducted. Rare malignant melanomas of the renal pelvis have been reported. Primary malignant lymphomas occur in the kidney and will be discussed with renal tumors (see p. 215).

Metastatic Tumors

Metastatic tumors involving the lumens of the renal pelves or ureters are exceedingly rare. An extension of renal carcinoma to the renal pelvis may occur. However, metastatic carcinomas from adjacent organs, such as the uterine cervix or endometrium in the female and the prostate in the male, may encase and compress the ureters. Rarely, carcinomas from distant sites may behave in a similar fashion. Such tumors may be diagnosed by transcutaneous aspiration biopsy (Luciani et al., 1987), which will be discussed in Chapter 7.

Results

Because of the relative rarity of tumors of the renal pelves and ureter, it is difficult to obtain a meaningful summary of results pertaining to the performance of cytologic techniques in the diagnosis of these tumors. Petersen (1992) summarized the existing literature and concluded that only about 40% of such tumors can be identified by cytology. Comparisons are difficult to make because of the disparity of techniques and interpretation from one laboratory to another. In general, however, using adequate specimen collection, all or nearly all high-grade tumors may be recognized in voided urine (Eriksson and Johansson, 1976;

Mahadevia et al., 1983; Highman, 1986; Oldbring et al., 1989). Oldbring, et al. also documented that tumor DNA ploidy plays a major role in cytologic recognition, with aneuploid tumors being much more likely to be recognized than diploid tumors, well in keeping with the results pertaining to the cytology of bladder tumors (see p. 124).

MONITORING OF PATIENTS AFTER CYSTECTOMY FOR BLADDER CANCER

Ileal Conduit

As has been repeatedly emphasized in this chapter, synchronous or metachronous urothelial carcinomas may occur throughout the lower urinary tract. If radical cystectomy is the treatment of choice for bladder cancer, the ureters are implanted into a conduit constructed of a segment of the ileum, the ileal bladder.

The normal cellular components of the urine sediment from ileal bladders were described on p. 42 and illustrated in Figure 3-3. Urothelial cancer cells are easily differentiated from the cells derived from the lining of an ileal conduit: they are much larger and have a crisp, well demarcated cytoplasm and large, irregular coarsely granular, hyperchromatic nuclei (Fig. 6-13). The malignant tumor is usually localized

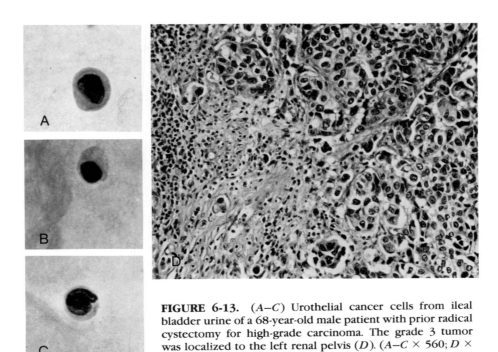

FIGURE 6-13. (*A–C*) Urothelial cancer cells from ileal bladder urine of a 68-year-old male patient with prior radical cystectomy for high-grade carcinoma. The grade 3 tumor was localized to the left renal pelvis (*D*). (*A–C* × 560; *D* × 150.)

to the renal pelvis. In the absence of radiologic evidence of tumor, as is sometimes the case, a careful catherization of the two ureters may be required to localize the lesion.

It is of interest that primary tumors of the urothelial type may sometimes also occur in the ileal conduit (Banigo et al., 1975; Grabstald, 1974).

Transplantation of Ureters into the Sigmoid Colon

For a variety of reasons this is sometimes the preferred way to create urinary diversion. As discussed on p. 99, the sigmoid colon in contact with urine is susceptible to the development of neoplastic lesions, ranging from polyps to carcinomas. In such patients sigmoidoscopy is the follow-up procedure of choice.

BIBLIOGRAPHY

Baird, S. S., Bush, L., and Livingstone, A. G.: Urethrectomy subsequent to total cystectomy for papillary carcinoma of the bladder. Case reports. J. Urol., *74*, 621–625, 1955.

Banigo, O. G., Waisman, J., and Kaufman, J. J.: Papillary (transitional) carcinoma in an ileal conduit. J. Urol., *114*, 626–627, 1975.

Barrasso, R., De Brux, J., Croissant, O., and Orth, G.: High prevalence of papillomavirus-associated penile intraepithelial neoplasia in sexual partners of women with cervical intraepithelial neoplasia. New Engl. J. Med., *317*, 916–923, 1987.

Batata, M. A., Whitmore, W. F., Jr., Hilaris, B. S., Tokita, N., and Grabstald, H.: Primary carcinoma of ureter: a prognostic study. Cancer, *35*, 1626–1632, 1975.

Bengtsson, U., Angervall, L., Ekman, H., and Lehman, H.: Transitional cell tumors of the renal pelvis in analgesic abusers. Scand. J. Urol. Nephrol., *2*, 145–150, 1968.

Bhagavan, B. S., Tiamson, E. M., Wenk, R. E., Berger, B. W., Hamamoto, G., and Egglestone, J. C.: Nephrogenic adenoma of the urinary bladder and urethra. Human Path., *12*, 907–916, 1981.

Bibbo, M., Gill, W. B., Harris, M. J., Lu, C. T., Thomsen, S., and Wied, G. L.: Retrograde brushing as a diagnostic procedure of ureteral, renal pelvic and renal calyceal lesions. A preliminary report. Acta Cytol., *18*, 137–141, 1974.

Brenner, D. W., and Schellhammer, P. F.: Upper tract urothelial malignancy after cyclophosphamide therapy. A case report and literature review. J. Urol., *137*, 1226–1227, 1987.

Bretton, P. R., Herr, H. W., Whitmore, W. F., Jr., Badalament, R. A., Kimmel, M., Provet, J., Oettgen, H. F., Melamed, M. R., and Fair, W. R.: Intravesical bacillus Calmette-Guerin therapy for in situ transitional cell carcinoma involving the prostatic urethra. J. Urol., *141*, 853–856, 1989.

Cantrell, B. B., Leifer, G., Deklerk, D. P., and Eggleston, J. C.: Papillary adenocarcinoma of the prostatic urethra with clear cell appearance. Cancer, *48*, 2661–2667, 1981.

Ceccini, S., Cipparone, I., Confortini, M., Scuderi, A., Meini, L., and Piazzesi, G.: Urethral cytology of cytobrush specimens. A new technique for detecting subclinical human papillomavirus infection in men. Acta Cytol., *32*, 314–317, 1988.

Chasko, S. B., Gray, G. F., and McCarron, J. P.: Urothelial neoplasia of the upper urinary tract. *In* Sommers, S. C., Rosen, P. P. (Eds.): Pathology Annual, Part 2. New York, Appleton-Century-Crofts, 1981;127–153.

Cordonnier, J. J., and Spjut, H. J.: Urethral occurrence of bladder carcinoma following cystectomy. J. Urol., *87*, 398–403, 1962.

Cullen, T. H., Popham, R. R., and Voss, H. J.: Urine cytology and primary carcinoma of the renal pelvis and ureter. Austr. N. Z. J. Surg., *41*, 230–236, 1972.

Culp, O. S., Utz, D. C., Harrison, E. G., Jr.: Experience with ureteral carcinoma in situ detected during operations for vesical problems. J. Urol., *97*, 679–682, 1967.

Dabbs, D. J.: Cytology of pyelitis cystica. A case report. Acta Cytol., *36*, 943–945, 1992.

Eriksson, O., and Johansson, S.: Urothelial neoplasms of the upper urinary tract. A correlation between cytologic and histologic findings in 43 patients with urothelial neoplasms of the renal pelvis or ureter. Acta Cytol., *20*, 20–25, 1976.

Foot, N. C., and Papanicolaou, G. N.: Early renal carcinoma in situ detected by means of smears of fixed urinary sediment. J. A. M. A., *139*, 356–358, 1949.

Fralick, R. A., Malek, R. S., Goellner, J. R., and Hyland, K. M.: Urethroscopy and urethral cytology in men with external genital condyloma. Urology, *43*, 361–364, 1994.

Fromowitz, F. B., Steinbok, M. L., Lautin, E. M., Friedman, A. C., Kahan, N., Bennett, M. J., and Koss, L. G.: Inverted papilloma of the ureter. J. Urol., *126*, 113–116, 1981.

Giacomini, G., Bianchi, G., and Moretti, D.: Detection of sexually transmitted diseases by urethral cytology, the ignored male counterpart of cervical cytology. Acta Cytol., *33*, 11–15, 1989.

Gill, W. B., Lu, C. T., and Thomsen, D.: Retrograde brushing: A new technique for obtaining histologic and cytologic material from ureteral, renal pelvic, and renal calyceal lesions. J. Urol., *109*, 573–578, 1973.

Gillenwater, J. Y., and Burros, H. M.: Unusual tumors of the female urethra. Obstet. Gynecol. *31*, 617–620, 1968.

Gowing, N. F.: Urethral carcinoma associated with cancer of the bladder. Br. J. Urol., *32*, 428–438, 1960.

Grabstald, H.: Carcinoma of ileal bladder stoma. J. Urol., *112*, 332–334, 1974.

Grabstald, H.: Tumors of the urethra in men and women. Cancer, *32*, 1235–1236, 1973.

Grabstald, H., Hilaris, B., Henschke, U., and Whitmore, W. F.: Cancer of the female urethra. J. A. M. A., *197*, 835–842, 1966.

Grabstald, H., Whitmore, W. F., Jr., and Melamed, M. R.: Renal pelvic tumors. J. A. M. A., *218*, 845–854, 1971.

Grace, D. D., Taylor, W. N., and Winter, C. C.: Carcinoma of the renal pelvis: a 15-year review. J. Urol., *98*, 566–569, 1968.

Grussendorf-Conen, E. I., Deutz, F. J., and de Villers, E. M.: Detection of human papillomavirus-6 in primary carcinoma of the urethra in men. Cancer, *60*, 1832–1835, 1987.

Harrison, J. H., Bostford, T. W., and Tucker, M. R.: The use of urinary sediment in the diagnosis and management of neoplasms of the kidney and bladder. Surg. Gyn. Obstet., *92*, 129–139, 1951.

Highman, W. J.: Transitional carcinoma of the upper urinary tract: a histological and cytopathological study. J. Clin. Path. *39*, 297–305, 1986.

Howley P. M.: Role of the human papillomarvirus in human cancer. Cancer Res, *51*, 5019s–5022s, 1991.

Johansson, S., Angervall, L., Bengtson, U., and Wahlquist, L.: Uroepithelial tumors of the renal pelvis associated with abuse of phenacetin-containing analgesics. Cancer, *33*, 743–753, 1974.

Johnson, D. E., and Guinn, G. A.: Surgical management of urethral carcinoma occurring after cystectomy. J. Urol., *103*, 314–316, 1970.

Kakizoe, T., Fujita, J., Murase, T., Matsumoto, K., and Kishi, K.: Transitional cell carcinoma of the bladder in patients with renal pelvic and ureteral cancer. J. Urol., *124*, 17–19, 1980.

Katz, J. I., and Grabstald, H.: Primary malignant melanoma of the female urethra. J. Urol., *116*, 454–457, 1976.

Khan, A. U., Farrow, G. M., Zincke, H., Utz, D. C., and Greene, L. F.: Primary carcinoma in situ of the ureter and renal pelvis. J. Urol., *121*, 681–683, 1979.

Kobayashi, S., Ohmori, M., Miki, H., Hirata, K., and Shimada, K.: Exfoliative cytology of a primary carcinoma of the renal pelvis. A case report. Acta Cytol., *29*, 1021–1025, 1985.

Koss, L. G.: Diagnostic Cytology and Its Histopathologic Bases. 4th Ed. Philadelphia, J. B. Lippincott, 1992.

Koss, L. G., and Durfee, G. R.: Unusual patterns of squamous epithelium of uterine cervix; cytologic and pathologic study of koilocytotic atypia. Ann. N.Y. Acad. Sci., *63*, 1245–1261, 1956.

Koss, L. G., Nakanishi, I., and Freed, S. Z.: Nonpapillary carcinoma in situ and atypical hyperplasia in cancerous bladders. Further studies of surgically removed bladders by mapping. Urology, *9*, 442–455, 1977.

Levine, R. U., Crum, C. P., Herman, E., Silvers, D., Ferenczy, A. and Richart, R. M.: Cervical papillomavirus infection and intraepithelial neoplasia: A study of male sexual partners. Obstet. Gynecol., *64*, 16–20, 1984.

Linker, D. G., and Whitmore, W. F.: Ureteral carcinoma in situ. J. Urol., *113*, 777–780, 1975.

Liwnicz, B. H., Lepow, H., Schutte, H., Fernandez, R., and Caberwal, D.: Mucinous adenocarcinoma of the re-

nal pelvis: Discussion of possible pathogenesis. J. Urol., *114*, 306–310, 1975.

Lomax-Smith, J. D., and Seymour, A. E.: Neoplasia in analgesic nephropathy. A urothelial field change. Am. J. Surg. Pathol., *4*, 565–572, 1980.

Luciani, L., Scappini, P., Pusiol, T., and Piscioli, F.: The role of aspiration cytology in the management of ureteral obstruction in patients with known cancer. Cancer, *59*, 1936–1946, 1987.

Mahadevia, P. S., Karwa, G. L., and Koss, L. G.: Mapping of urothelium in carcinomas of the renal pelvis and ureter. A report of nine cases. Cancer, *51*, 890–897, 1983.

Malek, R. S., Goellner, J. R., Smith, T. F., Espy, M. J. and Cupp, M. R.: Human papillomavirus infection and intraepithelial, in situ, and invasive carcinoma of the penis. J. Urol., *42*, 159–170, 1993.

Malmgren, R. A., Soloway, M. S., Chu, E. W., DelVecchio, P. R., and Ketcham, A. S.: Cytology of ileal conduit urine. Acta Cytol., *15*, 506–509, 1971.

McDougal, W. S., Cramer, S. F., and Miller, R.: Invasive carcinoma of renal pelvis following cyclophosphamide therapy for nonmalignant disease. Cancer, *48*, 691–695, 1981.

Meis, J. M., Ayala, A. G., and Johnson, D. E.: Adenocarcinoma of the urethra in women. Cancer, *60*, 1038–1052, 1987.

Melicow, M. M., and Tannenbaum, M.: Endometrial carcinoma of uterus masculinus (prostatic utricle). Report of 6 cases. J. Urol., *106*, 892–902, 1971.

Mihatsch, M. J., Torhost, J., Steinmann, E., Hofer, H., Stickelberger, M., Bianchi, L., Berneis, K., and Zollinger, H. U.: The morphologic diagnosis of analgesic (phenacetin) abuse. Path. Res. Pract., *164*, 68–79, 1979.

Mitsudo, S., Nakanishi, I., and Koss, L. G.: Paget's disease of the penis and adjacent skin. Its association with fatal sweat gland carcinoma. Arch. Pathol. Lab. Med., *105*, 518–520, 1981.

Murphy, M. W., Fu, Y. S., Lancaster, W. D., and Jenson, A. B.: Papillomavirus structural antigen in condyloma acuminatum of the male urethra. J. Urol., *130*, 84–85, 1983.

Murphy, W. M., von Buedinger, R. P., and Poley, R. W.: Primary carcinoma in situ of the renal pelvis and ureter. Cancer, *34*, 1126–1130, 1974.

Naib, Z. M.: Exfoliative cytology of renal pelvic lesions. Cancer, *14*, 1085–1087, 1961.

Ohkawa, M., Sugata, T., Hisazumi, H., Ishikawa, Y., and Mukawa, A.: Primary carcinoma in situ of the ureter: A case report. J. Urol., *132*, 1184–1185, 1984.

Oldbring, J., Hellsten, S., Lindholm, K., Mikulowski, P., and Tribukait, B.: Flow DNA analysis in the characterisation of carcinoma of the renal pelvis and ureter. Cancer, *64*, 2141–2145, 1989.

Palvio, D. H. B., Andersen, J. C., and Falk, E.: Transitional cell tumors of the renal pelvis and ureter associated with capillosclerosis indicating analgesic abuse. Cancer, *59*, 972–976, 1987.

Petersen, R. O.: Urologic Pathology. 2nd Ed. Philadelphia, J. B. Lippincott, 1992.

Petkowic, S. D.: Treatment of bilateral renal pelvic and ureteral tumors. A review of 45 cases. Europ. Urol., *4*, 397–400, 1978.

Peven, D. R., and Hidvegi, D. F.: Clear-cell adenocarcinoma of the female urethra. Acta Cytol., *29*, 142–146, 1985.

Piper, J. M., Tonascia, J., and Matanoski, G. M.: Heavy phenacetin use and bladder cancer in women aged 20 to 49 years. N. Engl. J. Med., *313*, 292–295, 1985.

Potts, I. F., and Hirst, E.: Inverted papilloma of the bladder. J. Urol., *90*, 175–179, 1963.

Richie, J. P., and Skinner, D. G.: Carcinoma in situ of the urethra associated with bladder carcinoma: The role of urethrectomy. J. Urol., *119*, 80–81, 1978.

Sacks, S. A., Waisman, J., Apfelbaum, H. B., Lake, P., and Goodwin, W. E.: Urethral adenocarcinoma (possibly originating in the glands of Littré). J. Urol., *113*, 50–55, 1975.

Sarnacki, C. T., McCormack, L. J., Kiser, W. S., Hazard, J. R., McLaughlin, T. C., and Belovich, D. M.: Urinary cytology and clinical diagnosis of urinary tract malignancy: A clinicopathologic study of 1,400 patients. J. Urol., *106*, 761–764, 1971.

Schade, R. O. K., Serck-Hanssen, A., and Swinney, J.: Morphological changes in the ureter in cases of bladder carcinoma. Cancer, *27*, 1267–1272, 1971.

Schellhammer, P. F., Whitmore, W. F., Jr.: Urethral meatal carcinoma following cystourethrectomy for bladder carcinoma. J. Urol., *115*, 61–64, 1976.

Schiff, H. I., Finkel, M., and Schapira, H. E.: Transitional cell carcinoma of the ureter, associated with cyclophosphamide therapy for benign disease. A case report. J. Urol., *128*, 1023–1024, 1982.

Sedlacek, T. V., Cunnane, M., and Carpiniello, V.: Colposcopy in the diagnosis of penile condyloma. Am. J. Obstet. Gynecol., *154*, 494–496, 1986.

Sharma, T. C., Melamed, M. R., Whitmore, W. F., Jr.: Carcinoma in situ of the ureter in patients with bladder carcinoma treated by cystectomy. Cancer, *26*, 583–587, 1970.

Sharpe, J. R., Duffy, G., and Chin, J. L.: Intrarenal bacillus Calmette-Guerin therapy for upper urinary tract carcinoma in situ. J. Urol., *149*, 457–460, 1993.

Sherwood, T.: Upper urinary tract tumours following bladder carcinoma: Natural history of urothelial neoplastic disease. Br. J. Rad., *44*, 137–141, 1971.

Smart, J. G.: Renal and ureteric tumours in association with bladder tumours. Br. J. Urol., *36*, 380–390, 1964.

Stragier, M., Desmet, R., Denys, H., Vergison, R., and Vanvuchelen, J.: Primary carcinoma in situ of renal pelvis and ureter. Brit. J. Urol., *52*, 401, 1980.

Sylsora, H. O., Diamond, H. M., Kaufman, M., Straus, F., and Lyon, E. S.: Primary carcinoid tumor of the urethra. J. Urol., *114*, 150–153, 1975.

Syrjänen, K., Gissmann, L., and Koss, L. G. (Eds.): Papillomaviruses and Human Disease. Berlin, Heidelberg, New York, Springer Verlag, 1987.

Tyler, D. E.: Stratified squamous epithelium in the vesical trigone and urethra: findings correlated with the menstrual cycle and age. Am. J. Anat., *111*, 319–325, 1962.

Wagle, D. G., Moore, R. H., and Murphy, G. P.: Primary carcinoma of the renal pelvis. Cancer, *33*, 1642–1648, 1974.

Wolinska, W. H., Melamed, M. R., Schellhammer, P. F., Whitmore, W. F., Jr.: Urethral cytology following cystectomy for bladder carcinoma. Am. J. Surg. Pathol., *1*, 225–234, 1977.

Wolinska, W. H., and Melamed, M. R.: Urinary conduit cytology. Cancer, *32*, 1000–1006, 1973.

Young, R. H., and Scully, R. E.: Clear cell adenocarcinoma of the bladder and urethra: a report of three cases and review of the literature. Am. J. Surg. Path., *9*, 816–826, 1985.

PART II

The Prostate, Kidney, Adrenal, Pararenal, and Retroperitoneal Spaces

CHAPTER 7

The Prostate

The primary purpose of securing tissue—or cell samples—from the prostate is the diagnosis of prostatic carcinoma. Traditionally, the first suspicion of prostatic cancer is obtained by palpation, and this method still occupies an important place in the diagnosis of this disease. In recent years, the determination of the serum level of prostate specific antigen (PSA) has been extensively used for screening. Levels of PSA above normal (1 to 4 ng/ml) are suggestive of a prostatic disorder. The normal levels are age-dependent and are higher in men over the age of 60 (Oesterling et al., 1993). Markedly elevated levels of PSA (above 20 ng/ml) are usually strongly suggestive of a prostatic carcinoma (Catalona et al., 1991). Moderate elevations, however, particularly in the range of 4 to 15 ng/ml may be due to a broad variety of disorders, whether benign or malignant. In patients with elevated PSA and absence of a palpable tumor, an ultrasound examination, using a transrectal probe, is often conducted. Ultrasound may reveal small prostatic lesions that are not accessible to palpation but may be biopsied. Regardless of the level of PSA or ultrasound findings, the diagnosis of prostatic carcinoma must be confirmed by morphologic evidence before a therapeutic decision can be reached.

Carcinoma of the prostate is a common disease, affecting primarily elderly males. In one early study, it was shown that at least 20% of males age 50 and above who died of other causes harbored occult prostatic carcinoma (Edwards et al., 1953). It is now estimated that from 20–100% of males living to the age of 75 years and dying of other causes will have microscopic foci of carcinoma in their prostates (summary in Petersen, 1992). Death from prostatic carcinoma is comparatively infrequent. For 1994, the American Cancer Society projected that 200,000 males in the United States would be diagnosed as having prostate cancer but only about 38,000 would die of it (Boring et al., 1994). The stage of the disease is not considered in such statistics. It is likely, therefore, that the annual prevalence rate of 200,000 cases includes all stages of disease, many of the carcinomas being incidental findings in prostatic chips and some discovered by biochemical or ultrasound detection methods. If one were to calculate a ratio of occult to clinically manifest prostatic cancer, it would likely be on the order of 10:1, assuming that there are, at this time (1994) in the United States, about 4 million living males over the age of 75, that half of them have occult carcinoma, and that only 200,000 of them will have the diagnosis established. The ratio of occult carcinoma to death from prostatic cancer, based on the same reasoning, would be approximately 40:1. Similar conclusions have been reached by Gittes (1991). While these figures represent only estimates, they strongly suggest that not all cancers of the prostate have the same behavior and clinical outcome. Such observations raise serious questions as to whether incidentally discovered, small, prostatic carcinomas should be treated at par with clinically overt disease. In fact, it has been repeatedly shown that conservative treatment, particularly in the elderly male, results in excellent long-term survival with a good quality of life, particularly if the carcinoma is well differentiated (Adolfsson et al., 1992; Johansson et al., 1992; Chodak et al., 1994). DNA ploidy of the tumor may also be of significant prognostic value (see Chap. 9). In spite of these reservations, recent data suggest that in the United States surgical resection or radiotherapy for prostatic carcinomas has increased nearly six-fold since 1984 (Lu-Yao et al., 1993), even though the benefits of these therapies are unclear and the consequences may rob the patient of a good quality of life (Wasson et al., 1993). Several voices have been raised against this "American prostatic holocaust" (Koss, 1993) suggesting a more conservative approach to incidentally observed small prostatic cancers (Whitmore, 1993). In fairness, it must be reported that in a study of 157 patients with radical prostatectomies for occult carcinomas, 37% of the tumors were advanced with capsular penetration (Epstein et al., 1994). Even this information, however, casts limited light on the survival of these patients, the effectiveness of the therapy, and the quality of life. These still unresolved issues require further long-term prospective studies, because they have a major impact on a substantial segment of the male population. DNA ploidy measurements and other morphometric parameters of prognostic value in prostatic carcinoma are discussed in Chapter 9. Current studies of molecular genetic parameters are discussed in Chapter 11.

HISTOLOGIC RECALL

Recent studies of the adult prostate, mainly by McNeil (1968, 1981) recognized five histologically distinct regions: (1) an anterior zone, composed mainly of a fibromuscular stroma with few glands; (2) a central zone, surrounding the ejaculatory ducts, corresponding to the middle lobe in previous nomenclature; (3) a peripheral zone, composed of simple glands and loose stroma; (4) a zone composed of periurethral glands in the proximal, membranous part of the urethra; and (5) the zone also known as the transition zone, which contains glands that terminate in the distal prostatic urethra. About 25% of prostatic carcinomas originate in the anterior periurethral transition zone. The peripheral zone, which comprises the posterior lobe of the prostate, is the site of origin of about 70% of prostatic carcinomas. About 5% of carcinomas originate elsewhere in the prostate (McNeil et al., 1988). Benign prostatic hypertrophy originates mainly in the anterior transition zone.

The prostate is composed of glands that are lined by a single layer of cuboidal or columnar cells with clear cytoplasm, surrounded by a layer of basal cells (see Fig. 7-8D). There is considerable controversy about the presence of peripheral myoepithelial cells in histologic material, but there is little doubt that they exist in cytologic samples (see p. 173). The basal cells stain with antibodies to high molecular weight keratin filaments (keratin 903). The reaction is often negative in prostatic carcinoma (Hedrick and Epstein, 1989). The prostatic ducts are lined by cuboidal to columnar cells with granular cytoplasm arranged in a single layer. The terminal portions of the prostatic ducts may be lined by urothelium. The prostatic glands often contain condensed secretions (corpora amylacea) that may become calcified ("prostatic stones"). The prostatic cells secrete prostatic acid phosphatase and prostate-specific antigen. The documentation of these activities by immunochemistry is often helpful in the identification of metastatic prostatic carcinoma. Melanin-producing cells (melanocytes) may be occasionally identified in prostatic glands and stroma (Aguilar et al., 1982).

In recent years, the presence of cells with endocrine features capable of producing several polypeptide hormones such as serotonin, human chorionic gonadotropin, prolactin, and glucagon has been demonstrated in normal prostate and in benign prostatic hypertrophy (Abrahamsson et al., 1986; Aprikian et al., 1993; Di Sant'Agnese, 1992). Such cells are scarce in prostatic carcinoma. The significance of the neuroendocrine cells in the prostate is not understood at the time of this writing (1994). Conceivably these cells contribute to the normal function of the prostate and its hormonal dependence.

The *seminal vesicles* are composed of convoluted tubules terminating in the ejaculatory duct. The tubules are lined by cuboidal to columnar epithelial cells with yellow granular cytoplasmic pigment. The nuclei of such cells are often markedly enlarged and hyperchromatic (Arias-Stella and Tokano-Moron, 1958; Kuo and Gomez, 1981; see Fig. 7-10A). Such cells may mimic cancer cells. The seminal vesicles are a repository of spermatozoa and their precursor cells, often accompanied by macrophages.

TARGETS OF CYTOLOGIC INVESTIGATION

Benign Disorders

There are a few benign conditions affecting the prostate that occasionally may be identified by cytology. Acute prostatitis due to staphyloccocci and other bacterial agents, including *Neisseria gonorrhoeae*, is fairly common. Rarely, Chlamydia and Actinomycosis have been observed (deSouza et al., 1985). *Tri-*

chomonas vaginalis may be identified (Gardner et al., 1986). Fungal infections due to blastomycosis (Inoshita et al., 1983) and coccidioidomycosis (Price et al., 1982) have been described. Cryptoccosis of the prostate has been repeatedly observed (O'Connor et al., 1965; Brooks et al., 1965). More recently, prostatic cryptococcosis has been identified as an important manifestation of AIDS (Lief and Sarfarazi, 1986; Larsen et al., 1989).

Chronic granulomatous prostatitis secondary to tuberculosis is occasionally observed (O'Dea et al., 1978). Similar granulomas may occur in patients treated with bacille Calmette-Guérin for bladder cancer (Oates et al., 1986) and after a surgical procedure (Eyre et al., 1986). Nonspecific granulomatous prostatitis of unknown etiology is characterized by granulomas morphologically similar to those occurring in rheumatoid nodules: areas of hyaline necrosis are surrounded by palisading epithelioid and occasional giant cells (Kelalis et al., 1965; Schmidt, 1965). Eosinophilic granulomas are observed in people with asthma or other forms of allergy (Kelalis et al., 1964). Granulomatous prostatitis may cause stone-hard prostate enlargement and thus may clinically mimic prostatic carcinoma. The lesions can be identified in aspirated material. Prostatic infarcts may also be mistaken for cancer (Baird et al., 1950). Further, such lesions may cause diagnostic problems because of atypical squamous metaplasia that may be observed in adjacent prostatic tissue (Mostofi and Morse, 1951; see also p. 177).

Benign prostatic hypertrophy (hyperplasia) is a common disorder of elderly men. A glandular form with increase in the number of prostatic glands is most frequently observed (see Fig. 7-8*D*). A fibromuscular form, in which the stroma of the prostate is increased, is probably the early form of this disorder (Franks, 1954). Neither form can be diagnosed from cytologic samples because the component cells have no abnormal characteristics.

Atypical Prostatic Hyperplasia (Adenosis)

Under the term "adenosis" Brawn (1982) described a nodular lesion composed of small prostatic glands, difficult to differentiate from a focus of carcinoma. The lesion has been since discussed under the term of "atypical hyperplasia." Bostwick et al. (1993) discussed at length the identification criteria for this lesion with uncertain results (Koss, 1993). The presence of nucleoli in at least some of these lesions casts some doubt on their identity. It is possible that in cytologic material some of the "atypical" smears may correspond to this entity (see p. 180).

Prostatic Carcinoma

Prostatic adenocarcinomas are the principal target of cytologic investigation.

The common prostatic carcinomas originate mainly in the acini and the terminal ducts of the prostatic glands. As discussed above, about 25% of prostatic carcinomas originate in the periurethral transition zone, about 70% in the posterior zone, and 5% elsewhere in the prostate. The tumors are classified according to the configuration of the glands, the relationship of the malignant glands to each other and to the stroma, and their cellular makeup, into three basic groups: well-differentiated, moderately well-differentiated, and poorly differentiated carcinomas (Mostofi, 1975). A more elaborate classification of prostatic carcinomas was proposed by Gleason et al. (1979). Gleason's classification is based on recognition of five patterns, reflecting increased degrees of anaplasia. If two different patterns are present, the grading is the sum of the two. Gleason's grades 2 or 3 correspond to the well-differentiated prostatic carcinomas. Gleason's grades 4 through 6 correspond to the moderately differentiated, and grades 7 and above to the poorly differentiated tumors.

The well-differentiated tumors are composed of glands that differ little from normal except for their cellular makeup and distribution. The cells lining the malignant gland have enlarged, often irregularly configured, nuclei and readily visible nucleoli. In my judgment, easily recognized nucleoli are a definite evidence of a malignant gland, even though it is sometimes proposed that borderline or atypical but not malignant prostatic lesions may also show enlarged nucleoli (Bostwick et al., 1993). The malignant glands vary in size and may be irregularly distributed in the stroma (see Fig. 7-14*A*). It has been proposed that the *absence of staining* of the basal cells with an antibody to high molecular weight keratin (keratin 903) is helpful in identifying cancerous glands in difficult cases (Hedrick and Epstein, 1989).

Moderately differentiated carcinomas show greater crowding of the malignant glands of variable sizes lined by cells with conspicuous nuclear abnormalities in the form of enlargement, hyperchromasia, and prominent nucleoli. The nucleocytoplasmic ratio is clearly shifted in favor of the nuclei.

Poorly differentiated carcinomas are composed of poorly formed glands or may become predominantly solid (see Fig. 7-17*C*). The cells have obvious malignant features. We have observed a few such tumors in younger men in their 50s with a very rapid downhill course. In one of these cases, the initial diagnosis of cancer was rendered in the sediment of voided urine because of a synchronous presence of a carcinoma in situ of the bladder (unpublished data). A similar case was described by Nguen-Ho et al. (1994).

There is good evidence that prostatic carcinomas originating in the anterior (transition) zone of the prostate are better differentiated and less aggressive than tumors originating in the posterior zone. The latter have a higher rate of spread beyond the prostate (McNeil et al., 1988; Greene et al., 1991).

There has been a great deal of discussion in reference to precancerous lesions of prostatic carcinoma, variously known as "dysplasia" (McNeil, 1988) or prostatic intraepithelial neoplasia (PIN) (Epstein, 1989; Bostwick et al., 1993). Briefly, atypical glands and terminal ducts are observed in areas of the prostate adjacent to or remote from documented carcinomas (Quinn et al., 1990). The cells lining the areas of high-grade PIN have some of the characteristics of prostatic carcinoma, to wit nuclear enlargement and visible nucleoli. The terminal ducts may also show a papillary proliferation of the lining. The prognostic significance of such lesions, when observed in prostatic biopsies, remains unknown but calls for additional biopsies and close surveillance of patients (see comments on atypical hyperplasia, p. 180).

Staging of Prostatic Carcinoma

Staging of prostatic carcinoma provides information on the spread of the tumor within or beyond the prostate and is, therefore, of major prognostic significance, particularly in conjunction with tumor grading and measurements of DNA ploidy. In the United States, the stages are designated by letters A, B, C, D, although the international TNM classification system (T = tumor, N = lymph nodes, M = metastases) may also be used.

Stage A. The tumor is clinically occult and is diagnosed by microscopic examination. Stage A_1, tumor is limited to no more than 15% of the tissues; Stage A_2, tumor is diffuse.

Stage B. The tumor is palpable but confined to the prostate. Stage B_1, tumor limited to one lobe; Stage B_2, tumor present in both lobes.

Stage C. The palpable tumor has extended beyond the capsule of the prostate but is localized to periprostatic area. Stage C_1, tumor without spread to seminal vesicles; Stage C_2, tumor involving seminal vesicles.

Stage D. The tumor has metastasized. Stage D_1, tumor metastatic to regional lymphocytes; Stage D_2, distant metastases are present.

The international TNM staging system of prostatic carcinoma is similar to the system used in the United States, with minor modifications.

Stage T_1—microscopically diagnosed occult carcinoma

Stage T_{1a}—three or fewer foci of carcinoma

Stage T_{1b}—more than three foci of carcinoma

Stage T_2—palpable tumor confined to prostate

Stage T_{2a}—tumor in one lobe, less than 1.5 cm in greatest diameter; normal tissue on at least 3 sections

Stage T_{2b}—tumor greater than 1.5 cm in diameter or in both lobes

Stage T_3—tumor invades the apex of prostate, the prostatic capsule, bladder neck, seminal vesicles but is mobile

Stage T_4—tumor is fixed and invasive to adjacent structures

The N component is divided into N_1, indicating metastases to a single lymph node, 2 cm or less in diameter; N_2, tumor metastatic to multiple lymph nodes, none greater than 5 cm in diameter; N_3, lymph node metastases greater than 5 cm in diameter.

The M component indicates distant metastases: M_0, no metastases; M_1, distant metastases.

The staging is particularly important in offering the patient a choice of therapies, as discussed on p. 164.

Uncommon Types of Prostatic Carcinoma

A number of uncommon types of prostatic carcinoma have been described. Because of the limited significance of these tumors in cytologic evaluation of the prostate, only a few key references are provided in the bibliography.

CARCINOMAS OF PROSTATIC DUCTS

Carcinomas of the prostatic ducts are uncommon tumors that may mimic comedo carcinomas of the breast or have a papillary configuration (Dube et al., 1973; Greene et al., 1979). Many of these tumors also have components of the ordinary prostatic carcinoma and have a similar prognosis, except for lesser response to hormonal manipulation. The differential diagnosis must always include urothelial carcinomas, particularly carcinoma in situ, extending to the prostatic ducts, which, in my experience, is much more common (see p. 77).

SQUAMOUS CARCINOMA

There is a handful of reported cases of squamous carcinoma (Gray and Marshall, 1975).

MUCINOUS ADENOCARCINOMA

Many of these tumors have a mucin-producing component and a component of ordinary prostatic carcinoma (Epstein and Lieberman, 1985). There is no significant difference in the prognosis of these tumors (Ro et al., 1990).

ADENOID CYSTIC CARCINOMA

These are exceedingly uncommon tumors, mimicking salivary gland tumors—probably a morphologic variant of ordinary prostatic carcinoma (Young et al., 1988).

ENDOCRINE CARCINOMAS

Carcinomas with evidence of endocrine activity have been described in the prostate as in all other organs (Rojas-Corona et al., 1987; Almagro, 1985). There are no documented behavioral differences of these tumors.

SMALL CELL CARCINOMAS

These very rare tumors akin to oat cell carcinoma are probably of various origins, because only a few had a documented endocrine component (Ro et al., 1987). A small cell component may appear early or late in the natural history of prostatic carcinoma but always indicates a rapid downhill course (Tetu et al., 1987).

CARCINOSARCOMA

These are exceedingly rare malignant tumors, combining features of a carcinoma and spindle cell sarcoma. The prognosis is poor (Wick et al., 1989).

Sarcomas of Prostate

The most common type of sarcoma of prostate is embryonal rhabdomyosarcoma of childhood, identical to bladder tumors (see Chap. 5).

Adult prostatic sarcomas are rare and are for the most part leiomyosarcomas. Rhabdomyosarcomas, osteogenic sarcomas, and angiosarcomas have been reported (MacKenzie et al., 1968; Mostofi and Price, 1973).

METHODS OF INVESTIGATION

Sediment of voided urine after prostatic massage, spontaneously voided urine, and thin needle aspiration biopsy of the prostate are the principal methods of cytologic investigation of the prostate. The three methods are discussed below.

Urinary Sediment After Prostatic Massage

Prostatic massage is usually administered for therapeutic rather than diagnostic purposes. However, in the 1950s attempts were made to use this technique for the diagnosis of occult prostatic carcinoma in normal men (Riaboff, 1954; Richardson et al., 1954). Voided urine sediment, collected after a rigorous prostatic massage, was the medium of diagnosis. Although the results of the study were essentially negative and the project was abandoned, it provided an opportunity to study cells derived from the prostate. Other observers used the prostatic massage technique for diagnosis of prostatic carcinoma in men with enlarged or clinically suspect prostates (Frank et al., 1954, 1958; Bamforth, 1958; Clarke and Bamford, 1960; Garret and Jassie, 1976). The results were modestly encouraging, but the method has now been replaced with direct aspirates and biopsies.

Prostatic Cells in Urinary Sediment After Prostatic Massage

BENIGN DISORDERS

Benign prostatic epithelial cells of normal or hyperplastic prostate origin appear as flat, tightly packed, cohesive clusters of polygonal small cells with small, uniform, spherical nuclei and a moderate amount of basophilic cytoplasm. The borders of the clusters are usually sharply demarcated (Fig. 7-1). The exact origin of such cells cannot be ascertained: they are derived either from the acini or, more likely, from prostatic ducts. The absence of nucleoli, the uniform sizes of the nuclei, and the cohesive nature of the clusters are all landmarks of benign epithelium. Prostatic concretions in the form of spherical, sometimes laminated, bodies are fairly common.

Besides epithelial prostatic cells, the sediment usually contains spermatozoa in various stages of maturation (Fig. 7-2A) and macrophages with ingested spermatozoa (Fig. 7-2B). Characteristically, the heads of the spermatozoa are within the cytoplasm of the macrophages and the flagella remain outside. One can also observe cells of seminal vesicle origin, some of them with large, hyperchromatic nuclei, characterized by cytoplasmic granules of brown pigment (lipofuscin) (Fig. 7-3). For further discussion of seminal vesicle cells in prostatic aspirates, see p. 175.

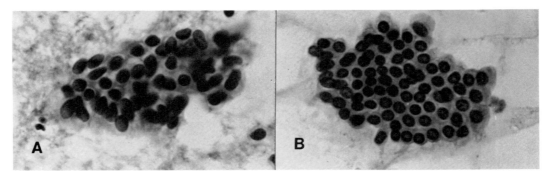

FIGURE 7-1. Urinary sediment after prostatic massage. Two clusters of benign epithelial prostatic cells, originating either in the acini or in the small ducts. Note the cohesive appearance of the clusters and the sharply demarcated periphery. In *A* some of the cells appear elongated (*A,B* × 560. From Koss, L. G.: Diagnostic Cytology and Its Histopathologic Bases. 4th Ed. Philadelphia, J.B. Lippincott, 1992.)

PROSTATIC CARCINOMA

Prostatic cancer cells may be observed in urine sediment obtained after massage, usually in patients with diffusely enlarged prostate or palpable tumors. The cancer cells are usually small and spherical, and are provided with scanty, sometimes vacuolated basophilic cytoplasm, spherical nuclei, and readily visible nucleoli. When such cells are dispersed and few in number, they are difficult to identify and may be confused with small macrophages or even atypical lymphocytes. Fortunately, in most cases the cells form small clusters in which the cells are superimposed on one another. When multiple clusters of monotonous cancer cells are observed, as in Figure 7-4, their origin in the prostate may be strongly suspected, particularly if there is clinical evidence of prostatic enlargement. In unclear clinical situations, however, it is advisable to secure tissue confirmation because similar cancer cells may sometimes reflect metastatic cancer of other primary origin.

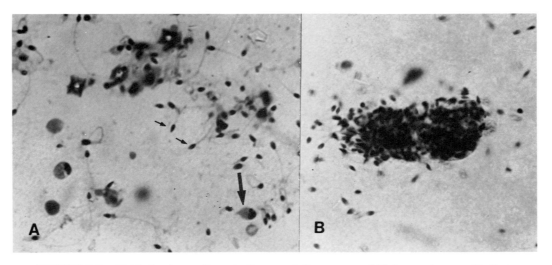

FIGURE 7-2. Voided urine sediment after prostatic massage. (*A*) Spermatozoa with their characteristic dense heads and slender flagella (*small arrows*) and their precursor cells (spermatogonia), seen as small cells with peripheral nuclei and often somewhat elongated, basophilic cytoplasm (*large arrow*). (*B*) A macrophage with numerous engulfed spermatozoa. Numerous spermatozoa may be seen in the background (*A,B* × 560. Modified from Koss, L. G.: Diagnostic Cytology and Its Histopathologic Bases. 4th Ed. Philadelphia, J.B. Lippincott, 1992.)

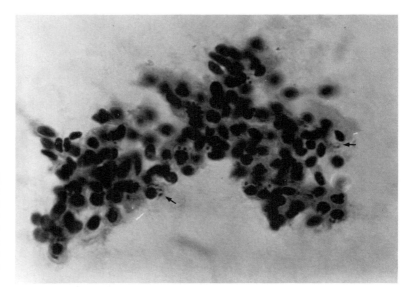

FIGURE 7-3. Voided urine sediment after prostatic massage. A large cluster of epithelial cells derived from the seminal vesicles, recognizable by granules of cytoplasmic pigment (*small arrows*) (× 560). (Modified from Koss, L. G.: Diagnostic Cytology and Its Histopathologic Bases. 4th Ed. Philadelphia, J.B. Lippincott, 1992.)

In some cases, the cancer cells are somewhat larger and may have a columnar shape and spherical nuclei with visible nucleoli (Fig. 7-5). It is the presence of the nucleoli that should direct the attention of the examiner in the direction of the prostate. A biopsy confirmation of the diagnosis is strongly advised.

Voided Urine

Spontaneously voided urine is usually submitted to the laboratory for reasons unrelated to prostatic disease, and the finding of cells derived from the prostate or seminal vesicles in the sediment is a surprise. On further investigation, virtually all of such patients have evidence of a prostatic disorder, and in some of them a prostatic palpation has been performed. Voided urine is not recommended as a primary medium of diagnosis of prostatic disease.

Cells of Prostatic Origin in Voided Urine

BENIGN DISORDERS

It is exceedingly uncommon to observe normal prostatic cells or evidence of benign disorders affecting prostate in spontaneously voided urine. On very rare occasions, the presence of *Trichomonas vaginalis* may suggest prostatic involvement by this common parasite. The gray-green oval organisms, measuring from 10 to 20 μm in greatest diameter and having an eccentric nucleus and flagella, may be sometimes identified. Prostatic trichomoniasis is an important source of trichomoniasis in women. For further de-

scription and discussion of this organism as a pathogenic agent in women, see Koss, 1992.

Voided urine obtained after intercourse may contain spermatozoa and seminal vesicle cells. More often such cells are observed after prostatic massage and in direct aspirates.

PROSTATIC CARCINOMA

Finding and identifying cells of prostatic carcinoma in voided urine sediment is a rare event. The cancer cells may form small clusters but are usually dispersed. Their appearance is identical to cancer cells after prostatic massage, described above (see Figs. 7-4 and 7-5). In the absence of clinical data, the cells may be easily overlooked and their origin is difficult to guess. Voided urine sediment is clearly not a recommended method of diagnosis of prostatic diseases.

There is an important caveat in the diagnosis of prostatic carcinoma either in voided urine or in the urinary sediment after prostatic massage. Even though the prostate may be clinically suspect of harboring a carcinoma, *the cancer cells may reflect a synchronous carcinoma of the bladder.* We have repeatedly observed urothelial carcinomas in situ in patients with prostatic enlargement. Thus, a confirmation of the site of origin of cancer cells is important, particularly because synchronous tumors of bladder and prostate may occur (see also comments on p. 107). De la Rosette, et al. (1993) reported on incidental cancer of the bladder diagnosed in urinary sediment of patients with symptoms of prostatism (see p. 107).

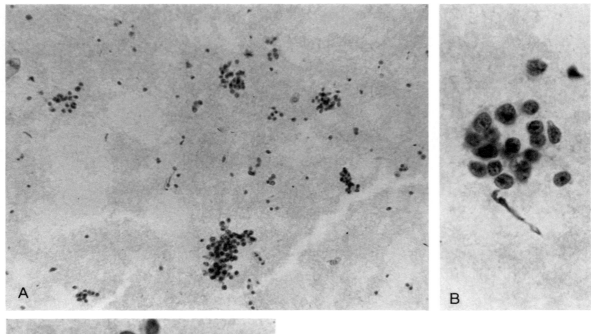

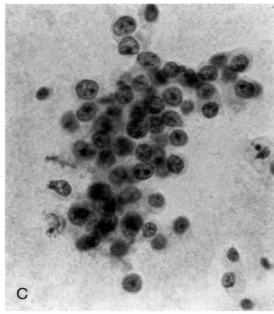

FIGURE 7-4. Prostatic carcinoma cells in voided urine. The elderly patient had an advanced, moderately differentiated carcinoma of the prostate. This observation is exceptional. (*A*) Low-power view of urinary sediment showing multiple clusters of small cells. (*B,C*) High-power view of the clusters. The cancer cells are small, uniform in size, and have a scanty, barely visible rim of cytoplasm, better seen in *C.* The nuclei are generally spherical, somewhat hyperchromatic, and provided with small but well visible nucleoli (*A* × 150, *B,C* × 560).

Aspiration Biopsy of the Prostate

Several methods of biopsy of the prostate have evolved since 1930. The method of "needle puncture and aspiration" was first suggested by Ferguson in 1930. The current two modalities of prostate sampling are the thin (fine) needle aspiration biopsy and a pistol-type core biopsy with instruments suitable for sampling either palpable lesions or lesions localized by ultrasound. Many urologists prefer to use the core biopsy instrument because of the relative ease with which the procedure can be employed (Brenner et al., 1990; Narayan et al., 1991). Still, thin needle aspiration biopsy with the Franzén instrument has its proponents, as it is often more informative than the tissue core biopsy. Furthermore, the prostatic aspiration

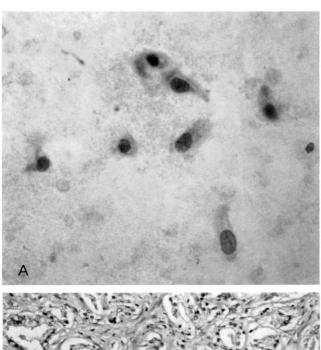

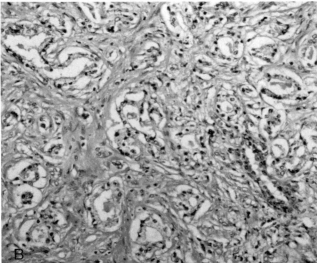

FIGURE 7-5. Voided urine sediment after prostatic massage. (*A*) Prostatic carcinoma cells of columnar configuration. (*B*) Histologic section of prostatic carcinoma in the same case (*A* × 560; *B* × 150).

smear is a much better medium than a tissue biopsy for measurements of DNA (Ackerman and Miller, 1977; see also Chap. 9).

The Aspiration Biopsy Procedure

The *instrument* devised by Franzén et al. in 1960 consists of a needle guide with a funnel-like, enlarged opening to facilitate the introduction of the needle. The guide is provided with a ring for the index finger and an adjustable thenar plate for placement in the palm of the hand. A specially constructed thin needle of appropriate length, attached to a syringe with a single hand grip (Franzén's syringe), completes the apparatus (Fig. 7-6*A*).

THE PROCEDURE

The prostate is palpated and the target area(s) identified. With the patient in a lithotomy position, the operator places the needle guide on the gloved hand, making sure that the tip of the index finger is free. The needle guide should fit snugly onto the operator's palm, and the position of the thenar plate must be adjusted and secured by the screw that fastens it to the needle guide (Fig. 7-6*B*). A rubber finger cot is then

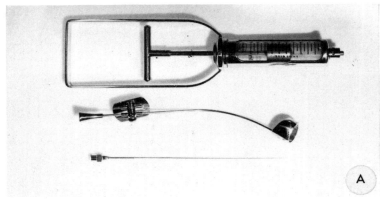

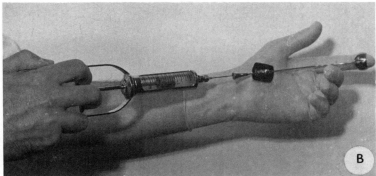

FIGURE 7-6. (*A*) The apparatus invented by Franzén for prostatic aspirations—see text for description. (*B*) The position of the needle guide and the needle in the operator's hand. For description of procedure, see text.

rolled over the finger holding the needle guide tip. This serves two purposes: (1) it assists in holding the guide onto the finger; (2) it minimizes the contamination of the needle guide (and thus of the needle) by lubricant or fecal material. The patient's anus is lubricated with sterile lubricant, and the index finger with the needle guide introduced until the patient's prostate, with the previously identified area of interest, is palpated (Fig. 7-7). At this point the needle is introduced. The needle is so constructed that only about 1 cm of its tip is free. Further extension of the needle is prevented by a thickened portion of the needle shaft that does not fit into the guide.

The needle is inserted into the prostate through the rectal wall, and a vacuum is created within the syringe. Several rapid to-and-fro movements of the needle within the palpable abnormalities are executed. It is important to aspirate the lesions repeatedly by partial withdrawal and reinsertion of the tip of the needle, which *must remain within the prostate during this procedure.*

Prior to withdrawal of the syringe, *the pull on the grip of the syringe must be released and the pressure equalized.* Otherwise, rectal contents will be aspirated during withdrawal of the syringe and the procedure will be of no diagnostic value.

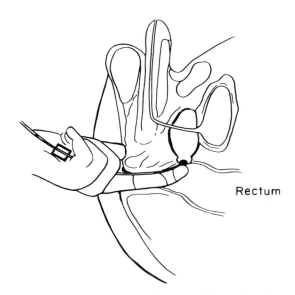

Rectum

FIGURE 7-7. Position of the tip of the index finger with needle guide in reference to the palpable prostatic nodule.

After removal, the needle is detached from the syringe, a new vacuum is created in the syringe, the needle is reattached, and the contents of the syringe are expelled onto two to four clean slides, making sure that not more than one tiny drop of the material is placed on each slide. Smears are prepared by placing another clean slide on the drop of expelled material until an even, thin spread is achieved. The smears are either air-dried for May-Gruenwald-Giemsa or similar staining or are immediately placed in 95% ethanol fixative prior to staining with the Papanicolaou method. The syringe and the needle are then rinsed with the fixative, and this material is used for the preparation of additional cytocentrifuge slides. In our laboratories Papanicolaou stain gives satisfactory results. Other observers use air-dried material stained with May-Gruenwald-Giemsa or similar stains. For further comments on techniques of smear preparation, see Ljung, 1992.

If more than one area of the prostate is of interest, new needle(s) and syringe(s) should be kept handy. After the completion of the first aspirate, *with the operator's index finger still in the rectum,* the finger is redirected to the next abnormality and the aspiration procedure is repeated, using a new needle. An attempt to redirect the same needle while inserted into the prostate can result in extensive tissue damage and hemorrhage.

Contraindications and Complications

Experienced observers agree unanimously that *only prostates with palpable abnormalities should be aspirated.* The primary targets should be palpable nodules regardless of size, but diffusely enlarged prostates can also be aspirated as they may sometimes harbor occult carcinomas.

Acute or subacute prostatitis are the principal contraindications to aspiration. The aspiration may cause a febrile reaction, bacteremia, or even a Gram-negative septicemia. Patients with rheumatic or rheumatoid arthritis appear to be at high risk for a febrile reaction. However, Esposti et al. (1975) indicated that in 10% of patients with a past history of prostatitis, carcinoma was diagnosed on aspiration.

Serious complications in the form of severe septicemia, one with a fatal outcome, were reported by Zajicek (1979) in four of several thousand patients investigated by thin needle aspiration biopsy. Other complications such as transient hematospermia, transient hematuria, and epididymitis were observed in 0.4% of over 3,000 patients. A case of perineal seeding of prostatic carcinoma after a needle aspiration was reported by Addonizio and Kapoor (1976). In general, the procedure appears to be safe for the majority of patients. In over 3,000 prostate aspirations carried out at Montefiore Medical Center, Bronx, New York, no complications were observed.

Targets of Aspiration Biopsy

The following entities must be considered in the evaluation of prostatic aspirates: (1) inflammatory disorders (nonspecific acute or chronic prostatitis and granulomatous prostatitis); (2) hyperplasia; (3) infarcts; (4) adenocarcinoma (of acinar or ductal origin); and (5) rare tumors of prostatic origin, tumors of adjacent organs invading the prostate, and metastases from distant sites.

The relatively small number of diseases resulting in palpatory abnormalities renders the evaluation of prostatic aspirates relatively uncomplicated. For all practical purposes, the most important target of aspirates is the diagnosis of prostatic adenocarcinoma and the determination of its grade of differentiation.

CYTOLOGY OF ASPIRATES

Benign Cell Populations

Prostatic Glands and Ducts

As stated above, normal prostate should not be aspirated. However, essentially normal cells are aspirated from patients with benign prostatic hyperplasia (Fig. 7-8D). Cells of prostatic glands or acini form cohesive, flat sheets of uniform cells with central round or oval nuclei and clear, basophilic cytoplasm (Fig. 7-8 A,B). The cell membranes are readily observed, are well demarcated, and form an orderly "honeycomb" pattern. The nuclei are of even sizes with finely granular, evenly distributed chromatin. The nucleoli are either absent or tiny and barely visible (Fig. 7-8C). Although the existence of myoepithelial cells around the prostatic acini is disputed (see p. 164), such cells may be recognized in smears by their small, spindly, darkly-stained nuclei, which either adhere to the periphery of the epithelial cell clusters or overlap the clusters (Fig. 7-8C). We have not identified any endocrine cells in prostatic aspirates (see p. 164). Prostatic concretions, the so-called corpora amylacea, are commonly seen (Fig. 7-8E).

Common Cellular Contaminants

Transrectal thin-needle aspirates of the prostate may yield cells from adjacent organs, usually as a result of procedural errors at the time of aspiration. Cells of rectal mucosa and seminal vesicles are most frequently seen.

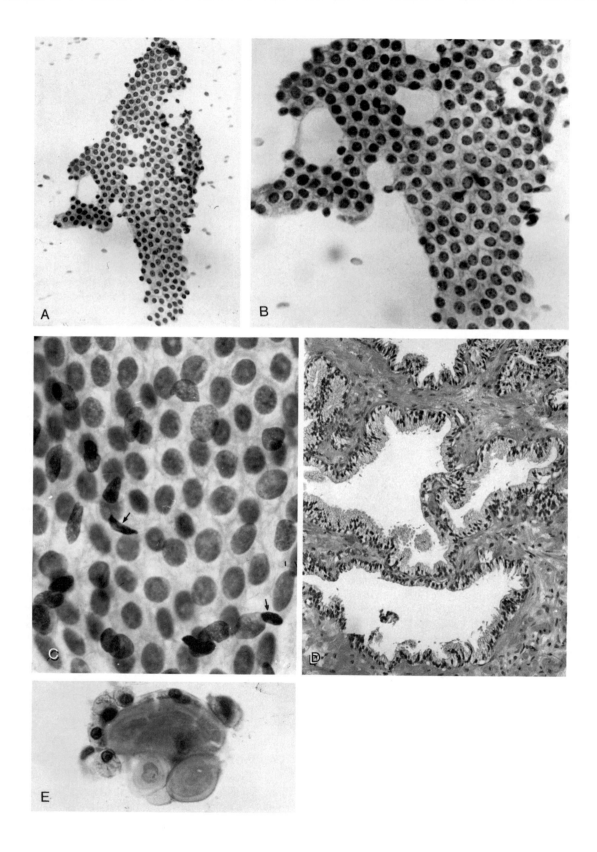

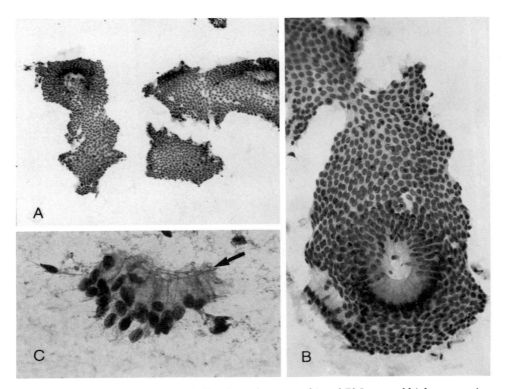

FIGURE 7-9.   Prostatic aspirate. Cells of rectal mucosa. (*A* and *B*) Low- and high-power view of sheets of rectal epithelial cells. In *B* a central gland formation may be noted. *C* shows a small cluster of detached columnar epithelial cells with peripheral nuclei and mucus secretion on the luminal surface (*arrow*). (*A* × 100; *B* × 200; *C* × 400.)

THE CELLS OF RECTAL MUCOSA

Cells of rectal mucosa are aspirated if the operator does not equalize the syringe negative pressure before withdrawing the needle from the prostate. Such cells are columnar, mucus-secreting cells with small, peripheral nuclei. In smears, these cells, which are much larger than the prostatic cells, may form large, cohesive sheets with a "honeycomb" appearance. Within these sheets, glandular structures may be observed (Fig. 7-9 *A,B*). At the periphery of the clusters, the columnar cells may form a palisade arrange-

ment. Detached rectal epithelial cells are of columnar configuration, and have uniform, small oval nuclei located in the basal portion of the cell. The cytoplasm is clear and transparent. Mucus secretion may be observed at the luminal border of the cells (Fig. 7-9C).

CELLS FROM THE SEMINAL VESICLES

The seminal vesicles may be inadvertently penetrated during the prostatic aspiration. The aspirate may show the contents of the seminal vesicles and cells derived from their epithelial lining. The epithe-

----

FIGURE 7-8.   Prostatic aspirate. Benign epithelial cells. Low- (*A*) and high-power (*B*) view of benign prostatic epithelial cells. The cells form flat, cohesive clusters wherein cell borders are well seen and form a honeycomb pattern, best seen in *B* (see also Fig. 7-1). (*C*) Higher power view of another benign cell cluster. The nuclei are centrally located, finely granular, and uniformly spherical. There are no visible nucleoli. Several comma-shaped or spindly, dark nuclei may be observed (*small arrows*). Such nuclei are of myoepithelial cell origin. (*D*) Histologic section of benign prostatic hyperplasia, corresponding to *C*. (*E*) Prostatic concretions, surrounded by macrophages. (*A* × 200; *B* × 400; *C* × 800; *D* × 150; *E* × 500. Modified from Koss, L. G., Woyke, S., and Olszewski, W.: Aspiration Biopsy. Cytologic Interpretation and Histologic Bases. 2nd Ed. New York, Igaku-Shoin, 1992.)

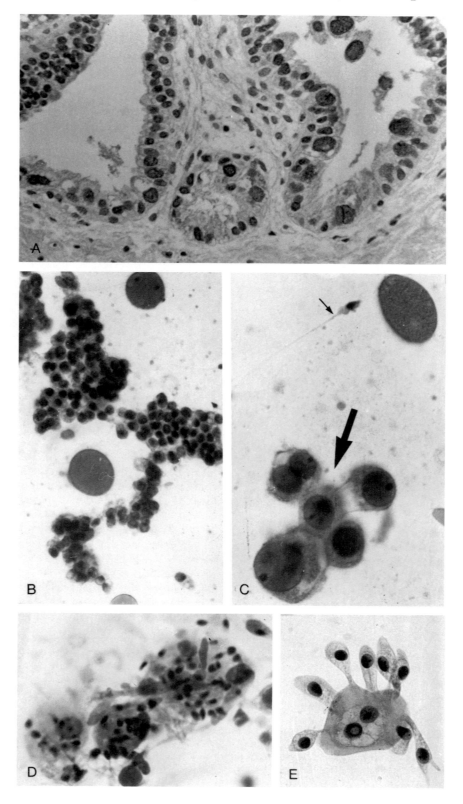

lial cells derived from the lining of the seminal vesicles are larger than the cells of normal prostatic glands and have an oval, triangular, or cylindrical shape (Fig. 7-10A). In aspirates, these cells may appear singly but usually form clusters, accompanied by globules of inspissated secretions (Fig. 7-10B). Some of the epithelial cells have large, homogeneous hyperchromatic nuclei of variable sizes, occasionally four or eight times larger than normal prostatic nuclei, reflecting polyploidy (Fig. 7-10C). Such nuclei appear opaque and diffusely hyperchromatic, sometimes with coarse chromatin texture. There are no visible nucleoli. The cytoplasm is abundant and vacuolated and contains the characteristic coarse, granular, brown-yellow lipofuscin pigment (see also Fig. 7-4). Spermatids, spermatozoa, and macrophages containing ingested sperm are a common accompaniment of seminal vesicle cells (Fig. 7-10D).

Seminal vesicle cells, particularly when they occur singly, are an important source of a potential diagnostic error, because they may be mistaken for cells of an anaplastic cancer. The presence of cytoplasmic pigment and of accompanying spermatozoa usually allows for an easy differential diagnosis.

UROTHELIAL CELLS

The accidental penetration of the tip of the needle into the urethra or the bladder may occur and may result in aspiration of urothelial cells. These are very large, flat, often multinucleated superficial cells (umbrella cells) and smaller, often elongated or polygonal urothelial cells from the depth of the epithelium (Fig. 7-10E; see also Chap. 2). Occasionally cells of urothelial carcinoma extending into prostatic ducts may be observed. This may be particularly important in the presence of occult or known carcinoma in situ of the bladder as it may lead to recognition of extension of the process into the prostate (see pp. 77 and 107).

SQUAMOUS CELLS

Squamous cells in deep prostatic aspirates may originate in squamous epithelium of the urethral lining or in patches of squamous epithelium lining the bladder. In prostatic infarcts the adjacent prostatic glands and ducts may also undergo squamous metaplasia that may be atypical (Mostofi and Morse, 1951; Koss et al., 1992). In such cases the cytology may be misleading because the aspirate may show atypical squamous cells (see below and Fig. 7-11C).

In patients with prostatic cancer treated with estrogens and related substances, the lining of the cancerous glands often becomes squamous (Fig. 7-11A). The aspirated squamous cells are of the intermediate type and are rich in glycogen, which may fill the cytoplasm and displace the nucleus to the periphery (Fig. 7-11B). Such cells closely resemble the "navicular" cells observed in vaginal and cervical smears of pregnant women (see p. 30). Cells aspirated from actively growing squamous epithelium, for example, from an area adjacent to an infarct, display large, somewhat hyperchromatic nuclei provided with visible nucleoli. The cytoplasm is abundant and either basophilic or eosinophilic, often showing cytoplasmic extensions (Fig. 7-11C). Such cells are significantly larger than the prostatic cells and mimic the so-called "repair reaction" sometimes observed in endocervical smears (Koss, 1992).

GANGLION CELLS AND MEGAKARYOCYTES

Prostatic aspirates performed by inexperienced operators may result in inadvertent aspiration of ganglion cells from the periprostatic plexus (Fig. 7-12). Rarely, the tip of the needle may penetrate the sacrum and bone marrow cells may be observed in the aspirate, the most conspicuous cells being the large multilobate megakaryocytes (Greenebaum, 1988).

Prostatitis

It has been emphasized above that prostatitis is one of the contraindications to prostatic aspiration biopsy. Nonetheless, there are clinical situations in which prostatitis may mimic, and thus must be differentiated from, prostatic carcinoma. For this reason, a description of the dominant cytologic features is given below.

FIGURE 7-10. (A) Histologic section of a seminal vesicle with numerous large, polyploid epithelial cells. (B–D) Aspirate of seminal vesicles. B shows a sheet of small epithelial cells and several spherical globules of inspissated secretions. (C) A cluster of seminal vesicle cells (*large arrow*) with homogeneous, dark, very large nuclei and dark pigment granules in the cytoplasm. A spermatozoon (*small arrow*) and a globule of inspissated secretions are also shown. (D) Spermatozoa and macrophages (see also Fig. 7-3). (E) A cluster of urothelial cells in prostatic aspirate. A binucleated umbrella cell (*center*) with several epithelial cells from the deeper epithelial layer attached is shown. (A × 350; B × 450; C × 1,000; D × 800; E × 400. B–E modified from Koss, L. G., Woyke, S., and Olszewski, W.: Aspiration Biopsy. Cytologic Interpretation and Histologic Bases. 2nd Ed. Igaku-Shoin, New York, 1992.)

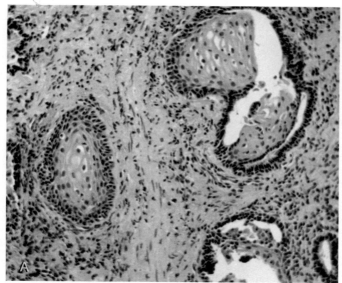

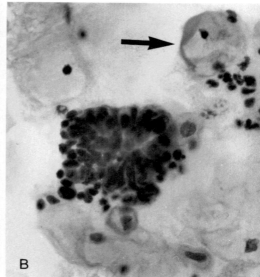

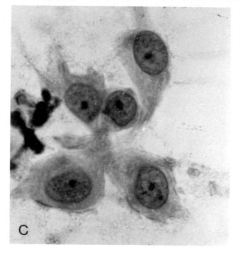

FIGURE 7-11. Squamous metaplasia of prostate in patients treated with estrogens and estrogen substitutes. (*A*) Histologic section of prostatic carcinoma treated with Stilbestrol, showing extensive squamous metaplasia of cancerous glands. (*B*) Prostatic aspirate. A cluster of prostatic cancer cells, surrounded by numerous squamous cells. Several of the squamous cells show cytoplasmic deposits of glycogen, pushing the nuclei to the periphery (*arrow*). These are the so-called navicular cells. (*C*) Prostatic aspirate. A small cluster of immature squamous cells aspirated from an area of squamous metaplasia (patient treated with estrogens for prostatic carcinoma). (*A* × 150; *B* × 560; *C* × 1,000. *C* modified from Koss, L. G., Woyke, S., and Olszewski, W.: Aspiration Biopsy. Cytologic Interpretation and Histologic Bases. 2nd Ed. New York, Igaku-Shoin, 1992.)

ACUTE PROSTATITIS

Acute inflammation of the prostate is usually attributable to gonococcal infection and occasionally to other microorganisms. Acute prostatitis may sometimes follow a surgical intervention such as cystoscopy. The inflammatory reaction may be diffuse or circumscribed and may result in abscess formation. The clinical features of acute prostatitis are usually very characteristic and do not require morphologic confirmation. In the rare instances when an aspiration is performed, the cytologic pattern is that of an acute inflammatory process. Thus, there is evidence of necrosis, a large population of neutrophils accompanied by macrophages, and a few sheets of epithelial cells.

The epithelial cells often show evidence of necrosis such as cytoplasmic vacuoles and nuclear pyk-

nosis. Occasionally, reactive epithelial cells may show enlarged nuclei and conspicuous nucleoli. Although the presence of nucleoli within prostatic epithelial cells is of great significance in the diagnosis of prostatic carcinoma, the background of smears in acute prostatitis, showing evidence of purulent exudate and necrosis, should prevent the false diagnosis of cancer. *In fact, the cytologic diagnosis of prostatic carcinoma must be avoided or rendered with extreme care if the smears show evidence of inflammation.*

CHRONIC AND NON-SPECIFIC GRANULOMATOUS PROSTATITIS

The aspirates of chronic prostatitis are characterized by a variety of cellular components. Besides lymphocytes and plasma cells, macrophages with

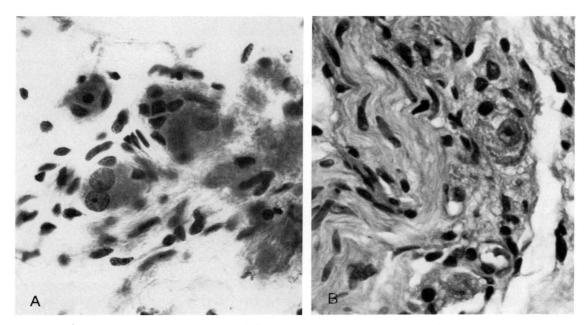

FIGURE 7-12. Prostatic aspirate. (*A*) Ganglion cells with double nuclei and prominent nucleoli, surrounded by strands of spindly cells, possibly nerve fibers (× 560). (*B*) Section of a transrectal core biopsy in the same case, with a ganglion cell embedded within a nerve bundle. It was postulated that this tissue fragment originated in the capsule of the prostate. (Photographs courtesy of Dr. Ellen Greenebaum. Modified from Greenebaum, E.: Megakaryocytes and ganglion cells mimicking cancer in fine needle aspiration of the prostate. Acta Cytol., *32*, 504, 1988, with permission.)

foamy cytoplasm, as well as multinucleated giant cells of foreign body or Langhans' type may be observed (Fig. 7-13). The epithelial cells are usually arranged in small clusters with evenly distributed nuclei. Occasionally, epithelial cells display some atypia. Again, the diagnosis of prostatic cancer must be avoided in the presence of inflammation.

GRANULOMATOUS PROSTATITIS CAUSED
BY SPECIFIC ORGANISMS

Tuberculous prostatitis may be identified in aspirated material by the presence of necrotic material and clusters of elongated, slender epithelioid cells accompanied by giant cells of Langhans' type (Koss et al.,

FIGURE 7-13. Aspirate of chronic prostatitis. A small cluster of benign prostatic cells (*small arrow*) is accompanied by leukocytes and macrophages, one of which is multinucleated and resembles a Langhans' giant cell (*large arrow*) (× 400). (Modified from Koss, L. G., Woyke, S., and Olszewski, W.: Aspiration Biopsy. Cytologic Interpretation and Histologic Bases. 2nd Ed. New York, Igaku-Shoin, 1992.)

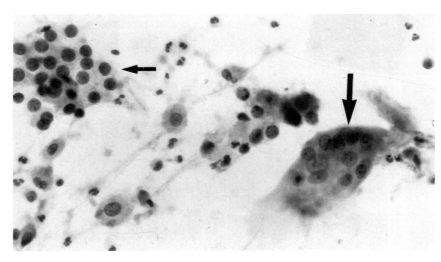

1992). The diagnosis must be confirmed by bacteriologic study. Tubercles have also been observed in the prostates of patients treated with bacille Calmette-Guérin for tumors of the urinary bladder (see p. 48 and Oates et al., 1988). For a description of the cytologic findings, see p. 47.

So far we have not observed in aspirates any cases of prostatitis secondary to other specific organisms, such as fungi (see p. 165).

Hyperplasia of Prostatic Glands (Benign Prostatic Hypertrophy)

The typical smears in prostatic glandular hyperplasia contain epithelial cells arranged in monolayered cohesive sheets and in clusters (see Fig. 7-8 A–C). The sheets are composed of closely fitting polygonal cells with distinctly outlined cytoplasmic borders resulting in a honeycomb configuration. The small, round, central nuclei of these cells are evenly distributed without crowding or overlapping. The nuclei have fine, granular, evenly distributed chromatin with few chromocenters and either no visible nucleoli or, at most, tiny, inconspicuous nucleoli. The cytoplasm is pale and finely granular. The small, oval, or spindly hyperchromatic nuclei of myoepithelial cells occasionally may be observed at the periphery or within the sheets of epithelial cells. At times the aspirates may contain a few benign squamous cells corresponding to foci of squamous metaplasia. Scarce inflammatory cells, mainly lymphocytes and plasma cells, may be present and reflect a chronic inflammatory reaction that may also be observed in histologic material. Occasionally the smears contain small fragments of prostatic stroma composed of spindly, elongated cells with elongated nuclei. Sharp, pointed ends of the nuclei suggest fibroblasts, whereas blunt, rounded ends are most consistent with smooth muscle cells.

ATYPICAL HYPERPLASIA

On rare occasions the sheets and the clusters of epithelial cells are atypical. While the cells are still cohesive, the cell borders may be somewhat blurred and the nuclei may become slightly larger and more hyperchromatic. Very small nucleoli may be observed under high dry power objective or with oil immersion. Such sheets are not diagnostic of carcinoma per se, but must trigger the search for single cancer cells with more classic features such as hyperchromatic, large nuclei and readily discernible nucleoli. If no cancer cells can be identified, the atypia should be reported and further investigation suggested. For further comments, see p. 165 and below under prostatic intraepithelial neoplasia (PIN).

Prostatic Carcinoma

Properly obtained thin needle aspirates of carcinoma of the prostate are usually rich in cancer cells that are either dispersed or arranged in irregular clusters (Fig. 7-14B). The relative proportion of cells in clusters to dispersed cells depends on the degree of tumor differentiation and varies from patient to patient. With increasing grade of the tumor, the proportion of single cancer cells increases.

The cell clusters are generally characterized by overlapping of cells, which, under low power, gives them a thick, crowded, three-dimensional appearance (Fig. 7-14 B,C). On closer scrutiny the relationship of the cells within the clusters is disturbed and lacks the orderly "honeycomb" appearance of evenly spaced cells with well-demarcated cell borders that characterizes benign prostatic cells. The periphery of the cancerous clusters is often loosely structured, with single cells becoming readily detached during smear preparation, a testimony to the poor adhesiveness of cancer cells. The small, dark nuclei of the myoepithelial cells, commonly observed in benign conditions, are virtually never seen in clusters of cancer cells.

The cell changes in prostatic cancer are best studied in single dispersed cells or in small cell clusters, in which there is an obvious change in the nucleocytoplasmic ratio in favor of the enlarged nuclei. Furthermore, the nuclei are often hyperchromatic with coarsely granular chromatin and are provided

FIGURE 7-14. Histologic presentation and aspirate of a moderately well-differentiated prostatic adenocarcinoma. (*A*) Histologic presentation: the tumor is composed of malignant glands. (*B*) Low-power view of aspiration smear to show numerous, irregularly structured clusters of superimposed malignant cells. (*C*) A somewhat higher power view of the squared area of *B* to document the multilayered configuration of the cluster and numerous dispersed small clusters (*arrow*) and single cancer cells. (*D*) A high-power view of the cluster marked with an arrow in *C*. Note the wreath-like arrangement of cancer cells around a lumen (microglandular complex). The characteristic nuclear features of prostatic carcinoma are well shown: nuclear enlargement, irregular contour, hyperchromasia, and the presence of prominent nucleoli in coarsely granular nuclei. (*A* × 300; *B* × 100; *C* × 300; *D* × 800. Modified in part from Koss, L. G., Woyke, S., and Olszewski, W.: Aspiration Biopsy. Cytologic Interpretation and Histologic Bases. 2nd Ed. New York, Igaku-Shoin, 1992.)

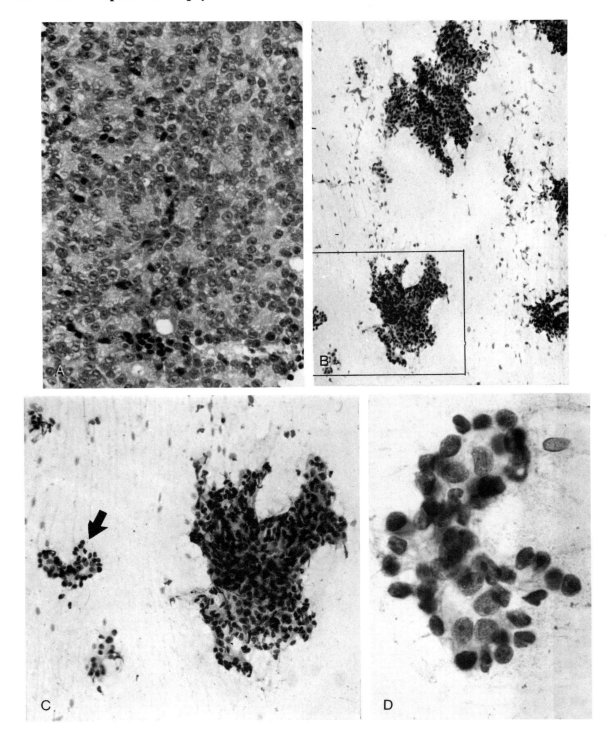

TABLE 7-1
Differential Diagnosis of Prostatic Cancer

	Benign hyperplasia	Well-Differentiated Carcinoma	Moderately Differentiated Carcinoma	Poorly Differentiated Carcinoma
Cell clusters	Flat, cohesive	Rarely flat and cohesive, often thick	Usually thick, loose	Rare, thick
Honeycombing	Conspicuous	Rare	Absent	Absent
Myoepithelial cell nuclei	Present	Exceptional	None	None
Detached single epithelial cells	Few with normal nuclei	Few with abnormal nuclei	About equally represented as clusters, abnormal nuclei	Dominant, highly abnormal nuclei
Nuclei	Round, oval, about equal in size, homogeneous	Hyperchromatic, enlarged	Hyperchromatic, large	Hyperchromatic and bizarre
Nucleoli	Absent or tiny	Present	Conspicuous	Conspicuous
Mitoses	Absent	Exceptional	Present	Conspicuous, often abnormal

(From Koss, L. G., Thin-needle aspiration biopsy of the prostate. Urol. Clin. N. Am. *11*, 237–251, 1984.

with conspicuous, sometimes multiple nucleoli of various sizes (Fig. 7-14*D*). The presence of enlarged nucleoli is one of the most secure morphologic features of prostatic carcinoma, which, however, should be supported by other evidence before the diagnosis is unequivocally established. Table 7-1 summarizes the principal points of differential diagnosis of benign and malignant prostatic lesions.

Significant morphologic differences may be observed in aspirates according to grade of tumor.

WELL-DIFFERENTIATED ADENOCARCINOMA

Aspirates of well-differentiated adenocarcinomas (Gleason's grade 2 to 3), tumors which in tissue sec-

tions shows very well-formed glands, are the principal source of diagnostic difficulty. In rare cases the cancer cells may form flat sheets with well-demarcated cell borders forming a "honeycomb" pattern, distinguished from benign cells only by the enlarged nuclei with readily visible nucleoli. Occasionally, the use of an oil-immersion lens is helpful in ascertaining the presence of large nucleoli. In such cases the search for detached cancer cells or small cell clusters with nuclear features of cancer is mandatory (Fig. 7-15). In the absence of single cancer cells, the diagnosis of carcinoma should be held in abeyance until additional cytologic or histologic evidence is secured.

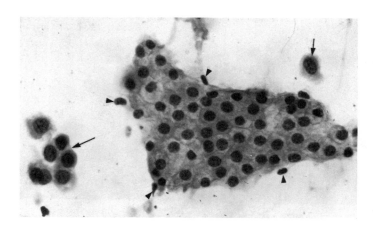

FIGURE 7-15. Aspirate of prostatic carcinoma. The dominant cell cluster shows the honeycomb arrangement of cells, characteristic of benign prostatic epithelium and several myoepithelial cells (*arrowheads*). The only abnormality is slight nuclear enlargement and hyperchromasia (see also Fig. 7-8*B*). The detached cell clusters (*arrows*) show significant nuclear enlargement and hyperchromasia. Such smears are suspicious of prostatic carcinoma but may also reflect the presence of prostatic intraepithelial neoplasia (PIN, see p. 185). (× 400. Modified from Koss, L. G., Woyke, S., and Olszewski, W.: Aspiration Biopsy. Cytologic Interpretation and Histologic Bases. 2nd Ed. New York, Igaku-Shoin, 1992.)

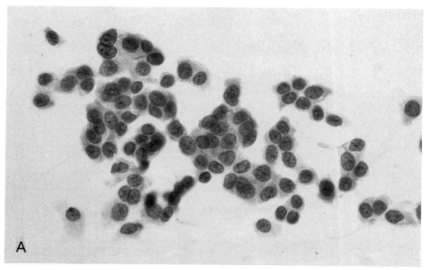

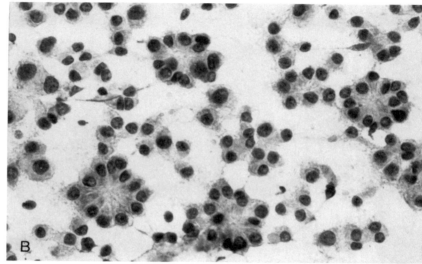

FIGURE 7-16. Aspirates of well-differentiated prostatic adenocarcinomas. Examples of microglandular complexes. In *A* the lumen is empty. Note the conspicuous small nucleoli. In *B* the lumen is filled with the cytoplasm of the cancer cells. Note the wreath-like arrangement of the nuclei forming the periphery of the microglandular complexes. (× 400. Modified from Koss, L. G., Woyke, S., and Olszewski, W.: Aspiration Biopsy. Cytologic Interpretation and Histologic Bases. 2nd Ed. New York, Igaku-Shoin, 1992.)

Fortunately, such cases are rare. More commonly, the well-differentiated carcinomas are characterized by the so-called *microglandular complexes,* described by Franzén et al. (1960), Esposti (1966), and Zajicek (1979). A microglandular complex is a loosely arranged, approximately circular cluster of cells centered around a vaguely defined lumen. The lumen is either empty or filled with poorly defined cytoplasmic extensions of the cells. The nuclei, which are arranged in a wreath-like fashion around the periphery of the lumen, are always larger than normal, often hyperchromatic, and are usually provided with conspicuous nucleoli (Figs. 7-14*D,* 7-16). The association of large, thick clusters of atypical cells with microglandular complexes is diagnostic of well-

differentiated prostatic carcinoma, even in the absence of single cells. With experience the microglandular complexes alone are sufficient for diagnosis.

MODERATELY AND POORLY DIFFERENTIATED ADENOCARCINOMA

Aspirates from cancers of this type cause little diagnostic difficulty. As noted in Table 7-1, the difference between moderately differentiated carcinoma (Gleason's grade 4 to 6) and poorly differentiated carcinomas (Gleason's grade 7 or higher) is based mainly on the presence of cancer cell clusters, which are frequent in moderately differentiated tumors (Fig. 7-17) and few in number or absent in poorly differentiated tumors (Fig. 7-18). The morphologic features of

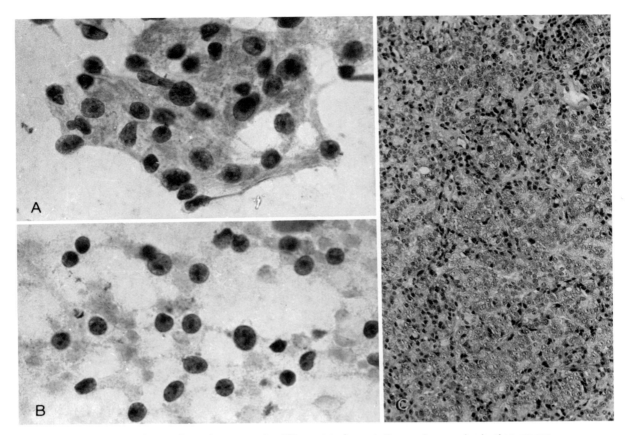

FIGURE 7-17.   Moderately to poorly differentiated prostatic carcinoma. Aspiration smear and tissue pattern. (*A*) A cluster of cancer cells with marked nuclear variability and poorly preserved, wispy cytoplasm. (*B*) Isolated nuclei of cancer cells. The remnants of the poorly preserved cytoplasm appear as grayish areas around the nuclei. (*C*) Tissue section. (*A,B* × 800; *C* × 150. Modified from Koss, L. G., Woyke, S., and Olszewski, W.: Aspiration Biopsy. Cytologic Interpretation and Histologic Bases. 2nd Ed. New York, Igaku-Shoin, 1992.)

cancer are usually obvious because of great variability in size and configuration of cancer cells with conspicuous nuclear abnormalities. Nuclear hyperchromasia and coarse texture of the chromatin are the rule. Mitotic figures, sometimes abnormal, are fairly common. Various bizarre cell abnormalities, such as cell-in-cell arrangement, may be observed (Fig. 7-18). The differential diagnosis comprises the rare metastatic cancers or cancers of adjacent organs invading the prostate.

Among the latter, one must signal high-grade carcinomas of the bladder, which may invade the prostate along the prostatic ducts. In fact, simultaneous carcinomas of the bladder and the prostate are not at all rare in our experience, and in such patients the problems of differential diagnosis may become ex-

tremely difficult even with ample tissue evidence, let alone in an aspirate.

CARCINOMAS OF PROSTATIC DUCTS

There is limited information on the cytologic presentation of carcinomas originating in prostatic ducts, perhaps because of the rarity of these tumors (Dube et al., 1973; Greene et al., 1979). Also, many of these tumors may have an acinar component lined by cells identical with the ductal tumors. There are no documented differences in cytologic presentation between the ductal and the acinar tumors.

Of somewhat greater interest is the invasion of prostatic ducts by occult urothelial carcinomas that can be mistaken for primary prostatic duct cancer. The urothelial cancer cells usually occur singly and

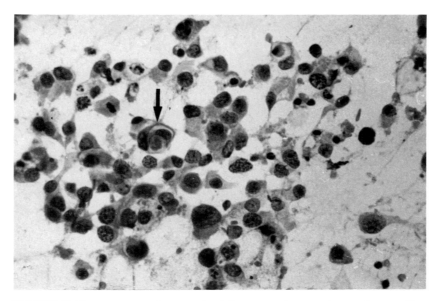

FIGURE 7-18. Aspirate of a poorly differentiated prostatic carcinoma. The smear is characterized by dispersed, conspicuously abnormal cancer cells. Note the cell-in-cell arrangement (*arrow*). ($\times$ 400.)

have a sharply demarcated periphery and large, hyperchromatic nuclei. It is common for these cells to have an eosinophilic cytoplasm, suggestive of an epidermoid component, quite different from cells of prostatic carcinoma. (For further description of urothelial cancer cells, see Chapter 5.)

PROSTATIC INTRAEPITHELIAL NEOPLASIA (PIN) (PROSTATIC "DYSPLASIA")

As discussed on p. 166, much recent writing has been dedicated to the recognition of precursor lesions of prostatic carcinoma. The cytologic presentation of prostatic intraepithelial neoplasia (PIN) is unknown. It may well be that the cytologic patterns observed in atypical hyperplasia (see above) correspond to PIN (see Fig. 7-15). It is also possible that PIN was present in some of the rare cases of benign prostatic hyperplasia with aneuploid DNA pattern (see p. 270). The issue is obviously important, but many years of follow-up of untreated patients may be required before the prognostic significance of these abnormalities becomes clear.

Cytologic Grading of Prostatic Carcinomas

Grading and staging of prostatic cancers may have significant therapeutic and clinical implications. The Swedish experience suggests that asymptomatic patients with very well-differentiated adenocarcinomas, particularly those with a diploid DNA pattern, derive limited benefit from any form of treatment and are best left alone (see also comments on p. 164 and Chapter 9). Patients with low-stage, moderately well-differentiated cancers may benefit from various forms of therapy, although a small proportion of these patients will have occult lymph node metastases. Patients with high-grade cancers usually respond to treatment only with temporary improvements.

Grading may be performed on aspiration smears according to the criteria outlined above. Thus, Esposti (1971), using a purely morphologic approach, was able to document that 5-year survival of patients depended significantly on cytologic grade: it was about 70% for 131 patients with well-differentiated carcinoma and only 10% for 73 patients with poorly differentiated carcinoma.

Objective Analysis of Prostatic Cancer Cells

The morphologic criteria of tumor grading, even if rigorously applied, are subjective and carry with them limited reproducibility. For this reason, objective assessment of features of tumors or the cells derived from them would be of obvious benefit. The bibliography for this chapter lists numerous papers pertaining to various modes of assessment of prostatic carcinomas; the various modalities of morphometric analysis and of DNA ploidy patterns of prostatic tumors are discussed in Chapter 9.

Other Tumors

Cancer of the Bladder

Prostatic aspiration may provide information on the spread of urothelial carcinoma to the prostate. This is particularly important for carcinoma in situ of the bladder, which may extend to prostatic ducts (see p. 77 and Fig. 5-7). Deep aspirates of the prostate may reveal the presence of urothelial cancer cells in prostatic ducts. As described in Chapter 5, in some of these cases the primary carcinoma in situ, usually located in the epithelium of the trigone, may be occult and difficult to document. The close relationship between prostatic enlargement and carcinoma in situ, first described by Barlebo and Sørensen (1972), must be kept in mind when prostatic aspirates yield urothelial cancer cells. The opposite is also true: a significant proportion of patients with urothelial bladder cancer also have prostatic carcinomas, usually occult (Mahadevia et al., 1986). The issue of routine prostatic aspirates in all patients with urothelial carcinoma should be considered.

OTHER CARCINOMAS

I do not know of any descriptions of the cytologic presentation of rare and unusual primary prostatic carcinomas, such as squamous carcinomas, adenoid cystic carcinomas, carcinosarcomas, and endocrine carcinomas. Such tumors have been seen and described in other organs, however (Koss et al., 1992). A case of small cell carcinoma was described by Nguen-Ho et al. (1994). The small cancer cells, observed in urine sediment, had no distinguishing features from similar tumors of other organs.

SARCOMAS

Most sarcomas of the prostate are embryonal rhabdomyosarcomas occurring in childhood. The cytologic presentation of such tumors is discussed on p. 110.

In adults, sarcomas are very rare. There are a few case reports describing prostatic sarcomas in cytologic preparations. Müller and Wunsch (1981) described a case of osteosarcoma. The smear of the tumor contained fragments of osteoid tissue that facilitated the diagnosis. Three cases of leiomyosarcoma have been described: two by Müller and Wunsch and one by Cookingham and Kumar (1985). All cases were characterized by bizarre cancer cells that were elongated and thus were unlikely to represent a carcinoma. Both sets of authors stress the similarity of the sarcoma cells to those of seminal vesicles (see p. 175).

There is also a case of a prostatic rhabdomyosarcoma in an adult described by Yao et al. (1988). The precise identity of the malignant cells could not be established in smears. The tissue diagnosis required immunohistochemistry.

Effects of Treatment

Effects of treatment with estrogenic substances can be followed in aspirates. Under the impact of the drugs, the prostatic cancer cells undergo a dramatic metamorphosis to squamous cells containing large amounts of cytoplasmic glycogen. Such cells are readily seen in smears (see p. 177 and Fig. 7-11 *A,B*). Their presence has little prognostic value.

DIAGNOSTIC EFFICACY OF PROSTATIC ASPIRATES

In order to determine the efficacy of prostatic aspirates, the smears have to be compared with adequate tissue evidence or with biochemical and clinical evidence of disease, which may require lengthy follow-up. This evidence is not always available for prostatic carcinoma. The largest series of 350 documented cases was presented by Esposti in 1974. There were 9 (4.3%) negative smears in 210 patients with subsequently documented prostatic carcinoma and 5 (3.6%) "false-positive" diagnoses among 140 patients with benign disease. In some of the latter group of patients, the evidence was incomplete and the presence of occult cancer could not be ruled out.

The results from Montefiore Medical Center, based on experience with 1,683 prostatic aspirates, and summarized by Suhrland et al. (1988) suggest that when prostatic aspirations are performed by inexperienced practitioners, such as house officers without adequate guidance or supervision, approximately one third to one half of the aspirations yield inadequate samples. On the other hand, a positive cytologic finding was diagnostic of cancer even in the absence of initial tissue confirmation. There were 10 such cases seen between the years 1983 and 1986. All but one, who died, were ultimately shown to have prostatic carcinoma, even though several years were occasionally required to confirm the diagnosis. Atypical or even suspicious cytologic findings were not necessarily diagnostic of prostatic cancer. In these two categories the experience of the pathologist played a more important role than the quality of the sample.

In the same paper the issue of prostatic aspirations as a means of screening for occult prostatic carcinoma was also addressed. The results were not encouraging: only 2 of 18 patients with stage A disease, ultimately documented by tissue findings, were considered to have abnormal cells in the aspirate.

Thus, prostatic aspiration has some limitations as a clinical diagnostic test. The enthusiastic accounts of the validity of the method must be tempered by the selection of patients and experience of the operator and of the pathologist. There is little doubt that in patients with clinical suspicion of prostatic carcinoma the method is reliable. In patients without palpatory findings the value of the method still needs to be clarified.

On the other hand, the clear advantage of prostatic aspiration is the sampling of a larger area of the prostate, when compared with the core biopsies. The smear also offers a better target for DNA analysis than a tissue biopsy (see Chap. 9).

BIBLIOGRAPHY

Abrahamsson, P. A., Waldstrom, L. B., Alumets, J., Falkmer, S., and Grimelius, L.: Peptide-hormone and serotonin-reactive cells in normal and hyperplastic prostate glands. Path. Res. Pract. 181, 675–683, 1986.

Ackermann, R., and Miller, H. A.: Retrospective analysis of 645 simultaneous perineal punch biopsies and transrectal aspiration biopsies for diagnosis of prostatic carcinoma. Eur. Urol., 3, 29–34, 1977.

Addonizio, J. C., and Kapoor, S. N.: Perineal seeding of prostatic cancer after needle biopsy. Urology, 8, 513–515, 1976.

Adolfsson, J., Carstensen, J., and Løwhagen, T.: Deferred treatment in clinically localized prostatic carcinoma. Brit. J. Urol., 69, 183–187, 1992.

Adolfsson, J., Ronstrom, L., Herlund, P., Løwhagen, T., Carstensen, J., and Tribukait, B.: The prognostic value of modal deoxyribonucleic acid in low grade, low stage untreated prostate cancer. J. Urol., 144, 1404–1407, 1990.

Adolfsson, J., and Tribukait, B.: Evaluation of tumor progression by repeated fine needle biopsies in prostate adenocarcinoma: modal deoxyribonucleic acid value and cytological differentiation. J. Urol., 144, 1408–1410, 1990.

Aguilar, M., Gaffney, E. F., and Finnerty, D. P.: Prostatic melanosis with involvement of benign and malignant epithelium. J. Urol., 128, 825–827, 1982.

Ajzen, S. A., Goldenberg, S. L., Allen, G. J., Cooperberg, P. L., Chan, N. H., and Jones, E. C.: Palpable prostatic nodules: Comparison of US and digital guidance for fine-needle aspiration biopsy. Radiology, 171, 521–523, 1989.

Alfthan, O., Klintrup, H. E., Koivuniemi, A., and Taskinen, E.: Cytological aspiration biopsy and Vim-Silverman biopsy in the diagnosis of prostatic carcinoma. Ann. Chir. Fenn, 59, 226–229, 1970.

Allsbrook, W. C. J., and Simms, W. W.: Histochemistry of the prostate. Hum. Pathol., 23, 297–305, 1992.

Almagro, U. A.: Argyrophilic prostatic carcinoma: case report with literature review on prostatic carcinoids and 'carcinoid-like' prostatic carcinoma. Cancer, 55, 608–614, 1985.

Amberson, J. B., and Koss, L. G.: Measurements of DNA as a prognostic factor in prostatic carcinoma. In Karr, J. P., Coffey, D. S., Gardner, W., Jr. (Eds): Prognostic Cytometry and Cytopathology of Prostate Cancer. New York, Elsevier, 1988, 281–286.

Angell, A., and Resnick, M. I.: Prostatic ultrasound for the early detection of prostate cancer. Cancer Treat. Res., 46, 1–13, 1989.

Aprikian, A. G., Cordon-Cardo, C., Fair, W. R., and Reuter, V. E.: Characterisation of neuroendocrine differentiation in human benign prostate and prostatic adenocarcinoma. Cancer, 71, 3952–3965, 1993.

Arias-Stella, J., and Tokano-Moron, J.: Atypical epithelial changes in the seminal vesicle. Arch. Pathol., 66, 761–766, 1958.

Auer, G., and Zetterberg, A.: The prognostic significance of nuclear DNA content in malignant tumors of breast, prostate and cartilage. In Koss, L. G., and Coleman, D. V. (Eds.): Advances in Clinical Cytology, vol. 2. New York, Masson USA, 1985, 123–134.

Baird, H. H., McKay, H. W., and Kimmelstiel, P.: Ischemic infarction of the prostate gland. South. Med. J., 43, 234–240, 1950.

Bamforth, J.: Cytological diagnosis of prostatic carcinoma. Ann. Roy. Coll. Surg. Eng., 23, 248–264, 1958.

Barlebo, S., and Sorensen, B. L.: Flat epithelial changes in the urinary bladder in patients with prostatic hypertrophy. Scand. J. Urol. Nephrol., 6 (Suppl. 15), 121–128, 1972.

Bauer, W. C., McGavran, M. H., and Carlin, M. R.: Unsuspected carcinoma of prostate in suprapubic prostatectomy specimens; clinicopathological study of 55 consecutive cases. Cancer, 13, 370–378, 1960.

Bentley, E. M., Mallery, W. R., Mueller, J. J., Anderson, M. C., Schott, A. W., Flegel, G., and Still, R.: Fine needle aspiration of the prostate gland in the community hospital. A predictive value analysis. Acta Cytol., 32, 499–503, 1988.

Bichel, P., Frederiksen, P., Kjaer, T., Thomessen, P., and Vindeløv, L. L.: Flow microfluorometry and transrectal fine needle biopsy in the classification of human prostatic carcinoma. Cancer, 40, 1206–1211, 1977.

Bishop, D., and Oliver, J. A.: A study of transrectal aspiration biopsies of the prostate with particular regard to prognostic evaluation. J. Urol., 117, 313–315, 1977.

Bissa, N. K., Rountree, G. A., and Sulieman, J. S.: Factors affecting accuracy and morbidity in transrectal biopsy of the prostate. Surg. Gynecol. Obstet., 145, 869–872, 1977.

Black, W. C., and Welch, H. G.: Advances in diagnostic imaging and overestimation of disease prevalence and the benefits of therapy. N. Engl. J. Med., 328, 1237–1243, 1993.

Blute, M. L., Nativ, O., Zincke, H., Farrow, G. M., Therneau, T., and Lieber, M. M.: Pattern of failure after radical retropubic prostatectomy for clinically and pathologically localized adenocarcinoma of the prostate: influence of tumor deoxyribonucleic acid ploidy. J. Urol., 142, 1262–1265, 1989.

Boring, C. C., Squires, T. S., Tong, T., and Montgomery,

S.: Cancer statistics, 1994. CA, Cancer J. Clin., *44*, 7–26, 1994.

Bostwick, D. G., Amin, M. B., Dundore, P., Marsh, W., and Schultz, D. S.: Architectural patterns of high-grade prostatic intraepithelial neoplasia. Hum. Path., *24*, 298–310, 1993.

Bostwick, D. G., Srigley, J., Grignon, D., et al.: Atypical adenomatous hyperplasia of the prostate: Morphologic criteria for its distinction from well-differentiated carcinoma. Hum. Path., *24*, 819–832, 1993.

Brawn, P. N.: Adenosis of prostate. A dysplastic lesion that can be confused with prostatic adenocarcinoma. Cancer, *49*, 826–833, 1982.

Brawn, P. N.: The dedifferentiation of prostate carcinoma. Cancer, *52*, 246–251, 1983.

Brawn, P.: Histologic features of metastatic prostate cancer. Hum. Pathol., *23*, 267–272, 1992.

Brawn, P. N.: Interpretation of Prostate Biopsies. Biopsy Interpretation Services. New York, Raven Press, 1983.

Brawn, P. N., Ayala, A. G., von Eschenbach, A. C., Hussey, D. H., and Johnson, D. E.: Histologic grading study of prostate adenocarcinoma: The development of a new system and comparison with other methods. A preliminary study. Cancer, *49*, 525–532, 1982.

Brawn, P., Kuhl, D., Johnson, C. I., Pandya, P., and McCord, R.: Stage D1 prostate carcinoma: The histologic appearance of nodal metastases and its relationship to survival. Cancer, *65*, 538–543, 1990.

Brenner, D. W., Schlossberg, S. M., Ladaga, L. E., Schellhammer, P. F., and Fillion, M. B.: Comparison of transrectal fine-needle aspiration cytology and core needle biopsy in diagnosis of prostate cancer. Urology, *35*, 381–384, 1990.

Brooks, M. H., Scheere, P. P., and Linman, J. W.: Cryptococcal prostatitis. J.A.M.A., *192*, 639–641, 1965.

Cantrell, B. B., Leifer, G., Deklerk, D. P., and Eggleston, J. C.: Papillary adenocarcinoma of the prostatic urethra with clear cell appearance. Cancer, *48*, 2661–2667, 1981.

Catalona, W. J., Smith, D. S., Ratliff, T. L., and Basler, J. W.: Detection of organ-confined prostate cancer is increased through prostate-specific antigen-based screening. J.A.M.A., *270*, 948–954, 1993.

Catalona, W. J., Smith, D. S., and Ratliff, T. L., et al.: Measurement of prostate-specific antigen in serum as a screening test for prostate cancer. N. Engl. J. Med., *324*, 1156–1161, 1991.

Chodak, G. W., Thisted, R. A., Gerber, G. S., Johansson, J. A., Adolfsson, J., Jones, G. W., Chisholm, G. D., Moskovitz, B., Livne, P. M., and Warner, J.: Result of conservative management of clinically localised prostate cancer. N. Engl. J. Med., *330*, 242–248, 1994.

Clarke, B. G., and Bamford, S. B.: Cytology of prostate gland in diagnosis of cancer. J.A.M.A., *172*, 1750–1753, 1960.

Cookingham, C. L., and Kumar, N. B.: Diagnosis of prostatic leiomyosarcoma with fine needle aspiration biopsy. Acta Cytol., *29*, 170–172, 1985.

Couture, M. L., Freund, M., Katubig, C. P., Jr.: The isola-

tion and identification of exfoliated prostate cells from human semen. Acta Cytol., *24*, 262–267, 1980.

De la Rosette, J. J. M., Hubregtse, M. R., Wiersma, A. M., and Debruyne, F. M. J.: Value of urine cytology in screening patients with prostatitis syndrome. Acta Cytol., *37*, 710–712, 1993.

DeGaetani, C. F., and Treutini, G. P.: Atypical hyperplasia of the prostate. A pitfall in the cytologic diagnosis of carcinoma. Acta Cytol., *22*, 483–486, 1978.

Denton, S. E., Walk, W. L., Jacobson, J. M., and Kettunen, R. C.: Comparison of the perineal needle biopsy and the transurethral prostatectomy in the diagnosis of prostate carcinoma. An analysis of 300 cases. J. Urol., *97*, 127–129, 1967.

de Souza, E., Katz, D. A., Dworzak, D. L., and Longo, G.: Actinomycosis of the prostate. J. Urol., *133*, 290–291, 1985.

Detjer, S. W., Moul, J. W., Cunningham, R. E., McLeod, D. G., Noguchi, P. D., Lynch, J. H., and Jones, R. V.: Prognostic significance of DNA ploidy in carcinoma of prostate. Urology, *33*, 361–366, 1989.

deVere White, R. W., Deitch, A. D., Tesluk, H., Lamborn, K. R., and Meyers, F. J.: Prognosis in disseminated prostate cancer as related to tumor ploidy and differentiation. World J. Urol., *8*, 47–50, 1990.

Di Sant'Agnese, P. A.: Neuroendocrine differentiation in carcinoma of the prostate: diagnostic, prognostic, and therapeutic implications. Cancer, *70*, 254–268, 1992.

Diamond, D. A., Berry, S. J., Umbricht, C., Jewett, H. J., and Coffey, D. S.: Computerized image analysis of nuclear shape as a prognostic factor for prostatic cancer. Prostate, *3*, 351–355, 1982.

Droese, M., and Voeth, C.: Cytologic features of seminal vesicle epithelium in aspiration biopsy smears of the prostate. Acta Cytol., *20*, 120–125, 1976. .

Dube, V. E., Farrow, G. M., and Greene, L. F.: Prostatic adenocarcinoma of ductal origin. Cancer, *32*, 402–409, 1973.

Edwards, C. N., Steinhorsson, E., and Nicholson, D.: Autopsy study of latent prostatic cancer. Cancer, *6*, 531–554, 1953.

Efremides, S. C., Dan, S., Nieburgs, H., and Mitty, H. A.: Carcinoma of the prostate: Lymph node aspiration for staging. A.J.R., *136*, 489–492, 1981.

Epstein, J. I.: Prostate Biopsy Interpretation. New York, Raven Press, 1989.

Epstein, J. I., Berry, S. J., and Egglestone, J. C.: Nuclear roundness factor: A predictor of prognosis in untreated stage A2 prostate cancer. Cancer, *54*, 1666–1671, 1984.

Epstein, J. I., Cho, K. R., and Quinn, B. D.: Relationship of severe dysplasia to stage A (incidental) adenocarcinoma of the prostate. Cancer, *65*, 2321–2327, 1990.

Epstein, J. I., and Lieberman, P. H.: Mucinous adenocarcinoma of prostate gland. Am. J. Surg. Path., *9*, 299–308, 1985.

Epstein, J. I., Walsh, P. C., Carmichel, M., and Brendler, C. B.: Pathologic and clinical findings to predict tumor extent of nonpalpable (stage T1c) prostate cancer. J.A.M.A., *271*, 368–374, 1994.

Epstein, N. A.: Prostatic carcinoma: Correlation of histologic features of prognostic value with cyto-morphology. Cancer, 38, 2071–2077, 1976.

Epstein, N. A.: Prostatic biopsy. A morphologic correlation of aspiration cytology with needle biopsy histology. Cancer, 38, 2078–2087, 1976.

Esposti, P. L.: Cytologic diagnosis of prostatic tumors with the aid of transrectal aspiration biopsy: A critical review of 1,110 cases and a report of morphologic and cytochemical studies. Acta Cytol., 10, 182–186, 1966.

Esposti, P. L.: Cytologic malignancy grading of prostatic carcinoma by transrectal aspiration biopsy: a five-year follow-up study of 469 hormone-treated patients. Scand. J. Urol. Nephrol., 5, 199–209, 1971.

Esposti, P. L., Elman, A., and Norlen, H.: Complications of transrectal aspiration biopsy of the prostate. Scand. J. Urol. Nephrol., 9, 208–213, 1975.

Esposti, P. L., Estborn, B., and Zajicek, J.: Determination of acid phosphatase activity in cells of prostatic tumours. Nature, 188, 663–664, 1960.

Esposti, P. L.: Aspiration biopsy cytology in the diagnosis and management of prostatic carcinoma. Stockholm, Stahl and Accidenstryck, 1974.

Eyre, R. C., Aaronsson, A. G., and Weinstein, B. J.: Palisading granulomas of the prostate associated with prior prostatic surgery. J. Urol., 136, 121–122, 1986.

Faul, P.: Prostata-Zytologie. Darmstadt, Dr. Dietrich Steinkopff Verlag, 1975.

Faul, P., and Schniedt, E.: Cytologic aspects of diseases of the prostate. Int. Urol. Nephrol, 5, 297–310, 1973.

Ferguson, R. S.: Prostatic neoplasms: Their diagnosis by needle puncture and aspiration. Am. J. Surg., 9, 507–511, 1930.

Fleming, C., Wasson, J. H., Albertsen, P. C., et al.: A decision analysis of alternative treatment strategies for clinically localized prostatic cancer. J.A.M.A., 269, 2650–2658, 1993.

Fordham, M. V. P., Burge, A. H., Matthews, J., Williams, G., and Cooke, T.: Prostatic carcinoma cell DNA content measured by flow cytometry and its relation to clinical outcome. Br. J. Surg., 73, 400–403, 1986.

Forsslund, G., and Zetterberg, A.: Ploidy level determination in high-grade and low-grade malignant variants of prostatic carcinoma. Cancer Res., 5014, 4281–4285, 1990.

Fowler, J. E., and Whitmore, W. F.: The incidence and extent of pelvic lymph node metastases in apparently localized prostatic cancer. Cancer, 47, 2941–2945, 1981.

Frank, I. N.: Cytologic evaluation of prostatic smear in carcinoma of prostate. J. Urol., 73, 128–138, 1955.

Frank, I. N., Benjamin, J. A., and Sergerson, J. E.: Cytologic examination of semen. Fertil. Steril., 5, 217–226, 1954.

Frank, I. N., and Scott, W. W.: Cytodiagnosis of prostatic carcinoma; follow-up study. J. Urol., 79, 983–988, 1958.

Franks, L. M.: Benign nodular hyperplasia of the prostate: a review. Ann. Roy. Coll. Surg., 14, 92–106, 1954.

Franzén, S., Giertz, G., and Zajicek, J.: Cytological diagnosis of prostatic tumors by transrectal aspiration biopsy: A preliminary report. Br. J. Urol., 32, 193–196, 1960.

Frederiksen, P., Thommesen, P., Kjaer, T. B., and Bichel, P.: Flow cytometric DNA analysis in fine needle aspiration biopsies from patients with prostatic lesions: Diagnostic value and relation to clinical stages. Acta Pathol Microbiol., 86, 461–464, 1978.

Gardner, W. A., Culberson, D. E., and Bennett, B. D.: Trichomonas vaginalis in the prostate gland. Arch. Pathol. Lab. Med., 110, 430–432, 1986.

Garret, M., and Jassie, M.: Cytologic examination of post prostatic massage specimens as an aid in diagnosis of carcinoma of the prostate. Acta Cytol., 20, 126–131, 1976.

Gittes, R. F.: Carcinoma of the prostate. N. Engl. J. Med., 324, 236–245, 1991.

Gleason, D. F., and The Veterans Administration Cooperative Urological Research Group: Histologic grading and clinical staging of prostatic carcinoma. In Tannenbaum, M. (Ed.): Urologic Pathology: The Prostate. Philadelphia, Lea & Febiger, 1979, pp. 171–197.

Goerttler, K., Ehemann, V., Tschahargane, C., and Stoeher, M.: Monodispersal and deoxyribonucleic acid analysis of prostatic cell nuclei. J. Histochem. Cytochem., 25, 560–564, 1977.

Gray, G. F., Jr. and Marshall, V. F.: Squamous carcinoma of the prostate. J. Urol., 113, 736–738, 1975.

Greene, D. R., Taylor, S. R., Wheeler, T. M., and Scardino, P. T.: DNA ploidy by image analysis of individual foci of prostate cancer: a preliminary report. Cancer Res., 51, 4084–4089, 1991.

Greene, D. R., Wheeler, T. M., Egawa, S., Dunn, J. K., and Scardino, P. T.: A comparison of the morphologic features of cancer arising in the transition zone and in the peripheral zone of the prostate. J. Urol., 146, 1069–1076, 1991.

Greene, L. F., Farrow, G. M., Ravits, J. M., and Tomera, F. M.: Prostatic adenocarcinoma of ductal origin. J. Urol., 121, 303–305, 1979.

Greenebaum, E.: Megakaryocytes and ganglion cells mimicking cancer in fine needle aspiration of the prostate. Acta Cytol., 32, 504–508, 1988.

Greenwald, P., Damon, A., Kirmss, V., and Polan, A. K.: Physical and demographic features of men before developing cancer of the prostate. J. Nat. Cancer Inst., 53, 341–346, 1974.

Grenwald, P., Kirmss, V., Polan, A. K., and Dick, V. S.: Cancer of prostate among men with benign prostatic hyperplasia. J. Nat. Cancer Inst., 53, 335–340, 1974.

Harbitz, T. B.: Endocrine disturbances in men with benign hyperplasia and carcinoma of the prostate. Acta Path. Microbiol. Scand., A244, 1–13, 1974.

Hedrick, L., and Epstein, J. I.: Use of keratin 903 as an adjunct in the diagnosis of prostatic carcinoma. Am. J. Surg. Path., 13, 389–396, 1989.

Helpap, B.: Cell kinetics and cytological grading of prostatic carcinoma. Virchows Arch (Pathol. Anat.), *393*, 205–214, 1981.

Helpap, B., and Otten, J.: Histologisch-cytologisches Grading von uniformen und pluriformen Prostatacarcinome. Pathologe, *3*, 216–222, 1982.

Hendry, W. F., and Williams, J. P.: Transrectal prostatic biopsy. Br. Med. J., *4*, 595–597, 1971.

Henke, R. P., Kruger, E., Ayhan, N., Hubner, D., and Hammerer, P.: Numerical chromosomal aberrations in prostate cancer: correlation with morphology and cell kinetics. Virchow's Arch. (A), *422*, 61–66, 1993.

Hodge, K. K., McNeal, J. E., Terris, M. K., and Stamey, T. A.: Random systematic versus directed ultrasound guided transrectal core biopsies of the prostate. J. Urol., *142*, 71–75, 1989.

Hodge, K. K., McNeal, J. E., and Stamey, T. A.: Ultrasound guided transrectal core biopsies of the palpably abnormal prostate. J. Urol., *142*, 66–70, 1989.

Hostetter, A. L., Pedersen, K. V., Gustafsson, B. L., Manson, J. C., and Boeryd, B. R. G.: Diagnosis and localization of prostate carcinoma by fine needle aspiration cytology and correlation with histologic whole-organ sections after radical prostatectomy. Am. J. Clin. Pathol., *94*, 693–697, 1990.

Hutchinson, M. L., Schultz, D. S., Stephenson, R. A., Wong, K. L., Harry, T., and Zahnizer, D. J.: Computerized microscopic analysis of prostate fine needle aspirates: Comparison with breast aspirates. Analyt. Quant. Cytol. Histol., *11*, 105–110, 1989.

Inoshita, T., Youngberg, G. A., Boelen, L. J., and Langston, J.: Blastomycosis presenting with prostatic involvement: report of 2 cases and review of the literature. J. Urol., *130*, 160–162, 1983.

Johansson, J. E., Adami, H. O., Andersson, S. O., Bergstrom, R., Krusemo, U. B., and Kraaz, W.: High 10-year survival rate in patients with early, untreated prostatic cancer. J.A.M.A., *267*, 2191–2196, 1992.

Jones, E. C., McNeal, J., Bruchovsky, N., and de Jong, G.: DNA content in prostatic adenocarcinoma. A flow cytometry study of the predictive value of aneuploidy for tumor volume, percentage Gleason grade 4 and 5, and lymph node metastases. Cancer, *66*, 752–757, 1990.

Kallioniemi, O. P., Visakorpi, K., Holli, K., Heikkinen, A., Isola, J., and Koivula, T.: Improved prognostic impact of S-phase values from paraffin embedded breast and prostate carcinoma after correcting for nuclear slicing. Cytometry, *12*, 413–421, 1991.

Kaufman, J. J., Rosenthal, M., and Goodwin, W. E.: Methods of diagnosis of carcinoma of the prostate: A comparison of clinical impression, prostatic smear, needle biopsy, open perineal biopsy and transurethral biopsy. J. Urol., *72*, 450–465, 1954.

Kaye, K. W., and Horwitz, C. A.: Transrectal fine needle biopsy of the prostate: Combined histological and cytological technique. J. Urol., *139*, 1229–1231, 1988.

Kelalis, P. P., Greene, L. F., Harrison, E. G., Jr.: Granulomatous prostatitis: a mimic of carcinoma of the prostate. J.A.M.A., *191*, 287–389, 1965.

Kelalis, P. P., Harrison, E. G., Jr., and Greene, L. F.: Allergic granulomas of the prostate in asthmatics. J.A.M.A., *18*, 963–967, 1964.

Kenny, G. M., and Hutchinson, W. B.: Transrectal ultrasound study of prostate. Urology, *32*, 401–402, 1988.

Kline, T. S.: Aspiration biopsy cytology of the prostate: Theme and variations. (Editorial). J. Urol., *140*, 802, 1988.

Kline, T. S.: Guides to Clinical Aspiration Biopsy: Prostate. New York, Igaku-Shoin, 1985.

Kline, T. S., Kelsey, D. M., and Kohler, F. P.: Prostatic carcinoma and needle aspiration biopsy. Am. J. Clin. Pathol., *67*, 131–133, 1977.

Kline, T. S., Kohler, F. P., and Kesley, D. M.: Aspiration biopsy cytology. Its uses in diagnosis of lesions of prostate gland. Arch. Pathol. Lab Med., *106*, 136–139, 1982.

Klotz, L. H., Shaw, P. A., and Srigley, J. R.: Transrectal fine-needle aspiration and Tru-Cut needle biopsy of the prostate: a blinded comparison of accuracy. Can. J. Surg., *32*, 287–289, 1989.

Koivuniemi, A., and Tyrkko, J.: Seminal vesicle epithelium in fine needle aspiration biopsies of the prostate as a pitfall in the cytologic diagnosis of carcinoma. Acta Cytol., *20*, 116–119, 1976.

Koss, L. G.: Atypical hyperplasia and other abnormalities of prostatic epithelium. (Editorial). Human Path., *24*, 817–818, 1993.

Koss, L. G.: Diagnostic Cytology and Its Histopathologic Bases, 4th Ed. Philadelphia, J. B. Lippincott, 1992.

Koss, L. G.: The puzzle of prostatic carcinoma (Editorial). Mayo Clin. Proc., *63*, 193–197, 1988.

Koss, L. G., and Czerniak, B.: Image analysis and flow cytometry of tumors of prostate and bladder. With a comment on molecular biology of urothelial tumors. *In* Weinstein, R., and Gardner, W. A., Jr. (Eds.): Pathology and Pathobiology of the Urinary Bladder and Prostate. Baltimore, Williams & Wilkins, 1992.

Koss, L. G., Woyke, S., and Olszewski, W.: Aspiration biopsy. Cytologic Interpretation and Histologic Bases. 2nd Ed. New York and Tokyo, Igaku-Shoin, 1992.

Koss, L. G., Woyke, S., Schreiber, K., Kohlberg, W., and Freed, S. Z.: Thin-needle aspiration biopsy of the prostate. Urol. Clin. N. Am., *11*, 237–251, 1984.

Kuo, T., and Gomez, L. G.: Monstrous epithelial cells in human epididymis and seminal vesicles. A pseudomalignant change. Am. J. Surg. Pathol., *5*, 483–490, 1981.

Lamm, D. L., Stogdill, W. D., Stogdill, B. J., and Crispen, R. G.: Complications of bacillus Calmette-Guerin immunotherapy in 1278 patients with bladder cancer. J. Urol., *135*, 272–274, 1986.

Larsen, R. A., Bozzette, S., McCutchan, A., Chiu, J., Leal, M., and Richman, D. D.: Persistent cryptococcus neoformans infection of the prostate after successful treatment of meningitis. Ann. Int. Med., *111*, 125–128, 1989.

Lee, F., Siders, D. B., Torp-Pedersen, S. T., Kirscht, J. L., McHugh, T. A., and Mitchell, A. E.: Prostate cancer: transrectal ultrasound and pathology comparison. A preliminary study of outer gland (Peripheral and Central Zones) and inner gland (Transition Zone) cancer. Cancer, 67, 1132–1142, 1991.

Lee, S. E., Currin, S. M., Paulson, D. F., and Walther, P. J.: Flow cytometric determination of ploidy in prostatic adenocarcinoma: A comparison with seminal vesicle involvement and histopathological grading as a predictor of clinical recurrence. J. Urology, 140, 769–774, 1988.

Leistenschneider, W., and Nagel, R.: Atlas of Prostatic Cytology. Berlin and New York, Springer, 1984.

Leistenschneider, W., and Nagel, R.: The cytologic differentiation of prostatitis. (In German). Pathol. Res. Pract., 165, 429–444, 1979.

Lieber, M. M.: Prostatic dysplasia: Significance in relation to nuclear DNA ploidy studies of prostate adenocarcinoma. Urology, 34 (Suppl.), 43–48, 1989.

Lief, M., and Sarfarazi, F.: Prostatic cryptococcosis in acquired immunodeficiency syndrome. Urology, 28, 318–319, 1986.

Lin, B. P. C., Davies, W. E. L. and Harmata, P. A.: Prostatic aspiration cytology. Pathology, 11, 607–614, 1979.

Linsk, J. A., Axelrod, H. D., Solyn, R., and Delaverdac, C.: Transrectal cytologic aspiration in the diagnosis of prostatic carcinoma. J. Urol., 108, 455–459, 1972.

Ljung, B. M.: Techniques of aspiration and smear preparation. In Koss, L. G., Woyke, S., Olszewski, W.: Aspiration Biopsy. Cytologic Interpretation and Histologic Bases. 2nd Ed. New York, Igaku-Shoin, 1992, pp. 12–30.

Ljung, B. M., Cherrie, R., and Kaufman, J. J.: Fine needle aspiration biopsy of the prostate gland: a study of 103 cases with histological follow-up. J. Urol., 135, 955–958, 1986.

Lu-Yao, G. L., McLerran, D., Wasson, J., and Wennberg, J. E.: An assessment of radical prostatectomy. Time trends, geographic variation, and outcomes. J.A.M.A., 269, 2633–2636, 1993.

MacKenzie, A. R., Sharma, T. C., Whitmore, W. F., Jr., and Melamed, M. R.: Non-extirpative treatment of myosarcomas of the bladder and prostate. Cancer, 28, 329–334, 1971.

MacKenzie, A. R., Whitmore, W. F., Jr., and Melamed, M. R.: Myosarcomas of the bladder and prostate. Cancer, 22, 833–843, 1968.

Macoska, J. A., Micale, M. A., Sakr, W. A., Benson, P. D., and Wolman, S. R.: Extensive genetic alterations in prostate cancer revealed by dual PCR and FISH analysis. Genes, Chromosom. Cancer, 8, 88–97, 1993.

Mahadevia, P. S., Koss, L. G., and Tar, I. J.: Prostatic involvement in bladder cancer: Prostate mapping in 20 cystoprostatectomy specimens. Cancer, 58, 2096–2102, 1986.

Maksem, J. A., Johenning, P. W., and Galang, C. F.: Prostatitis and aspiration biopsy cytology of prostate. Urology, 32, 263–268, 1988.

Marshall, S.: Prostatic needle biopsy: A simple technique for increasing accuracy. J. Urol., 142, 1023, 1989.

McIntire, T. L., Murphy, W. M., Coon, J. S., Chandler, R. W., Schwartz, D., Conway, S., and Weinstein, R. S.: The prognostic value of DNA ploidy combined with histologic substaging for incidental carcinoma and the prostate gland. Am. J. Clin. Pathol., 89, 370–373, 1988.

McNeil, J. E., and Bostwick, D. G.: Intraductal dysplasia: A premalignant lesion of the prostate. Hum. Pathol., 17, 555–561, 1986.

McNeil, J. E.: Normal and pathologic anatomy of the prostate. Urology (Suppl), 17, 11–16, 1981.

McNeil, J. E.: Regional morphology and pathology of the prostate. Am. J. Clin. Path., 49, 347–357, 1968.

McNeil, J. E.: The significance of duct-acinar dysplasia in prostatic carcinogenesis. The Prostate, 13, 91–102, 1988.

McNeil, J. E., and Bostwick, D. G.: Intraductal dysplasia: a premalignant lesion of the prostate. Hum. Path., 17, 64–71, 1986.

McNeil, J. E., Redwine, E. A., Freiha, F. S., and Stamey, T. A.: Zonal distribution of prostatic adenocarcinoma. Correlation with histologic pattern and direction of spread. Am. J. Surg. Path., 12, 897–906, 1988.

McNeil, J. E., Villers, A. A., Redwine, E. A., Freiha, F. S., and Stamey, T. A.: Capsular penetration in prostate cancer. Significance for natural history and treatment. Am. J. Surg. Path., 14, 270–277, 1990.

Meisels, A., and Ayotte, D.: Cells from the seminal vesicles: Contaminants of the V-C-E smear. Acta Cytol., 20, 211–219, 1976.

Melicow, M. M., and Tannenbaum, M.: Endometrial carcinoma of uterus masculinus (Prostatic utricle). Report of 6 cases. J. Urol., 106, 892–902, 1971.

Micale, M. A., Sanford, J. S., Powell, I. J., Sakr, W. A., and Wolman, S. R.: Defining the nature of cytogenetic events in prostatic adenocarcinoma: paraffin FISH vs. metaphase analysis. Cancer Genet. Cytogenet., 69, 7–12, 1993.

Miller, G. J., and Shikes, J. L.: Nuclear roundness as a predictor of response to hormonal therapy of patients with stage D2 prostatic carcinoma. In Karr, J. P., Coffey, D. S., and Gardner, W. (Eds.): Prognostic Cytometry and Cytopathology of Prostate Cancer. New York, Elsevier, 1988, pp. 349–354.

Miller, J., Horsfall, D. J., Marshall, V. R., Rao, D. M., and Leong, A. S-Y.: The prognostic value of deoxyribonucleic acid flow cytometric analysis in stage D2 prostatic carcinoma. J. Urol., 145, 1192–1196, 1991.

Moller, J. T.: Transrectal cytological aspiration biopsy in prostatic disease. Int. Urol. Nephrol., 9, 235–240, 1977.

Moller, J. L., Partin, A. W., Lohr, D. W., and Coffey, D. S.: Nuclear roundness factor measurement for assessment of prognosis of patients with prostatic carcinoma. I. Testing of digitization system. J. Urol., 139, 1080–1084, 1988.

Montgomery, B. T., Nativ, O., Blute, M. L., Farrow, G. M., Myers, R. P., Zincke, H., Therneau, T. M., and Lieber, M. M.: Stage B Prostate adenocarcinoma. Flow cytometric nuclear DNA ploidy analysis. Arch. Surg., 125, 327–331, 1990.

Mostofi, F. K.: Grading of prostatic carcinoma. Cancer Chemother. Reports, *59,* 111–117, 1975.

Mostofi, F. K.: and Morse, W. H.: Epithelial metaplasia in 'prostatic infarction.' Arch. Path., *51,* 340–345, 1951.

Mostofi, F. K., and Price, E. B.: Tumors of the Male Genital System. Atlas of Tumor Pathology, second series, Fascicle 8. Washington D.C., Armed Forces Institute of Pathology, 1973.

Mulholland, S. W.: A study of prostatic secretion and its relation to malignancy. Proc. Mayo Clin., *6,* 733–735, 1931.

Muller, H. A., and Wunsch, P. H.: Features of prostatic sarcoma in combined aspiration and punch biopsies. Acta Cytol., *25,* 480–484, 1981.

Murphy, G. P.: The diagnosis and detection of urogenital cancers. Cancer, *47,* 1193–1199, 1981.

Murphy, G. P. and Whitmore, W. F.: A report of the workshop on the current status of the histologic grading of prostate cancer. Cancer, *44,* 1490–1494, 1979.

Nagle, R. B., Brawer, M. K., Kittelson, J., and Clark, V.: Phenotypic relationships of prostatic intraepithelial neoplasia to invasive prostatic carcinoma. Am. J. Path., *138,* 119–128, 1991.

Narayana, A. S., Loening, S., Weimer, G. W., and Culp, D. A.: Sarcoma of the bladder and prostate. J. Urol., *119,* 72–76, 1978.

Narayan, P., Jajodia, P., and Stein, R.: Core biopsy instrument in the diagnosis of prostate cancer: superior accuracy to fine needle aspiration. J. Urol., *145,* 795–797, 1991.

Nativ, O., and Lieber, M. M.: Prostatic carcinoma: Prognostic importance of static and flow cytometric nuclear DNA ploidy measurements. J. Urol., 178–183, 1991.

Nativ, O., Myers, R. P., Farrow, G. M., Therneau, T. M., Zincke, H., and Lieber, M.: Nuclear deoxyribonucleic acid ploidy and serum prostate specific antigen in operable prostatic carcinoma. J. Urol., *144,* 303–306, 1990.

Nativ, O., Winkler, H. Z., Raz, Y., Therneau, T., Farrow, G. M., Myers, R. P., Zincke, H., and Lieber, M. M.: Stage C prostatic adenocarcinoma: flow cytometric nuclear DNA ploidy analysis. Mayo Clin. Proc., *64,* 911–919, 1989.

Nemoto, R., Kawamura, H., Miyakawa, I., Uchida, K., Hattori, K., Koiso, K., and Harada, M.: Immunohistochemical detection of proliferating cell nuclear antigen (PCNA/cyclin) in human prostate adenocarcinoma. J. Urol., *149,* 165–169, 1993.

Nguen-Ho, P., Nguen, G. K., and Villanueva, R. R.: Small cell anaplastic carcinoma of the prostate. Report of a case with positive urine cytology. Diagn. Cytopathol., *10,* 159–161, 1994.

Nienhaus, H.: Aspiration cytology of prostatic carcinoma. Cancer Res., *60,* 53–60, 1977.

Nowels, K., Kent, E., Rinsho, K., and Oyasu, R.: Prostate specific antigen and acid phosphatase-reactive cells in cystitis cystica and glandularis. Arch. Pathol. Lab. Med., *112,* 734–737, 1988.

Oates, R. D., Stilmant, M. M., Freedlund, M. C., and Siroky, M. B.: Granulomatous prostatitis following ba-cillus Calmette-Guérin immunotherapy of bladder cancer. J. Urol., *140,* 751–754, 1988.

O'Connor, M. H., Foushee, J. H., and Cox, C. E.: Prostatic cryptococcosis: A case report. J. Urol., *94,* 160–163, 1965.

O'Dea, M. J., Moore, S. B., and Greene, L. F.: Tuberculous prostatitis. Urology, *11,* 483–485, 1978.

Oesterling, J. E., Jacobsen, S. J., Chute, C. G., Guess, H. A., Girman, C. J., Panser, L. A., and Lieber, M. M.: Serum prostate-specific antigen in a community-based population of healthy men. Establishment of age-specific reference ranges. J.A.M.A., *270,* 860–864, 1993.

Palazzo, J. P., Ellison, D., and Petersen, R. O.: DNA content in prostate adenocarcinoma. Correlation with Gleason score, nuclear grade and histologic subtypes. J. Urol. Path., *1,* 283–292, 1993.

Partin, A. W., Carter, H. B., Epstein, J. I., and Coffey, D. S.: The biology of prostate cancer: new and future directions in predicting tumor behavior. *In* Weinstein, R. S., and Gardner, W. A. (Eds.): Pathology and Pathobiology of the Urinary Bladder and Prostate. pp. 198–218. Baltimore, Williams & Wilkins, 1992.

Partin, A. W., Walsh, A. C., Pitcock, R. V., Mohler, J. L., Epstein, J. I., and Coffey, D. S.: A comparison of nuclear morphometry and Gleason grade as a predictor of prognosis in stage A2 prostate cancer. A critical analysis. J. Urol., *142,* 1254–1258, 1989.

Pedersen, S. T., Lee, F., Littrup, P. J., Siders, D. B., Kumasaka, G. H., Solomon, M. H., and McLeary, R. D.: Transrectal biopsy of the prostate guided with transrectal US: Longitudinal and multiplanar scanning. Radiology, *170,* 23–27, 1989.

Petersen, R. O.: Urologic Pathology, 2nd Ed. Philadelphia, J. B. Lippincott, 1992.

Pontes, J. E., Wajsman, Z., Huben, R. P., Wolf, R. M., and Englander, L. S.: Prognostic factors in localized prostatic carcinoma. J. Urol., *134,* 1137–1139, 1985.

Price, M. J., Lewis, E. L., and Carmalt, J. E.: Coccidioidomycosis of prostate gland. Urology, *19,* 653–655, 1982.

Quinn, B. D., Cho, K. R., and Epstein, J. I.: Relationship of severe dysplasia to stage B adenocarcinoma of the prostate. Cancer, *65,* 2328–2337, 1990.

Ragde, H., Aldape, H. C., and Bagley, C. M.: Ultrasound-guided prostate biopsy. Urology, *32,* 503–506, 1988.

Ramzy, I., and Larson, V.: Prostatic duct carcinoma: Exfoliative cytology. Acta Cytol., *21,* 417–420, 1977.

Razvi, M., Firfer, R., and Berkson, B.: Occult transitional cell carcinoma of the prostate presenting as skin metastasis. J. Urol., *113,* 734–735, 1975.

Reuter, H. J., and Schuck, W.: Die Nadelbiopsie der Prostata zur zytologischen Karzinomdiagnostik. Erfahrungen an 1500 Fallen. Z. Urol. Nephrol., *64,* 857–862, 1971.

Rheinfrank, R. E., and Nulf, T. H.: Fine needle aspiration biopsy of the prostate. Endoscopy, *1,* 27–32, 1969.

Riaboff, P. J.: Detection of early prostatic and urinary tract cancer in asymptomatic patients 50 years of age and over; preliminary report. J. Urol., *72,* 62–66, 1954.

Richardson, H. L., Durfee, G. R., Day, E., and Papanicolaou, G. N.: Role of cytology in detection of early prostatic cancer. *In* Homburger, F., and Fishman, W. H. (Eds.): The Laboratory Diagnosis of Cancer of the Prostate. Boston, Tufts Medical School, 1954.

Ritchie, A. W. S., Layfield, L. J., Turcillo, P., and deKernion, J. B.: The significance of atypia in fine needle aspiration cytology of the prostate. J. Urol., *140*, 761–764, 1988.

Ro, J. Y., Grignon, D. J., Ayala, A. G., Fernandez, P. L., Ordonez, N. G., and Wishnow, K. I.: Mucinous adenocarcinoma of the prostate: histochemical and immunohistochemical studies. Human Path., *21*, 593–600, 1990.

Ro, J. Y., Tetu, B., Ayala, A. G., and Ordonez, N. G.: Small cell carcinoma of the prostate. II. Immunohistochemical and electron microscopic study of 18 cases. Cancer, *59*, 977–982, 1987.

Rojas-Corona, R. R., Chen, L. Z., and Mahadevia, P. S.: Prostate carcinoma with endocrine features: a report of a neoplasm containing multiple immunoreactive hormonal substances. Am. J. Clin. Path., *88*, 759–762, 1987.

Ronstrom, L., Tribukait, B., and Esposti, P. L.: DNA pattern and cytological findings in fine-needle aspirates of untreated prostatic tumors. A flow-cytofluorometric study. Prostate, *2*, 79–88, 1981.

Ruebush, T. K. I., McConville, J. H., and Calia, F. M.: A double-blind study of trimethoprim-sulfamethoxazole prophylaxis in patients having transrectal needle biopsy of the prostate. J. Urol., *122*, 492–494, 1979.

Rupp, M., O'Hara, B., McCollough, L., Saxena, S., and Olchiewski, J.: Prostatic carcinoma cells in urine specimens. Cytopathology, *5*, 164–170, 1994.

Schmidt, J. D.: Non-specific granulomatous prostatitis. Classification review and report of cases. J. Urol., *94*, 607–615, 1965.

Schnürer, L. B., Fritjofsson, A., Lindgren, A., Magnuson, P. H., and Petersson, S.: Fine needle versus coarse needle in punction diagnosis of prostatic carcinoma. Acta Pathol. Microbiol. Scand., *76*, 150–160, 1969.

Shankey, T. V.: Urologic cancers. Chap. 16 in Bauer, K. D., Duque, R. E., Shankey, T. V. (Eds.): Clinical Flow Cytometry. Principles and Applications. Baltimore, Williams & Wilkins, 1993.

Shimada, H., Misugi, K., Sasaki, Y., Iizuka, A., and Nishihira, H.: Carcinoma of the prostate in childhood and adolescence: Report of a case and review of the literature. Cancer, *46*, 2534–2542, 1980.

Smith, F. L., Bibbo, M., Schoenberg, H. W., and Chodak, G. W.: Transrectal aspiration biopsy of the prostate: The importance of atypia. J. Urol., *140*, 766–768, 1988.

Spieler, P., Gloor, F., Egle, N., and Bandhauer, K.: Cytologic findings in transrectal aspiration biopsy on hormone and radiotreated carcinoma of the prostate. Virchows Arch. (Pathol. Anat.), *372*, 149–159, 1976.

Sprenger, E., Michaelis, W. E., Vogt-Schaden, M., and Otto, C.: The significance of DNA flow-through fluorescence cytophotometry for the diagnosis of prostate carcinoma. Beitr. Pathol., *159*, 292–298, 1976.

Sprenger, E., Volk, L., and Michaelis, W. E.: The significance of nuclear DNA measurements in the diagnosis of prostatic carcinomas. Beitr. Pathol., *153*, 370–378, 1974.

Staehler, W., Ziegler, H., and Volter, D.: Zytodiagnostik der Prostata. Grundriss und Atlas. Stuttgart, F. K. Schattauer Verlag, 1975.

Stege, R., Lundh, B., Tribukait, B., Pousette, A., Carlstrom, K., and Hasenson, M.: Deoxyribonucleic acid ploidy and the direct assay of prostatic acid phosphatase and prostate specific antigen in fine needle aspiration biopsies as diagnostic methods in prostatic carcinoma. J. Urol., *144*, 299–302, 1990.

Stenkvist, B., and Olding-Stenkvist, E.: Cytological and DNA characteristics of hyperplasia/inflammation and cancer of the prostate. Eur. J. Cancer, *263*, 261–267, 1990.

Stephenson, R. A., James, B. C., Gay, H., Fair, W. R., Whitmore, W. F., Jr., and Melamed, M. R.: Flow cytometry of prostate cancer: relationship of DNA content to survival. Cancer Res., *47*, 2504–2507, 1987.

Suhrland, M. J., Deitch, D., Schreiber, K., Freed, S., and Koss, L. G.: Assessment of fine needle aspiration as a screening test for occult prostatic carcinoma. Acta Cytol., *32*, 495–498, 1988.

Tanner, F. H., and McDonald, J. R.: Granulomatous prostatitis: Histologic study of a group of granulomatous lesions collected from prostate glands. Arch Pathol., *36*, 358–370, 1943.

Tetu, B., Ro, J. Y., Ayala, A. G., Johnson, D. E., Logothetis, C. G., and Ordonez, N. G.: Small cell carcinoma of the prostate: I. A clinicopathologic study of 20 cases. Cancer, *59*, 1803–1809, 1987.

Tisell, L. E., and Salander, H.: The lobes of human prostate. Scand. J. Urol. Nephrol., *9*, 185–191, 1975.

Tribukait, B.: DNA flow cytometry in carcinoma of the prostate for diagnosis, prognosis and study of tumor biology. Acta Oncologica, *30*, 187–192, 1991.

Tribukait, B.: Flow cytometry in surgical pathology and cytology of tumors of the genito-urinary tract. *In* Koss, L. G., and Coleman, D. V. (Eds.): Advances in Clinical Cytology, Vol. 2. New York, Masson USA, 1984, pp. 163–189.

Tribukait, B.: Flow cytometry in assessing the clinical aggressiveness of genito-urinary neoplasms. World J. Urol., *5*, 108–122, 1987.

Waisman, J., and Mott, L. J. M.: Pathology of neoplasms of the prostate gland. *In* Skinner, D. G., and de Kernion, J. B. (Eds.): Genitourinary Cancer. Philadelphia, W. B. Saunders, 1978, pp. 310–343.

Wasson, J. H., Cushman, C. C., Bruskewitz, R. C., Littenberg, B., Mulley, A. G. J., and Wennberg, J. E.: A structured literature review of treatment for localized prostate cancer. Arch. Fam. Med., 487–493, 1993.

Whitmore, W. F., Jr.: Management of clinically localized prostatic cancer. An unsolved problem. J.A.M.A., *269*, 2676–2677, 1993.

Wick, M. R., Young, R. H., Malvesta, R., Beebe, D. S., Hansen, J. J., and Dehner, L. P.: Prostatic carcinosarcomas: clinical, histologic, and immunohistochemical data on two cases, with review of the literature. Am. J. Clin. Path., *92,* 131–139, 1989.

Williams, J. P.: Transrectal fine-needle biopsy in diagnosing prostatic cancer. London Clin. Med. J., *9,* 39–43, 1968.

Williams, J. P., Still, B. M., and Pugh, R. C. B.: The diagnosis of prostatic cancer. Cytological and biochemical studies using the Franzén biopsy needle. Br. J. Urol., *39,* 549–554, 1967.

Wilson, J. O.: The pathogenesis of benign prostatic hyperplasia. Am. J. Med., *68,* 745–756, 1980.

Winkler, H. Z., Rainwater, L. M., Myers, R. P., Farrow, G. M., Therneau, T. M., Zincke, H., and Lieber, M. M.: Stage D1 prostatic adenocarcinoma: significance of nuclear DNA ploidy patterns studied by flow cytometry. Mayo Clin. Proc., *63,* 103–112, 1988.

Yao, J. C. T., Wang, W. C. C., Tseng, H. H., and Hwang, W. S.: Primary rhabdomyosarcoma of the prostate. Diagnosis by needle biopsy and immunocytochemistry. Acta Cytol., *32,* 509–512, 1988.

Young, R. H., Frierson, H. F., Jr., Mills, S. E., Kaiser, J. S., Talbot, W. H., and Bhan, A. K.: Adenoid cystic-like tumor of the prostate gland: a report of two cases and review of the literature on 'adenoid cystic carcinoma.' Am. J. Clin. Path., *89,* 49–56, 1988.

Zajicek, J.: The aspiration biopsy smear. *In* Koss L. G.: Diagnostic Cytology and Its Histopathologic Bases. 3rd Ed. Philadelphia, J. B. Lippincott, 1979, pp. 1001–1109.

Zajicek, J.: Aspiration Biopsy Cytology, Part 2: Cytology of Infradiaphragmatic Organs. Basel, S. Karger, 1979.

Zetterberg, A.: Stability of diploid genome in carcinoma of the prostate with long follow up. WHO consensus meeting on prostatic carcinoma, Stockholm, 1993.

Zetterberg, A., and Esposti, P. L.: Cytophotometric DNA-analysis of aspirated cells from prostatic carcinoma. Acta Cytol., *20,* 46–57, 1976.

Zetterberg, A., and Esposti, P. L.: Prognostic significance of nuclear DNA levels in prostatic carcinoma. Scand. J. Urol. Nephrol. (Suppl), *55,* 53–58, 1980.

CHAPTER 8

Renal, Pararenal, Adrenal, and Retroperitoneal Lesions

Except for lesions of the kidney and renal pelves that are sometimes accessible to cytologic examination using voided urine, brushings, or retrograde washings, the transcutaneous aspiration biopsy is the method of choice for diagnostic assessment of abdominal organs, discussed in this chapter. The aspiration biopsy requires roentgenologic guidance in the form of either computed tomography or ultrasound, the latter technique being useful only for lesions larger than 2 cm in diameter.

TECHNIQUE OF TRANSCUTANEOUS ASPIRATION OF ABDOMINAL ORGANS

Instruments

Needles

An assortment of stainless steel needles, measuring from 10 to 20 cm in length, gauges 22 to 25, must be at hand. Because the smaller caliber needles may bend when crossing the subcutaneous tissue and the muscle before reaching the target, it is often advisable to use caliber 18 or 19 needle guides with an obturator in place, or an 18-gauge spinal tap needle with a stylet to reach the target. The obturators or stylets are then removed and replaced with the thin needle to perform the aspiration.

Syringes

Disposable plastic syringes with an eccentric tip, 10- or 20-ml in size, are used for aspiration. Single-grip syringe holders, which are sometimes very useful in aspirating palpable lesions, are of limited use. Rosenblatt (1992) advocated the use of both hands to insert the needle guide or the spinal needle.

Other Instruments and Supplies

To reach the kidney, the adrenal, and the retroperitoneum, it is often advisable to perform a 2- to 3-mm skin incision to facilitate the introduction of the needle guide or the spinal needle. Therefore, disposable scalpel blades and scalpel handles should be secured in advance. Other supplies include an antiseptic solution, gauze, and a cutaneous anesthetic such as lidocaine, to be used in pain-sensitive patients. Sterile gloves and towels are also needed. A supply of clean glass slides and coverslips is essential. It is also advisable to have at hand a bottle or bottles with staining solutions of one of the rapid stains (discussed in Chapter 1 on pp. 12 and 13) for a preliminary assessment of the sample under a microscope. In institutions where aspiration procedures of abdominal organs are common, it is helpful to have all the sterile instruments and other supplies prepared in advance on a tray or a cart, thus avoiding a frantic search at the time of the procedure.

Patient Preparation

It is important to determine the clotting parameters and to rule out any serious blood disorders prior to the aspiration procedure. It is also important to explain the procedure to the patient and to secure an informed consent. In general the acceptance of the procedure is very good, so long as care has been taken to keep the patient informed and reasonably comfortable.

The Aspiration Procedure

Both modern ultrasound instruments and computed tomography machines offer a two-dimensional view of the target lesion and display computer-generated coordinates in terms of angle of entry and depth of the lesion. Thus, it is possible to calculate the optimal site and angle of entry of the needle in advance. The position of the tip of the needle before aspiration can be verified with computed tomography and on new ultrasound machines.

After placing the patient in the most advantageous position, which generally means using the posterior or lateral approach for the kidney or the adrenal, the skin is cleaned and draped, and the local anesthetic applied. The operator, wearing sterile gloves, makes a small skin incision and introduces the needle guide or the spinal needle into the target. As the target is reached, the operator usually feels a change in tissue consistency. An additional scan may be taken to verify the position of the tip of the needle. The obturator or stylet is then removed and a thin needle is advanced to the target.

The aspiration procedure consists of several (4 to 20) rapid to-and-fro movements of the tip of the needle within the target to loosen up the cells. The movements of the needle should remain in the same plane, as any attempt to change the direction of the needle may result in hemorrhage within the tumor. *If it is desirable to sample another area of the lesion, the needle guide and the needle should be withdrawn to the level of subcutaneous tissue and reinserted at a different angle.* This maneuver is sometimes difficult to perform; in such cases the aspiration procedure must be repeated, using the same skin incision and a different angle of entry.

The syringe is then attached to the needle and, by withdrawing the barrel of the syringe to the level of 5 or 10 ml, a negative pressure is applied to aspirate the loosened fragments into the *lumen of the needle. Except for the aspiration of the cysts* with a large fluid content, *the syringe should not contain any visible tissue fragments.* If tissue fragments or cells reach the barrel of the syringe they usually become irretrievably lost. *The negative pressure must be equalized by releasing the barrel of the syringe,* and the syringe should be detached from the needle, *before the needle is withdrawn.* It is preferable to leave the needle guide, if one is used, in place, thus facilitating the

next aspiration procedure, should one be needed because the first sample was inadequate.

Checking the Adequacy of the Aspiration

Except for cyst contents, which are visible to the naked eye, the next step in the procedure is the verification of the quality of the aspirated material. The syringe with the barrel withdrawn is reattached to the needle, and a drop of the contents is expelled on one or more clean microscopic slides, prepared in advance. A smear is prepared by placing a cover slip or by using another slide to flatten the drop of material. There are several different techniques of smear preparation; the interested reader is referred to the contribution by Ljung (1992) wherein these techniques are described in great detail. It is advisable to verify the contents of the aspiration by staining the first smear with one of the rapid stains, described on pp. 12 and 13. If the cell content is inadequate, the aspiration procedure may be repeated immediately.

Processing of Material

If the smear appears to have an adequate cell content, the remaining smears may be either fixed for staining with the Papanicolaou stain, or left to air dry, before fixation in methyl alcohol and application of the May-Gruenwald-Giemsa or another hematologic stain. If it is suspected that the lesion may require immunostaining—for example, a malignant lymphoma—it is advisable to prepare a few additional smears for freezing or fixation in acetone. Alternatively the contents of the syringe may be expelled into one of the cell-preserving media, such as the Hanks' balanced salt solution or a bone marrow transport medium (for example, RPMI 1640, manufactured by Gibco, Grand Island, NY 14072) for preparation of multiple slides, using the cytocentrifuge technique (see Chapter 1 for description). If tissue fragments can be secured, they can be processed as microbiopsies (cell blocks) by fixation in buffered formalin and embedding in paraffin (see p. 12). The cell block technique is very useful, as it often provides additional information about the pattern of the lesion and offers the option of multiple histologic sections for immunostaining or other special procedures.

For additional details on the technical procedures and processing options in aspiration biopsy, the reader is referred to the book Aspiration Biopsy: Cytologic Interpretation and Histologic Bases (Koss et al., 1992).

Complications of the Abdominal Aspiration Biopsy

The dangers of the intra-abdominal aspiration biopsy procedure appear to be minimal, in the absence

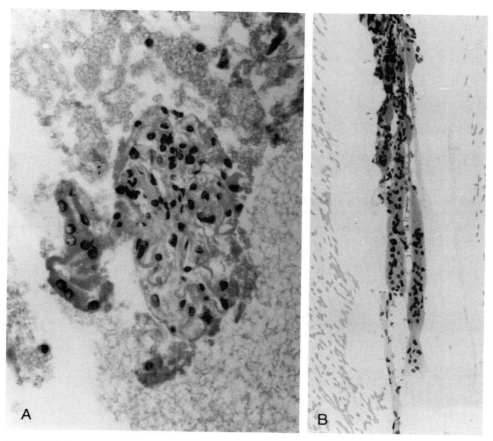

FIGURE 8-1. Renal aspirate. (*A*) Cell block. Normal renal glomerulus with an attached fragment of a proximal convoluted tubule. (*B*) Smear. Distal convoluted tubules. (*A* × 560; *B* × 150)

of a debilitating disease or a blood dyscrasia. The question of damaging vital organs or vessels interposed between the skin and the target lesion has been extensively debated. Experience has shown that perforations of a viscus, a major blood vessel, or even the aorta by the small-caliber needle has no practical consequence. There are only very few reported cases of peritonitis or intra-abdominal hemorrhage, usually in patients at high risk. We have not seen any such mishaps in many thousands of transcutaneous abdominal aspirations performed to date. The only complication we have observed was a perforation of a distended gallbladder (Courvoisier gallbladder) in a hepatic aspiration (Koss et al., 1992). *Tumor seeding* in the needle tract is also exceptional—perhaps a dozen such cases in all organs have been observed worldwide. There are several reports pertaining to seeding of tumors after aspirates of renal carcinomas (Gib-

bons et al., 1977; Kiser et al., 1986; Wehle and Grabstald, 1986). In most of these cases, large-caliber needles were used. The chance of tumor seeding is very low with small-caliber needles.

THE KIDNEY

Histologic Recall

Knowledge of the complex structure of the kidney is rarely necessary in the interpretation of cytologic material. In aspirated material renal glomeruli and tubules occasionally may be observed but rarely, if ever, interfere with the diagnosis (Fig. 8-1). The differentiation of *adrenal* cortical cells from tumors of renal origin may be sometimes troublesome, as discussed on p. 219.

Indications

Space-occupying lesions of the kidney and its surrounding areas, whether discovered in symptomatic patients or as an incidental finding, may be the target of cytologic studies. By far the most common lesions subjected to cytologic analysis are renal cysts and renal tumors.

Most renal carcinomas can be identified by clinical and roentgenologic means, such as ultrasound, computed tomography, and angiography, the latter to document the tumor "blush." Hence, the principal benefits of the aspiration technique are in cases in which the exact nature of a lesion cannot be determined by the customary approaches (Pilotti et al., 1988). Thus, preoperative cytologic diagnosis is applicable mainly to unusual renal and perirenal lesions such as angiomyolipomas, renal carcinomas without a "blush," renal oncocytomas, metastatic tumors, and juvenile and adult Wilms' tumors (nephroblastomas).

Other Methods of Investigation

Voided Urine

It is occasionally possible to recognize renal carcinoma cells and, on the rarest occasion, cells of other renal tumor types in the urinary sediment, when the tumors have invaded the renal pelvis (see p. 201). Because the diagnostic yield of the sediment of voided urine is unpredictable, the *transcutaneous aspiration biopsy technique* is the technique most commonly used. Early observers performed aspirations of renal cysts using palpation or retrograde pyelography as a guide (Dean, 1939). Today, as described above, the aspiration procedures are performed using ultrasound or computed tomography guidance. These techniques can also be used for transcutaneous evacuation of contents of renal cysts.

Benign Lesions of Kidney and Perirenal Tissues

Aspiration biopsy technique is applicable to the diagnosis of a number of benign lesions affecting the kidney and the perirenal tissue.

Renal Cysts

Simple acquired renal cysts belong to the earliest targets of aspiration. In 1939 Dean described a number of cases of aspirates of solitary renal cysts, using a large caliber needle and a glass syringe. The lesions were localized either by palpation or by intravenous pyelography. The same procedure may be applied to-day, except for progress in roentgenologic or ultrasound localization techniques. It is debatable whether cysts in polycystic kidneys should ever be aspirated, unless there is a suspicion of a tumor; thus the procedure is limited to the aspiration of either solitary or multiple acquired cysts. The latter (and renal carcinomas) may also occur in patients undergoing dialysis (Dunhill et al., 1977; Hughson et al., 1980). In fact, end-stage renal disease is considered a high risk factor for renal cancer (Bretan et al., 1986). Most cysts are asymptomatic and usually are an incidental finding, except for those cysts that for reasons of rupture, infection, or hemorrhage may cause pain. As a point of caution, renal carcinomas may become cystic (Pollack et al., 1982), and carcinomas may be associated with or occur within benign cysts (Levine et al., 1964; Anderson et al., 1977; Ambrose et al., 1977; Navarri et al., 1981; Silva and Childers, 1989). A case of a large aneurysm of the renal artery mimicking a cyst has been described by Hantman et al. (1982).

HISTOLOGY AND CYTOLOGIC FINDINGS

Most acquired renal cysts are lined by a simple cuboidal epithelium. Occasionally a papillary proliferation of the epithelial lining may be observed. The lumen of the cyst often contains desquamated epithelial cells and, quite often, macrophages. The aspirated fluids are usually clear, straw-colored, sometimes murky or brown.

The corresponding cytologic findings consist of scattered small epithelial cells, usually few in number, but sometimes forming clusters (Color Plate 8-1A). The epithelial cells sometimes may show pyknotic nuclei, but very rarely any significant nuclear abnormalities. Occasionally cells resembling renal tubular cells may be noted. The dominant feature of most smears is usually an accumulation of macrophages with single or double peripheral nuclei, surrounded by abundant, finely vacuolated cytoplasm (Fig. 8-2). Occasionally the nuclei of the macrophages may appear large and may show central nucleoli. Very rarely, however, are these findings sufficiently important to warrant a suspicion of cancer. Hemosiderin accumulation may be occasionally observed as the result of a hemorrhage.

A rare finding in hemorrhagic cysts is the presence of spherical structures of variable sizes with spoke-like striations of the outer ring, resembling Liesegang rings described by Sneige et al., 1988. These presumably crystalline structures may be derived from hemoglobin.

There are two situations in which cyst contents may require either a very careful follow-up, another aspiration, or even a surgical exploration: if the aspirated cyst content is bloody (in the absence of a

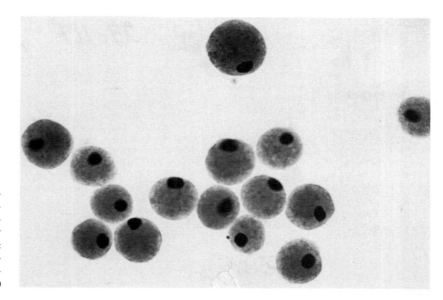

FIGURE 8-2. Aspirate of a renal cyst. Macrophages with finely vacuolated cytoplasm, sometimes referred to as "foamy cells." ($\times$ 600; from Koss, L. G.: Diagnostic Cytology and Its Histopathologic Bases. 4th Ed. Philadelphia, J.B. Lippincott, 1992.)

known trauma to the vessels) and contains atypical cells or if the smear shows papillary epithelial fragments that may suggest a proliferative process of cyst lining. Such findings are exceptional, provided that one is aware of the fact that renal carcinomas may occur in cysts and that such tumors may sometimes masquerade as cysts (Ambrose et al., 1977; Bruun and Nielsen, 1986; Ljungberg et al., 1990). The cytologic findings in renal carcinomas are described on p. 201.

Renal Abscess

Renal abscesses are usually symptomatic and may occur as a consequence of pyelonephritis. The aspirate usually shows necrotic material and polymorphonuclear leukocytes, characteristic of pus.

Angiomyolipoma

This rather uncommon renal tumor with frequent perirenal extension may occur as an isolated event in otherwise normal patients (usually women) or as multiple small bilateral lesions in patients with tuberous sclerosis, the latter being characterized by mental retardation, epilepsy, and sebaceous adenomas of the skin (Bennington and Beckwith, 1975; Brodsky and Garnick, 1989; Silva and Childers, 1989). Angiomyolipoma may be recognized on computed tomography because of the characteristic clear areas corresponding to fat (Bosnik et al., 1988). Histologically the lesion is composed of fatty tissue, thick-walled blood vessels, and bundles of smooth muscle (Fig. 8-3 *C,D*). The latter may show significant variations in nuclear sizes. Lymph node involvement by tumor

has been reported (Ro et al., 1990). We have observed an invasion of vena cava by the tumor in a 16-year-old patient with a negative follow-up of 12 years.

In smears of aspirated material the characteristic feature of the tumor is tissue fragment, accompanied by few single cells or isolated nuclei. The presence of fat cells is usually conspicuous and serves to identify the nature of the tumor, a clue that is particularly valuable in the presence of substantial nuclear abnormalities in the smooth muscle cells. Such nuclei may be significantly enlarged and hyperchromatic, thus mimicking a malignant tumor (Fig. 8-3). The cytologic features combined with the findings in computed tomography usually allow an accurate cytologic identification of the lesion. Similar observations were reported by Sant et al., 1990 and by Koss et al., 1992. On very rare occasions, angiomyolipoma may be associated with renal carcinoma (Blute et al., 1988; Taylor et al., 1989).

Other Benign Lesions

Xanthogranulomatous pyelonephritis, and *malakoplakia* may occasionally form space-occupying renal lesions, and it is likely that sooner or later aspiration biopsy of these lesions will take place. To the best of my knowledge, no such cases have been reported to date. Das et al. (1992) reported the results of ultrasound-guided renal aspirates in 19 patients, clinically suspected of *renal tuberculosis.* In 16 of these patients, the diagnosis was confirmed by culture. In 15 of these 16 patients, the cytologic findings disclosed granulomas represented by epithelioid cells, accompanied by Langhans' type giant cells and/or

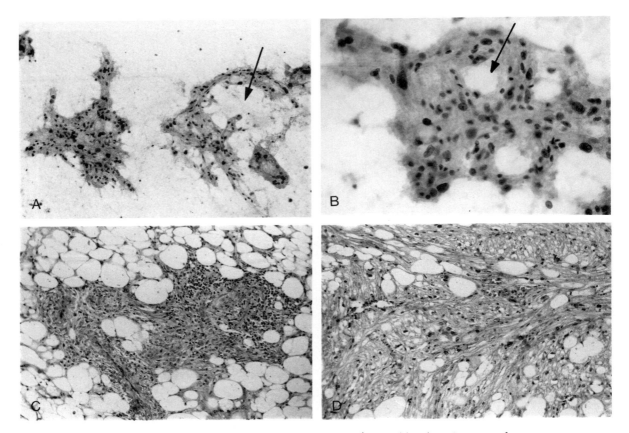

FIGURE 8-3. Angiomyolipoma of left kidney in a 34-year-old, otherwise normal, woman. Aspirate (*A,B*) and histologic pattern (*C,D*). (*A*) Low-power view of the aspirate, showing compact fragments of tissue, composed of spindly cells. In one of the clusters a central core of fat cells may be seen (*arrow*). (*B*) A high-power view of the spindly (smooth muscle) cells, showing significant variability in nuclear sizes and hyperchromasia. The clear spaces (*arrow*) represent fat cells. (*C*) Low-power view of the histology of the resected tumor, showing a mixture of fat and spindly cells with occasional thick-walled blood vessels. (*D*) A high-power view of the smooth muscle and fat in the same tumor. (*A,C* × 150; *B,D* × 400. Photographs courtesy of Professor S. Woyke.)

necrosis. The aspirated material could also be used for bacterial cultures with positive results in 7 patients. Cytologic presentation of tuberculosis is discussed on p. 47 and of malakoplakia on p. 65.

Renal Cortical Adenomas

Before the era of contemporary imaging, these small lesions were usually recognized as an incidental finding at autopsy (Bell, 1950). Nowadays computed tomography may occasionally contribute to the discovery of these tumors in asymptomatic patients. It was arbitrarily proposed by Bell (1950) that the diameter of 3 cm separates benign adenomas from small renal carcinomas capable of metastases, but this view is increasingly questioned. It has been pointed out that there are no fundamental histologic differences between "adenomas" and renal carcinomas. Further,

it has been shown that lesions less than 3 cm in diameter are occasionally capable of metastases. On the other hand, larger renal carcinomas may be free of metastases (summaries in Bennington and Beckwith, 1975, and Petersen, 1992). For this reason, Bennington and Beckwith proposed that renal "adenomas" are "small renal carcinomas that have not yet produced metastases." This view, however, has been challenged by cytogenetic observations that documented a different set of chromosomal abnormalities (trisomy of chromosome 7, absence of chromosome Y) in adenomas than in carcinomas, which are characterized by changes in the short arms of chromosomes 3 and 5 (Cin et al., 1989). Kovacs (1993) also expressed the view that renal cortical adenomas may be distinguished from small renal carcinomas by cytogenetic features.

The cytologic presentation of the two lesions is, however, identical and is described below.

Juxtaglomerular Cell Tumor

These are very rare renal cortical tumors composed of richly vascularized tubules and sheets of small epithelial cells, first described by Kihara et al. (1968). These tumors are derived from modified smooth muscle cells producing renin and hence renin-induced hypertension with a high urinary potassium loss (Squires et al., 1984; Abbi et al., 1993). The tumors may be mistaken for cortical adenomas. There is no description of the cytologic presentation of these tumors.

Oncocytomas

These tumors are described below (see p. 207).

MALIGNANT TUMORS OF THE KIDNEY

Renal Carcinoma

Renal carcinoma is the most common malignant tumor of the kidney. A familial occurrence associated with a specific abnormality on chromosome 3 has been described (Cohen et al., 1979). In most instances, however, the disease appears to be sporadic. Hematuria is the most common symptom, but weight loss, fever, erythrocytosis, anemia, hypercalcemia, hepatic dysfunction, and amyloidosis may also occur.

Renal carcinomas have a variable and often puzzling behavior. Some tumors reach large sizes without forming metastases, whereas in some cases, the tumors metastasize widely from a small, clinically occult primary (summary in Petersen, 1992). Metastases to bone, lung, or brain may occur many years after nephrectomy. Some renal carcinomas may invade the renal veins and from there the inferior vena cava, sometimes extending into the right atrium of the heart. Hemorrhage and necrosis within the tumor may lead to cavity formation.

Renal carcinomas display a variety of histologic patterns. The *classical pattern* consists of clear cells with abundant cytoplasm filled with delicate vacuoles containing glycogen and lipids, and a central, slightly hyperchromatic nucleus provided with a small but clearly visible nucleolus. The clear cells may be arranged in solid sheets, cords, or tubule-like structures. In other tumors the cytoplasm of the predominant cells is denser, more granular and eosinophilic, and the nuclear abnormalities may be more conspicuous. Such tumors often display hemorrhagic necrosis and may be cystic. A *tubular pattern* composed of smaller, cuboidal cells and a papillary pattern are also recognized. I have also seen a pattern in which the cancer cells resembled oncocytes lining tubular structures.

Thoenes et al. (1985, 1986) proposed a classification of renal carcinomas into a chromophil and a chromophobe group, the latter characterized by pale cytoplasm, distinct cell membranes, and positive staining with Hale's acid colloidal iron. Ultrastructurally, this group is characterized by the presence of numerous cytoplasmic vesicles. The chromophobe renal tumors appear to have specific chromosomal abnormalities (Kovacs, 1993). This classification has had no documented bearing on tumor behavior (except papillary carcinomas—see below) and has limited bearing on cytologic diagnosis.

One of the immunocytologic peculiarities of renal cell carcinoma is its reactivity with antibodies to keratin and vimentin (Domagala et al., 1988). This coexpression of intermediate filaments is sometimes observed in epithelial tumors of endometrial, ovarian, and mammary origin, but because it is very rare in other carcinomas, it may serve to identify the primary origin of metastatic tumors of renal origin if the primary tumor is occult (Domagala and Osborn, 1992).

Renal carcinomas may have a *papillary-cystic configuration*. In such tumors the core of the papillae may contain large macrophage-like cells. Psammoma bodies may also be observed in tumors of this type. The prognosis of this group of tumors appears to be more favorable than that of clear cell carcinomas (Boczko et al., 1979). Kovacs (1989) and Kovacs et al. (1989) observed genetic differences between the common renal carcinomas and the papillary tumors. The latter failed to show any abnormalities on chromosome 3 but had a gain of an extra chromosome 17.

There is a rare, highly aggressive variant of renal carcinoma with highly abnormal spindly tumor cells, imitating sarcomas, known as *sarcomatous carcinoma* (Farrow et al., 1968; Ro et al., 1987). Carcinomas of the collecting tubules have also been described. These tumors are mainly distinguished by their origin in the renal medulla. Their microscopic identification is, at best, very difficult (Kennedy et al., 1990).

Cytologic Presentation

VOIDED URINE

Although several observers have claimed that between 25% and 50% of renal carcinomas can be recognized in the voided urine sediment (Meisels, 1963; Umiker, 1964; Piscioli et al., 1983) this has not been my experience. In fact, I have seen few cases in which unequivocal cancer cells of renal parenchymal origin could be identified in urine sediment, usually in high-grade, large tumors (Figs. 8-4 and 8-5). Such cells are fairly large, spherical or elongated (Fig. 8-4) and have abundant, transparent, sometimes vacuolated cyto-

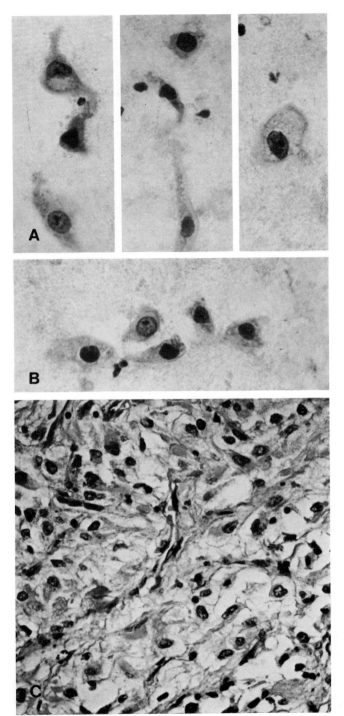

FIGURE 8-4. Voided urine sediment in renal carcinoma. (*A* and *B*) Cancer cells with fairly abundant cytoplasm, relatively small nuclei, some containing nucleoli. The recognition of such cells is difficult. (*C*) Section of renal carcinoma, showing a mixture of clear and spindly cells. (*A,B* × 560; *C* × 350. From Koss, L. G.: Diagnostic Cytology and Its Histopathologic Bases. 4th Ed. Philadelphia, J.B. Lippincott, 1992.)

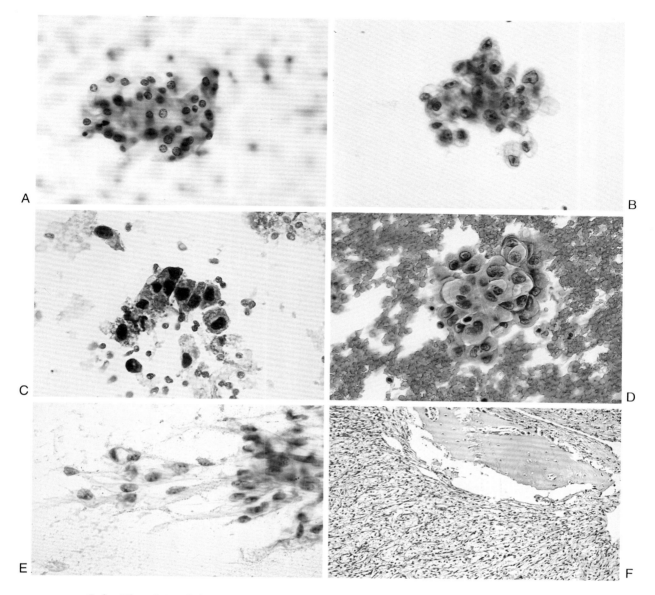

Color Plate 8-1. (*A*) Renal cyst. A cluster of benign epithelial cells. (*B*) Renal carcinoma—voided urine. A cluster of cancer cells with vacuolated cytoplasm, large, finely granulated nuclei, and prominent nucleoli. (*C,D*) Renal carcinoma, masquerading as a renal pelvic tumor, in retrograde washings. (*C*) Smear of sediment with numerous cancer cells with hyperchromatic nuclei and foamy cytoplasm. (*D*) Cell block, showing a fragment of tumor. (*E,F*) Occult renal carcinoma, metastatic to a rib. (*E*) Aspirate of the metastatic lesion. Note the elongated cancer cells, mimicking a sarcoma—a common event in renal cancer. (*F*) Histologic section of the metastatic focus, showing renal carcinoma. The primary tumor was a small carcinoma of right kidney. (*A–E* × 160; *F* × 40 enlarged about × 2.5)

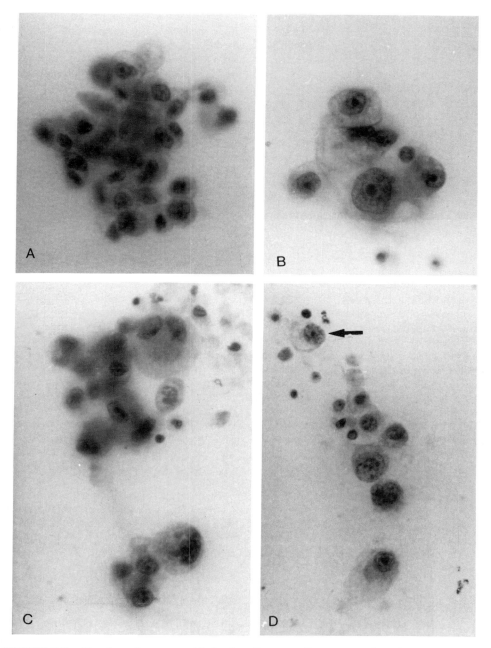

FIGURE 8-5. Renal carcinoma—voided urine. Cancer cells occur singly and in clusters. (*A*) Cluster of medium-sized cancer cells with clear, abundant cytoplasm. Nucleoli are readily visible in most vesicular nuclei. (*B*) Large cancer cells with clear, vacuolated cytoplasm and large, granular nuclei with very large nucleoli. (*C*) A less conspicuous cluster of smaller cancer cells. (*D*) Medium-sized cancer cells, some with conspicuous nucleoli (*arrow*), some with lobulated nuclei. The small cells in this photograph are presumably renal tubular cells. (*A–D* × 560)

plasm. The nuclei are vesicular and contain large, single nucleoli. In favorable cases, clusters of such cells may be observed (Fig. 8-5, Color Plate 8-1*B*). Because of the difficulties in recognizing such cells as of renal origin, it is advisable to have supporting radiologic evidence of a renal abnormality.

To facilitate the recognition of renal carcinoma in voided urine, Hajdu et al. (1971) proposed the use of fat stain such as Sudan IV; in fact, in the initial study, 14 of 20 patients with cells staining for fat were shown to harbor renal carcinoma. Subsequently, however, Mount et al. (1973) failed to confirm these results.

On a rare occasion, *retrograde washings* may document the presence of a renal carcinoma, masquerading as a tumor of renal pelvis (Color Plate 8-1*C,D*).

ASPIRATION BIOPSY

Aspirates of renal carcinomas, composed of clear or granular cells, or a mixture of these cell types, often contain much blood and considerable necrosis. Within this background abundant tumor cells are usually seen and readily identified. Although the common histologic pattern of clear cell carcinoma of the kidney may appear quasi-benign, the cells aspirated therefrom are clearly abnormal. The cancer cells are either dispersed or form clusters and, occasionally, gland-like arrangements. The cancer cells are large, and have abundant, mainly eosinophilic, cytoplasm that is often filled with numerous small vacuoles or granules. The nuclei vary in size, and, although usually not markedly hyperchromatic (with some exceptions), are large and have a coarse chromatin pattern. The nucleoli are readily seen, and, in some cancer cells, are multiple, markedly enlarged, and of irregular shape (Figs. 8-6, 8-7). Intranuclear cytoplasmic inclusions are sometimes observed (Fig. 8-8*A, inset*). Other tumor cells of similar size and configuration have a granular, more opaque, sharply demarcated, eosinophilic cytoplasm. The two cell types—the cells with vacuolated or granular cytoplasm—are often seen in the same smear. In some tumors the cancer cells tend to be elongated and may mimic the spindly configuration of cells in a sarcoma (Fig. 8-8). Such cells may also occur in metastatic foci, a common source of diagnostic errors (Color Plate 8-1*E,F;* Koss et al., 1992). When bizarre, spindly cancer cells dominate the cytologic presentation, the possibility of a *sarcomatous carcinoma* must be considered. We have seen very few aspirates from *tubular carcinomas*. In such cases, the cancer cells were smaller and had scanty cytoplasm without the characteristic vacuoles. The nuclear features were also somewhat different because of conspicuous hyperchromasia that obscured the presence of nucleoli.

In many conventional renal carcinomas the cytologic presentation is surprisingly complex, inasmuch as the various cell types may occur side by side (see Fig. 8-6). The sources of such cellular diversity are not always evident in conventional tissue sections, and multiple tissue blocks may have to be processed to identify the areas of the tumor composed of unusual cell types.

In *poorly differentiated renal cell carcinomas,* most cancer cells in aspirates may be quite small and occur singly and in small clusters. Such cells have large, hyperchromatic nuclei and scanty, clear cytoplasm. In histologic sections such tumors are composed of tightly packed small cancer cells with scanty, sometimes clear cytoplasm (Fig. 8-9). In still other tumors the high degree of vascularity will be reflected by the presence of capillary vessels.

The cytologic presentation of *papillary-cystic carcinomas* is quite characteristic: the tumor cells are large, and have a delicate, basophilic, slightly granular cytoplasm, and round, large, rather pale nuclei with finely granular chromatin and large central nucleoli (Fig. 8-10). The cancer cells occur singly or in small, flat clusters and are usually accompanied by numerous macrophages of variable sizes. The latter are characterized by faintly vacuolated, delicate cytoplasm and small, usually single but sometimes multiple, nuclei. Cancer cells and macrophages may be quite similar, and the distinction between them must be based on nuclear and nucleolar size rather than any other features. The macrophages have been traced to the cores of the papillae, and their presence in a renal aspirate must signal the possibility of a papillary carcinoma.

A rare type of renal carcinoma originating in collecting ducts (*Bellini duct carcinoma*) has been described (summary in Kennedy et al., 1990). There has been no reported experience with cytologic presentation of this tumor.

Grading of Renal Cell Carcinomas

The prognosis of renal cancer depends on the stage and grade of the disease. The Scandinavian investigators established a system of cytologic grading based on nuclear features (Zajicek, 1979; Arner et al., 1965). In well-differentiated tumors the cells resembled the cells of convoluted tubules, the nuclei were uniform in size, and the nucleoli were small. In poorly differentiated carcinomas, conspicuous nuclear abnormalities were present. The moderately well-differentiated carcinomas were intermediate between the two extremes. Preoperative radiotherapy was given to patients with poorly differentiated tumors, a practice generally not followed in the United States. Although I have not attempted to grade renal carcino-

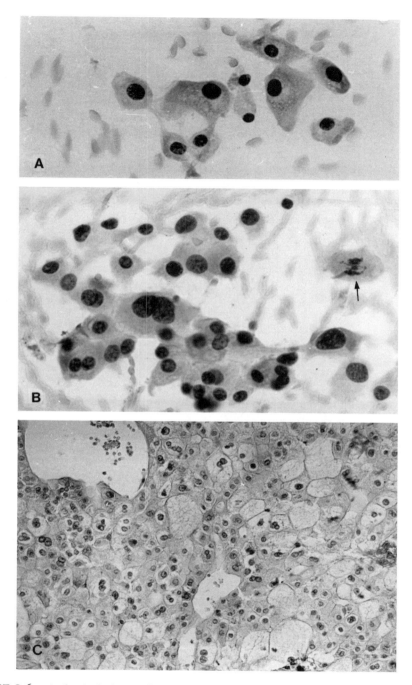

FIGURE 8-6. A classical clear cell carcinoma of kidney—aspiration biopsy. Cytologic presentation (*A,B*) and tissue pattern (*C*). (*A,B*) The cancer cells are large, of variable sizes, and are provided with large, hyperchromatic, sometimes multiple nuclei. The abundant cytoplasm contains fine vacuoles. (*C*) Histologic appearance of the primary tumor. (*A,B* × 560; *C* × 300. From Koss, L. G., Woyke, S., and Olszewski, W.: Aspiration Biopsy. Cytologic Interpretation and Histologic Bases. 2nd Ed. New York, Igaku-Shoin, 1992.)

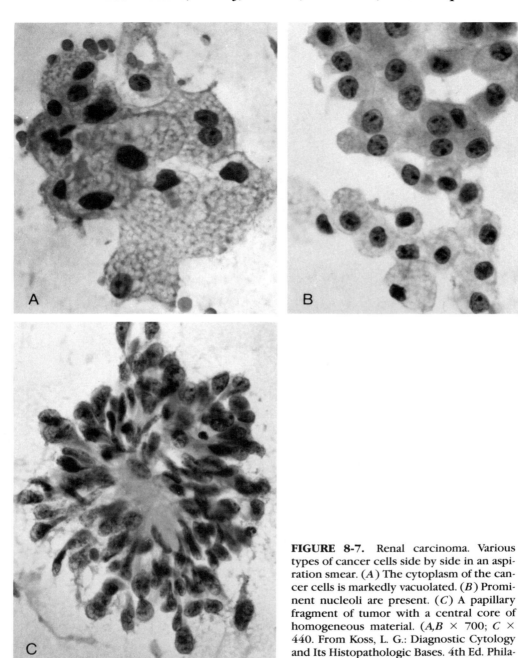

FIGURE 8-7. Renal carcinoma. Various types of cancer cells side by side in an aspiration smear. (*A*) The cytoplasm of the cancer cells is markedly vacuolated. (*B*) Prominent nucleoli are present. (*C*) A papillary fragment of tumor with a central core of homogeneous material. (*A,B* × 700; *C* × 440. From Koss, L. G.: Diagnostic Cytology and Its Histopathologic Bases. 4th Ed. Philadelphia, J. B. Lippincott, 1992.)

mas, the variety of cytologic patterns encountered, even among the best differentiated renal cancers, would indicate serious limitations to any objective cytologic grading systems. It is of interest that DNA measurements of renal carcinomas in retrospective flow cytometric studies produced conflicting results. On the other hand, the size of the cancer cell nuclei may be of prognostic value in stage I tumors; the prognosis was better if the average nuclear size was below 3.2 μm in diameter (Tosi et al., 1986). For further comments on DNA ploidy and morphometry, see Chapter 9.

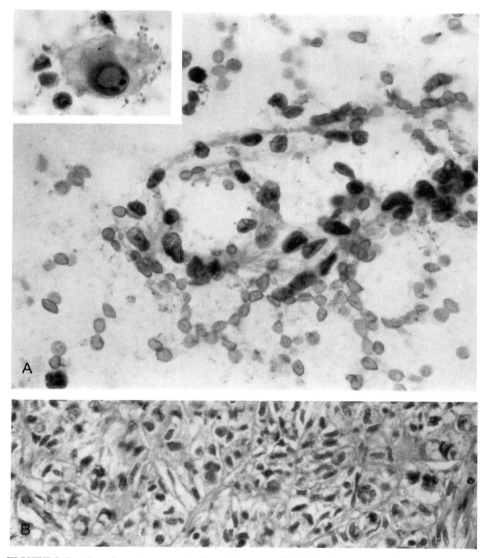

FIGURE 8-8. Renal carcinoma, spindly cell pattern. (*A*) Spindly cancer cells in an aspiration smear. *Inset:* A cancer cell with an intranuclear cytoplasmic inclusion. (*B*) Histologic section of the same case. (*A* and *inset* × 700; *B* × 440)

Renal Oncocytomas (Tubular Adenomas With Oncocytic Features)

Although renal oncocytomas are generally thought to be benign, there is sufficient uncertainty about the behavior of these tumors to discuss them with malignant tumors of the kidney. These solid renal tumors have an excellent prognosis, unlike the common forms of renal carcinoma (Klein and Valensi, 1976; Lieber et al., 1981; Barnes and Beckman, 1983;

Davis et al., 1991). The tumors are composed of sheets and trabeculae of large cells with granular, eosinophilic cytoplasm and large, often multiple, irregularly shaped hyperchromatic and pyknotic nuclei (Fig. 8-11*E,F*). In electron microscopy the cytoplasm of the tumor cells is filled with numerous mitochondria (Fig. 8-11*G*). The tumors may reach considerable size and may be multiple (Hamperl, 1962). Recurrences and metastases have been rarely observed, usually in tumors that combine some features

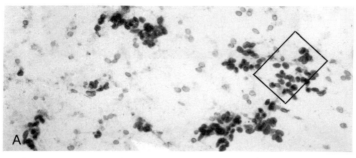

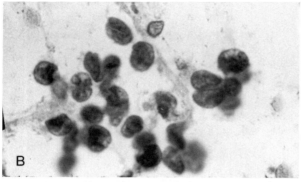

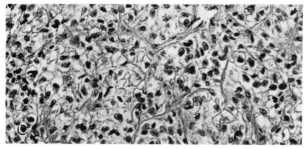

FIGURE 8-9. Poorly differentiated renal carcinoma, composed of small cells. (*A*) Low-power view of the aspiration smear. The squared area in *A* is shown in *B*. (*B*) High-power view of the small cancer cells with scanty cytoplasm and irregular, hyperchromatic nuclei. (*C*) Histologic appearance of the same tumor. (*A* × 200; *B* × 1,000; *C* × 300. Photographs courtesy of Professor S. Woyke.)

of an oncocytoma with those of a more conventional carcinoma (Rodriguez et al., 1980; Lieber et al., 1981). It is of note that many oncocytomas are aneuploid (see page 273). Angiography of oncocytomas usually reveals an avascular or hypovascular renal lesion (Sos et al., 1976).

Cytologic Presentation

In a case reported by Rodriguez et al. (1980), the aspiration smear contained large tumor cells singly and in small clusters (Fig. 8-11*A*–*C*). The sharply demarcated cells had abundant granular cytoplasm and large, spherical or ovoid, smoothly outlined, pyknotic, single or multiple nuclei. The cytologic appearance was unlike any other renal neoplasm or normal renal tissue. In some of the other cases reported to date, cell pleomorphism and nuclear atypia were noted (Nguyen et al., 1985). Whether such cases

should be classified as "pure" oncocytomas or as one of the transitional forms to renal carcinoma is not clear.

Nephroblastoma (Wilms' Tumor)

Nephroblastoma is seen almost exclusively in young children and very rarely in adolescents and adults (Bennington and Beckwith, 1975; Beckwith, 1986, 1989). Some of the young patients may first present with metastases to regional lymph nodes, lungs, and liver, or the tumor may be detected as an incidental abdominal mass. Histologically, these mixed malignant neoplasms contain elements of embryonal epithelium mimicking tubules and glomeruli, elements of sarcoma, usually rhabdomyosarcoma, and undifferentiated tumor cells.

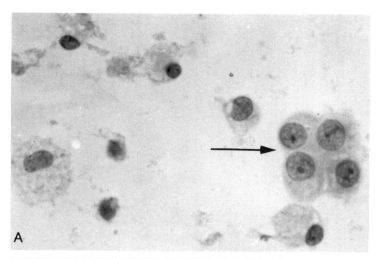

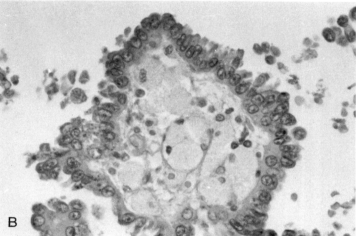

FIGURE 8-10. Papillary carcinoma of kidney. (*A*) The aspiration smear shows a small cluster of cancer cells with prominent nucleoli in finely granular nuclei (*arrow*). The cytoplasm is abundant. Several large macrophages are seen in the background. (*B*) Histologic appearance of the same tumor. (*A* × 700; *B* × 440. Modified from Koss, L. G.: Diagnostic Cytology and Its Histopathologic Bases. 4th Ed. Philadelphia, J.B. Lippincott, 1992.)

Several years ago, the prognosis of Wilms' tumor, particularly if diagnosed in an advanced stage of the disease, was considered hopeless. With advances in surgery and radio- and chemotherapy, there has been a dramatic change in the outcome of treatment (Beckwith, 1989). It has been shown, though, that the outcome depends not only on stage of the disease but also on histologic pattern. Tumors with foci of marked cytologic abnormality (anaplasia) and those composed mainly of sarcomatous stroma had an unfavorable outcome (Beckwith and Palmer, 1978). Still, even in tumors with favorable prognosis, relapses may occur. The unfavorable factors pertain mainly to extension of the tumor beyond its capsule or invasion of the kidney or renal vessels (Weeks et al., 1987). Because the outcome is much more favorable in resectable tumors still limited to the kidney (Stage I), an early cytologic diagnosis may contribute to salvage of the patients.

Cytologic Presentation

VOIDED URINE

The finding of cancer cells derived from a nephroblastoma is a rare event, usually observed in patients with large tumors that may have invaded the renal pelvis. Still, voided urine is the easiest to secure and the least invasive of diagnostic procedures and should be tried in the young patients suspected of harboring the disease, sometimes with rewarding results.

An example of such an examination is shown in Figure 8-12. Tightly packed clusters of small cancer cells with hyperchromatic nuclei and scanty cytoplasm (Fig. 8-12*A*,*B*), corresponded to the poorly dif-

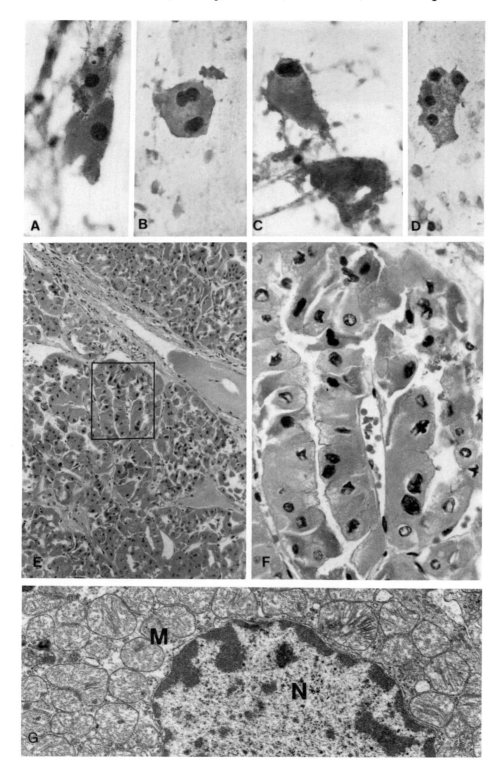

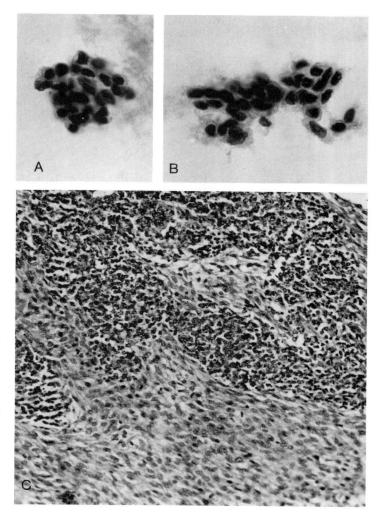

FIGURE 8-12. Nephroblastoma (Wilms' tumor). Voided urine sediment in a 9-year-old child with a renal mass and subsequent diagnosis of nephroblastoma. (*A,B*) Tightly knit clusters of small cancer cells with hyperchromatic nuclei and scanty, sometimes columnar-shaped, cytoplasm. (*C*) A histologic section of the tumor, showing the sarcomatous element composed of clear spindly cells and the undifferentiated epithelial element composed of small, dark cells, the latter corresponding to the findings in the urinary sediment. (*A,B* × 560; *C* × 150)

ferentiated epithelial cell component in the surgically removed tumor (Fig. 8-12*C*). The differential diagnosis in children includes other small cell cancers, such as Ewing's sarcoma, neuroblastoma, or a malignant lymphoma. In none of these tumors, however, is the tumor cell clustering as dominant as in Wilms' tumor. Knowledge of clinical data is, of course, essential in diagnosis.

TRANSCUTANEOUS ASPIRATION BIOPSY

Transcutaneous aspiration biopsy is much more secure than voided urine in the diagnosis of Wilms' tumors.

The complex structure of Wilms' tumors is usually reflected in the aspirated material. The smears often contain large fragments of tissue wherein one can

FIGURE 8-11. Renal oncocytoma. Aspiration biopsy, histology of tumor and ultrastructural features. (*A–D*) Aspirate. *A,B,* and *C* show large, oncocytic tumor cells with the characteristic large pyknotic nuclei and granular, markedly eosinophilic cytoplasm. (*D*) This photograph most likely represents a cluster of renal tubular cells. (*E,F*) Low- and high-power view of the tumor composed of strands of large, eosinophilic cells with pyknotic nuclei. (*G*) An electron micrograph of a tumor cell, showing the cytoplasm filled with mitochondria (*M*). N = nucleus. (*A–D* × 360; *E* × 80; *F* × 360; *G* × 8,000. Modified from Rodriguez, C. A., et al. Renal oncocytoma. Preoperative diagnosis by aspiration biopsy. Acta Cytol. *24,* 355, 1980, with permission.)

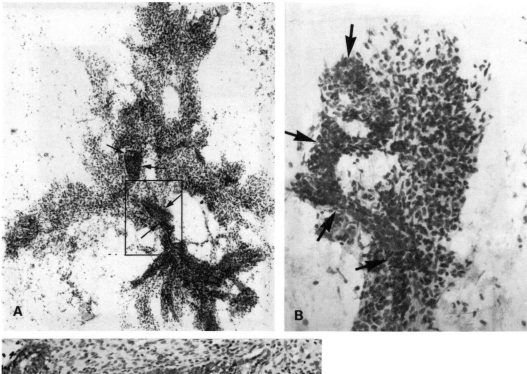

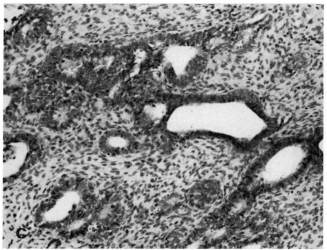

FIGURE 8-13. Aspiration biopsy of a nephroblastoma (Wilms' tumor) in a boy, age 11 months. (*A,B*) Classical presentation of a Wilms' tumor in smears. (*A*) The aspirate contained a large fragment of tissue with darker staining, tubular areas (*arrows*) corresponding to tubules observed in the tumor. (*B*) A higher magnification of the squared area in *A*, showing the tightly packed tubular structures (*arrows*), surrounded by small spindly cells, corresponding to the tumor stroma. (*C*) Histologic section of the same tumor, showing tubular structures, surrounded by stromal cells. (*A* × 70; *B,C* × 150. Modified from Koss, L. G., Woyke, S., and Olszewski, W.: Aspiration Biopsy. Cytologic Interpretation and Histologic Bases. 2nd Ed. New York, Igaku-Shoin, 1992.)

distinguish tubular aggregates of tightly packed, small epithelial cells surrounded by small tumor cells (blastema cells) corresponding to the undifferentiated stroma (Figs. 8-13, 8-14). In some cases, spindle-shaped stromal cells are the dominant feature of the aspirate (Fig. 8-15). The spindly cells are characterized by a delicate, elongated cytoplasm. The nuclei of these cells are usually also elongated, but some may assume spherical shapes.

The epithelial cells are small, cuboidal, or columnar, with scanty cytoplasm. They may be recognized mainly because of their occurrence in multi-layered tubular clusters corresponding to tumor tubules (Figs. 8-13*B*, 8-14*B,D*). Other features of note include the occasional presence of smooth and striated muscle cells and of bizarre, large, malignant cells.

Not all of these cell types are seen in all cases, but

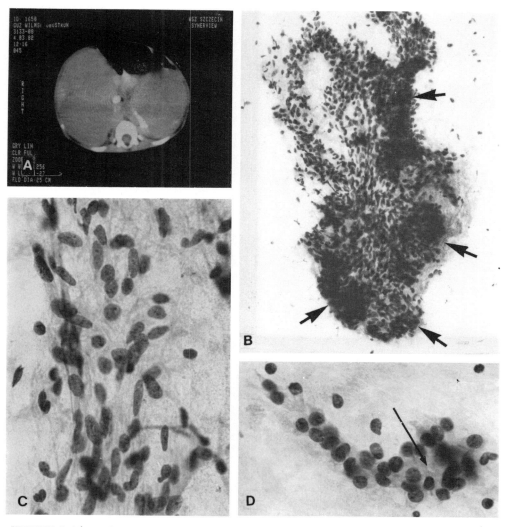

FIGURE 8-14. Bilateral nephroblastomas (Wilms' tumors) in a 5-month-old boy. (*A*) Computed tomography of the abdomen showing bilateral renal masses. (*B*) Typical aspirate of nephroblastoma showing a large cell cluster composed of spindly cells and several dark-staining, compact areas (*arrows*), corresponding to the epithelial components of the tumor. (*C*) High magnification of the loosely arranged, spindly stromal cells. (*D*) A tubular structure with a lumen (*arrow*). (*B* × 150; *C,D* × 400. Modified from Koss, L. G., Woyke, S., and Olszewski, W.: Aspiration Biopsy. Cytologic Interpretation and Histologic Bases. 2nd Ed. New York, Igaku-Shoin, 1992.)

in the clinical setting of these tumors the diagnosis is usually quite easy. Perhaps the only significant point of differential diagnosis is neuroblastoma, which is usually readily recognized by the characteristic rosette formation and neurofilaments (see p. 221).

Wilms' tumors in adults are very rare. In one such case, occurring in a 54-year-old man, the predominant cell pattern in the aspirate was similar to that of a small cell carcinoma, with cancer cells forming loosely structured clusters (Fig. 8-16). The differential diagnosis included a malignant lymphoma or a small cell carcinoma, either primary or metastatic. The surgical biopsy was interpreted as adult Wilms' tumor. In spite of multiple pulmonary metastases, the patient

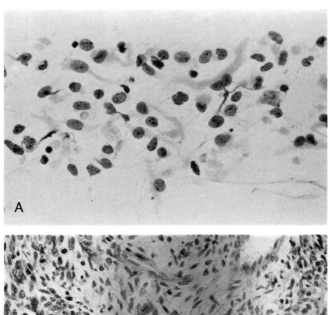

FIGURE 8-15. Wilms' tumor composed primarily of stromal cells, similar to fibroblasts, in a 4-year-old boy. (*A*) The aspiration smear is composed mainly of elongated, spindly quasi-benign–looking cells, corresponding to the dominant histologic feature of the tumor, shown in (*B*). (*A* × 400; *B* × 250. Modified from Koss, L. G., Woyke, S., and Olszewski, W.: Aspiration Biopsy. Cytologic Interpretation and Histologic Bases. 2nd Ed. New York, Igaku-Shoin, 1992.)

responded dramatically, though temporarily, to a chemotherapeutic regimen suitable for Wilms' tumor.

Rare Malignant Tumors

Clear Cell Sarcoma

Clear cell sarcoma of kidney (bone metastasizing renal tumor of childhood) has been now separated from Wilms' tumors because of its unique histologic make-up, unusual behavior, and poor prognosis (Marsden et al., 1980; Haas et al., 1984; Wood et al., 1990). The tumors are composed of sheets of small cells with clear cytoplasm and display a marked propensity to skeletal metastases. Katz (1991) described the tumor cells in aspirated material as occurring in clusters, having uniform nuclei, and showing cytoplasmic vacuolization. The example in Color Plate 8-2*A,B* is from a metastatic tumor to the bone in a 4-year-old child.

Malignant Rhabdoid Tumor

This entity, with a very poor prognosis, has also been separated from Wilms' tumors, although its pathogenesis is unknown (Beckwith and Palmer, 1978; Sotelo-Avila et al., 1986; Weeks et al., 1989). Similar tumors have been observed in locations other than the kidney (summary in Parham, 1994). The small tumor cells often contain eosinophilic cytoplasmic deposits, resembling those observed in embryonal rhabdomyosarcoma (Weeks et al., 1989). Ultrastructural studies (Haas et al., 1981; Parham et al., 1994) disclosed that the cytoplasmic inclusions in these tumors are not composed of myofibrils but of aggregates of intermediate filaments, mainly vimentin. Parham et al. (1994) suggested that these tumors be considered "poorly differentiated neoplasms with rhabdoid features." There is a report of the cytologic presentation of this rare tumor (Drut, 1990). Katz (1991) described the tumor cells as sheets of "monotonous population of oval to round cells" with central

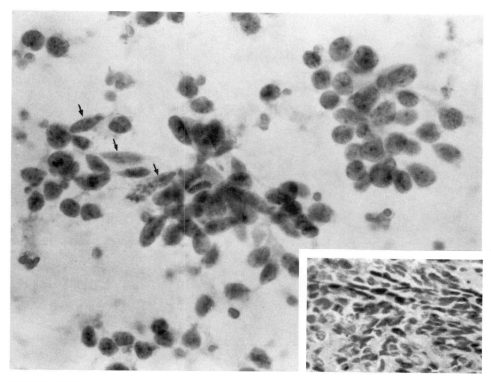

FIGURE 8-16. Wilms' tumor in a 54-year-old man. Aspiration biopsy smear and histologic features. The aspirate was characterized by clusters of numerous small cancer cells with pale nuclei and prominent nucleoli. Some of the tumor cells were elongated (*small arrows*), corresponding to the dominant feature of the tumor in the histologic material, shown in *inset*. (*Smear* × 700; *inset* × 440)

or eccentric nuclei with finely granular chromatin and variable number of nucleoli. The plasmacytoid appearance of the tumor cells was stressed. Of note was the strongly positive cytokeratin stain in tumor cells (Color Plate 8-2*C,D*).

Sarcomas

Sarcomas of childhood were described above. In adults, sarcomas constitute less than 1% of malignant neoplasms of the kidney. They include leiomyosarcoma (the most common type), liposarcoma, rhabdomyosarcoma, malignant lymphoma, and hemangiopericytoma (Farrow et al., 1968; Brodsky and Garnick, 1989). Sano and Koprowska (1965) reported a case of a primary malignant lymphoma of the kidney, identified in voided urine. None of the other tumors have been reported in aspirated material to date.

For further comments on cytologic presentation of rhabdomyosarcoma and malignant lymphoma in voided urine, see Chapter 5.

Renal Pelvic Carcinomas

Carcinomas of the renal pelvis frequently present with hematuria and ipsilateral pain. The cytologic presentation of these tumors in urine and other sampling techniques pertaining to the lower urinary tract have been discussed in Chapter 6. Occasionally, invasive urothelial tumors are thought to be of renal origin and are aspirated.

The cytologic presentation in aspirates depends on tumor grade and differentiation. The well-differentiated urothelial carcinomas shed tumor cells of variable sizes, characterized by sharply demarcated cytoplasm and large, irregular, markedly hyperchromatic, sometimes pyknotic nuclei. The cytoplasm is often eosinophilic in Papanicolaou stain. In such tumors, cells mimicking umbrella cells are sometimes recognized.

Cells of poorly differentiated carcinomas lack the characteristic cytoplasmic or structural features. They are characterized by large, hyperchromatic, often

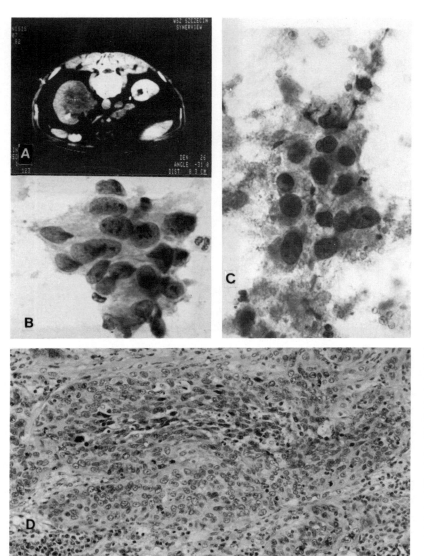

FIGURE 8-17. Poorly differentiated carcinoma of renal pelvis. (*A*) Computed tomography: a tumor in the right renal pelvis is marked with a faint cross. (*B,C*) Aspirate. There are two clusters of cancer cells of medium size, characterized mainly by irregular, hyperchromatic nuclei, some of which are pyknotic. The cytoplasm is poorly preserved. (*D*) Histologic section of primary tumor. (*B,C* × 400; *D* × 150. From Koss, L. G., Woyke, S., and Olszewski, W.: Aspiration Biopsy. Cytologic Interpretation and Histologic Bases. 2nd Ed. New York, Igaku-Shoin, 1992.)

pyknotic nuclei, surrounded by scanty, sometimes frayed cytoplasm (Fig. 8-17).

The differential diagnosis between renal parenchymal tumors and urothelial cancer of renal pelvic origin is relatively simple if both tumor types are well represented: the vacuolated cytoplasm and the large size of renal carcinoma cells differ markedly from the sharply circumscribed urothelial cancer cells. In poorly differentiated tumors, however, the distinction may not be easy and may not be solved until the surgical specimen is available. In difficult cases, immunocytochemistry may be helpful (see Chapter 10). Other tumor types such as primary squamous and adenocar-

cinomas of renal pelves are uncommon, and we have not seen such tumors in aspirates (see Chapter 6).

Metastatic Carcinoma in Kidney

The kidney occasionally is the site of metastatic cancers from other organs, such as the lung, breast, colon, or thyroid, as well as malignant melanomas and lymphomas. The kidneys may also be involved in contiguity by cancer from adjacent organs, such as the adrenals and the peritoneum, including lymphomas. The aspiration biopsy cytology of these lesions is the same as that of the primary neoplasms (Koss et al., 1992).

ASPIRATION OF RENAL TRANSPLANTS

Monitoring of renal transplants with voided urine sediment was discussed in Chapter 4. Direct aspirations of the transplanted kidneys may also provide guidance on their status. The technique allows the study of the population of lymphocytes: a predominance of T-lymphocytes over B-lymphocytes strongly suggests that a rejection may be threatening the transplanted kidney. The estimation of T- and B-lymphocytes may be performed by flow cytometry (see Chapter 9) or by immunologic microscopic techniques (von Willebrand, 1985).

THE ADRENAL

Histologic Recall

The adrenal glands are small organs capping the cranial poles of the kidneys. The adrenal cortex is composed of cuboidal cells arranged in layers known as the zona glomerulosa, zona fasciculata, and zona reticularis. The cells have eosinophilic, faintly vacuolated, cytoplasm and centrally located nuclei of variable sizes. Giant nuclei may occasionally occur, particularly in children (Koss, 1992). The medulla, which is a part of the autonomic nervous system, is composed of epithelium-like cells with basophilic cytoplasm, arranged in spherical groups (Zellballen), or short cords in an intimate relation to blood capillaries. With potassium bichromate fixation, most of the cells of the adrenal medulla contain brown cytoplasmic granules and hence are known as chromaffin cells or pheochromocytes. Sympathetic ganglion cells, singly or in small groups, also occur in the medulla.

Methods of Investigation

Until refinement of visualizing techniques was achieved, the diagnosis of adrenal abnormalities was based mainly on measuring the endocrine hormonal activity of the glands by biochemical analysis. Currently, a transcutaneous needle aspiration biopsy of the adrenal glands adds yet another dimension to the clinical and biochemical background. The normal adrenal glands can be visualized by computed tomography, but only with difficulty by sonography. Space-occupying lesions of the adrenal can be visualized

with either method, but have to be at least 3 cm in diameter for sonography to be effective. The lesions that do not give any specific radiologic clues are the targets for aspiration biopsies. The diagnostic options include benign or malignant primary lesions and metastatic cancer.

Lesions of the Adrenal Cortex

Benign Tumors

CORTICAL ADENOMAS

The most common tumor of the adrenal is the adrenal cortical adenoma, which is usually an incidental finding of no clinical significance. These tumors are composed of one or more nodules of adrenal cortical cells without any distinguishing microscopic features. Most cortical adenomas are about 1 cm in diameter, but much larger tumors may be observed. As in normal adrenal cortex, isolated, large hyperchromatic nuclei may be observed. Occasionally, cortical adenomas (or hyperplasias) have an intense hormonal activity and cause Cushing's syndrome or hyperaldosteronism (Conn's syndrome). Unfortunately, the morphology of functioning and nonfunctioning adenomas is identical, and an aspirate is unlikely to clarify the endocrine status of the neoplasm.

Cytologic Presentation. Smears of adrenal cortical adenoma are cellular, containing cohesive clusters and dispersed adrenal cortical cells with abundant, eosinophilic, finely granular cytoplasm and uniform, usually vesicular but sometimes somewhat pyknotic, nuclei. Many of the nuclei are eccentric (Fig. 8-18). Such cells somewhat resemble normal hepatocytes in size and configuration, and care must be taken in aspirates of the right adrenal to make sure that the needle has not been erroneously placed in the liver. However, other components of the hepatic aspirates (cytoplasmic bile granules, bile duct cells) are not present in adrenal aspirates.

OTHER BENIGN TUMORS

The cytologic features of adrenal cysts and of myelolipomas have been described by several observers. *Adrenal cysts'* content consisted of fluid with a few leukocytes, macrophages, and cortical epithelial cells (Scheibl et al., 1977).

Myelolipomas are asymptomatic tumors without any known malignant potential that are composed of fat with evidence of hematopoiesis, best recognized as nucleated precursors of erythrocytes (erythroblasts) and megakaryocytes. Until the era of contemporary

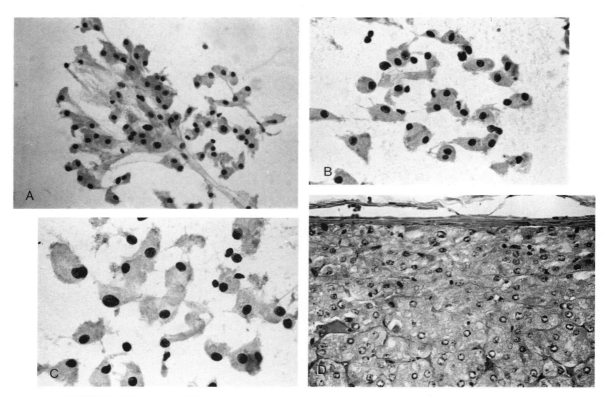

FIGURE 8-18. Large (10 cm in diameter) benign adrenal cortical adenoma: aspiration smear and histology of tumor in a 92-year-old woman. (*A,B*) Sheets and dispersed large epithelial cells, characteristic of this lesion. (*C*) A somewhat higher power view of the smear. Note the abundant faintly granular eosinophilic cytoplasm of the component cells and dark nuclei with some variability in size. A binucleated cell may be noted. (*D*) The histologic section of the fully encapsulated tumor. (*A,B* × 250; *C* × 400; *D* × 200)

roentgenology, myelolipomas were usually incidental findings at surgery or at autopsy. They may now be discovered as an incidental finding in computed tomography of abdominal organs, and their recognition has become important in order to avoid unnecessary surgery, which has been performed on some patients (Noble et al., 1982; de Blois and deMay, 1985). The lesion is easily recognized in transcutaneous aspirations, showing a mixture of fat and hematopoietic cells. The easiest to recognize are the large, multilobate megakaryocytes (Katz, et al., 1984; Pinto, 1985; de Blois and DeMay, 1985).

Adrenal Cortical Carcinoma

Most of these very rare tumors are large, either encapsulated or invasive, and often show necrosis and hemorrhage. Histologically, they have an alveolar, trabecular, or solid pattern. The cytoplasm of the tumor cells is often abundant, vacuolated, or compact, and the nuclei are usually enlarged and hyperchromatic. Some of the tumors resemble cortical adenoma, whereas others are completely undifferentiated. However, the behavior of these tumors need not be reflected in their make-up. The histologic separation of a cortical adenoma and a well-differentiated cortical carcinoma may be difficult, unless there is supporting clinical evidence of recurrence or metastases. Large size of the tumor as well as necrosis, atypia, numerous mitotic figures, and invasion of vessels favor carcinoma (Page et al., 1985).

CYTOLOGIC PRESENTATION

The cytologic features of adrenal cortical carcinoma were illustrated by a few observers who described

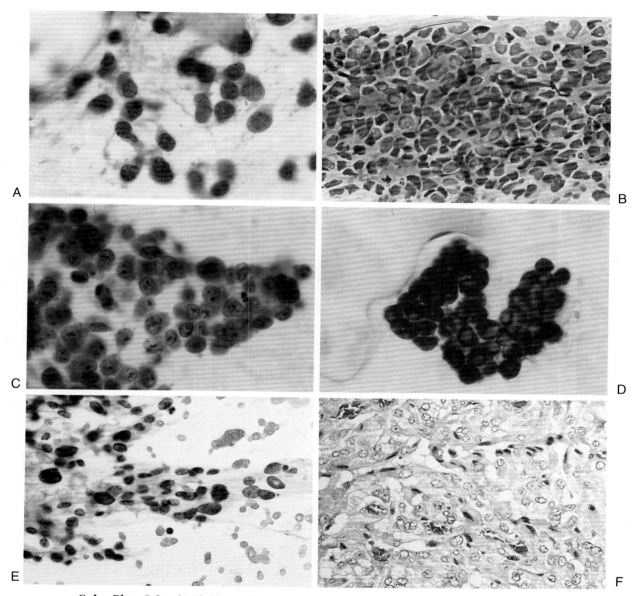

Color Plate 8-2. (*A,B*) Clear cell sarcoma of kidney in a 4-year-old child. (*A*) The aspirate of bone metastasis shows small tumor cells with basophilic cytoplasm and peripheral nuclei. (*B*) A fragment of metastatic tumor. (Photographs courtesy of Dr. Ruth Katz, M. D. Anderson Cancer Center, Houston, Texas.) (*C,D*) Malignant rhabdoid tumor. (*C*) The aspirate shows a sheet of malignant cells with abundant cytoplasm and spherical nuclei with nucleoli. (*D*) The tumor cells show a strongly positive reaction to cytokeratin. (Photographs courtesy of Dr. Ruth Katz, M. D. Anderson Cancer Center, Houston, Texas.) (*E,F*) Retroperitoneal pheochromocytoma in a 43-year-old patient with severe hypertension. (*E*) The aspiration smears are composed mainly of spindly cells occurring singly or in clusters. Note the variability in the sizes of the hyperchromatic nuclei. (*F*) Section of the primary tumor with considerable cytologic atypia. (*A,C,D* × 260; *B* approximately 160; *E* × 160; *F* × 100, enlarged about × 2.5.)

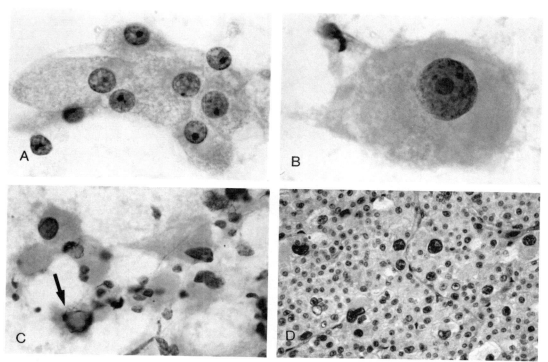

FIGURE 8-19. Recurrent adrenal cortical carcinoma in a 40-year-old woman, 18 months after removal of primary tumor. (*A–C*) aspiration smear; (*D*) histology of the tumor. (*A*) Tumor cells arranged in a cohesive cluster, closely resembling normal cortical cells. (*B*) A tumor giant cell with a large, hyperchromatic nucleus and a huge nucleolus. (*C*) A cluster of poorly preserved tumor cells with hyperchromatic nuclei and one with a suggestion of an intranuclear cytoplasmic inclusion (*arrow*). (*D*) Histologic appearance of tumor. Note the numerous tumor giant cells with large, sometimes multiple, hyperchromatic nuclei. (*A,B* × 800; *C* × 400; *D* × 250. Case courtesy of Professor S. Woyke. Modified from Koss, L. G., Woyke, S., and Olszewski, W.: Aspiration Biopsy. Cytologic Interpretation and Histologic Bases. 2nd Ed. New York, Igaku-Shoin, 1992.)

large, often multinucleated tumor cells with large, hyperchromatic nuclei and large nucleoli (Zajicek, 1979; Levin, 1981; Zornoza, 1981). In a personal case of a recurrent, moderately differentiated cortical carcinoma, the smears contained small cells with abundant vacuolated cytoplasm and round nuclei, similar to those of cortical adenoma (Fig. 8-19*A*), and larger cells with large, often hyperchromatic nuclei with huge nucleoli (Fig. 8-19*B*). There were numerous poorly preserved, presumably necrotic tumor cells, often with large, somewhat pyknotic nuclei (Fig. 8-19*C*). The recurrent tumor (Fig. 8-19*D*) resembled an adrenal cortical adenoma, except for the presence of numerous giant cells with very large, occasionally multiple nuclei. It must be stressed once again that neither the cytologic nor the histologic fea-

tures of these rare tumors are of prognostic value. Nuclear hyperchromasia and enlargement may also occur in cells of the normal adrenal cortex and in benign adenomas (Koss, 1992). Thus, the diagnosis of adrenocortical carcinoma may prove difficult, even with growing experience.

Zajicek (1979) emphasized considerable similarities between renal carcinomas and adrenal cortical carcinomas. In my judgment, these similarities are more evident in histologic material (and are reflected in the old name [hypernephroma] for renal tumors) than in cytologic samples. As described on p. 204, the diversity of cancer cells in most renal parenchymal carcinomas is diagnostic of these tumors. A surgical intervention will clarify the origin of these tumors in debatable cases.

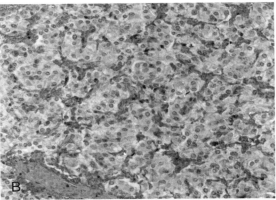
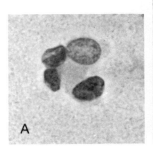

FIGURE 8-20. Common cytologic presentation of pheochromocytoma. (*A*) The tumor cells are fairly uniform and their cytoplasm is poorly preserved. The nuclei appear bland. (*B*) The retroperitoneal tumor is composed of the characteristic *Zellballen,* surrounded by a network of capillaries. (*A* × 700; *B* × 175.) For a different cytologic presentation, see Color Plate 8-2 *E,F.*

Tumors of the Adrenal Medulla

Pheochromocytoma

Pheochromocytomas, or paragangliomas, are tumors of the adrenal medulla, the retroperitoneal space, or other sites in which paraganglia may occur, for example the urinary bladder. These tumors may be associated with excessive catecholamine production and with paroxysmal or sustained hypertension. In its familiar form the tumor may be associated with multiple endocrine neoplasms such as medullary carcinoma of the thyroid, parathyroid adenomas and neurofibromas (multiple endocrinopathies of several types, Sipple's syndrome) (Schimke et al., 1968; Webb et al., 1980). The behavior of a pheochromocytoma cannot be determined on morphologic grounds, and some of them may produce metastases. The diagnosis is usually supported by the biochemical demonstration of increased serum and urine levels of catecholamines and their metabolites. Grossly, the tumors vary in size, are usually red in color because of a rich blood supply, and, if placed in a bichromate-containing fixative, turn brown in color, hence the name chromaffin tumors.

Histologically, pheochromocytomas in their classic form are composed of tightly knit nests of large cells (Zellballen) with granular cytolplasm (Fig. 8-20*B*). The nuclei are vesicular and are provided with small nucleoli. The cell nests are surrounded by a dense network of capillaries. It is quite common to observe single bizarre, large cells with single or multiple, sometimes hyperchromatic, nuclei dispersed throughout the tumor. This feature is common to all endocrine tumors, and it has no bearing on behavior or prognosis. Less often, parts of the tumor may be composed of spindly or polygonal cells that may appear to be very atypical and, in fact, may mimic a spindle cell

sarcoma. The endocrine features of this group of tumors may be documented by electron microscopy, which usually discloses the presence of osmiophilic, dark cytoplasmic endocrine granules, bound by a single membrane. The functional nature of these granules may be documented by immunocytochemistry with appropriate antibodies. Staining with an antibody to chromogranin is commonly used to document the presence of the endocrine granules. Staining with antibodies to various polypeptide hormones may reveal the actual product of secretion of these tumors (see Chapter 10).

CYTOLOGIC PRESENTATION

Aspirates of pheochromocytoma are usually represented by clusters of approximately cuboidal epithelial cells of similar sizes (Fig. 8-20*A*). The nuclei, of equal sizes, are spherical, vesicular, and provided with small nucleoli. The cytoplasm is usually poorly preserved. These cells represent the cell nests (Zellballen) seen in histology. Sometimes, however, the presence of giant tumor cells with single or multiple hyperchromatic nuclei may suggest a malignant epithelial tumor. This finding must be assessed in light of the clinical presentation, and it does not necessarily indicate that the pheochromocytoma will behave in a malignant fashion. In some tumors the presence of highly abnormal spindle cells, suggesting a sarcoma, may be noted (Color Plate 8-2*E,F*). If the tumor is located within the adrenal the diagnosis of pheochromocytoma is usually secure, particularly if supported by clinical and biochemical data. In retroperitoneal tumors the diagnosis of the specific tumor type may have to be withheld, pending a histologic examination of the tissue. Although no accidents have been recorded in aspiration of an adrenal or retroperitoneal pheochromocytoma, there are reports of attacks of acute hypertension during aspirates of ca- rotid body tumor, a closely related neoplasm. Thus, if a pheochromocytoma is suspected on clinical and bio- chemical grounds, the aspiration procedure should be performed with appropriate caution.

Neuroblastoma

Neuroblastomas are tumors derived from primitive nerve cells and are usually observed in infants and children, very rarely in adults. Their most common primary location is the adrenal medulla, but similar tumors may occur in the cerebellum and sometimes in other primary sites. Retinoblastoma is a very similar tumor affecting the eyes; retinoblastomas are associ- ated with a defect in the growth inhibitory Rb gene that may have a familial distribution. Neuroblastomas may metastasize very early and widely in the course of the disease, and many patients are first seen be- cause of metastases. The tumors secrete catechol- amines and their metabolites, notably vanillylman- delic acid (VMA) and homovanillic acid, which may be observed in urine and support strongly the diag- nosis (Evans et al., 1987). Histologically, this highly malignant tumor of the adrenal medulla is composed of undifferentiated small cells, often forming rosettes with delicate neurofibrils filling the lumen. Until some years ago these tumors were nearly always fa- tal. Today, with a combination of chemotherapy and, sometimes, radiotherapy, at least 60% of the children can be salvaged. The tumor produces N-*myc* on- cogene, and titration of this oncogene appears to be of prognostic value (Brodeur et al., 1984; Seeger et al., 1985).

CYTOLOGIC PRESENTATION

The aspiration smears are cellular and contain nu- merous small tumor cells that are somewhat larger than small lymphocytes. The cells have round or slightly oval nuclei with granular chromatin and one or two small nucleoli. The cells are either dispersed or form loosely structured clusters without nuclear molding. In most cases the cells form rosette-like structures, the center of which is filled with delicate neurofibrils (Fig. 8-21). Similar fibrils are often seen within the loosely structured cell clusters. The recog- nition of neuroblastoma is based on the presence of neurofibrils and rosettes in an appropriate clinical set- ting. Other small cell malignant tumors of childhood may sometimes mimic neuroblastoma in metastatic sites. Thus, Ewing's sarcomas, embryonal rhab- domyosarcomas, primitive neuroepithelial tumors (PNETs), and lymphomas (sometimes combined as the "small, round, blue-cell" malignant tumors of childhood) may have a somewhat similar cytologic presentation (Koss et al., 1992). In the rare situation

when a differential diagnosis is needed, the search for neurofibrils and, if necessary, immunocytology may be of help in solving the problem.

In the very rare neuroblastomas in older patients, the differential diagnosis includes malignant lympho- mas and, exceptionally, metastatic oat cell carcino- mas, usually of pulmonary origin. Neither tumor forms rosettes. Cell molding, common in oat cell car- cinoma, does not occur in either neuroblastoma or malignant lymphoma.

Ganglioneuroblastoma and Ganglioneuroma

Ganglioneuroblastomas are uncommon tumors combining the features of a neuroblastoma with the presence of mature ganglion cells. There is evidence that the ganglion cells may represent a differentiation and maturation process occurring in neuroblastomas. Some neuroblastomas may differentiate fully into ma- ture ganglion cells, resulting in a ganglioneuroma. In ganglioneuromas, only ganglion cells are observed.

CYTOLOGIC PRESENTATION

In aspirates of ganglioneuroblastomas the presence of the large ganglion cells with their cytoplasmic ex- tensions and neurofibrils, next to the small cells of the neuroblastoma, are diagnostic of this tumor type (Fig. 8-22).

Metastatic Tumors

We have seen several aspirates of metastases from various primary sites to the adrenal. The most com- mon were metastases of lung cancer in men and breast cancer in women. Metastases of renal carcinoma and malignant melanoma have also been described (Berk- man et al., 1984; Katz et al., 1984; Pagani, 1984; Mitchell et al., 1985). In all cases seen by us, the cytologic presentation of a metastatic tumor was eas- ily distinguished from that of adrenal cells. The diag- nosis is often aided by the clinical history and by the computed tomography scan: metastatic tumors often affect both adrenals, whereas primary adrenal tumors (with some exceptions, such as neuroblastoma in chil- dren and some pheochromocytomas), are usually con- fined to one gland.

THE RETROPERITONEUM

The retroperitoneal space is of major interest in urologic pathology and cytopathology as a site of pri- mary tumors and tumorous conditions and of metasta- ses from tumors of the genitourinary tract. Aspiration biopsy cytology has significantly modified the diag- nostic approach to retroperitoneal lesions because of

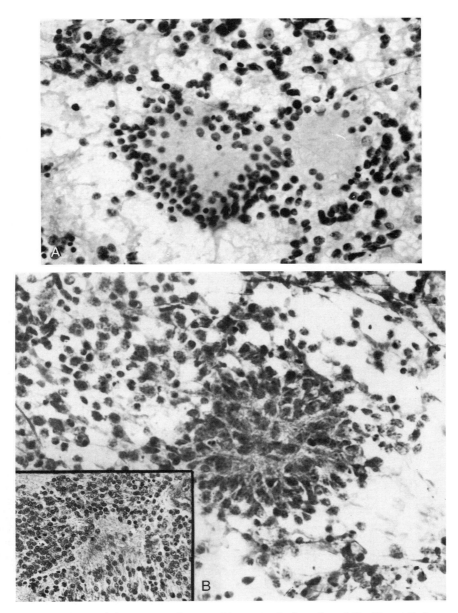

FIGURE 8-21. (*A*) Aspirate of a neuroblastoma of adrenal medulla. The cells form the characteristic rosettes with a center filled with delicate neurofibrils. (*B*) An aspirate of metastatic neuroblastoma in a lymph node. The rosette-like arrangement of the small cells is characteristic of the tumor. *Inset:* Histologic appearance of the metastatic tumor. Note the center of the rosette filled with neurofilaments. (*A* × 400; *B* × 450; *inset* × 100. *A* courtesy of Professor S. Woyke. *B* from Koss, L. G., Woyke, S., and Olszewski, W.: Aspiration Biopsy. Cytologic Interpretation and Histologic Bases. 2nd Ed. New York, Igaku-Shoin, 1992.)

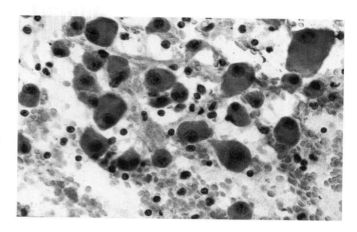

FIGURE 8-22. Aspirate of a ganglioneuroblastoma in a 19-month-old boy. The smear shows a mixture of large ganglion cells and small cells, representing the component of neuroblastoma (× 300). (From Koss, L. G., Woyke, S., and Olszewski, W.: Aspiration Biopsy. Cytologic Interpretation and Histologic Bases. 2nd Ed. New York, Igaku-Shoin, 1992.)

the very low risk of the transcutaneous approach, obviating the need of an exploratory laparotomy in many but not all cases. The best results of the transcutaneous approach are with metastatic tumors and staging of genitourinary cancers, for example, with testicular tumors, or recurrent lymphomas. In many primary tumors, aspiration cytology may offer a preliminary diagnosis that may allow better planning of therapy. Still, cytologic sampling of the primary tumor may be deceptive, and the preliminary diagnosis may have to be modified in histologic material. Also, typing of primary malignant lymphomas may be limited by the size of the sample. In spite of these caveats, transcutaneous aspiration is the procedure of choice in the evaluation of retroperitoneal space-occupying lesions. The fundamental principles of the aspiration biopsy techniques were described above.

Special Features of Retroperitoneal Aspiration

The first attempts at aspiration of retroperitoneal organs were based on lymphangiographic visualization of lymph nodes by Göthlin in 1976. With the introduction of ultrasound and computed tomography, these became the methods of choice as a guide to transcutaneous aspirations. Ultrasound can only be used if the size of the lesion is at least 3 cm in diameter. Skilled operators can aspirate smaller lesions with computed tomography.

Space-occupying lesions located above the pelvic brim are best aspirated through the posterior approach. For lesions within the bony pelvis, the approach is anterior and transperitoneal. The method described for aspiration of the abdominal organs (see p. 195) is used: a needle guide is inserted before the introduction of the needle. Although care should be

exercised to avoid the large vessels and the intestine, the complications of an incidental perforation of these organs are vanishingly small. Intra-abdominal hemorrhage or peritonitis occurring as a consequence of the aspiration of the retroperitoneal space must be exceptional, and no cases have been seen in many hundreds of aspirations performed at the Montefiore Medical Center.

Benign Lesions

There are few benign disorders of the retroperitoneal space that call for evaluation by aspiration biopsy. Although various primary benign tumors are known to occur, such as lipomas, leiomyomas and hemangiomas, they are rarely of sufficient size to be aspirated. We observed one example of *retroperitoneal neurilemoma*. The tumor type was readily recognized because of the cohesive nature of the clusters and the presence of dark lines, corresponding to palisading of nuclei (the so-called Verocay bodies, Fig. 8-23). We have not observed other benign retroperitoneal tumors to date. Inflammatory processes, such as tuberculosis and mycoses, and in some countries, parasitic infections (for example, *Paragonimus westermanni* infection in Korea) may occur. I have not seen an example of it in aspirated material and, to the best of my knowledge, none have been described (Katz, 1991).

One benign condition that may be aspirated is *hyperplasia of retroperitoneal lymph nodes*. The smears show a mixture of lymphoid cells in various stages of maturation, accompanied by large macrophages with phagocytized debris (tingible body macrophages, Fig. 8-24). The latter cells may also occur in Burkitt's lymphoma (see below).

The causes of hyperplasia of retroperitoneal lymph

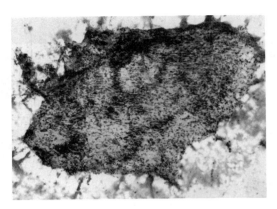

FIGURE 8-23. An aspirated fragment of a mediastinal neurilemoma with the characteristic dark lines, corresponding to nuclear palisading (Verocay bodies) (× 56).

nodes are often unclear. The condition may mimic a malignant lymphoma (Fig. 8-25) and aspiration biopsy may be helpful in differentiating between these two conditions.

Primary Malignant Tumors

Pheochromocytoma

Because pheochromocytomas sometimes display malignant behavior, they are listed here. The histo-

logic and cytologic presentation of these tumors was discussed on p. 220.

Malignant Lymphomas

Non-Hodgkin's lymphomas and Hodgkin's disease may be primary or recurrent in the retroperitoneal space.

Non-Hodgkin's Lymphomas

The reader is referred to other sources for a detailed discussion of histologic and cytologic presentation of the non-Hodgkin's lymphomas (Koss, 1992; Koss et al., 1992). For the purposes of this discussion, a brief summary of the current classification scheme is given.

Non-Hodgkin's lymphomas (NHL) may be subdivided into two principal groups, one derived from B-lymphocytes and one from T-lymphocytes.

B-cell lymphomas are much more common than T-cell lymphomas, and are for the most part characterized by monoclonal formation of immunoglobulins (kappa or lambda) and by specific cell receptors that can be visualized with appropriate antibodies (e.g., CD19, CD20, CD22).

T-cells may be recognized with antibodies CD2, CD3, CD4, CD7, and CD8. The CD4 positive cells are helper cells, and CD8 positive cells are suppressor cells, both being affected in AIDS. In malignant T-cell lymphomas, one or more of the markers for normal T-cells is usually missing.

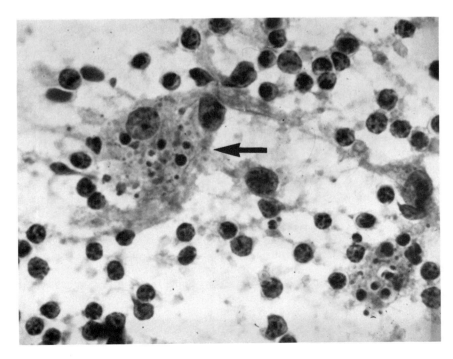

FIGURE 8-24. Aspirate of a hyperplastic lymph node. The smear contains lymphocytic cells of various sizes, reflecting stages of maturation. Large macrophages containing phagocytized debris (tingible body macrophages—*arrow*) are evident (× 900).

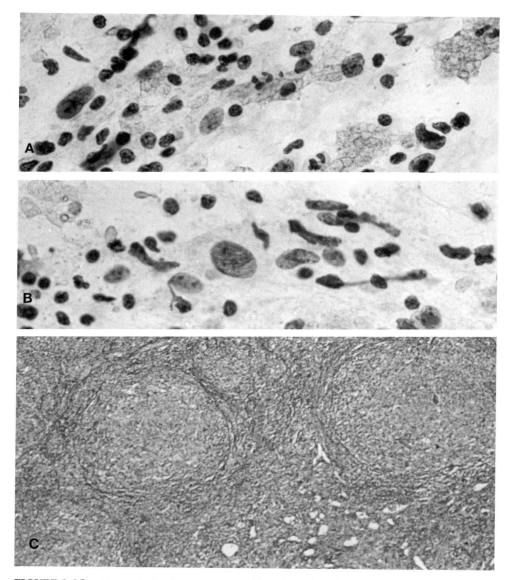

FIGURE 8-25. Hyperplasia of retroperitoneal lymph nodes. There was a clinical suspicion of a malignant lymphoma in a 54-year-old woman. The lesion regressed spontaneously after biopsy. (*A,B*) Aspiration smear showing lymphocytes of various sizes and macrophages with vacuolated cytoplasm. (*C*) Histologic section of a lymph node obtained by exploratory laparotomy. (*A,B* × 700; *C* × 70).

Non-Hodgkin's lymphomas may retain the basic follicular configuration of normal lymph nodes (follicular lymphomas) or lose it (diffuse lymphomas). Cell sizes (maturation) and nuclear configuration, correlated with clinical outcome, has led to the classification of these disorders given in Table 8-1, the so-called Working Formulation.

In the United States, the frequency of the three groups of NHL was given as 35% for low-grade, 63% for intermediate-grade and 2% for high-grade. The survival patterns of treated patients also correlated well with the Working Formulation: 5–7 years, 2–5 years, and 0.5–2 years, respectively (Scarin, 1989).

TABLE 8-1
Working Formulation of Non-Hodgkin's Lymphomas

Low-Grade (Best Prognosis)

Small lymphocytic, plasmacytoid
Follicular mixed (small and large cleaved cells)

Intermediate-Grade (Intermediate Prognosis)

Follicular, predominantly large cell
Diffuse, small cleaved cells
Diffuse, small and large cells
Diffuse, large cells (cleaved or noncleaved)

High-Grade (Poor Prognosis)

Large cell, immunoblastic
Lymphoblastic
Small, noncleaved cells
Burkitt's lymphoma

CYTOLOGIC PRESENTATION

The common feature of aspirates of non-Hodgkin's lymphomas is the dominance of dispersed, single cells, usually similar to each other in size and configuration within the same smear. Further classification depends on the type and configuration of the cells and their nuclei (see below). There are some exceptions to the cardinal rule: in poorly prepared, thick smears, the cells may form thick clusters. Some rare types of lymphoma, such as the Ki-1 type, the rare histiocytic type, and some large cell types, mainly of T-cell lineage, may not only form tumor cell clusters but also display significant variability in cell size and configuration. In such cases, the cytologic differentiation of a large cell lymphoma from a metastatic carcinoma may be very difficult and usually requires immunocytochemical studies and accurate knowledge of clinical data to establish the correct diagnosis. Incidentally, such diagnostic problems may occur in histologic material as well. The cytologic features of the most important types of malignant lymphomas are described below. For a detailed analysis of cytologic findings, the reader is referred to Koss et al., 1992.

SMALL CELL LYMPHOMAS

Well-Differentiated, Small Cell Lymphomas. Such tumors of good general prognosis and long-term survival of patients are characterized by smears composed of dispersed cells of equal sizes, somewhat larger than resting lymphocytes (Fig. 8-26). The nuclei may sometimes display a granular arrangement of chromatin (*cellules grumelées*) and small nucleoli.

The cytoplasm is very scanty and barely visible. Identical cytologic presentation may occur in chronic lymphocytic leukemia.

Variants. Cells of small cell lymphomas may show eccentric nuclei with cartwheel arrangement of chromatin, similar to plasma cells (plasmacytoid variant) or nuclei with an indentation or crease (cleaved cell variant [Fig. 8-26C]).

LARGE CELL LYMPHOMAS

The diagnosis of cancer is usually easy in large cell lymphomas. The cancer cells are large, usually dispersed, and show clearly abnormal nuclei (Fig. 8-27). The cytoplasm is scanty but sometimes easier to identify than in small cell lymphomas. In air-dried smears stained with one of the hematologic stains (such as May-Gruenwald-Giemsa) the background of the smear often shows numerous fragments of bluish-staining material, the so-called lymphoglandular bodies (Linsk and Franzén, 1982). The bodies are fragments of the fragile cytoplasm of lymphocytic cells and represent a useful artifact caused by the smear preparation technique that separates malignant lymphomas from anaplastic carcinomas (see Fig. 8-27).

Large cell lymphomas of T-cell type often display convoluted and lobulated nuclei (Fig. 8-28). Ki-1 lymphomas are uncommon, highly malignant neoplasms, characterized by large, bizarre, sometimes multinucleated cancer cells, reacting with a unique antibody of the same name. These tumors (and other large cell lymphomas) often present a problem in the differential diagnosis with large cell anaplastic carcinomas of various origins. As a rule of thumb, carcinoma cells form multilayered aggregates, whereas cells of malignant lymphoma are dispersed. There are, however, many exceptions to this rule. In such cases the presence of lymphoglandular bodies (see above) may be of help. Most often, however, immunocytochemical studies are necessary to identify tumor type (Tani et al., 1989; Yazdi and Burns, 1991).

An important form of retroperitoneal lymphoma is *Burkitt's lymphoma*, usually observed in children. The tumor is characterized by moderate size lymphoma cells, accompanied by numerous tingible body macrophages that account for the "starry sky" appearance in tissue sections (Fig. 8-29). As has been described on p. 223, tingible body macrophages are commonly observed in aspirates of hyperplastic lymph nodes, albeit with a vastly different background (compare Fig. 8-24 with Fig. 8-29B). Still, errors in diagnosis may occur unless close attention is paid to cytologic details and clinical history. Air-dried smears, stained with May-Gruenwald-Giemsa stain

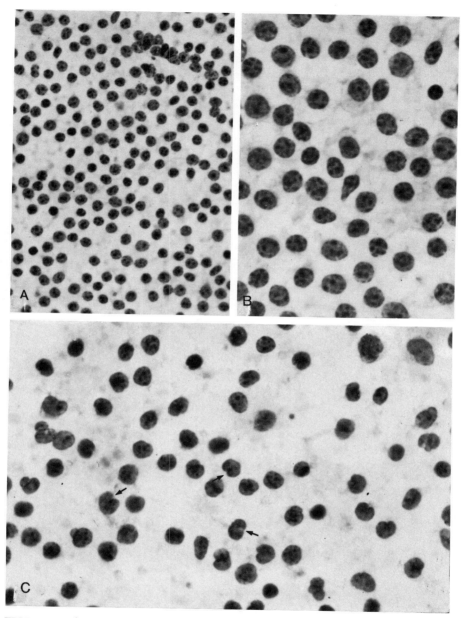

FIGURE 8-26. Aspirates of small cell, well-differentiated lymphomas. Low- (*A*) and high-power (*B*) view of the same aspiration smear to show the uniform, dispersed cell population. In *B* the granularity of some of the nuclei is shown. (*C*) Small cleaved cell lymphoma. Note the characteristic nuclear indentations (*arrows*). (*A* × 450; *B,C* × 900. Photographs courtesy of Professors S. Woyke and W. Olszewski.)

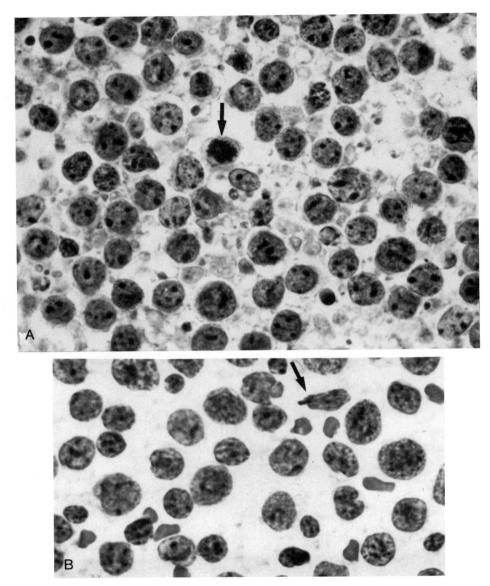

FIGURE 8-27.   Aspirates of a large cell lymphoma. (*A*) The large, dispersed nuclei show irregularities in contour and prominent, large, irregular, frequently multiple nucleoli. A mitotic figure is indicated by arrow. The cytoplasm is poorly preserved and is seen in the background as dispersed fragments, the "lympho-glandular bodies." This artifact is useful in differentiating a malignant lymphoma from an anaplastic carcinoma. (*B*) Another large cell lymphoma. Large size of the dispersed nuclei, some showing nipple-like projections (*arrow*) is characteristic of this tumor type. (*A,B* × 900. *A* modified from Koss, L. G., Woyke, S., and Olszewski, W.: Aspiration Biopsy. Cytologic Interpretation and Histologic Bases. 2nd Ed. New York, Igaku-Shoin, 1992. *B* modified from Koss, L. G.: Diagnostic Cytology and Its Histopathologic Bases. 4th Ed. Philadelphia, J.B. Lippincott, 1992.)

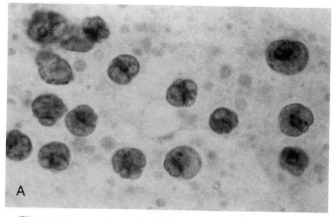

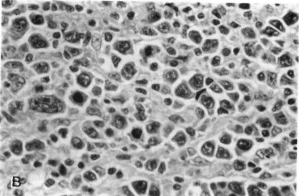

FIGURE 8-28. A large cell T-cell lymphoma. (*A*) The aspirate smear shows markedly lobulated and convoluted nuclei. (*B*) The biopsy of the lymph node shows large tumor cells of variable sizes. (*A* × 900, *B* × 450. Photographs courtesy of Professor S. Woyke.)

may reveal, in tumor cells, cytoplasmic vacuoles, quite characteristic of this tumor type (Fig. 8-29*C*).

Hodgkin's Disease

This common form of malignant lymphoma may occur in the retroperitoneum either as a primary event or as a recurrence. The key cell in the diagnosis of Hodgkin's disease is the Reed-Sternberg (RS) cell, characterized by two or more large nuclei, sometimes arranged in a "mirror image" fashion, each provided with a huge nucleolus. The background of the RS cells depends on the type of the disease. In the "lymphocytic predominance" type, the RS cells are found among mature lymphocytes. In the common "mixed cellularity" type, the RS cells are usually numerous and are accompanied by large mononuclear cells with large nuclei and nucleoli (Hodgkin's cells), large multinucleated cells with clear cytoplasm (lacunar cells), macrophages, and eosinophils. In the "nodular sclerosis" and "lymphocytic depletion" types the characteristic cell types remain the same, although their pro-

portions may vary significantly. Obtaining adequate diagnostic material from the nodular sclerosis type of disease is sometimes very difficult. In smears, the subdivision of the types of Hodgkin's disease is rarely possible.

CYTOLOGIC PRESENTATION

In smears, the classical RS cells are readily recognized because of their large size and two or more nuclei, each provided with a huge nucleolus (Fig. 8-30). The classical RS cells may be accompanied by mononucleated cells with similar nuclear features (Hodgkin's cells), by cells with smaller nuclei and a large, perinuclear clear zone (lacunar cells), and by elongated small cells with clear cytoplasm—the epithelioid cells (Fig. 8-31*A*). Cells with hyperlobulated nuclei ("popcorn cells") may also be recognized mainly in the so-called nodular, lymphocytic dominance type (Fig. 8-31*B*). The background of the smears depends on the type of Hodgkin's disease. Abundant lymphocytes may be observed in the lym-

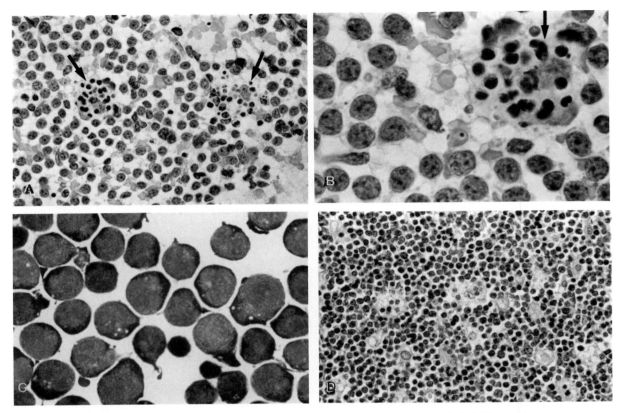

FIGURE 8-29. Retroperitoneal Burkitt's lymphoma in an 8-year-old girl. (*A*) The aspirate, viewed under low power, displays two very large tingible body macrophages (*arrows*) surrounded by cells of a malignant lymphoma. (*B*) High-power view of the same smear to demonstrate the significant nuclear abnormalities in the lymphoma cells. Note large, multiple nucleoli and creases in nuclear chromatin. One of the tingible body macrophages is seen (*arrow*). (*C*) Same case, air-dried smear stained with May-Grünwald-Giemsa. The characteristic cytoplasmic vacuoles may be observed. (*D*) Tissue section, same case. The "starry sky" appearance of the tumor is shown. (*A* × 300; *B,C* × 1,000; *D* × 250. Modified from Koss, L. G., Woyke, S., and Olszewski, W.: Aspiration Biopsy. Cytologic Interpretation and Histologic Bases. 2nd Ed. New York, Igaku-Shoin, 1992.)

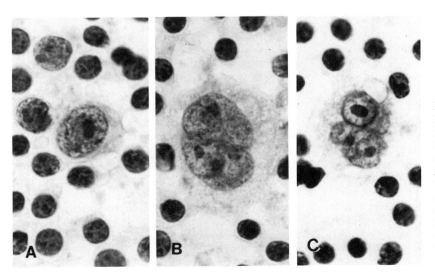

FIGURE 8-30. Aspirate of Hodgkin's disease. (*A*) A large mononucleated cell with a large nucleolus, the so-called Hodgkin's cell. (*B,C*) Reed-Sternberg (RS) cells. In *B* a typical binucleated cell with "mirror image" nuclei and large nucleoli is shown. In *C* the RS cell is multinucleated. (× 1,200. From Koss, L. G.: Diagnostic Cytology and Its Histopathologic Bases. 2nd Ed. Philadelphia, J.B. Lippincott, 1992.)

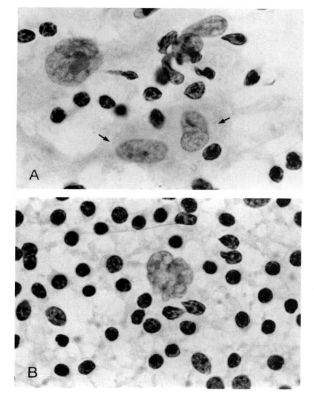

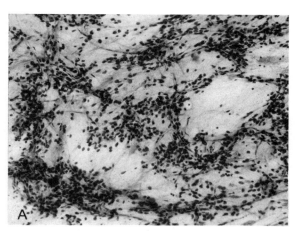

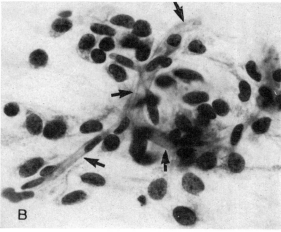

FIGURE 8-31. Various aspects of Hodgkin's disease in aspiration smears. (*A*) A single RS cell is accompanied by several epithelioid cells. (*B*) The so-called "popcorn cell" with a pale, hyperlobulated nucleus is shown against a background of lymphocytes, characteristic of nodular, lymphocytic dominance form of this disease. (*A,B* × 900. Photographs courtesy of Professor S. Woyke.)

phocytic predominance type (Fig. 8-31*B*). Eosinophilic polymorphonuclear leukocytes and epithelioid cells are common in all other types of Hodgkin's disease.

Retroperitoneal Sarcomas

A variety of sarcomas other than malignant lymphomas may occur in the retroperitoneal space. Katz (1991) lists ten different types of sarcoma and a number of teratoid tumors, such as the endodermal sinus tumor and malignant teratomas. Katz also states that the final diagnosis in such cases should be based on histologic findings on the surgically resected or biopsied tumor.

I observed a few retroperitoneal sarcomas, studied by aspiration cytology, in which a tentative cytologic diagnosis could be confirmed by tissue analysis. *Myx-*

oid liposarcoma may be recognized by the presence of cells with vacuolated cytoplasm, sometimes resembling mature fat cells, clustering around numerous branching capillary vessels, so characteristic of this type of tumor (Fig. 8-32).

A *leiomyosarcoma* is shown in Figure 8-33. The aspirate consisted mainly of elongated nuclei of variable sizes (Fig. 8-33*A*), not fully reflecting the level of cell abnormality seen in the histologic sections of the tumor (Fig. 8-33*B*).

Cytologic presentation of rhabdomyosarcomas has been discussed in Chapter 5 on p. 110.

FIGURE 8-32. Aspirate of a myxoid liposarcoma. (*A*) Low-power view of the smear to show the dense network of capillaries with tumor cells attached. (*B*) A branching capillary (*arrows*), surrounded by tumor cells. The characteristic vacuolization of the cytoplasm cannot be seen in this photograph. (*A* × 100; *B* × 400. Modified from Koss, L. G., Woyke, S., and Olszewski, W.: Aspiration Biopsy. Cytologic Interpretation and Histologic Bases. 2nd Ed. New York, Igaku-Shoin, 1992.)

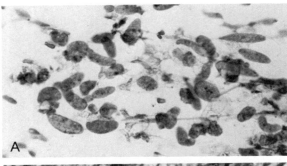

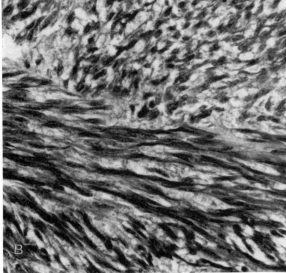

FIGURE 8-33. Retroperitoneal leiomyosarcoma. (*A*) Smear of aspirate showing elongated tumor nuclei of various sizes. Small nucleoli may be noted. (*B*) Histologic section of the same tumor, showing a high grade leiomyosarcoma. (*A,B* × 600. From Koss, L. G.: Diagnostic Cytology and Its Histopathologic Bases. 4th Ed. Philadelphia, J. B. Lippincott, 1992.)

METASTATIC TUMORS

Perhaps the most important role in aspiration biopsy of the retroperitoneal space, in urologic practice, is in staging of cancers. The presence of retroperitoneal metastases, be they in lymph nodes or in soft tissue, is of prime importance in planning treatment of these tumors. Tumors of the prostate and testes are the primary target of these investigations, but sometimes urothelial tumors of bladder and renal pelvis are included.

Prostatic Carcinomas

The cytologic presentation of prostatic carcinomas was discussed in Chapter 7. Nearly all metastatic tumors are of the poorly differentiated type (see Figs. 7-17 and 7-18). Recognition of their site of origin may be very difficult in the absence of clinical data. Immunocytochemistry documenting the presence of prostatic acid phosphatase is usually very helpful in tumor identification. Prostate-specific antigen may not be expressed in poorly differentiated carcinoma (see Chapter 10).

Testicular Tumors

In the United States primary testicular tumors are very rarely aspirated, although in Sweden this diagnostic procedure is often used with excellent preoperative diagnostic results (Zajicek, 1979; Linsk and Franzén, 1989). A detailed description of the histologic and cytologic presentation of testicular lesions may be found in Koss et al., 1992.

On the other hand, recognition of retroperitoneal metastases of testicular tumors is of great significance in staging and planning the optimal treatment. The principal testicular tumor types that may give retroperitoneal metastases are therefore described.

Seminoma

Seminoma is observed in young males, with diminishing frequency to the age of 40. Such tumors may also be observed in undescended testes (sometimes as seminomas *in situ*) or may be a component of complex malignant teratomas. The tumors are composed of sheets of large, monotonous tumor cells with clear, glycogen-rich cytoplasm and large nuclei, provided with large nucleoli (Fig. 8-34C). There are two important ancillary features that are helpful in the identification of this tumor. Lymphocytes, sometimes forming large aggregates, are a common component of the tumor. Granulomas, composed of epithelioid cells and multinucleated giant cells, are common in primary and metastatic sites. Sometimes primary tumors are occult and may be discovered only after the identification of retroperitoneal lymph node metastases. Thus, the recognition of this tumor type in aspirated material may be very important. Such a case is illustrated in Figure 8-34.

The cytologic appearance of aspirated material corresponds to the histologic pattern. The smears contain large dispersed nuclei of tumor cells with prominent nucleoli with only occasional fragments of cytoplasm attached (Fig. 8-34A,B). Numerous lymphocytes may be found in the background of the smear. The fragility

FIGURE 8-34. Occult, nonpalpable seminoma of testis in a 35-year-old man with primary manifestation as a retroperitoneal mass. Following the cytologic diagnosis, the small primary tumor in the left testis was discovered by ultrasound. (*A*) Retroperitoneal aspirate. The smear shows a mixture of dispersed, large, clear tumor cell nuclei with prominent nucleoli. Numerous lymphocytes form the background. (*B*) High-power view of tumor nuclei with small fragments of cytoplasm attached. Several lymphocytes are also seen. (*C*) Histologic section of testicular tumor. Note sheets of large tumor cells and an aggregate of lymphocytes. (*A* × 400; *B* × 800; *C* × 300. Modified from Koss, L. G., Woyke, S., and Olszewski, W.: Aspiration Biopsy. Cytologic Interpretation and Histologic Bases. 2nd Ed. New York, Igaku-Shoin, 1992.)

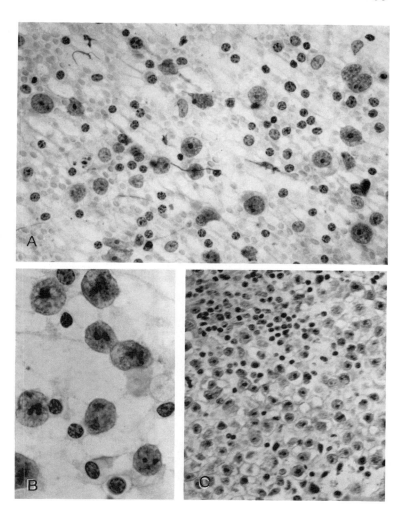

of the cytoplasm of the tumor cells results in a diagnostically useful artifact in air-dried, May-Gruenwald-Giemsa (MGG) stained smears: the fragments of the cytoplasm often form a linear pattern of denser and lighter stripes, known as "tigroid pattern" (Fig. 8-35). Such patterns may also be observed in other testicular tumors, such as embryonal carcinomas (Linsk and Franzén, 1989).

Occasionally epithelioid cells and multinucleated giant cells, the components of tumor granulomas, may be observed (Fig. 8-36). In fact, in my experience, the finding of multinucleated macrophages among tumor cells in young men is suggestive of a seminoma.

ATYPICAL ANAPLASTIC SEMINOMAS

Atypical anaplastic seminomas have the same basic structure as a classical seminoma, except for a marked pleomorphism of tumor cells. An aspirate is shown in Figure 8-37.

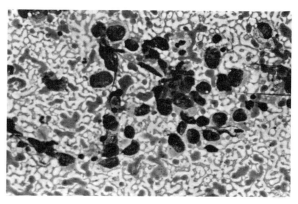

FIGURE 8-35. Air-dried aspirate of a seminoma, stained with May-Gruenwald-Giemsa. Note the peculiar linear pattern ("tigroid pattern"), sometimes observed in other testicular tumors as well (× 250). (Case courtesy of Dr. Mark Suhrland, Montefiore Medical Center.)

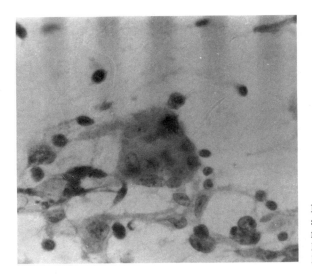

FIGURE 8-36. Seminoma of testis. Fixed aspirate, showing a multinucleated giant cell, surrounded by a few poorly preserved elongated cells, most likely epithelioid cells (× 560). (Case courtesy of Dr. Mark Suhrland, Montefiore Medical Center.)

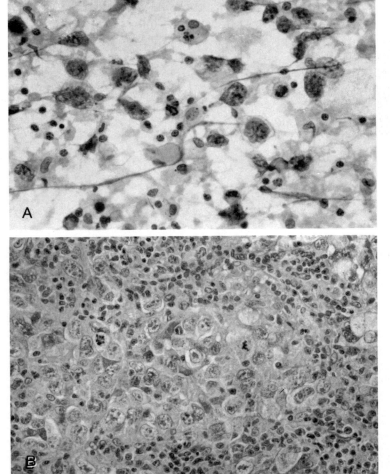

FIGURE 8-37. An aspirate and tissue section of an atypical (anaplastic) seminoma. (*A*) Note marked variability of tumor nuclei, when compared with classical seminoma, shown in Fig. 8-34*A*. (*B*) Tissue section, showing marked polymorphism of tumor cells and aggregates of lymphocytes. Compare with Fig. 8-34*C*. (*A* × 300; *B* × 200. Modified from Koss, L. G., Woyke, S., and Olszewski, W.: Aspiration Biopsy. Cytologic Interpretation and Histologic Bases. 2nd Ed. New York, Igaku-Shoin, 1992.)

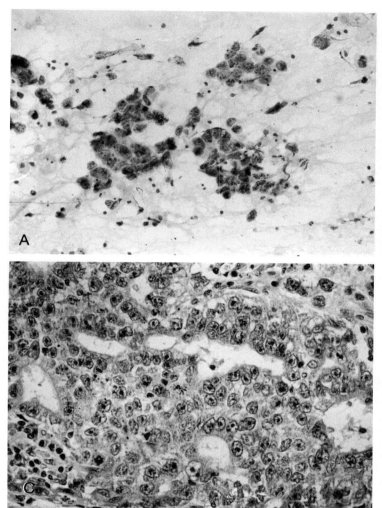
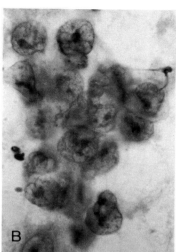

FIGURE 8-38. Embryonal carcinoma of testis. (*A*) In the aspiration smear the cancer cells
form clusters. (*B*) The structure of the nuclei is well shown:
note the clear, finely granular
chromatin and large, irregular
nucleoli. (*C*) Histologic section of the tumor. (*A* × 300;
B × 800; *C* × 300. Photographs
courtesy Professor S. Woyke.)

Embryonal Carcinoma

Embryonal carcinoma, a common malignant tumor
of the testes, is characterized by sheets and strands of
large malignant cells, sometimes forming glandular
structures (Fig. 8-38*C*). The tumor is capable of production of various polypeptide hormones, such as
chorionic gonadotropin and carcino-embryonic antigen, extensively used in clinical evaluation.

The cytologic appearance of embryonal carcinoma
differs significantly from seminomas, inasmuch as the
large cancer cells form clusters, although dispersed
cells may also be observed in the background (Fig.
8-38*A*). The nuclear features are similar to seminomas: the nuclei are large, with a finely granular
chromatin and very large nucleoli (Fig. 8-38*B*). The

cytoplasm is fragile and may form the same "tigroid
pattern" seen in seminomas.

Yolk-sac Tumors (Endodermal Sinus Tumors)

Yolk-sac tumors are much more common in the
ovary than in the testis. They are characterized by
glandular structures with papillary projections (Fig.
8-38*B*). The cells are capable of production of alpha-
fetoprotein that may be elevated in the serum. The
deposits of alpha-fetoprotein may be observed as
hyaline, periodic acid-Schiff (PAS)–positive globules
within the gland lumina but also as spherical deposits
in the cancer cells.

In an example of this tumor, metastatic to the retro-

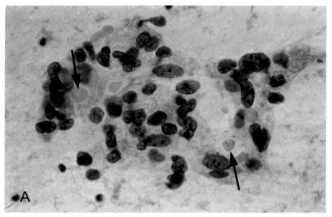

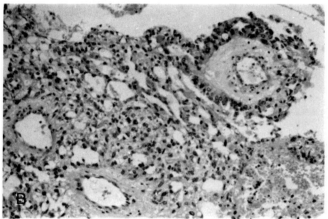

FIGURE 8-39. Metastatic yolk-sac tumor (endodermal sinus tumor) of testis. (*A*) Aspirate of the retroperitoneal space showing a poorly formed cluster of cancer cells. Note the pale globules of alpha-fetoprotein (*arrows*). (*B*) Histologic section of the original tumor of the right testis in a 26-year-old man. Note the poorly formed glandular structures and the papillary projections. (*A* × 400; *B* × 125. Modified from Koss, L. G., Woyke, S., and Olszewski, W.: Aspiration Biopsy. Cytologic Interpretation and Histologic Bases. 2nd Ed. New York, Igaku-Shoin, 1992.)

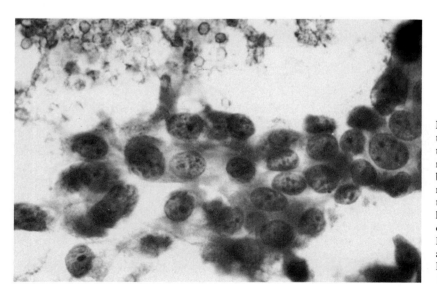

FIGURE 8-40. Metastatic urothelial carcinoma to retroperitoneal lymph nodes. The diagnosis of a carcinoma is obvious because of the marked nuclear abnormalities and cohesiveness of the cluster. The patient had a high-grade urothelial carcinoma of the bladder (× 700). (From Koss, L. G.: Diagnostic Cytology and Its Histopathologic Bases. 4th Ed. Philadelphia, J.B. Lippincott, 1992.

peritoneal space, the cancer cells formed poorly structured clusters (Fig. 8-39*A*). Within the cytoplasm, the diagnostic globular deposits of alpha-fetoprotein could be observed.

Teratomas

Teratomas of the testis contain elements of seminoma, embryonal carcinoma, and mesenchymal components, such as cartilage.

Regardless of the degree of differentiation, all testicular teratomas are malignant. We have not observed these tumors in the retroperitoneal space.

Other Metastatic Tumors

Urothelial carcinomas of bladder, ureter, or renal pelvis may metastasize to the retroperitoneal lymph nodes.

Urothelial carcinomas form clusters of large tumor cells, usually with crisply outlined cytoplasm and hyperchromatic nuclei with prominent multiple nucleoli (Fig. 8-40). Occasionally the large flat, multinucleated umbrella cells may be identified, a most helpful diagnostic hint.

Other carcinomas, such as those of the uterine cervix, endometrium, colon, or breast, may also occur in the retroperitoneal space. Because these tumors do not fall within the realm of urologic disorders, the reader is referred to other sources for a detailed description of the cytologic presentation of these tumors (Koss, 1992; Koss et al., 1992).

BIBLIOGRAPHY

Kidney
Adrenal
Retroperitoneum

Kidney

Abbi, R., McVicar, M., Teichberg, S., Fish, L., and Kahn, E.: Pathologic characterization of a renin-secreting juxtaglomerular cell tumor in a child and review of the pediatric literature. Ped. Pathol., *13,* 443–451, 1993.

Alanen, K. A., Tyrkko, J. E. S., and Nurmi, M. J.: Aspiration biopsy cytology of renal oncocytoma. Acta Cytol., *29,* 859–862, 1985.

Ambrose, S. S., Lewis, E. L., O'Brien, D. P., III, Walter, K. N., and Ross, J. R.: Unsuspected renal tumors associated with renal cysts. J. Urol., *117,* 704–707, 1977.

Anderson, J. D., Lieber, M., and Smith, R. B.: Latent adenocarcinoma in renal cysts. J. Urol., *118,* 861–862, 1977.

Arner, O., Blanck, D., and von Schreeb, T.: Renal adenocarcinoma. Morphology-grading of malignancy-prognosis. Acta Chir. Scand., *346,* 11–51, 1965.

Baish, H., Koppel, G., and Otto, U.: DNA analysis in renal neoplasia. *In* Eble, J. N. (Ed.): Tumors and Tumor-like

Conditions of the Kidney and Ureter. New York, Churchill Livingstone, 1990, pp. 250–251.

Bander, N. H.: Monoclonal antibodies: state of the art. J. Urol., *137,* 603–612, 1987.

Banner, B. F., Erstoff, M. S., Bahnson, R. R., Titus-Erstoff, L., and Taylor, S. R.: Quantitative DNA analysis of small renal cortical neoplasms. Human Path., *22,* 247–253, 1991.

Barnes, C. A., and Beckman, E. N.: Renal oncocytoma and its congeners. Am. J. Clin. Pathol., *79,* 312–318, 1983.

Baum, S., Rabinowitz, P., and Malloy, W. A.: The renal scan as an aid in percutaneous renal biopsy. J.A.M.A., *195,* 913–915, 1966.

Beckwith, J. B.: Renal neoplasms of childhood. *In* Sternberg, S. S. (Ed.): Diagnostic Surgical Pathology. New York, Raven Press, 1989, pp. 1331–1353.

Beckwith, J. B.: Wilms' tumor and other renal tumors of childhood: An update. J. Urol., *136,* 320–324, 1986.

Beckwith, J. B., and Palmer, N. F.: Histopathology and prognosis of Wilms' tumor. Results of the national Wilms' tumor study. Cancer, *41,* 1937–1948, 1978.

Bell, E. T.: Tumors of the Kidney. *In* Bell, E. T. Renal Diseases. Philadelphia, Lea and Febiger, 1950.

Bennington, J. L., and Beckwith, J. B.: Tumors of the Kidney, Renal Pelvis and Ureter. Atlas of Tumor Pathology, Second series, fascicle 12. Washington, D.C., Armed Forces Institute of Pathology, 1975.

Blute, M. L., Malek, R. S., and Segura, J. W.: Angiomyolipoma. Clinical metamorphosis and concepts for management. J. Urol., *139,* 20–24, 1988.

Boczko, S., Fromovitz, F. B., and Bard, R. H.: Papillary adenocarcinoma of the kidney: a new perspective. Urology, *14,* 491–495, 1979.

Bolton, W. K., Vaughan, E. D., Jr.: A comparative study of open surgical and percutaneous renal biopsies. J. Urol., *117,* 696–698, 1977.

Bosnik, M. A., Megibon, A. J., Hubrick, D. H., Horii, S., and Raghavendra, B. N.: CT-diagnosis of renal angiomyolipoma. The importance of detecting small amounts of fat. A.J.R., *151,* 491–501, 1988.

Bretan, P. N., Jr., Bush, M. P., Hricak, H., and Williams, R. D.: Chronic renal failure: a significant risk factor in the development of acquired renal cysts and renal cell carcinoma. Cancer, *57,* 1871–1879, 1986.

Brodsky, G. L., and Garnick, M. D.: Renal tumors in the adult patient. *In* Tisher, C. C., and Brenner, B. M. (Eds.): Renal Pathology. Philadelphia, J. B. Lippincott, 1989, pp. 1467–1504.

Bruun, E., and Nielsen, K.: Solitary cyst and clear cell adenocarcinoma of the kidney: report of two cases and review of the literature. J. Urol., *136,* 449–451, 1986.

Chin, J. L., Pontes, J. E., and Frankfurt, O. S.: Flow cytometric deoxyribonucleic acid analysis of primary and metastatic human renal cell carcinoma. J. Urol., *133,* 582–585, 1985.

Cin, P. T., Gaeta, J., Huben, R., Li, F. P., Prout, G. R., and Sandberg, A. A.: Renal cortical tumors: cytogenetic characterisation. Am. J. Clin. Path., *92,* 408–414, 1989.

Cohen, A. J., Li, F. P., Berg, S., Marchetto, D. J., Tsai, S., Jacobs, S. C., and Brown, R. S.: Hereditary renal-cell carcinoma associated with a chromosomal translocation. New Engl. J. Med., *301,* 592–595, 1979.

Conrad, M. R., Sanders, R. C., and Mascardo, A. D.: Perinephric abscess aspiration using ultrasound guidance. Am. J. Roentgenol., *128,* 459–464, 1977.

Das, K. M., Vaidyanathan, S., Rajwanshi, A., and Indudhara, R.: Renal tuberculosis: diagnosis with sonographically guided aspiration cytology. Am. J. Radiol., *158,* 571–573, 1992.

Davis, C. J., Jr., Mostofi, F. K., Sesterhenn, I. A., and Ho, C. K.: Renal oncocytoma: Clinicopathologic study of 166 patients. J. Urogenital Path., *1,* 41–52, 1991.

Dean, A. L.: Treatment of solitary cyst of kidney by aspiration. Trans. Am. Assoc. Genitour. Surg., *32,* 91–95, 1939.

Dekmezian, R. H., Charnsangavej, C., Rava, P., and Katz, R. L.: Fine needle aspiration of kidney tumors in 105 patients: a cytologic and histologic correlation (Abstract). Acta Cytol., *29,* 931, 1985.

Domagala, W., Lasota, J., Wolska, H., Lubinski, J., Weber, K., and Osborn, H.: Diagnosis of metastatic renal cell and thyroid carcinomas by intermediate filament typing and cytology of tumor cell in fine needle aspirates. Acta Cytol., *32,* 415–421, 1988.

Domagala, W., and Osborn, M.: Immunocytochemistry. Chapter 3 *in* Koss, L. G., Woyke, S., and Olszewski, W. Aspiration Biopsy. Cytologic Interpretation and Histologic Bases. 2nd Ed. New York, Igaku-Shoin, 1992.

Drut, R.: Malignant rhabdoid tumor of kidney diagnosed by fine-needle aspiration cytology. Diagn. Cytopath., *6,* 124–126, 1990.

Drut, R., and Pollono, D.: Anaplastic Wilms' tumor. Initial diagnosis by fine needle aspiration. Acta. Cytol., *32,* 774–776, 1987.

Dunhill, M. S., Millard, P. R., and Oliver, D.: Acquired cystic disease of the kidneys: a hazard of long-term intermittent maintenance dialysis. J. Clin. Path., *30,* 868–877, 1977.

Eble, J. N.: Tumors and Tumor-like Conditions of the Kidney and Ureter. New York, Churchill-Livingstone, 1990.

Ekfors, T. O., Lipasti, J., Nurmi, M. J., and Eerola, B.: Flow cytometric analysis of the DNA profile of renal cell carcinoma. Pathol. Res. Pract. *182,* 58–62, 1987.

Farnsworth, W. V., Cohen, C., McCue, P. A., and DeRose, P. B.: DNA analysis of small renal cortical neoplasms. J. Urol. Path., *2,* 65–79, 1994.

Farrow, G. M., Harrison, E. G., Jr., and Utz, D. C.: Sarcomas and sarcomatoid and mixed malignant tumors of the kidney in adults. Cancer, *22,* 556–563, 1968.

Flint, A., and Cookingham, C.: Cytologic diagnosis of the papillary variant of renal cell carcinoma. Acta. Cytol., *31,* 325–329, 1987.

Furmann, S. A., Lasky, L. C., and Limas, C.: Prognostic significance of morphologic parameters in renal cell carcinoma. Am. J. Surg. Pathol., *6,* 663–665, 1982.

Gibbons, R. P., Bush, W. H., and Burnett, L. L.: Needle tract seeding following aspiration of renal cell carcinoma. J. Urol., *118,* 865–867, 1977.

Glentoj, A., and Partoft, S.: Ultrasound guided percutaneous aspiration of renal angiomyolipoma. Acta Cytol., *28,* 265–268, 1984.

Grignon, D. J., el-Naggar, A., Green, L. K., Ayala, A. G.,

Ro, J. Y., Swanson, D. A., Troncoso, P., McLemore, D., Giaccio, G. G., and Guinee, V. F.: DNA flow cytometry as a predictor of outcome in stage I renal cell carcinoma. Cancer, *63,* 1161–1165, 1989.

Haas, J. E., Bonadio, J. F., and Beckwith, J. B.: Clear cell sarcoma of kidney with emphasis on ultrastructural studies. Cancer, *54,* 2978–2987, 1984.

Haas, J. E., Palmer, N. F., Weinberg, A. G., and Beckwith, J. B.: Ultrastructure of malignant rhabdoid tumor of the kidney. A distinctive renal tumor of children. Hum. Pathol., *12,* 646–657, 1981.

Hajdu, S. I.: Exfoliative cytology or primary and metastatic Wilms' tumors. Acta Cytol., *15,* 339–342, 1971.

Hajdu, S. I., Foote, F. W., Jr.: Angiomyolipoma of kidney. Report of 27 cases and review of literature. J. Urol., *102,* 396–401, 1969.

Hajdu, S. I., and Hajdu, E. O.: Cytopathology of sarcomas and other nonepithelial malignant tumors. Philadelphia, W. B. Saunders, 1975.

Hajdu, S. I., and Koss, L. G.: Endometriosis of the kidney. Am. J. Obstet. Gynecol., *106,* 314–315, 1970.

Hajdu, S. I., Savino, A., Hajdu, E. O., and Koss, L. G.: Cytologic diagnosis of renal cell carcinoma with the aid of fat stain. Acta Cytol., *15,* 31–33, 1971.

Hamperl, H.: Benign and malignant oncocytoma. Cancer, *15,* 1019–1027, 1962.

Hantman, S. S., Barie, J. J., Glendening, T. B., Eisenberg, M. N., and Rapoport, K. D.: Giant renal artery aneurysm mimicking a simple cyst on ultrasound. J. Clin. Ultrasound, *10,* 136–139, 1982.

Hartman, D. S., Davis, C. J., Jr., Jahns, T., and Goldman, S. M.: Cystic renal cell carcinoma. Urology, *28,* 145–153, 1986.

Helm, C. W., Burwood, R. J., Harrison, N. W., and Melcher, D. H.: Aspiration cytology of solid renal tumors. Br. J. Urol., *55,* 249–253, 1983.

Hughson, M. D., Hennigar, G. R., and McManus, J. F. A.: Atypical cysts, acquired renal cystic disease, and renal cell tumors in end-stage dialysis kidney. Lab. Invest., *42,* 475–480, 1980.

Iversen, P., and Brun, C.: Aspiration biopsy of the kidney. Am. J. Med., *11,* 324–330, 1951.

Juul, N., Torp-Pedersen, S., Gronvall, S., Holm, H. H., Koch, F., and Larsen, H.: Ultrasonically guided fine needle aspiration biopsy of renal masses. J. Urol., *133,* 579–581, 1985.

Katz, R. L.: Kidney, adrenal, and retroperitoneum. *In* Bibbo, M. (Ed.). Comprehensive Cytopathology. Philadelphia, W. B. Saunders, 1991, pp. 771–805.

Kennedy, S. M., Merino, M. J., Linehan, W. M., Roberts, J. R., Robertson, C. N., and Neumann, R. D.: Collecting duct carcinoma of the kidney. Human Path., *21,* 449–456, 1990.

Kihara, I., Kitamura, S., Hoshino, T., Seida, H., and Watanabe, T.: A hitherto unreported vascular tumor of the kidney: a proposal of "juxtaglomerular cell tumor." Acta Path. Jap., *18,* 197–206, 1968.

Kiser, G. C., Totonchy, M., and Barry, J. M.: Needle tract seeding after percutaneous renal adenocarcinoma aspirate. J. Urol., *136,* 1292–1293, 1986.

Klein, M. J., and Valensi, Q. J.: Proximal tubular adenoma

of kidney with the so-called oncocytic features. Cancer, *38,* 906–914, 1976.

Kline, T. S.: Handbook of Fine Needle Aspiration Biopsy Cytology. 2nd Ed. New York, Churchill Livingstone, 1988.

Kloeppel, G., Knoefel, W. T., Baisch, H., and Otto, U.: Prognosis of renal cell carcinoma related to nuclear grade, DNA content, and Robson stage. Europ. Urol., *12,* 426–431, 1986.

Koss, L. G.: Diagnostic Cytology and Its Histopathologic Bases. 4th Ed., Philadelphia, J.B. Lippincott, 1992.

Koss, L. G., Woyke, S., and Olszewski, W.: Aspiration biopsy. Cytologic Interpretation and Histologic Bases. 2nd Ed. New York, Igaku-Shoin, 1992.

Kovacs, G.: Molecular differential pathology of renal cell tumours. Histopathology, *22,* 1–8, 1993.

Kovacs, G.: Papillary renal cell carcinoma. A morphologic and cytogenetic study of 11 cases. Am. J. Path., *134,* 27–34, 1989.

Kovacs, G., Wilkens, L., Papp, T., and Riese, W.: Differentiation between papillary and nonpapillary renal cell carcinomas by DNA analysis. J. Nat. Cancer Inst., *81,* 527–530, 1989.

Kristensen, J. K., Bartels, E., and Jorgensen, H. E.: Percutaneous renal biopsy under the guidance of ultrasound. Scand. J. Urol. Nephrol., *8,* 223–226, 1974.

Kristensen, J. K., Holm, H. H., Rasmussen, S. N., and Barlebo, H.: Ultrasonically guided percutaneous puncture of renal masses. Scand. J. Urol. Nephrol. (Suppl), *6,* 49–56, 1972.

Lang, E. K.: Renal cyst puncture and aspiration: A survey of complications. Am. J. Roentgenol., *128,* 723–727, 1977.

Lang, E. K.: Renal cyst structure studies. Urol. Clin. North. Am., *14,* 91–102, 1987.

Levine, S. R., Emmett, J. L., and Woolner, L. B.: Cyst and tumor occurring in the same kidney. J. Urol., *91,* 8–9, 1964.

Lieber, M. M., Tomera, K. M., and Farrow, G. M.: Renal oncocytoma. J. Urol., *125,* 481–485, 1981.

Linsk, J. A., and Franzén, S.: Aspiration cytology of metastatic hypernephroma. Acta Cytol., *28,* 250–260, 1984.

Linsk, J. A., and Franzén, S.: Clinical aspiration cytology. 2nd Ed. Philadelphia, J.B. Lippincott, 1989.

LiPuma, J. P.: The kidney. *In* Haaga, J. R., and Alfidi, R. J. (Eds.): Computed Tomography of the Whole Body. St. Louis, C. V. Mosby, 1988, pp. 1014–1073.

Ljung, B. M.: Techniques of aspiration and smear preparation. *In* Koss, L. G., Woyke, S., Olszewski, W.: Aspiration Biopsy. Cytologic Interpretation and Histologic bases. 2nd Ed. New York, Igaku-Shoin, 1992, pp. 12–30.

Ljungberg, B., Holmberg, G., Sjodin, J. G., Hietala, S. O., and Stenling, R.: Renal cell carcinoma in a renal cyst. J. Urol., *143,* 797–799, 1990.

Ljungberg, B., Stenling, R., and Roos, G.: DNA content in renal cell carcinoma with reference to tumor heterogeneity. Cancer, *56,* 503–508, 1985.

Mancilla-Jimenez, R., Stanley, R. J., and Blath, R. A.: Papillary renal cell carcinoma. A clinical, radiologic,

and pathologic study of 34 cases. Cancer, *38,* 2469–2480, 1976.

Marsden, H. B., and Lawler, W.: Bone-metastasizing renal tumour of childhood. Histopathology and clinical review of 38 cases. Virch. Arch. (A), *387,* 341–351, 1980.

Meier, W. L., Willscher, M. K., Novicki, D. E., and Pischinger, R. J.: Evaluation of perihilar and central renal masses using the Chiba needle. J. Urol., *121,* 414–416, 1979.

Meisels, A.: Cytology of carcinoma of kidney. Acta Cytol., *7,* 239–244, 1963.

Mount, B. M., Curtis, M., Marshall, K., and Husk, M.: Cytologic diagnosis of renal cell carcinoma. Urology, *2,* 421–425, 1973.

Murphy, W. M., Zambroni, B. R., Emerson, L. D., Moinuddin, S. M., and Lee, L. H.: Aspiration biopsy of the kidney in 152 cases: The value of simultaneously collected cytologic and histologic material in renal cancers. (Meeting abstract). Acta Cytol., *28,* 625, 1984.

Mussouris, H. F., Koss, L. G., Rosenblatt, R., and Kutcher, R.: The needle aspiration biopsy of abdominal organs. *In* Koss, L. G., and Coleman, D. V. (Eds.): Advances In Clinical Cytology, Vol. 2. New York, Masson, 1984, pp. 191–241.

Navarri, B. M., Ploth, D. W., and Tatum, R. K.: Renal adenocarcinoma associated with multiple cysts. J.A.M.A., *246,* 1808–1809, 1981.

Nguyen, G. K.: Aspiration biopsy cytology of renal angiomyolipoma. Acta Cytol., *28,* 261–264, 1984.

Nguyen, G. K.: Percutaneus fine needle biopsy cytology of the kidney and adrenal. Pathol. Annu., *22,* 163–191, 1987.

Nguyen, G. K., Amy, R. W., and Tsang, S.: Fine needle aspiration biopsy cytology of renal oncocytoma. Acta Cytol., *29,* 33–36, 1985.

Ogden, B. W., Beckman, E. N., Rodriguez, F. H., Jr.: Multicystic renal oncocytoma. Arch. Path. Lab. Med., *111,* 485–486, 1987.

Orell, S. R., Langlois, S. L., and Marshall, V. R.: Fine needle aspiration cytology in the diagnosis of solid renal and adrenal masses. Scand. J. Urol. Nephrol., *19,* 211–216, 1985.

Osborne, B. M., Brenner, M., Weltzer, S., and Butler, J. J.: Lymphomas presenting as a renal mass. Am. J. Surg. Path., *11,* 375–382, 1987.

Parham, D. M., Weeks, D. A., and Beckwith, J. B.: The clinicopathologic spectrum of putative extrarenal rhabdoid tumors. An analysis of 42 cases studied with immunohistochemistry and electron microscopy. Am. J. Surg. Path., *18,* 1010–1029, 1994.

Petersen, R. O.: Urologic Pathology. 2nd Ed. Philadelphia, J. B. Lippincott, 1992.

Pilotti, S., Rilke, F., Alasio, L., and Garbagnati, F.: The role of fine needle aspiration in the assessment of renal masses. Acta Cytol., *32,* 1–10, 1988.

Piscioli, F., Detassis, C., Polla, E., Pusiol, T., Reich, A., and Luciani, L.: Cytologic presentation of renal adenocarcinoma in urinary sediment. Acta Cytol., *27,* 383–390, 1983.

Pode, D., Meretik, S., Shapiro, A., and Caine, M.: Angiomyolipoma. Urology, *25,* 461–467, 1985.

Pollack, H. M., Banner, M. P., Arger, P. H., Peters, J., Mulhern, C. B. J., and Coleman, B. G.: The accuracy of gray-scale renal ultrasonography in differentiating cystic neoplasms from benign cysts. Radiology, *143*, 741–745, 1982.

Quijano, G., and Drut, R.: Cytologic characteristics of Wilms' tumors in fine needle aspirates. A study of ten cases. Acta Cytol., *33*, 263–266, 1989.

Ro, J. Y., Ayala, A. G., El-Nagger, A., Grignon, D., and Hogan, S. F.: Angiomyolipoma of kidney with lymph node involvement: DNA flow cytometric analysis. Arch. Path. Lab. Med., *114*, 65–67, 1990.

Ro, J. Y., Ayala, A. G., Sella, A., Samuels, M. L., and Swanson, D. A.: Sarcomatoid renal cell carcinoma: clinicopathologic correlations. A study of 42 cases. Cancer, *59*, 516–526, 1987.

Rodriguez, C. A., Buskop, A., Johnson, J., Fromowitz, F., and Koss, L. G.: Renal oncocytoma. Preoperative diagnosis by aspiration biopsy. Acta Cytol., *24*, 355–359, 1980.

Rosenblatt, R.: Imaging modalities as guides to percutaneous aspiration. *In* Koss, L. G., Woyke, S., and Olszewski, W. (Eds.): Aspiration Biopsy. Cytologic Interpretation and Histologic Bases. 2nd Ed. New York, Igaku-Shoin, 1992, pp. 39–54.

Sano, M. E., and Koprowska, I.: Primary cytologic diagnosis of a malignant renal lymphoma. Acta Cytol., *9*, 194–196, 1965.

Sant, G. R., Ayers, D. K., Bankoff, M. S., Micheson, H. D., Ucci, A. A., Jr.: Fine needle aspiration biopsy in the diagnosis of renal angiomyolipoma. J. Urol., *143*, 999–1001, 1990.

Schmidt, D., Wiedemann, B., Keil, W., Sprenger, E., and Harms, D.: Flow cytometric analysis of nephroblastomas and related neoplasms. Cancer, *58*, 2494–2500, 1986.

Shankey, T. V.: Urologic cancers. *In* Bauer, K. D., Duque, R. E., Shankey, T. V. (Eds.): Clinical Flow Cytometry. Principles and Applications. Baltimore, Williams & Wilkins, 1993.

Silva, F. G., and Childers, J. H.: Adult renal diseases. *In* Sternberg, S. S. (Ed.). Diagnostic Surgical Pathology. New York, Raven Press, 1989, pp. 1255–1330.

Sneige, N., Dekmezian, R., and Zaatari, G. S.: Liesegang-like rings in fine needle aspirates of renal/perirenal hemorrhagic cysts. Acta Cytol., *32*, 547–551, 1988.

Söderström, N.: Fine needle aspiration biopsy used as a direct adjunct in clinical diagnostic work. New York, Grune and Stratton, 1966.

Sos, T. A., Gray, G. F., Jr., and Baltaxe, H. A.: The angiographic appearance of benign oxyphilic adenoma. Am. J. Roentgenol. *127*, 717–722, 1976.

Sotelo-Avila, C., Gonzales-Crussi, F., de Mello, D., et. al.: Renal and extrarenal rhabdoid tumors in children: a clinicopathologic study of 14 patients. Semin. Diagn. Path., *3*, 151–163, 1986.

Squires, J. P., Ulbright, T. M., DeSchryver-Kaecskemeti, K., and Engleman, W.: Juxtaglomerular cell tumor of the kidney. Cancer, *53*, 516–523, 1984.

Takagi, M., Takakuwa, T., Ushigome, S., Nakata, K., Fujika, T., and Watanabe, A.: Sarcomatous variant of Wilms' tumors. Immunohistochemical and ultrastructural comparison with classical Wilms' tumor. Cancer, *59*, 963–971, 1987.

Taylor, R. S., Joseph, D. B., Kohaut, E. C., Wilson, E. B., and Bueschen, A. J.: Renal angiomyolipoma associated with lymph node involvement and renal cell carcinoma in patients with tuberous sclerosis. J. Urol., *141*, 930–932, 1989.

Taylor, S. R., and Nunez, C.: Fine needle aspiration biopsy in a pediatric population. Report of 64 consecutive cases. Cancer, *54*, 1449–1453, 1984.

Thoenes, W., Storkel, S. T., and Rumpelt, H. J.: Histopathology and classification of renal cell tumors (adenomas, oncocytomas, and carcinomas). The basic cytological and histopathological elements and their use for diagnosis. Path. Res. Pract., *181*, 125–143, 1986.

Thoenes, W., Storkel, S. T., and Rumpelt, H. J.: Human chromophobe cell renal carcinoma. Virch. Arch. (B), *48*, 207–217, 1985.

Tosi, P., Luzi, P., Baak, J. P. A., Mirraco, C., Santopietra, R., Vindigni, C., Mattei, F. M., Acconcia, A., and Massai, M. R.: Nuclear morphometry as an important prognostic factor in stage I renal cell carcinoma. Cancer, *58*, 2512–2518, 1986.

Umiker, W.: Accuracy of cytologic diagnosis of cancer of the urinary tract. Acta Cytol., *8*, 186–193, 1964.

von Schreeb, T., Abner, O., Skovsted, G., and Wikstad, N.: Renal adenocarcinoma: Is there a risk of spreading tumour cells in diagnostic puncture? Scand. J. Urol. Nephrol., *1*, 270–276, 1967.

von Schreeb, T., Franzén, S., and Ljungqvist, A.: Renal adenocarcinoma. Scand. J. Urol. Nephrol., *1*, 265–269, 1967.

von Willebrand, E.: Fine needle aspiration cytology of renal transplants: Background and present applications. Transplant Proc., *17*, 2071–2074, 1985.

Weeks, D. A., Beckwith, B., and Luckey, D. W.: Relapse-associated variables in stage I favorable histology Wilms' tumor: A report of the National Wilms' Tumor Study. Cancer, *60*, 1204–1212, 1987.

Weeks, D. A., Beckwith, J. B., and Mierau, G. W.: Rhabdoid tumor. An entity or a phenotype? Arch. Path. Lab. Med., *113*, 113–114, 1989.

Weeks, D. A., Beckwith, J. B., Mireau, G. W., and Luckey, D. W.: Rhabdoid tumors of the kidney. A report of 111 cases from the National Wilms' Tumor Study Pathology Center. Am. J. Surg. Pathol., *13*, 439–458, 1989.

Wehle, M. J., and Grabstald, H.: Contraindications to needle aspiration of solid renal mass: tumor dissemination by needle aspiration. J. Urol., *136*, 446–448, 1986.

Wood, D. P. Jr., Kay, R., and Norris, D.: Renal sarcoma of childhood. Urology, *36*, 73–78, 1990.

Zornoza, J., Handel, P., Lukeman, J. M., Jing, B. S., and Wallace, S.: Percutaneous transperitoneal biopsy in urologic malignancies. Urology, *9*, 395–398, 1977.

Adrenal

Abrams, H. L., Siegelman, S. S., Adams, D. F., Sanders, R., Finberg, H. J., Hessel, S. J., and McNeil, B. J.: Computed tomography versus ultrasound of the adrenal gland: a prospective study. Radiology, *143*, 121–128, 1982.

Akhtar, M., Ashraf, M., Sabbah, R., Bakry, M., and Nash, J. E.: Fine needle aspiration biopsy diagnosis of round cell malignant tumors of childhood: A combined light and electron microscopic approach. Cancer, *55*, 1805–1817, 1985.

Berkman, W. A., Bernardino, M. E., Sewell, C. W., Price, R. B., and Sones, P. J.: The computed tomography-guided adrenal biopsy. An alternative to surgery in adrenal mass diagnosis. Cancer, *53*, 2098–2103, 1984.

Brodeur, G. M., Seeger, R. C., Schwab, M., Varmus, H. E., and Bishop, J. M.: Amplification of N-myc in untreated human neuroblastoma correlates with advanced stage disease. Science, *224*, 1121–1124, 1984.

deBlois, G. G., and deMay, R. M.: Adrenal myelolipoma diagnosis by computed tomography-guided fine needle aspiration. Cancer, *55*, 848–850, 1985.

Epstein, A. J., Patel, S. K., and Petasnick, J. P.: Computerized tomography of the adrenal gland. J.A.M.A., *242*, 2791–2794, 1979.

Evans, A. E., D'Angio, G. J., Propert, K., Anderson, J., and Hann, H. W.: Prognostic factors in neuroblastoma. Cancer, *59*, 1853–1859, 1987.

Heaston, D. K., Handel, D. B., and Ashton, P. R.: Narrow gauge needle aspiration of solid adrenal masses. Am. J. Roentgenol., *138*, 1143–1148, 1982.

Javaheri, P., and Raafat, J.: Malignant pheochromocytoma of the urinary bladder: report of two cases. Brit. J. Urol., *47*, 401–404, 1975.

Katz, R. L.: Kidney, adrenal, and retroperitoneum. *In* Bibbo, M. (Ed.). Comprehensive Cytopathology. Philadelphia, W. B. Saunders, 1991, pp. 771–805.

Katz, R. L., Patel, S., Mackay, B., and Zornoza, J.: Fine needle aspiration cytology of the adrenal gland. Acta Cytol., *28*, 269–282, 1984.

Katz, R. L., and Shirkhoda, A.: Diagnostic approach to incidental adrenal nodules in the cancer patient. Results of a clinical, radiologic and fine needle aspiration study. Cancer, *55*, 1995–2000, 1985.

Koss, L. G.: Diagnostic Cytology and Its Histopathologic Bases. 4th Ed. Philadelphia, J.B. Lippincott, 1992.

Koss, L. G., Woyke, S., and Olszewski, W.: Aspiration biopsy. Cytologic Interpretation and Histologic Bases. 2nd Ed. New York, Igaku-Shoin, 1992.

Levin, N. P.: Fine needle aspiration and histology of adrenal cortical carcinoma. A case report. Acta Cytol., *25*, 421–424, 1981.

Ljung, B. M.: Techniques of aspiration and smear preparation. *In* Koss, L. G., Woyke, S., Olszewski, W.: Aspiration Biopsy. Cytologic Interpretation and Histologic bases. 2nd Ed. New York, Igaku-Shoin, pp. 12–30, 1992.

McCorkell, S. J., and Niles, N. L.: Fine needle aspiration of catecholamine-producing adrenal masses: a possible fatal mistake. Am. J. Radiol., *145*, 113–114, 1985.

Min, K. W., Song, J., Boesenberg, M., and Acebey, J.: Adrenal cortical nodule mimicking small round cell malignancy on fine needle aspiration. Acta Cytol., *32*, 543–546, 1988.

Mitchell, M. L., Ryan, F. P., and Shermen, R. W.: Pulmo-nary adenocarcinoma metastatic to the adrenal gland mimicking normal adrenal cortical epithelium on fine needle aspiration. Acta Cytol., *29*, 994–998, 1985.

Moussouris, H. F., Koss, L. G., Rosenblatt, R., and Kutcher, R.: Thin Needle Aspiration Biopsy of Abdominal Organs. *In* Koss, L. G., and Coleman, D. V. (Eds.): Advances in Clinical Cytology, Vol. 2. pp. 191–241. New York, Masson Publishing USA, 1984.

Noble, M. J., Montague, D. K., and Levin, H. S.: Myelolipoma: an unusual surgical lesion of the adrenal gland. Cancer, *49*, 952–958, 1982.

Nguyen, G. K.: Cytopathologic aspects of adrenal pheochromocytoma in a fine needle aspiration biopsy. Acta Cytol., *26*, 354–358, 1982.

Nguyen, G. K.: Percutaneous fine needle biopsy cytology of the kidney and adrenal. Pathol. Annu., *22*, 163–191, 1987.

Orell, S. R., Langlois, S. L., and Marshall, V. R.: Fine needle aspiration cytology in the diagnosis of solid renal and adrenal masses. Scand. J. Urol. Nephrol., *19*, 211–216, 1985.

Pagani, J. J.: Non-small cell lung carcinoma adrenal metastases. Computed tomography and percutaneous needle biopsy in their diagnosis. Cancer, *53*, 1058–1060, 1984.

Page, D. L., De Lellis, R. A., and Hough, A. J.: Tumors of the Adrenal. Atlas of Tumor Pathology, 2nd Series, Fascicle 23. Washington, D.C., The Armed Forces Institute of Pathology, 1985.

Pinto, M. M.: Fine needle aspiration of myelolipoma of the adrenal gland. Report of a case with computed tomography. Acta Cytol., *29*, 863–866, 1985.

Samaan, N. A., Hickey, R. C., and Shutts, P. E.: Diagnosis localisation, and management of pheochromocytoma: Pitfalls and follow-up in 41 patients. Cancer, *62*, 2451–2460, 1988.

Scheible, W., Coel, M., and Siemers, P. T.: Percutaneous aspiration of adrenal cysts. Am. J. Roentgenol, *128*, 1013–1016, 1977.

Schimke, R. N., Hartmann, W. H., Prout, I. E., et al.: Syndrome of bilateral pheochromocytoma, medullary thyroid carcinoma, and multiple neuromas: A possible regulatory defect in the differentiation of chromaffin tissue. N. Engl. J. Med., *279*, 1–7, 1968.

Seeger, R. C., Brodeur, G. M., Sather, H., Dalton, A., Siegel, S. E., Wong, K. Y., and Hammond, D.: Association of multiple copies of the N-myc oncogene with rapid progression of neuroblastoma. N. Engl. J. Med., *313*, 1111–1116, 1985.

Silverman, J. F., Dabbs, D. J., Ganick, D. J., Holbrook, C. T., and Geisinger, K. R.: Fine needle aspiration cytology of neuroblastoma, including peripheral neuroectodermal tumor, with immunocytochemical and ultrastructural confirmation. Acta Cytol., *32*, 367–376, 1988.

Webb, T. A., Sheps, S. G., and Carney, J. A.: Differences between sporadic pheochromocytoma and pheochromocytoma in multiple endocrine neoplasia, type 2. Am. J. Surg. Pathol., *4*, 121–126, 1980.

White, E. A., Schambelan, M., Rost, C. R., Biglieri, E. G., Moss, A. A., and Korobkin, M.: Use of computed tomography in diagnosing the cause of primary aldosteronism. N. Engl. J. Med., *303*, 1503–1507, 1980.

Wilson, R. A., and Ibanez, M. L.: A comparative study of 14 cases of familial and nonfamilial pheochromocytoma. Hum. Pathol., *9,* 181–188, 1978.

Yeh, H. C.: Sonography of the adrenal glands: Normal glands and small masses. Am. J. Roentgenol., *135,* 1167–1177, 1980.

Zajicek, J.: Aspiration Biopsy Cytology, Part 2: Cytology of Infradiaphragmatic Organs. Basel, S. Karger, 1979.

Zornoza, J., Handel, P., Lukeman, J. M., Jing, B. S., and Wallace, S.: Percutaneous transperitoneal biopsy in urologic malignancies. Urology, *9,* 395–398, 1977.

Zornoza, J., Ordonez, N., Bernadino, M. E., and Cohen, M. A.: Percutaneous biopsy of adrenal tumors. Urology, *18,* 412–417, 1981.

Retroperitoneum

Adler, O. B., and Engel, A.: CT guided transgluteal fine needle aspiration biopsy. Eur. J. Radiol., *7,* 101–102, 1987.

Bonfiglio, T. A., MacIntosh, P. K., Patten, S. F., Jr., Cafer, D. J., Woodworth, F. E., and Kim, C. W.: Fine needle aspiration cytopathology of retroperitoneal lymph nodes in the evaluation of metastatic disease. Acta Cytol., *23,* 126–130, 1979.

Brascho, D. J., Durant, J. R., and Green, L. E.: The accuracy of retroperitoneal ultrasonography in Hodgkin's disease and non-Hodgkin's lymphoma. Radiology, *125,* 485–487, 1977.

Bree, R. L., Jafri, S. Z., and Schwab, R. E.: Abdominal fine needle aspiration biopsies with CT and ultrasound guidance: techniques, results and clinical implications. Comput. Radiol., *8,* 9–15, 1984.

Bret, P. M., Fond, A., Casola, G., Farach, J., Bernacki, E. G., and Ellwood, R. A.: Abdominal lesions: a prospective study of clinical efficacy of percutaneous fine needle biopsy. Radiology, *159,* 345–346, 1986.

Cafferty, L. L., Katz, R., Ordonez, N. G., and Cabanillas, F. R.: Fine needle aspiration diagnosis of intraabdominal and retroperitoneal lymphomas by a morphologic and immunocytochemical approach. Cancer, *65,* 72–77, 1990.

Cochand-Priollet, B., Roger, B., Boccon-Gibod, J., Ferrand, J., Faure, B., and Blery, M.: Retroperitoneal lymph node aspiration biopsy in staging of pelvic cancer: a cytological study of 228 consecutive cases. Diagn. Cytopathol., *3,* 102–107, 1987.

Droese, M., Altmannsberger, M., Kehl, A., Lankisch, P. G., Weiss, R., Weber, K., and Osborn, M.: Ultrasound-guided percutaneous fine needle aspiration biopsy of abdominal and retroperitoneal masses. Accuracy of cytology in the diagnosis of malignancy, cytologic tumor typing and use of antibodies to intermediate filaments in selected cases. Acta Cytol., *28,* 368–384, 1984.

Dunnick, N. R., Fischer, R. I., and Chu, E. W.: Percutaneous aspiration of retroperitoneal lymph nodes in ovarian cancer. Am. J. Roentgenol., *135,* 109–113, 1980.

Edeiken-Monroe, B. S. E., and Zornoza, J.: Carcinoma of the cervix: Percutaneous lymph node aspiration biopsy. Am. J. Roentgenol., *138,* 655–657, 1982.

Efremides, S. C., Dan, S., Nieburgs, H., and Mitty, H. A.: Carcinoma of the prostate: Lymph node aspiration for staging. Am. J. Roentgenol. *136,* 489–492, 1981.

Ennis, M. G., and MacErlean, D. P.: Percutaneous aspiration biopsy of abdomen and retroperitoneum. Clin. Radiol., *31,* 611–616, 1980.

Glatstein, E., Guernsey, J. M., Rosenberg, S. A., and Kaplan, H. S.: The value of laparotomy and splenectomy in the staging of Hodgkin's disease. Cancer, *24,* 709–718, 1969.

Göthlin, J. H.: Percutaneous transperitoneal fluoroscopy. Guided fine needle biopsy of lymph nodes. Acta Radiol. (Diagn.), *20,* 660–664, 1979.

Göthlin, J. H.: Post-lymphographic percutaneous fine needle biopsy of lymph nodes guided by fluoroscopy. Radiology, *120,* 205–207, 1976.

Göthlin, J. H., and Hoiem, L.: Percutaneous fine needle biopsy of radiographically normal lymph nodes in the staging of prostatic carcinoma. Radiology, *141,* 351–354, 1981.

Hidai, H., Sakuramoto, T., Miura, T., Nakahashi, M., and Kikyo, S.: Needle tract seeding following puncture of retroperitoneal liposarcoma. Eur. Urol., *9,* 368–369, 1983.

Jan, G. M., and Mahajan, R.: Ultrasound guided percutaneous fine needle aspiration biopsy (FNAB) of intraabdominal and retroperitoneal masses. Indian J. Gastroenterol., *8,* 99–100, 1989.

Juul, N., Torp-Pedersen, S., and Holm, H. H.: Ultrasonically guided fine needle aspiration biopsy of retroperitoneal mass lesions. Br. J. Radiol., *57,* 43–46, 1984.

Katz, R. L.: Kidney, adrenal, and retroperitoneum. *In* Bibbo, M. (Ed.). Comprehensive Cytopathology. Philadelphia, W. B. Saunders, 1991, pp. 771–805.

Kinmoth, J. B.: Lymphography in man. Clin. Sci., *11,* 13–20, 1952.

Knelson, M., Haaga, J., Lazarus, H., Ghosh, C., Abdul-Karim, F., and Sorenson, K.: Computed tomography-guided retroperitoneal biopsies. J. Clin. Oncol., *7,* 1169–1173, 1989.

Koss, L. G.: Diagnostic Cytology and Its Histopathologic Bases. 4th Ed. Philadelphia, J.B. Lippincott, 1992.

Koss, L. G., Woyke, S., and Olszewski, W.: Aspiration biopsy. Cytologic Interpretation and Histologic Bases. 2nd Ed. New York, Igaku-Shoin, 1992.

Lagergren, C., and Friberg, S.: Aspiration biopsy of lymph nodes after lymphography. Proc. Swed. Soc. Med. Radiol., *5,* 14–15, 1976.

Ljung, B. M.: Techniques of aspiration and smear preparation. *In* Koss, L. G., Woyke, S., Olszewski, W.: Aspiration Biopsy. Cytologic Interpretation and histologic bases. 2nd Ed. New York, Igaku-Shoin, 1992, pp. 12–30.

MacIntosh, P. K., Thompson, K. R., and Barbaric, Z. L.: Percutaneous transperitoneal lymph node biopsy as a means of improving lymphographic diagnosis. Radiology, *131,* 647–649, 1979.

Morettin, L. B., Brown, R. W., Amparo, E. G., and Matteson, R.: Multiple simultaneous percutaneous needle biopsy (MSPNB) technique for masses of the abdomen and peritoneum. Eur. J. Radiol., *7,* 98–100, 1987.

Mugharbil, Z. H., Tannenbaum, M., and Schapira, H.: Retroperitoneal malignant fibrous histiocytoma: case report and literature review. Mt. Sinai. J. Med. (NY), *54,* 158–161, 1987.

Mussouris, H. F., Koss, L. G., Rosenblatt, R., and Kutcher, R.: The needle aspiration biopsy of abdominal organs. *In* Koss, L. G., and Coleman, D. V. (Eds.). Advances In Clinical Cytology, Vol. 2. New York, Masson Publishing USA, 1984.

Otal-Salaverri, C., Gonzalez-Campora, R., Hevia-Vazquez, A., Lerma-Puertas, E., and Galera-Davidson, H.: Retroperitoneal ganglioneuroblastoma. Report of a case diagnosed by fine needle aspiration cytology and electron microscopy. Acta Cytol., *33,* 80–84, 1989.

Pereiras, R. V., Meirers, W., Kunhardt, B., Troner, M., Hutson, D., Barkin, J. S., and Viamonte, M.: Fluoroscopically guided thin needle aspiration biopsy of the abdomen and retroperitoneum. Am. J. Roentgenol., *131,* 197–202, 1978.

Rosenblatt, R.: Imaging modalities as guides to percutaneous aspiration. *In* Koss, L. G., Woyke, S., and Olszewski, W. (Eds.): Aspiration Biopsy. Cytologic Interpretation and Histologic Bases. 2nd Ed. New York, Igaku-Shoin, 1992, pp. 39–54.

Scarin, A.: Non-Hodgkin's lymphoma. Adv. Int. Med., *34,* 209–242, 1989.

Tao, L. C., Negin, M. L., and Donat, E. E.: Primary retroperitoneal seminoma diagnosed by fine needle aspiration biopsy. A case report. Acta Cytol., *28,* 598–600, 1984.

Tani, E., Löwhagen, T., Nasiell, K., Ost, A., and Skoog, L.: Fine needle aspiration cytology and immunocytochemistry of large cell lymphomas expressing the Ki-1 antigen. Acta Cytol., *33,* 359–362, 1989.

Thomson, K. R., House, A. J. S., Gothlin, J. H., and Dolan, T. E.: Percutaneous lymph node aspiration biopsy: Experience with a new technique. Clin. Radiol., *28,* 329–332, 1977.

Valkov, I., and Bojikin, B.: Fine needle aspiration biopsy of abdominal and retroperitoneal tumors in infants and children. Diagn. Cytopathol., *3,* 129–133, 1987.

Yazdi, H. M., and Burns, B.: Fine needle aspiration biopsy of Ki 1 positive large-cell "anaplastic" lymphoma. Acta Cytol., *35,* 306–310, 1991.

Zornoza, J., Cabanillas, F. F., Altoff, T. M., Ordonez, N., and Cohen, M. A.: Percutaneous needle biopsy in abdominal lymphoma. Am. J. Roentgenol., *136,* 97–103, 1981.

Zornoza, J., Handel, P., Lukeman, J. M., Jing, B. S., and Wallace, S.: Percutaneous transperitoneal biopsy in urologic malignancies. Urology, *9,* 395–398, 1977.

Zornoza, J., Lukeman, J. M., Jing, B. S., Wharton, J. T., and Wallace, S.: Percutaneous retroperitoneal lymph node biopsy in carcinoma of the cervix. Gynecol. Oncol., *5,* 43–51, 1977.

Zornoza, J., Wallace, S., Goldstein, M., Lukeman, J. M., and Jing, B.: Transperitoneal percutaneous retroperitoneal lymph node aspiration biopsy. Radiology, *122,* 111–115, 1977.

PART III

Newer Techniques in the Assessment and Monitoring of Tumors of the Urinary Tract

CHAPTER 9

Quantitative and Analytical Techniques

Recent developments in analytical and molecular biologic techniques have been applied to the study of urologic tumors and cells derived therefrom, increasing the scope of the knowledge of objective parameters that may account for tumor behavior, hence prognosis. The principal techniques are *flow cytometry, image analysis,* and *morphometry,* discussed in this chapter; cyto- and histochemistry, discussed in Chapter 10; and molecular biologic techniques, discussed in Chapter 11.

The similarities and differences between the two principal quantitative analytical techniques, discussed in this chapter, are summarized in Table 9-1.

FUNDAMENTAL PRINCIPLES AND APPLICATIONS OF FLOW CYTOMETRY

Reduced to its simplest parameters, the technique of flow cytometry is based on the principle of measuring fluorescence of cells and/or cell components suspended in a mantle of fluid, passing (flowing) one by one across a source of fluorescent light, usually a laser (Fig. 9-1). Contemporary machines are highly automated and comparatively simple to use, following the manufacturer's instructions. By staining the cells with an appropriate fluorescent probe (fluorochrome), specifically and stoichiometrically binding to the cell component to be measured, the amount of fluorescence recorded will faithfully reflect the amount of the cell component present in the cell. The

technique allows rapid measurements of a large number (1000 to several million) of particles (such as cells) and the recording of the levels of fluorescence in each particle by a computer. The distribution of the

TABLE 9-1
Comparison of Image Analysis with Flow Cytometry

Features	Image Analysis	Flow Cytometry
Applicability to routine cytologic material or smears	Yes	No
Speed	Slow	Very fast
Correlation with cell morphology	Yes	Possible with cell sorters
Measurement of multiple morphologic parameters	Yes	No
Measurements of cell components such as DNA	Yes	Yes
Use of fluorescent probes	Yes*	Yes
Use of absorbent probes	Yes	No
Autoradiography	Yes	No
Bioassays quantitation	Yes[†]	Yes[‡]
Tissue analysis	Yes	No

*With new, laser-based microscopes
[†]With monoclonal antibodies and peroxidase-antiperoxidase reaction
[‡]With fluorescent tagging
(Modified from Koss, L.G.: Diagnostic Cytology and its Histopathologic Bases. 4th Ed. Philadelphia, J.B. Lippincott, 1992. Copyright L.G. Koss.)

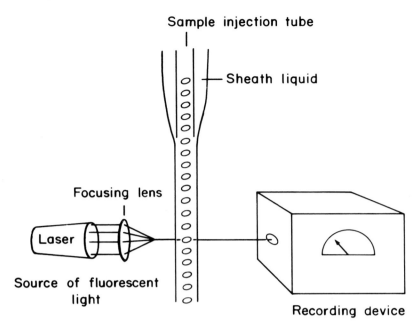

FIGURE 9-1.   Schematic representation of a flow cytometer. This much simplified diagram of a flow cytometer does not take into account the intricate system of prisms and dichroic mirrors that are an integral part of every machine but do not contribute to the understanding of the principles of the apparatus.

given cell component in a cell population can be displayed, usually in the form of a histogram or scattergram of distribution, by plotting the number of cells studied against the intensity of fluorescence encountered in this population, expressed as channel numbers, determined by the manufacturer (Fig. 9-2).

In addition to fluorescence, contemporary machines are capable of measuring several other cell features, such as volume and granularity. The machines are also capable of sorting subpopulations of cells with specific characteristics. Sorting is accomplished by using the printer droplet technique, in which the tiny droplets containing the cells, identified by a specific fluorescence profile, are electrically charged and deflected in a magnetic field. The selected droplets are collected in a separate container for further analysis or for cell culture.

By using two fluorochromes, each fluorescing at a different wavelength, and by splitting and adjusting the laser beam, simultaneous measurements of two or three cell components may be performed. Thus, the study of immunofluorescence and of the nucleic acid distribution can be combined or epithelial cells may be measured separately from lymphocytes. As an example, in our own work, using the appropriate anti-

bodies, we were able to correlate the expression of Ha-*ras* oncogene protein product (p21) and of the so-called CA1 antigen (Oxford antigen or epitectin) in cultured human cancer cells (Czerniak et al., 1984, 1987B), and in cells derived from urothelial tumors of the bladder (Czerniak et al., 1990) with DNA measurements. The relationship of the expression of these proteins during the various stages of the cell cycle could be elucidated (Fig. 9-3).

The most common applications of flow cytometry are in the area of immunology and in measurements of nucleic acids and other cell components in a population of cells. In immunologic studies the quantitation of an antigen expressed by a cell can be performed by measuring the fluorescence of one or more specific, usually monoclonal, antibodies tagged with a fluorescent molecule, such as fluorescein. For example, the immunologic characteristics of various subpopulations of T lymphocytes can be identified in such a system, a procedure helpful in evaluating patients with AIDS (Fig. 9-4).

Direct measurements of nucleic acids, notably DNA, can be performed by using a fluorescent probe that binds directly to the target molecule. DNA quantitation can be performed with a variety of intercalat-

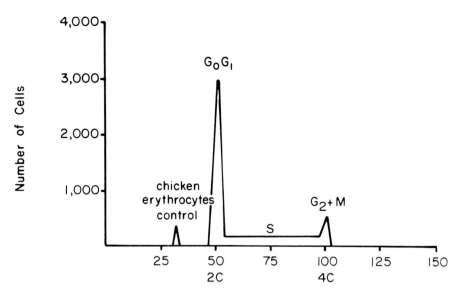

FIGURE 9-2. Basic structure of a histogram of DNA distribution in a normal (diploid) cycling cell population, generated by a flow cytometer. The diagram shows events in the cell cycle, indicated as G_0G_1, S, and G_2M, distributed along the abscissa marked in channel numbers (*e.g.,* 0–25–50). In this diagram, channel 50 position was arbitrarily selected as the center of the G_0G_1 peak. The intensity of fluorescence increases with channel numbers. Chicken erythrocytes (first peak left), served as control. For explanation of events in cell cycle, see text, p. 252 and Figure 9-5.

ing fluorescent compounds, *i.e.,* compounds that can be inserted into the double-stranded molecule of DNA and bind to the nucleotides. It is also possible to study single-stranded nucleic acids, such as RNA, by using appropriate probes (see below under Staining).

Preparation of Samples for Flow Cytometry

Flow cytometric techniques can be applied to cell suspensions, cultured cells, and, after suitable preparation, to fresh or paraffin-embedded tissue samples. Because flow cytometry is based on measurements of fluorescence intensity of individual cells, each "flowing" across the laser beam in a mantle of fluid, the principal objective of cell preparation for fluorescence measurements is a *suspension of single cells or particles*. The reason for this requirement is simple: the machines are unable to distinguish between a single particle and two or more particles stuck together; the signals generated by cell clusters result in an abnormally high level of fluorescence that may confound the measurements. Although contemporary machines are usually provided with computer soft-

ware that attempts to eliminate artifacts due to doublets or triplets (gating technique), it is still very important to achieve as clean a preparation as possible. Some machines now provide mathematical modeling to subtract aggregates from integrated histograms.

The task is relatively simple with fresh lymphocytes, other blood cells, or cultured cells, because they do not form solid cell attachments and usually can be studied directly after staining with the appropriate reagents (see below). Processing fresh tissue samples, however, may cause substantial difficulties, particularly in reference to epithelia and tumors derived therefrom. The epithelial cells are usually bound to each other by tough cell junctions, such as the desmosomes, and disrupting epithelial cell clusters is sometimes very difficult.

Methods of Preparation of Fresh Human Tissue and Epithelial Cell Samples

Fresh human tissue or cell samples (such as bladder washings) should be delivered to the laboratory in phosphate-buffered saline (PBS) or a similar physiologic solution for rapid processing. The bone marrow transport medium (RPMI 1640 with 10% calf serum and 14.3 units of sodium heparin/ml [Gibco,

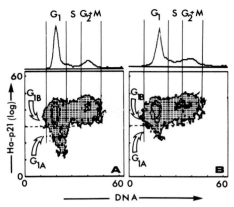

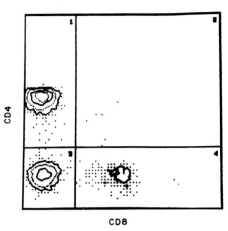

FIGURE 9-3. A scattergram of simultaneous flow cytometric measurements of the product of Ha-*ras* protein (Ha-p21) expression across the cell cycle in the human colon cancer cell line HT-29. The abscissa shows the distribution of DNA, again depicted as a histogram on top of the diagram as events in the cell cycle (G_1, $S, G_2 + M$). The ordinate shows the variable cell content of p21, which increases during the G_1 phase of the cell cycle. *A*, control cells; *B*, cells treated with prednisolone. In *B* the proportion of cells with low p21 content was decreased. (From Czerniak, B., Herz, F., Wersto, R. P., and Koss, L. G.: Modification of Ha-*ras* oncogene p21 expression and cell cycle progression in the human colonic cancer cell line HT-29. Cancer Res. *47*, 2826–2830, 1987, with permission.)

FIGURE 9-4. Scattergram of fluorescence, using a window technique, with antibodies characterizing the CD4 group of T-lymphocytes (helper cells) and the CD8 group of T-lymphocytes (suppressor cells). The quantitation of these two groups of lymphocytes in two of the windows is indicated on the diagram. The remaining lymphocytes are not characterized. Evaluation of T4 and T8 lymphocytes is important in assessing the immunologic status of patients with AIDS. (Diagram courtesy of Dr. Michael Prystowsky, Montefiore Medical Center/Albert Einstein College of Medicine, Bronx, NY.)

Grand Island, NY 14072]) is a suitable medium for transporting tissue or cell samples to the laboratory.

Tissue samples must be carefully and rapidly minced with a razor blade or a scalpel in a small shallow glass dish before further processing. Several methods can be used to achieve a single-particle suspension. The simplest method is one used by Tribukait in Stockholm (personal communication, 1993): centrifugation of minced tissue fragments results in a supernatant that contains a sufficient number of cells for one parameter measurement, such as DNA.

Syringing, or aspirating and reaspirating the sample through a small-caliber needle attached to a syringe, is a commonly used technique. The procedure is usually performed ten or more times. The resulting suspension must be filtered through a fine nylon mesh (pore size about 50 μm) to eliminate larger particles. While the method is usually effective in securing a large population of isolated nuclei, it usually fails in providing intact cells. The method also results in a very large amount of cell debris and often fails to disaggregate cell clusters or tissue fragments.

There are several other methods of preparation,

suitable only for measurements of nuclear parameters. These methods take advantage of the different response of the cell membrane and the nuclear membrane to acid or detergent treatment. The cell membranes and the cytoplasm are rapidly destroyed, whereas the nuclear membranes are quite resistant. The methods use an acid solution to strip the cytoplasm and prepare a suspension of nuclei. The first such method proposed was the CASC (citric acid and sodium citrate) method, using a mixture of citric and acetic acids (Koss et al., 1977). The use of other low pH solutions and of detergents has also been advocated (Krishan, 1975, Vindeløv et al., 1983), and these techniques have remained popular (see Appendix to this chapter for details).

Processing of Paraffin-Embedded Tissues

Hedley and his colleagues (1984) devised a method of processing paraffin-embedded tissue samples. Only samples fixed in buffered formalin or a related compound that stabilize DNA are suitable for such studies. Other fixatives, especially mercury-containing solutions, denature DNA and preclude accurate measurements. Sections of the selected paraffin block, usually 50 μm in thickness, are deparaffinized, rehydrated in a descending series of alcohols, and dissociated by proteolytic enzymes, resulting in a suspension of nuclei. Some aspects of this procedure can be automated in tissue processing machines, as described by Amberson and Wersto (see Appendix to this chapter). The method has the advantage of using archival tissues in patients with a known clinical outcome and has been very widely used in estimating the prognostic value of DNA ploidy. However, the measurements of DNA are often quite inaccurate, particularly in the assessment of aneuploid tumors. There is often a loss of nuclei with high DNA content, probably because of their size.

Staining of the Samples

Regardless of the target of flow cytometric measurements, whether immunologic or nucleic acids, extreme care must be exercised in the preparation of reagents. Because these reagents are by definition fluorescent compounds that may lose their fluorescent properties after exposure to light, many of the procedures have to be performed in darkness. It is also important to keep the stained samples in the dark before processing.

In reference to immune reagents, their suitability must be established by a method known as Western blotting, in which the specificity of the selected antibody to the target antigen is established by immunoelectrophoresis (see Fig. 9-14). Many of the commercially-sold antibodies may not be specific enough in the research laboratory, and their suitability must be confirmed before use. Labeling the antibody with a fluorescent molecule may also be difficult and, again, great care must be exercised in this regard.

In reference to nucleic acid staining, particularly DNA, there are several well established methods described with the use of the many compounds (probes) available for this purpose. Among the most widely used probes are propidium iodide (PI), ethidium bromide (EB), and 4′,6′ diamidinophenolindole (DAPI). To measure the fluorescence of these compounds (and, by implication, of the DNA), appropriate wave length of the laser beam, corresponding to maximal emission levels of the compound, must be selected. An essential step in the analysis of DNA is the preliminary use of RNAse, to eliminate RNA as it may cross-react with the dyes and alter the results.

Acridine orange (AO), a metachromatic fluorescent compound, forms different bonds with DNA and RNA and therefore can be used to measure both these components and their ratio, using two different wavelength of fluorescent light in the green and red range

(summary in Traganos et al., 1984). AO technique has been applied to bladder washings (Melamed et al., 1976). In a laboratory starting a flow cytometry program even the known methods must be tried until satisfactory results are achieved with control samples.

The interested reader is referred to the Appendix and to several published books and papers, listed in the bibliography, for a detailed description of the technical methods.

Controls

The use of control measurements to calibrate the machine and to establish the validity of the measurements in an unknown sample is an essential step in flow cytometry, as in any other measurement technique. The controls may be external or internal, *i.e.*, mixed with the sample to be measured. Many manufacturers provide external control samples in the form of a suspension of plastic spheres with known fluorescent properties for calibration of the machines. When working with cell suspensions and tissue samples it is also important to secure control samples with known properties, preferably from the same source. For example, in studying the characteristics of a human tumor, it is often helpful to secure a normal cell sample from the same patient, processed in an identical fashion. A suspension of benign lymphocytes freshly isolated from the peripheral blood may serve this purpose (Shackney et al., 1979). In measuring DNA, internal controls of the measurement may also be used. For example, mixing the unknown sample with nucleated chicken or trout erythrocytes with known and reasonably constant DNA content provides yet another security measure that the measurements are correct (Jakobsen, 1983; see Fig. 9-2).

Another approach to controls is the use of multiparameter flow cytometry on samples in which the benign cells, *e.g.*, lymphocytes, are identified with a specific antibody, in this example lymphocyte common antigen, CD 45. The position of the peak identified with this antibody becomes the diploid standard. Various permutations of this system may be attempted, using various antibodies.

A particularly difficult task is establishing controls for paraffin-embedded tissues. Obtaining control samples processed in an identical fashion is often very difficult. Samples of benign lymph nodes from the same patient and surgical procedure are the best controls, but these are often impossible to obtain. Lack of suitable controls often unfavorably affects published results.

In spite of these control measures it must be recognized that considerable variations exist in individuals and that each series of measurements should be repeatedly performed to establish the standard deviation of measurements (Koss et al., 1989; Wersto et al., 1991). In reference to DNA measurements it is also advisable to establish a range of normal measurements for any given histogram situation. In a large study of cell samples from colonic epithelium it has been documented that there is considerable patient-to-patient variability in the range of normal values (Wersto et al., 1988).

Significant variability of results among laboratories was also documented in a Bladder Cancer Cooperative Study, sponsored by the National Cancer Institute (Coon et al., 1988). Important differences were shown to exist in results of DNA measurements on identical samples of cultured or human cells, performed by five outstanding laboratories (Wheeless et al., 1989, 1991).

Measurements of DNA by Flow Cytometry

In recent years numerous investigators have directed their attention toward the potential value of DNA measurements in human tumors (summaries in Coon et al., 1988; Koss et al., 1989). The measurements take place in two forms: the determination of the *events in the cell cycle,* as a measure of cell proliferation, and of *DNA ploidy of tumors,* to determine the genetic makeup of a cell population in a tumor.

Events in the Cell Cycle

With a few notable exceptions, such as ganglion cells in the brain or heart muscle cells, the integrity of all living tissues is ensured by cell division, or mitotic activity, serving either to replace cells that die of senescence, apoptosis, or in combat, or in response to an appropriate stimulus. Mitotic activity in malignant tumors is often intense and sometimes abnormal. The events leading to cell division are known as the *cell cycle.* The cell cycle is a universal phenomenon, occurring in both normal and abnormal tissues. To ensure that the two daughter cells are endowed with the full genetic apparatus of the mother cell, hence the same amount of DNA, and, by implication, the same number of chromosomes, the cells destined to divide have to traverse a number of phases during which the amount of DNA will double. In recent years the biochemical and molecular bases of the cell cycle have begun to be unraveled, with the molecules known as cyclins implicated in the sequence of events (summary in Ohtsubo and Roberts [1993] and Murray and Hunt [1993]).

Nondividing cells are designated as G_0. Once the cells are committed to divide they enter the phase of the cell cycle known as G_1 (preparatory gap), followed by S (synthesis), G_2 (gap prior to mitosis), and M (mitosis). The duration of the normal human cell cycle from the onset of G_1 phase to the end of the mitotic division is about 18 hours. During the G_1 phase the cell accumulates RNA and proteins required for doubling of the amount of DNA. During the S-phase the amount of the DNA will gradually double. During the G_2 phase events preparatory to cell division (mitosis) take place. During mitosis (M phase) the cells divide into daughter cells.

It is evident from the above that the amount of DNA in G_2 and M phases of the cell cycle will be double the amount in G_0 and G_1 cells, with intermediate values seen in S-phase. In a proliferating cell population the distribution of the amounts of DNA in a histogram, based on analysis of 10,000 or more cells, will reflect cells in various stages of the cell cycle (Fig. 9-5). Such a histogram does not provide any information about individual cells but assesses the events in a population of cells. The analysis of the cell cycle events begins by assigning arbitrary dividing borders to the various segments of the histogram. Computer programs are available that will calculate the percentage of cells in each compartment (see Fig. 9-5B). The percentage of cells in S-phase will indicate the approximate proportion of cells in a given cell population that are synthesizing DNA. This may be important in human tumors, wherein the proportion of cells in the S-phase of cell cycle may serve as an index of proliferative activity.

In rapidly growing cell populations, such as cells in tissue culture, the duration of the G_1 phase may be relatively short and the proportion of cells in S-phase may be very high, reaching 20% (see Fig. 9-5). In normal human tissue the proportion of cells in S-phase varies, depending on the proliferative activity. Thus, in the colon, with its constant renewal of epithelial cells, the S-phase cells averaged slightly above 3% (Wersto et al., 1988), and it is generally lower in other tissues. In human cancer, high S-phase values may be observed. Although the estimates are often not accurate, they may serve *grosso modo* as a guide in the assessment of prognosis of a given tumor, when carefully compared with normal controls and with other tumors. Some of the sources of error in the assessment of the S-phase component may be vested in the characteristics of the histogram that are sometimes very difficult to interpret (see below in the section on histogram characteristics and interpretation). In tumors, abnormal cells that are not cycling may have a DNA content that falls within the range of S-phase of other cells.

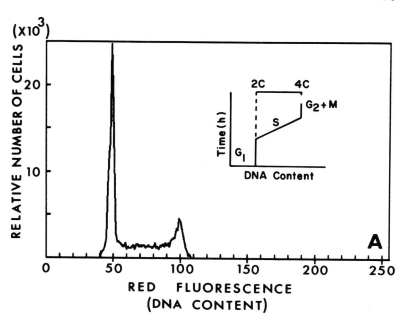

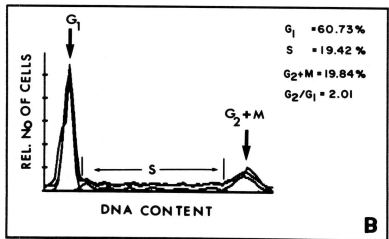

FIGURE 9-5. Histogram of DNA distribution of an actively cycling cell population (human leukemic cell line #L60) generated by flow cytometry, using propidium iodide as fluorochrome. (*A*) The DNA content is displayed as intensity of red fluorescence (corresponding to propidium iodide) measured in channel numbers on the abscissa (compare to Fig. 9-2). The ordinate shows the distribution of the number of cells in thousands. The inset translates the histogram into events in the cell cycle versus time. The inset shows the doubling of the DNA content as the cells traverse the S phase and reach the G_2M compartment. (*B*) Computer-generated analysis of the histogram shown in *A*. Two markers were placed to separate the S-phase cells from G_0G_1 and G_2M cells. The placement of the markers was computer generated. The proportion of cells in each compartment of the cell cycle is shown. In this example, a very large proportion of cells is in S-phase. (Diagram courtesy of Dr. Robert P. Wersto, Department of Pathology, Montefiore Medical Center/Albert Einstein College of Medicine, Bronx, NY.)

DNA Ploidy of Human Tumors

The term "ploidy" is used to define the DNA content of a given dominant cell population, on the assumption that the amount of DNA reflects the genetic make-up of this cell population, hence the number of chromosomes. Since direct cytogenetic studies of solid human tumors are extremely tedious, the rapid measurements of DNA by flow cytometry are a fair, even though sometimes not very precise, substitute that offers information of value.

Another concept of significance is the *stemline:* this is the dominant number of chromosomes per cell, in a population of cells (Fig. 9-6). Each normal human somatic cell has a constant number of 46 chromosomes. The cell population with these cytogenetic characteristics is defined as *diploid* or *euploid*. For germ cells, such as spermatozoa that each have only 23 chromosomes, the term *haploid* is used. Other terms reflect the number of chromosomes when referring to the diploid standard: cells with a number of chromosomes below 46 are *hypodiploid*. The *hyperdiploid* cells are further classified in numerous groups as shown in Figure 9-6.

The ploidy of cell populations may be approximately assessed in histograms of DNA distribution. The DNA ploidy (or, by implication, the stemline) is defined by the position of the first peak of the histo-

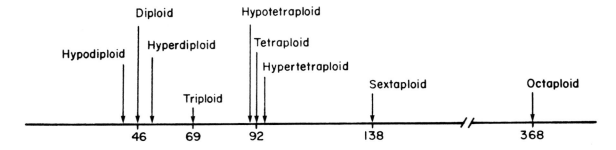

Number of Chromosomes

FIGURE 9-6. Designation of stem lines in human cancer according to the number of chromosomes per cell. (Modified from Koss, L. G.: Diagnostic Cytology and Its Histopathologic Bases. 4th Ed. Philadelphia, J.B. Lippincott, 1992.)

gram, containing non-cycling cells (G_0 cells) and cells in the G_1 phase of the cell cycle. In a normal human somatic cycling cell population this is the dominant peak, containing about 90% of all cells. This peak is designated as the *diploid peak* (corresponding to the diploid stemline of 46 chromosomes) and is assigned a channel number on the flow cytometer and in the histogram. The channel number corresponding to this peak position is used as a standard against which deviations from the normal histogram will be measured. For the purposes of this assessment the remaining phases of the cell cycle reflected in the histogram are ignored, unless there is a conspicuous increase in the number of cells in the second (G_2M) peak (see below). Some malignant tumors, such as many leukemias and lymphomas, and some solid human cancers show a normal or diploid distribution of DNA values or a diploid stemline. Studies using in situ hybridization with fluorescent chromosome probes (FISH technique) have documented that many of the "diploid" tumor cells have an abnormal chromosomal component (Hopman et al., 1988; Poddighe et al., 1992) (see also pp. 259, 264 and Chap. 11).

The diploid histograms are stable and vary less with time than aneuploid histograms. In many but not all human cancers, however, the number of chromosomes, and consequently the histograms of DNA distribution, will have abnormal values and are known as *aneuploid*. Such histograms are characterized by the presence of one or more dominant peaks of DNA distribution in abnormal channel locations in the histogram (Fig. 9-7). The aneuploid populations of cells may be cycling, and thus doubling their DNA component in the G_2M phases. The position of such G_2M peaks is again the double (in channel numbers) of the first aneuploid peak (see Fig. 9-7C,D). The location of

the abnormal peaks is defined by the DNA Index (DI), which is a ratio of the position of the aneuploid peak to the position of the normal diploid peak, expressed in channel numbers. For example, if the position of the normal diploid peak is in channel 50, and the position of the abnormal peak is in channel 60, the DI of the tumor will be 60:50, or 1.2 (Fig. 9-8). The designation of the abnormal peak in reference to the diploid peak again follows the rule established for stem lines: abnormal peaks below the diploid standard are *hypodiploid;* above the standard, *hyperdiploid*.

An increase in the number of cells in the G_2M peak above normal, which is rarely higher than 5–10%, is also abnormal. This finding indicates an abnormality characterized by doubling of the DNA, hence a *tetraploid* population of cells, presumably containing 92 chromosomes. As mentioned above, the normal proportion of cells in the G_2M peak varies from organ to organ, and it must be established by multiple measurements of the normal cell population. A maximum of 10% is commonly and arbitrarily accepted.

Histogram Characteristics and Interpretation

The quality of the histogram generated by flow cytometry is of paramount importance. The width of the dominant peak of the histogram is assessed by a *coefficient of variation* (CV). The CV is determined by dividing the mean channel number of the dominant peak by its standard deviation, determined by multiple measurements. The tighter the curve, the lower the CV. Although in theory an ideal peak should have a CV of 0, in reality a CV between 2% and 3% is usually observed in normal control cells, such as lym-

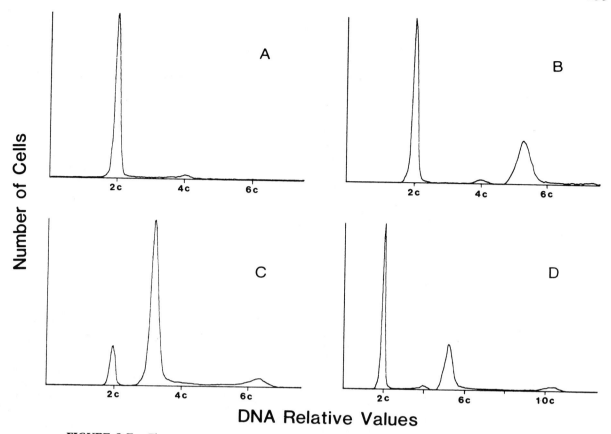

FIGURE 9-7. Flow cytometric histograms of urothelial bladder tumors. (*A*) superficially invasive tumor grade II with a normal (diploid) histogram; (*B*) a grade III invasive carcinoma with an aneuploid peak in hypertetraploid position; (*C*) a superficially invasive grade III tumor with an aneuploid peak in approximately triploid position—this cell population is cycling as it shows another peak in a position just above 6c; (*D*) a grade III invasive carcinoma with a cycling aneuploid cell population in hypertetraploid position and a corresponding G₂M peak above 10c. C refers to ploidy: 2c = diploid; 4c = tetraploid etc.
Special technique was used to demonstrate the G₂M aneuploid peaks in diagrams c and d. (Diagrams courtesy of Dr. Bernard Tribukait, Stockholm.)

phocytes (Fig. 9-9). Machine-generated variations in measurements and slight variations in the DNA content that occur even in control cells account for these observations. In tumors, depending on the technique of preparation and the specimen type, the CV of 6% is still acceptable. Data based on histograms with CV above 6% should be interpreted with caution, because the measurement may include two populations of cells with slightly different DIs (Wersto et al., 1991). CVs of 8% or more are not acceptable, and the results must be rejected.

Other measures of the histogram adequacy are *skewness* and *kurtosis*. These measures pertain to the shape of the curve and the flatness of the peak. If the curve is asymmetrical and its peak is flat, the possibility must be raised that it contains two populations of cells, not one.

The interpretation of "clean" histograms with a low CV and straight peak curves, either as diploid or aneuploid, is comparatively easy for experienced observers armed with appropriate computer software. In many instances, however, the DNA distribution of human tumors is complex and such histograms are difficult to interpret. The common difficulties are in

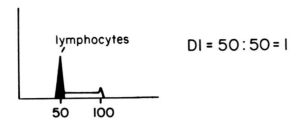

DI = 50 : 50 = 1

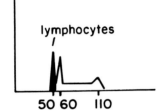

DI first peak = 60 : 50 = 1.2

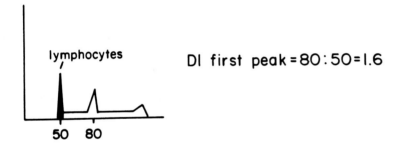

DI first peak = 80 : 50 = 1.6

FIGURE 9-8. Calculation of the DNA Index (DI). In this example, the position of the diploid peak (lymphocytes in black) was assigned to channel 50. In the top diagram the position of the first peak of the unknown cell population overlaps with lymphocytes, and hence the DI = 1 (diploid or euploid). The abnormal peaks in the central diagram are assigned to channel 60 and in the bottom diagram to channel 80. The DI is calculated at 1.2 and 1.6, respectively, and hence is aneuploid.

the assessment of the percentage of S-phase cells in histograms that have a large CV or a sloping shape of curves. In such histograms the placement of the markers for cell cycle analysis (see Fig. 9-5*B*) is entirely arbitrary and may result in S-phase differences of 10% or even 20% depending on the position of the markers. Also, in complex histograms, containing one diploid and one or more aneuploid cycling populations (or two or more aneuploid cycling populations), the estimation of S-phase based on histogram analysis becomes highly arbitrary, even with the use of mathematical modeling (Koss et al., 1989; Koss, 1992). Another potential source of difficulty in the analysis of S-phase is the presence of non-cycling abnormal cells.

For these reasons, alternate means of assessment of S-phase cells have been developed. Bromodeoxyuridine is a compound that is incorporated into DNA during the S-phase of the cell cycle, replacing the nucleotide thymidine. Using an antibody fluorescent to bromodeoxyuridine, it is possible to determine the proportion of cells in the S-phase of cell cycle (Schutte

et al., 1987; Gray and Mayall, 1985). Another method of analyzing the cell cycle is based on the analysis of an antibody to Ki67 protein that becomes activated in cycling cells (Wersto et al., 1988) and proliferating cell nuclear antigen (PCNA, see Chap. 10). The discovery of cyclins as enzymes participating in various aspects of cell cycle is likely to improve still further the analysis of cell cycle events (summary in Murray and Hunt, 1993).

Another source of difficulty in determining the events in the cell cycle (and tumor DNA ploidy as well—see below) is the cell population. Inevitably, the samples processed for flow cytometry contain a mixture of benign cells (such as leukocytes and endothelial cells) and tumor cells. By using various cell markers in a fluorescent mode, it is often possible to study the DNA distribution of a defined cell population. For example, the use of anti-keratin antibodies may make it possible to identify cells of urothelial carcinoma among other (benign) cells that do not contain keratin filaments (Fietz et al., 1985; Smeets et al., 1987; see also p. 264).

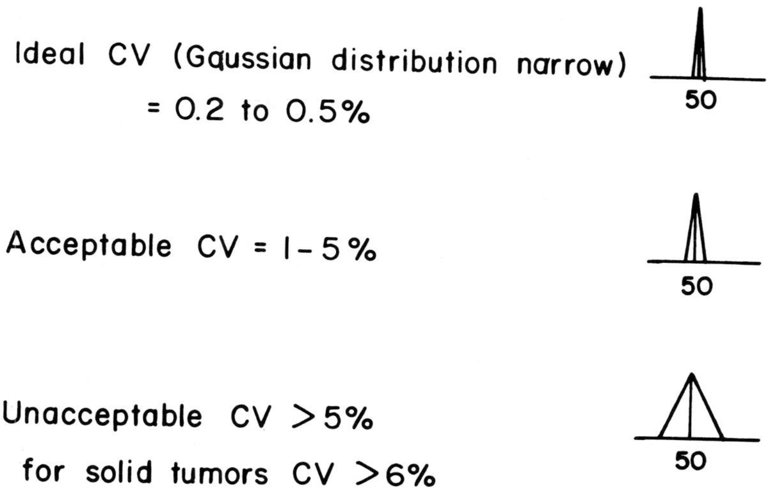

Ideal CV (Gaussian distribution narrow)
= 0.2 to 0.5%

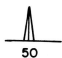

50

Acceptable CV = 1–5%

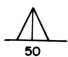

50

FIGURE 9-9. Coefficient of variation (CV) is calculated by dividing the channel number at the center of the first peak by its standard deviation.

Unacceptable CV >5%

for solid tumors CV >6%

50

Another difficulty pertains to the designation of the G_2M peak as abnormal. To do it well, one should establish by multiple measurements the range of normal. Arbitrarily, the G_2M peak containing more than 10% of cells is considered abnormal. The designation of a tumor as aneuploid, with only a slight deviation from normal (CV of 1.2, for example) may again be difficult if the curves are not neat and the CV of the measurements is above 3% or 4%.

The applications of flow cytometric techniques to tumors of the urinary tract are discussed below.

FUNDAMENTAL PRINCIPLES AND APPLICATIONS OF IMAGE ANALYSIS

Image analysis and image analysis–based cytophotometry are microscope-based techniques used in quantitative analysis of cells and their components in appropriately prepared smears and, to a lesser extent, tissue sections. When compared with flow cytometry, the techniques have the advantage of visual control of the material to be analyzed but are time consuming. The principal differences between the two approaches to cell analysis are shown in Table 9-1 on p. 247.

Basic Principles of Image Analysis

The principle of the system is the transformation of microscopic images into a set of objective, measurable optical or electrical parameters that can be subjected to mathematical analysis. In the early instruments, introduced in the 1930s and 1940s, the transformation of images was based on point-by-point measurements of the intensity of either *visible or fluorescent* transmitted light. Although the calculations were extremely tedious and time-consuming, a surprising amount of fundamental information on cell structure and function was generated by the pioneers of this method, notably Torbjørn Caspersson and his students in Stockholm. In recent years, significant progress has been made in constructing machines capable of analytical functions. The basic components of such a machine are: a microscope with good quality optics; an image acquisition system, usually a television camera recording in red, blue, and green; one or often two color television monitors (one to display the objects to be analyzed and the other to display the results of the analysis); and a personal computer with appropriate software and memory. Most machines are "user friendly" and provide screen displays indicating the sequential steps that are necessary to achieve the results to be displayed on the television monitor. Printers, usually provided with the machines, make it possible to record the results.

Such machines may be used for two basic purposes. One application provides measurements of cell components, for example DNA (cytophotometry). The other serves the purpose of objective classification of cells in reference to their biologic behavior, for example as cancer cells or benign cells (analytical cytometry). Regardless of the application of the machines, the processing of the microscopic images follows a well-established sequence of events:

- *Image acquisition*
- *Image digitization*
- *Scene segmentation*
- *Feature extraction*
- *Feature analysis*

Image Acquisition

The term "image acquisition" is self-explanatory. The selection of objects to be analyzed occurs under visual control. In most of the contemporary systems that are available, the object is captured instantly by the television camera and is displayed on the television monitor. A computer command is used to retain the object for future analysis.

Image Digitization

For the image to be analyzed by a computer, it has to be presented to the computer in numerical form. In early machines a point-by-point measurement of light transmission or absorbance was used. Each point of measurement was assigned an arbitrary value (Fig. 9-10). A sum total of the values, usually a histogram, represented the object. In contemporary machines the transformation occurs in the television camera, using the charge-coupled devices (CCD) that convert light intensity into electronic signals. The digitized images are stored in the computer for analysis and may be displayed in the form of a histogram of digital values.

Scene Segmentation

For the object (cell) to be analyzed it has to be separated from its environment. For example, if one is dealing with a cluster of cells and wishes to analyze only one, a separation of the selected cell must take place. In older machines the separation required a selection of cut-outs or matrices, fitting the contour of the selected cell. Now there are computer programs that perform this function but require the input of the operator to place markers separating cells.

Feature Extraction

From the digitized image one can extract values that serve the purpose of the analysis. For example, if one wishes to compare the features of cancer cells and benign cells of the same origin, numerical features pertaining to cell size, cell configuration, nuclear size, nuclear configuration, nuclear texture, and such features as the nucleo-cytoplasmic ratio, may be analyzed. Elaborate calculations and histogram analyses were required in the past to accomplish these goals. Computer programs available in most contemporary machines accomplish this function rapidly.

Feature Analysis

Depending on the purpose of the analysis, the features extracted may be analyzed for their similarities and differences. For example, the size, configuration, and texture of the nuclei, or a combination of these and other features, may be used in attempting to separate cancer cells from benign cells. If the purpose of the analysis is a measurement of a cell component, integrated values of the cell component, provided by the computer, may be displayed in the form of a histogram. If the measurement pertains to light absorption, Beer's law must be observed. The law states that the amount of light absorbed is *not* in direct proportion to the density of the object. In most machines an adjustment for Beer's law is built into the computer software.

Cytophotometry of DNA

Application to Smears

An extension of the concepts of image analysis is cytophotometry, which, in fact, was the first system of objective cell analysis developed. The concept of cytophotometry is based on measuring the density and size of cell nuclei in smears, usually stained with a DNA-specific Feulgen stain (see Chap. 1). In contemporary machines Beer's law is usually accounted for in the software of the computer that coordinates the function of the machines. The visually selected nuclei are captured and digitized, and their total density assessed. The summary results of the measurements are displayed on the computer monitor in the form of a histogram, adjusted in some machines for the approximate DNA content in picograms (Fig. 9-11). The histograms are usually based on a relatively small number of nuclei, from 100 to 500, with an average of about 200 per smear. The DNA values of individual nuclei are placed in compartments or "bins," approximately corresponding to their DNA content. Because the number of measurements and the number of bins are limited, the resulting histogram resembles an edifice constructed of building blocks and lacks the smoothness of the flow cytometric histogram.

Some machines are calibrated to determine the events in cell cycle, in a manner similar to that discussed for flow cytometers on p. 252. However, such determinations in cytophotometry are, at best, approximate because of the limited number of nuclei that are being measured. On the other hand, the histograms of DNA distribution usually allow a determination whether a cell population has a DNA content within normal limits or is abnormal.

The nuclei to be measured are selected under visu-

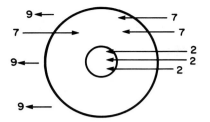 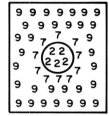

FIGURE 9-10. Principles of image digitization. Each point of the image (pixel) is assigned an arbitrary numerical value, according to the amount of light transmitted (or absorbed) by the target. The cell is represented by an array of numbers. In this example, 9 represents the clear background, 2 the optically dense nucleus, and 7 the transparent cytoplasm.

al control, with the operator's choice often directed at large nuclei. In this regard, cytophotometry offers certain selection advantages over flow cytometry wherein all nuclei in a sample must be measured. As a consequence, in measuring the DNA content of human samples such as cancer cells, small subpopulations of aneuploid cells that may remain unnoticed in flow cytometry can be identified (Fig. 9-12). The superiority of image analysis over flow cytometry in identifying aneuploid patterns has been repeatedly documented (Cornelisse and van Drier-Kulker, 1985; Schneller et al., 1987; Koss et al., 1989.)

A significant problem in cytophotometry of DNA is the identification and use of appropriate *controls*. Theoretically, one should find in a cell population at least some cells that are normal, such as normal leukocytes, fibroblasts, or epithelial cells for comparison with abnormal cells. In practice, the identification of benign cell nuclei in Feulgen-stained preparations is sometimes very difficult. Unfortunately, for most machines the nuclei of quiescent fixed lymphocytes are too compact to serve as diploid controls. In air-dried smears, however, the lymphocytes may be an acceptable control. Some manufacturers are providing standard controls in the form of an aliquot of animal cells with a known DNA content. The best control is the performance of every set of measurements in duplicate, using a different cell population, to make certain that the results are reproducible.

Application to Histologic Sections

Some contemporary machines offer the option of measuring DNA content in histologic sections 5 or 6 μm thick and stained with Feulgen stain. Because such sections contain cross sections rather than intact, whole nuclei, software is provided to compensate for the cutting artifact. The technique has been applied to tissue sections and biopsies of the prostate, and it allows for a rough estimation of the DNA content of a tumor as presumably diploid or aneuploid (Fig. 9-13). The technique is far from accurate and is certainly not suitable for a detailed analysis of histograms.

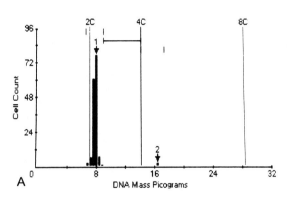

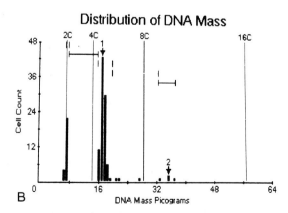

FIGURE 9-11. Examples of DNA histograms obtained with the CAS 200 machine (Cell Analysis Systems, 909 South Route 83, Elmhurst, IL 60126-4944). Both histograms pertain to aspiration biopsy smears of the breast stained with Feulgen stain. (*A*) Diploid histogram. (*B*) Tetraploid–aneuploid histogram with 3 dominant peaks: the diploid peak (left, not numbered), the tetraploid peak (numbered 1), and an octaploid peak (2), representing cycling tetraploid cells (compare to Fig. 5-16).

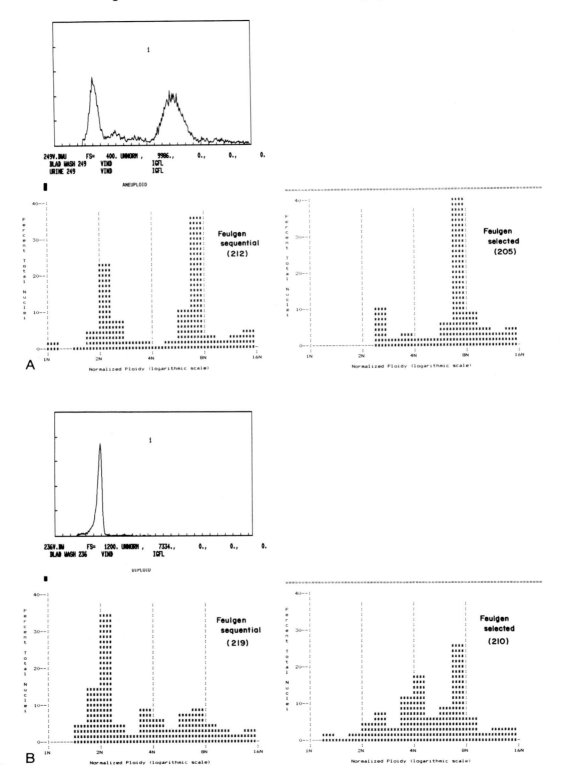

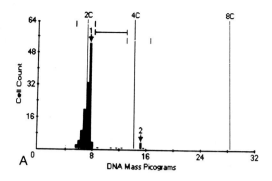

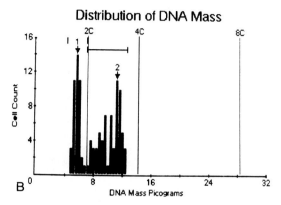

FIGURE 9-13. Histograms of DNA distribution in biopsies of prostatic carcinoma, cut at 5 μm, stained with Feulgen stain (CAS 200, Cell Analysis Systems, 909 South Route 83, Elmhurst, IL 60126-4944). (*A*) A diploid tumor. The distribution of the nuclei in the dominant diploid peak (*1*) is broader than in smears (compare with Fig. 9-11A). A small tetraploid peak is also noted (*2*). (*B*) An aneuploid tumor. The DNA values are widely distributed and a designation of a DNA index would be purely arbitrary (compare with Fig. 9-16).

DNA Ploidy Analysis and Fluorescent In Situ Hybridization (FISH) With Chromosomal Probes

Whether the DNA content of human tumors is studied by flow cytometry or image analysis, it does not necessarily reflect the genetic make-up of the

tumor. The use of the FISH technique with probes to various chromosomes has shown that chromosomal abnormalities may occur in tumors judged to be diploid (Poddighe et al., 1992). This was first shown by Hopman et al. (1988) in reference to tumors of the urinary bladder and by several observers in reference to tumors of the prostate (see p. 273). The application of the hybridization technique is still in its infancy as of the time of this writing (1994). For further comments on FISH, see Chapter 11.

Measuring Cell Products by Cytophotometry

There are no theoretical or technical problems with measuring almost any cell or tissue parameter that may be visualized by a light-absorbing or fluorescent stain. With the advent of cytochemical or fluorescent markers that can be attached to a broad variety of monoclonal and polyclonal antibodies, it is theoretically possible to measure any number of cellular antigens and cell components. Fluorescent technique, however, is not particularly well suited for cytophotometry because the systems are slow and the fluorescence may fade, sometimes rather rapidly. New microscopes, provided with laser light sources, may improve the situation (Kamentsky and Kamentsky, 1991). In my judgment, flow cytometry is superior in measuring fluorescent compounds, although it does not offer any information on their distribution within a cell, as microscopy does.

On the other hand, compounds brought into evidence by immunocytochemistry and visualized by one of the many chromatogenic substances are perfectly well suited for cytophotometric measurements. The customary medium used in such studies is the standard peroxidase-antiperoxidase reaction, used in immunocytochemistry. For example, using such systems it has been possible to obtain quantitative analysis of the estrogen and progesterone receptors and of oncogene products in breast cancer, and to compare these data with the DNA content of the same tumors (Bacus et al., 1988, 1989, 1990; Clark et al., 1989; Czerniak et al., 1989). In our laboratories it could be

FIGURE 9-12. Bladder washings. Comparison of flow cytometry (propidium iodide stained nuclei) with image analysis of Feulgen-stained cells. (*A*) An aneuploid tumor. Flow cytometry shows an abnormal histogram (*top*) with a huge aneuploid peak in the hyper-tetraploid region. Two histograms of Feulgen-stained cells obtained by image analysis are shown (*bottom*). On the left, sequential nuclei were measured; on the right, selected large nuclei were measured. It may be noted that the selection enhanced the aneuploid peak. (*B*) A bladder tumor that had a diploid histogram in flow cytometry (*top*). The image analysis histograms (*bottom*) show a clear aneuploid distribution of DNA values, again enhanced by selection of large nuclei.

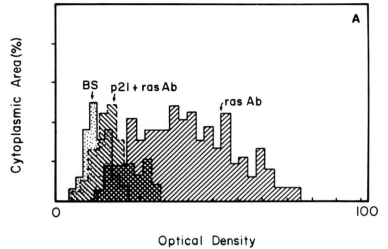

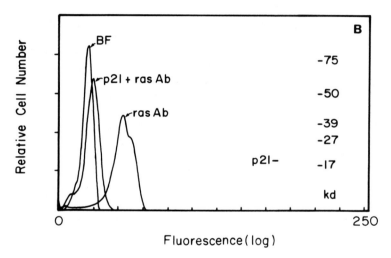

FIGURE 9-14. Quantitation of Ha-*ras* gene product (protein 21 or p21), using an appropriate antibody, in a human breast cancer cell line MCF 7-KO. The immunocytologic reaction was obtained with a peroxidase-antiperoxidase reaction in the cytoplasm of the cells. For flow cytometry, the antibody was tagged with fluorescein. The specificity of the antibody was tested with Western blotting (*bottom, right*) showing a band in the area of 21 kilodaltons, corresponding to p21. The measurements were performed with image analysis (*top*) and, after attaching a fluorescein tag to the antibody, by flow cytometry (*bottom*). The expression of the p21 is enhanced when compared with background measurements—background staining (BS) and background fluorescence (BF). The reaction is blocked by the addition of p21 (p21 + *ras* Ab). (From Czerniak, B., Herz, F., Wersto, R. P., et al.: Quantitation of oncogene products by computer-assisted image analysis and flow cytometry. J. Histochem. Cytochem., *38,* 463–466, 1990, with permission.)

documented that the expression of various oncogene products in cultured human cells could be measured, providing important information on the distribution of these compounds in cycling cells (Czerniak et al., 1987B, 1990). Careful measurements of oncogene product in cultured postmitotic human cells revealed that the distribution of the proteins is not equal between the daughter cells, with some receiving more and some less of the product (Czerniak et al., 1992). This observation explained the variability of the oncogene product content in cultured cells entering the cell cycle (see Fig. 9-3). Several precautions must be carefully observed before such measurements can be undertaken. The specificity of the antibody must be carefully established by performing Western blots with the antigen to be measured. The measurements must be carefully standardized and repeated several

times to establish the standard deviation and to eliminate possible errors (Fig. 9-14).

Discriminant Analysis of Cell Populations

One of the early goals of image analysis was objective classification of cells and their components. Prewitt and Mendelsohn (1966) were the first to propose this use of computerized images for blood cells, followed by Wied et al. (1968) who applied this technique to classification of images of cells in cervical smears, using a program known as Taxonomic Intracellular Analysis System (TICAS).

The TICAS program has been successfully applied to the discrimination among various classes of cells in cervical (Pap) smears (summary in Bahr et al., 1992). A number of dedicated instruments for automated image analysis of such samples have been devised (summary in Koss et al., 1994). The principle of these instruments was quite simple—for each cell population a number of features (parameters) was established, based on morphologic criteria such as cell size, nuclear size, nucleo-cytoplasmic ratio, and configuration of nuclear chromatin. These features (and combinations thereof) were then applied to cells in smears. The results of such studies were generally poor, mainly because of the problems with overlapped cells that were giving false alarms. The creation of a monolayer smear represents another set of problems that may be solved by current technology.

The options of automated analysis of cells in smears received a major boost with the application of computer software known as artificial intelligence and neural nets. These devices, which mimic the function of the eye–brain axis, are capable of separating out and analyzing cells of a specific type (such as cancer cells) for automated analysis or for display on television monitors for human analysis. The application of one such machine, based on these principles (the PAPNET system), has been shown to have a high degree of accuracy, comparable to human diagnostic performance in cervical smears (Koss et al., 1994).

Such instruments may soon become useful in urologic cytology.

MORPHOMETRY

Morphometry is closely related to image analysis, inasmuch as it attempts to identify cell characteristics and spatial relationships of cells to each other in a given microscopic field (Baak and Oort, 1983). The fields are visually selected to show the highest degree of abnormality, and hence, the technique cannot be considered objective or reproducible (Collan et al., 1987). The technique is primarily applicable to tissue sections and prognostic information has been obtained in carcinomas of the bladder, prostate, ovary, and endometrium, and in renal tumors.

APPLICATION OF ANALYTICAL TECHNIQUES IN UROLOGY

DNA Ploidy of Urothelial Tumors of the Bladder

DNA Ploidy in Fresh Tumor Tissue Samples

The first measurements of DNA distribution in bladder tumors stained by the Feulgen method were

performed by cytophotometry on tissue sections (Lederer et al., 1972). In that study, it was shown that grade I tumors were predominantly diploid, grade II tumors were diploid with an added tetraploid component, and grade III and IV tumors were uniformly aneuploid. These results were in keeping with contemporary measurements of DNA.

Numerous observers measured the DNA distribution in fresh tissue samples of urothelial tumors by flow cytometry. The largest experience is that of Tribukait (1984, 1987) who pointed out that most urothelial tumors grade 1 are diploid and nearly all urothelial tumors grade 3 (including flat carcinomas in situ) are aneuploid. Tumors grade 2 were almost equally divided into diploid and aneuploid categories (Table 9-2). The study of tumor ploidy according to clinical stages pointed out that diploid tumors are not likely to invade beyond the lamina propria, whereas nearly all deeply invasive tumors and carcinomas in situ are aneuploid.

It is of note, however, that among the aneuploid grade 2 tumors, about one half were tetraploid, whereas very few tetraploid tumors were deeply invasive (stage T3 and T4). This observation strongly suggests that tetraploid grade 2 tumors are less likely to invade the wall of the bladder than aneuploid tumors. The observation also suggests that tetraploidy may be an intermediate stage in the development of invasive, aneuploid tumors, as also noted for urothelial tumors of renal pelves (see p. 267).

The concordance of ploidy data between the deeply invasive cancers and carcinoma in situ forged yet another link between these two manifestations of bladder cancer (see Chap. 5). This link was further enhanced by a study of 290 primary exophytic bladder tumors and synchronous "random" biopsies of unaffected areas of bladder epithelium (Norming et al., 1989). In 69 of these patients, aneuploid patterns were observed in the peripheral epithelium, nearly always associated with identical DNA pattern in the primary tumors. Most of the latter were grade 3 tumors, with a few aneuploid grade 2 tumors. On the other hand, none of the 31 diploid grade 1 tumors showed aneuploidy in peripheral biopsies. Grade 2 tumors were once again divided into diploid and aneuploid: only 3 of 46 diploid tumors showed aneuploidy in peripheral biopsies, whereas 10 of 61 aneuploid tumors showed aneuploidy. This observation strongly supports the notion that aneuploid tumors are derived from aneuploid, flat epithelial abnormalities, as discussed in Chapter 5 on p. 82. In a more recent paper, Tribukait's group pointed out that the progression of carcinoma in situ to invasive cancer is linked to DNA multiploidy: carcinomas in situ with two aneuploid peaks (or stem lines) were shown to be more

TABLE 9-2
Frequency of Diploid and Aneuploid Cell Lines in 277 Untreated Bladder Carcinomas Related to Tumor Stage and Grade

Tumor Grade	Diploid	Aneuploid		Multiple	Total
		TETRAPLOID	NONTETRAPLOID		
Grade 0	2	—	—	—	2(1%)
Grade I	24(80%)	4(13%)	2(7%)	—	30(11%)
Grade II	56(52%)	22(21%)	22(21%)	7(6%)	107(38%)
Grade III	6(5%)	5(4%)	67(52%)	52(40%)	130(47%)
Adenocarcinoma	1(12%)		5(63%)	2(25%)	8(3%)
Total	89(32%)	31(11%)	96(35%)	61(22%)	277
Tumor Stage					
TaT1	82(51%)	25(16%)	40(25%)	13(8%)	160(58%)
T2	2(8%)	3(13%)	11(46%)	8(33%)	24(9%)
T3	5(9%)	1(2%)	29(51%)	22(38%)	57(20%)
T4		2(17%)	5(42%)	5(42%)	12(4%)
Tis			11(46%)	13(54%)	24(9%)
Total	89(32%)	31(11%)	96(35%)	61(22%)	277

Abbreviations: T_a = noninvasive papillary tumors
T_1 = papillary tumors extending into lamina propria
T_2 = tumors with superficial muscle invasion
T_3 = tumors with deep invasion
T_4 = deeply invasive tumors with metastases
Tis = flat carcinoma in situ
For definition of grades, see Chapter 5, p. 72.
(Modified from Tribukait, B.: Flow cytometry in surgical pathology and cytology of tumors of the genito-urinary tract. *In* Koss, L.G., and Coleman, D. [Eds.]: Advances in Clinical Cytology, Vol. 2. New York, Masson. 1984, with permission.)

likely to progress to invasive cancer than carcinomas in situ with a single aneuploid peak (Norming et al., 1992).

Cell suspensions obtained from bladder tumors contain a mixture of cells. Besides benign and malignant epithelial cells, the mixture contains lymphocytes, endothelial cells, and fibroblasts, all of which stain with the fluorescent probes and add to the complexity of the DNA histogram. For this reason, Ramaekers et al. (1984) proposed the use of antibodies identifying intermediate filaments in epithelial cells to eliminate non-epithelial cells from the histogram. The system was tested on bladder tumors with antibodies to keratin filaments (Feitz et al., 1985) with the gating technique, in which the histograms were constructed from cells in the keratin-positive "window," similar to the procedure used for lymphocyte typing (see Fig. 9-4). The resulting histograms of DNA distribution in bladder tumors were much more precise than the histograms obtained on the entire cell suspension. Still, the overall results of the study were quite similar to those cited above and did not significantly change the distribution of DNA ploidy values according to tumor grade or stage.

DNA ploidy values obtained by flow were also compared with cytogenetic make-up of bladder tumors (Wijkström et al., 1984; Smeets et al., 1987).

The difficulty of obtaining adequate chromosomal preparations from tumor cells was considerable and has been since complemented by the fluorescent in situ hybridization (FISH) technique, discussed in Chapter 11.

The original FISH studies cited above disclosed that chromosomal abnormalities may occur in some diploid tumors and are the rule in all non-diploid tumors, thus confirming the overall value of DNA ploidy measurements.

A still unresolved question is the significance of the S-phase cell compartment in the prognosis of bladder tumors. Because such measurements are not fully reliable in flow cytometry (see p. 252), immunocytologic techniques with antibodies to cell proliferation antigens, discussed in Chapter 10, may shed additional light on this problem.

Thus, DNA ploidy of urothelial tumors is of significant prognostic value. It is of major interest that the results of cytologic examination of voided urine correspond very closely to the ploidy distribution of urothelial tumors, as shown in Table 5-3. Aneuploid tumors are much more likely to shed identifiable cancer cells in urinary sediment than diploid tumors.

It is of added interest that certain biologic characteristics of urothelial tumors, such as the density of nuclear pores or the expression of CA antigen (epitectin), are related to ploidy of urothelial tumors. The density of the nuclear pores and the level of epitectin expression are higher in aneuploid than in diploid tumors (see Table 5-2 and p. 82). It is also of note that some immunologic data, discussed in Chapter 10, and some molecular biologic data, discussed in Chapter 11, may also be correlated with tumor ploidy and behavior.

DNA Ploidy Measurements in Paraffin-Embedded Tissue

The application of Hedley's method or one of its variants to measurements of DNA content of bladder tumors has the advantage of using archival material with known clinical outcome. In our own flow cytometric studies, the relationship of DNA ploidy measurements to stage and grade of bladder tumors essentially confirmed the observations by Tribukait and others reported above. High-grade invasive tumors were for the most part aneuploid, whereas low-grade noninvasive papillary tumors were for the most part diploid (Koss et al., 1989). The limitations of flow cytometry in paraffin-embedded samples were discussed on p. 250. Similar observations were reported using image analysis–based morphometry on nuclei secured from paraffin-embedded bladder tumors (Czerniak et al., 1992; see Chap. 11).

DNA Ploidy of Bladder Washings (Barbotage) in Urothelial Tumors

The technique of bladder washings was described on p. 4. Melamed and his group at Memorial Sloan-Kettering Cancer Center in New York pioneered the concept of flow cytometric measurements of DNA content of cells in bladder washings or barbotage as a guide to tumor behavior, hence prognosis (Melamed et al., 1976; Klein et al., 1982; Badalament et al., 1986, 1987). Another application of this technique was in monitoring patients treated by surgery or immunotherapy for bladder tumors (Klein et al., 1981; Stoiano-Coico et al., 1985; Bretton et al., 1989; Giella et al., 1992). The assumption of these studies was that aneuploid DNA pattern in urothelial cells was a poor prognostic sign that led to tumor recurrence or to invasion. For low-grade tumors that often failed to give an aneuploid pattern of DNA distribution, it was arbitrarily proposed that histograms with 15% or more cells above the diploid peak were suggestive of a possible recurrence. The ultimate goal of this study was to determine to what extent, if any, flow cytometry of bladder washings can replace cytology and cystoscopy as a guide to tumor recurrence or progression.

A group of investigators from five institutions, working under the auspices of the National Cancer Institute, USA, was convened to determine whether the reported observations were applicable to a large group of patients and could be recommended as a standard clinical procedure (Coon et al., 1988; Aamodt et al., 1992). The group made a number of observations that did not fully concur with the previous claims as to the value of the method. Although it could be confirmed that clearly aneuploid patterns of DNA usually corresponded to high-grade tumors (including carcinoma in situ), the reproducibility of results among the five institutions was only approximate (Wheeless et al., 1989, 1991). Furthermore, the group observed and reported false positive results in the absence of cancer (deVere White et al., 1986). Acute cystitis and drug treatment for benign disease were common sources of errors. It could also be shown that concurrent DNA analysis by cytophotometry often disclosed aneuploid patterns of DNA distribution in the absence of flow cytometric abnormalities (see Fig. 9-12B; Koss et al., 1989). The results were not surprising because similar performance of the two methods has also been observed in other targets, such as effusions (Schneller et al., 1987) and in breast cancer (Cornelisse and van Driel-Kulker, 1985). The selection of large nuclei in the image analysis mode may bring forth a minority proportion of cancer cells with a high DNA content. This subgroup may be lost in the very large number of cells studied by flow cytometry.

The conclusions of this work suggested that flow cytometric analysis of DNA content in bladder washings may be a valuable technique but should not be indiscriminately applied. Because of its inherent technical difficulties the procedure should be used only in competent laboratories with experienced personnel and in the presence of known bladder tumors (Wheeless et al., 1993). It was stressed that the value of flow cytometry was best judged in conjunction with clinical observations and that the abnormalities of a DNA histogram should *per se* not lead to any treatment decisions (Aamodt et al., 1992). In our experience, cytophotometry of Feulgen-stained cells in bladder washings may prove to be a better guide to diagnosis, treatment, and prognosis of bladder tumors than flow cytometry.

Flow Cytometric Analysis of DNA Ploidy of Voided Urine

Because of difficulties with securing adequate bladder washings in ambulatory patients, many attempts have been made to study the DNA distribution patterns in voided urine. Virtually all of these trials ended in failure, mainly because of poor preservation of cells. In 1988 a new sedimentation technique for processing of voided urinary sediments for flow cytometry was proposed by deVere White et al., apparently with good results, comparable to those obtained with bladder washings. Our experience with DNA

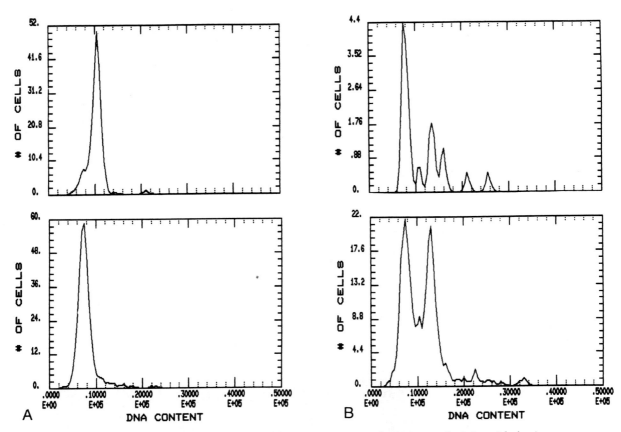

FIGURE 9-15.   Comparative results of DNA measurements by image analysis in voided urine sediment and the corresponding tumors. (*A*) Diploid smear (*top*) and primary tumor (*bottom*). The cytologic diagnosis was negative for tumor cells. (*B*) An aneuploid sediment (*top*) and primary tumor (*bottom*). The cytologic diagnosis was positive. (Modified from Koss, L. G., Eppich, E. M., Medler, K. H., and Wersto, R. P.: DNA cytophotometry of voided urine sediment: Comparison with results of cytologic diagnosis and image analysis. Anal. Quant. Cytol. Hist., *9,* 398–404, 1987, with permission.)

analysis of voided urine by flow cytometry has not been favorable. It may be that the technique of specimen collection or processing was faulty, but we were unable to duplicate the results reported by others.

Cytophotometric Analysis of DNA in Voided Urine

Direct measurements by cytophotometry of DNA values in Feulgen-stained urothelial cells in voided urine confirmed that DNA ploidy was related to cytologic diagnosis (Koss et al., 1987). In six cases of diploid tumors the DNA ploidy pattern in voided urine was also diploid, and the cytologic findings were either negative or atypical. In ten cases of aneuploid tumors, the urinary sediment was also aneuploid, and the cytologic diagnosis was either positive or suspicious (Fig. 9-15). There were, however, several non-concordant cases: in seven of them aneuploid

urine sediment resulted in negative or atypical cytologic diagnoses, and in three cases a positive or suspicious cytologic pattern could not be correlated with ploidy of the urinary sediment. An extensive investigation failed to reveal the reason for the discrepant cases, strongly suggesting that DNA measurements of cells in voided urine specimens are of limited value. In spite of that, commercial laboratories claim that this is an acceptable mode of identifying high-risk patients (Amberson et al., 1992). Although better technology may account for these results, extreme caution must be exercised in the interpretation of the results because of the poor preservation of the cells in voided urine. A major study from our laboratories has shown that the presence of human polyomavirus-infected cells commonly results in histograms with aneuploid DNA pattern (Koss et al., 1984), and this is yet another important source of major diagnostic errors in DNA cytophotometry of voided urine (see also p. 55).

DNA Ploidy of Other Histologic Types of Bladder Carcinoma

Adenocarcinomas

DNA ploidy of six adenocarcinomas of the bladder was reported by Tribukait (1984; see Table 9-2). One of the tumors was diploid; five were aneuploid. Because of lack of follow-up, the clinical significance of these observations is unknown.

Squamous Carcinomas

The DNA ploidy patterns of 100 squamous carcinomas from Egyptian sources were retrospectively studied by Shaaban et al. (1990), working in Tribukait's laboratory. Contrary to urothelial tumors, DNA ploidy offered no information of prognostic value in this group of tumors. Thirty of the 31 grade I well-differentiated diploid tumors were invasive, as were all but one grade II and grade III tumors, and all but one were aneuploid.

DNA Ploidy in Urothelial Tumors Other Than of the Urinary Bladder

Studies of DNA ploidy patterns in carcinomas of the renal pelves (Blute et al., 1988; Oldbring et al., 1989; Nativ et al., 1990) revealed the same distribution of DNA patterns as in similar tumors of the bladder. There was a good correlation with tumor grade, with most grade I tumors being diploid, most high-grade tumors aneuploid, and the grade II tumors about equally divided between diploid and aneuploid. The survival of patients closely followed tumor stage and the ploidy patterns. Patients with aneuploid tumors had a poor prognosis, those with diploid tumors had a very good survival, and patients with aneuploid-tetraploid tumors were intermediate between the other two groups.

It was stressed that for patients with grade 2, low-stage tumors, the ploidy was of important predictive value: patients with aneuploid tumors had poor survival. Corrado et al. (1991) essentially confirmed these findings.

Chromosomal Analysis of Bladder Tumors

As will be discussed in detail in Chapter 11, the pattern of chromosomal analysis in urothelial tumors of the bladder shows some differences between low-grade and high-grade tumors. Such differences have been explored in molecular genetic studies. A comparison of cytogenetic findings with DNA analysis of bladder tumors is discussed on p. 254. More importantly, perhaps, the application of the fluorescent in situ hybridization (FISH) technique using probes specific for individual chromosomes disclosed that even in diploid tumors with anticipated good behavior, chromosomal abnormalities may occur (Hopman et al., 1988; Poddighe et al., 1992). The issue is less important with regard to aneuploid tumors that by definition show significant and complex chromosomal rearrangement. Such studies, combined with molecular genetic analysis may provide additional parameters pertaining to tumor behavior. For further comments, see Chapter 11 and Color Plate 11-1.

Application of Image Analysis to Classification of Urothelial Cells in Voided Urine

In our laboratories, work was performed to analyze cells in the urinary sediment for purposes of automated diagnostic analysis of bladder cancer (Koss et al., 1975, 1977, 1980, 1983, 1984, 1987; Sherman et al., 1981, 1984, 1986).

The studies disclosed that, under favorable circumstances, computer-generated cell features are capable of identifying cancer cells and benign cells in the sediment of voided urine with a high degree of accuracy (Koss et al., 1975). There remained, however, a large group of difficult-to-classify cells that were considered to be "atypical." Based on computer algorithms, the atypical cells could be subdivided into two groups, one group associated with benign events and the other associated with cancer (Koss et al., 1977). Preliminary data suggested that the sediment could be utilized for an automated analysis, but the methods used were inaccurate, extremely slow, and not consistent with an efficient use of expensive optical and computer equipment (Koss et al., 1983; Sherman et al., 1981, 1986). The study, although of limited practical value, nevertheless laid the foundation for future applications of image analysis to classification of cells.

MORPHOMETRY

There are several studies on record that show that a morphometric analysis of histologic sections of urothelial tumors provides a guide to grading and prognosis (Baak and Oort, 1983; Blomjous et al.,

1989). As discussed on p. 263, the subjective selection of the fields robs this method of objectivity. Still, it offers interesting options in tumor grading, a notoriously difficult subjective task.

Prostatic Adenocarcinoma

Measurements of DNA in Prostatic Carcinoma

The issue of prostatic cancer progression and prognosis has become increasingly important with the current trend to identify small, presumably early tumors by screening for elevation of Prostatic Specific Antigen (PSA) and by ultrasound, as discussed in Chapter

7. The high frequency of discovery of these tumors raises the issue of treatment, particularly in younger men and men past the age of 70. Treatment of prostatic carcinoma by radical prostatectomy or by radiotherapy is not an innocuous procedure. The complications frequently include loss of sexual function and incontinence.

As was emphasized in Chapter 7, there has been a six-fold increase in the number of radical prostatectomy procedures performed from 1984 through 1990 in the United States (Lu-Yao et al., 1993), but the effects on quality of life and survival of the patients are not clear (Wasson et al., 1993). Although clinical staging and histologic grading are of prognostic value, little is known about the characteristics of small (stage A_1), occult prostatic cancers that come to light

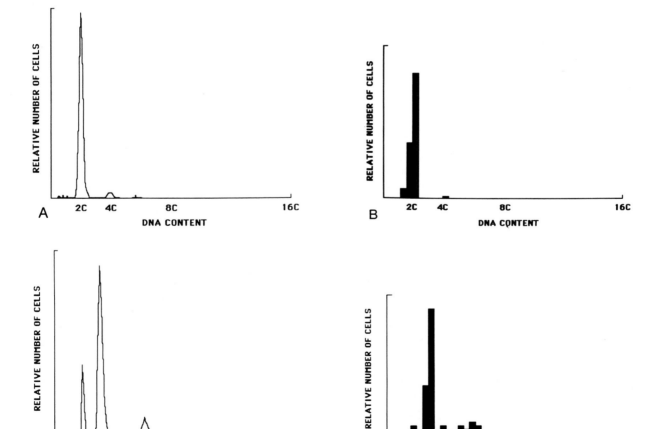

FIGURE 9-16.   DNA analysis of two prostatic carcinomas by flow cytometry (*left A,C*) and image analysis of aspiration smear (*right, B,D*). Top: diploid tumor (*A,B*), bottom: aneuploid tumor (*C,D*). (Photographs courtesy of Dr. James Amberson, Dianon Corp., 200 Watson Blvd., Stratford, CT 06497.)

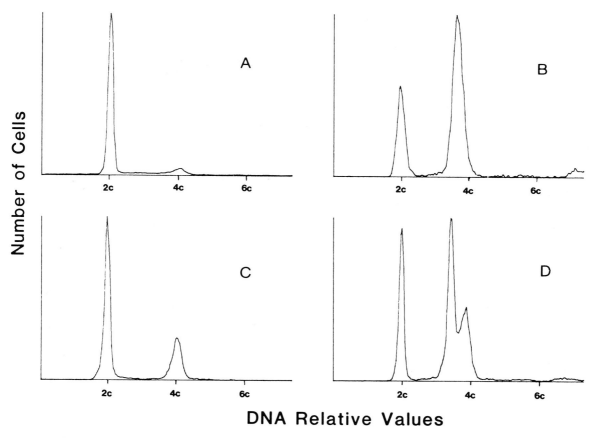

FIGURE 9-17. DNA patterns of prostatic carcinomas by flow cytometry. (*A*) diploid pattern from a benign prostate, (*B*) aneuploid tumor with a hypotetraploid second peak, (*C*) a tumor with a tetraploid peak, (*D*) tumor exhibiting two aneuploid cell lines. (From Tribukait, B. Flow cytometry in surgical pathology and cytology of tumors of the genito-urinary tract. *In* Koss, L. G., and Coleman, D. V. [Eds.]: Advances in Clinical Cytology, Vol. 2. New York, Masson, 1984, pp. 163–189, with permission.)

as a consequence of screening and that may lead to a radical surgical procedure. It is known from many sources that occult prostatic carcinoma is common, reaching 75% in some studies of men in the 8th decade of life who die of unrelated causes (summary in Petersen, 1992). It is quite clear, therefore, that at least some of the discovered prostatic cancers may not progress to clinical disease. The dilemma "to treat or not to treat" is a serious one that affects the lives of many people. At the time of this writing (1994) there are many research projects attempting to define the factors governing the behavior and prognosis of prostatic carcinoma. Interestingly, DNA ploidy of these tumors appears to be an important prognostic parameter, not only for small, occult prostatic carcinomas but also for advanced and even metastatic tumors.

DNA ploidy can be measured by image analysis on prostatic aspiration smears and, with a lesser degree of accuracy, on histologic sections of tumors and on histologic sections of prostatic biopsies (see p. 259 and Fig. 9-13). Flow cytometry may also be used on adequate prostatic aspirates or on fresh and paraffin-embedded tumor samples. In adequate material, the results of image analysis and flow cytometry are comparable (Fig. 9-16). Tribukait (1984) investigated the ploidy pattern of a large number of prostatic carcinomas and observed diploid, tetraploid, and aneuploid DNA patterns (Fig. 9-17). A correlation of these patterns with grade and stage of the disease are shown in Table 9-3.

It is immediately evident from Table 9-3 that with decreasing degree of differentiation and with increasing stage of the disease, there is an increase in tetraploid–aneuploid and aneuploid tumors. These

TABLE 9-3
DNA Ploidy of Prostatic Carcinoma by Grade (391 Patients) and Stage (500 Patients)

*Grading**	*Diploid*	*Tetraploid*	*Aneuploid*	*Total*
Well differentiated	79(61%)	44(34%)	6(5%)	129
Moderately well differentiated	41(21%)	104(55%)	46(24%)	191
Poorly differentiated	2(3%)	23(32%)	46(65%)	71
Total	122	171	98	391
Stage[†]				
T1	27(80%)	5(14%)	2(6%)	34
T2	51(34%)	72(49%)	25(17%)	148
T3	33(12%)	129(48%)	105(40%)	267
T4	1(2%)	18(36%)	32(62%)	51
Total	112	224	164	500

*Grading based on aspiration biopsies
[†]Staging: T1 = small tumor confined to prostate
         T2 = large tumor confined to prostate
         T3 = tumor extending beyond prostatic capsule
         T4 = tumor invading adjacent organs or metastatic
(Modified from Tribukait, B.: Flow cytometry in surgical pathology and cytology of tumors of the genito-urinary tract. *In* Koss, L.G., and Coleman, D.V. (Eds.): Advances in Clinical Cytology, Vol. 2. New York, Masson, 1984, with permission.)

data also strongly suggest that in the prostate, tetraploid tumors occupy an important position, accounting for a large proportion of tumors of moderate degree of differentiation and stage.

It was of further interest that in a 5-year follow-up study of 53 patients with prostatic carcinoma whose disease progressed, there was a change from diploid to tetraploid to aneuploid DNA pattern (Adolfsson and Tribukait, 1990). Zetterberg (1993) pointed out that, on the whole, a diploid pattern is stable over the years and that changes of DNA ploidy occur in only 10% to 15% of patients, most of whom have progressive disease.

We conducted a prospective flow cytometric analysis of DNA ploidy of prostatic cancers for a number of years. The samples for the study were obtained either by direct aspiration of the prostatic tumors (see Chap. 7) or by securing cell samples by aspiration from the freshly removed surgical specimen. The study, conducted at the Montefiore Medical Center in New York, aimed at small, sometimes occult prostatic cancers, incidentally discovered. The study encompassed 632 patients with adequate samples. There were 531 patients with benign prostatic hypertrophy and 101 patients with prostatic carcinoma, of whom 82 were evaluated. The distribution of DNA patterns in benign prostatic hyperplasia is shown in Table 9-4.

It may be noted that 11 samples, or 2% of this group, had abnormal DNA patterns in the absence of prostatic carcinoma. Extensive search of the surgical material failed to clarify the source of this abnor-

mality, which must therefore be considered to be a rare deviation from normal. Similar observations were reported by Deitch et al. (1989).

The analysis of 82 prostatic carcinomas according to stage of the disease is shown in Table 9-5.

It may be noted that the 34 prostatic carcinomas in stage A of the disease, representing small tumors still confined to the prostate, often an incidental finding, were diploid. Of the 29 larger tumors, palpable but still confined to the prostate (Stage B tumors), 24 (about 80%) were diploid, and 5 (20%) aneuploid. The 12 tumors extending beyond the capsule of the prostate without evidence of metastases (Stage C tumors) were evenly divided between diploid and aneuploid. All 7 prostatic carcinomas with metastatic spread (Stage D) were aneuploid. The actual outcome

TABLE 9-4
Prostate: Prospective Study of DNA Content Benign Prostatic Hypertrophy

DNA Histograms	*n*
Diploid	520 (100%)
Nondiploid	11 (2%)*

*No cancer found in extensive studies of chips.
(Modified from Amberson, J.B., and Koss, L.G.: Measurements of DNA as a prognostic factor in prostatic carcinoma. *In* Karr, J.P., Coffey, D.S., and Gardner, W., Jr. [Eds.]: Prognostic Cytometry and Cytopathology of Prostate Cancer. pp. 281–286. New York, Elsevier, 1988.)

TABLE 9-5

Prostate: Prospective Study, Correlation of DNA Ploidy with Stages of Prostatic Carcinoma*

	n	Intraprostatic		Disseminated	
		A	B	C	D
Diploid	64	34(0)	24(22)	6	
Nondiploid	18		5(5)	6(2)	7(7)
Total	82				

*Numbers in parentheses are patients with clinical evidence of disease.
(Modified from Amberson, J.B., and Koss, L.G.: Measurements of DNA as a prognostic factor in prostatic carcinoma. *In* Karr, J.P., Coffey, D.S., and Gardner, W., Jr. [Eds.]: Prognostic Cytometry and Cytopathology of Prostate Cancer. pp. 281–286. New York, Elsevier, 1988.)

of the disease in these patients is not known because of insufficient follow-up time.

The prospective study, briefly summarized above, was supplemented by a retrospective study, based on paraffin-embedded blocks of prostatic carcinoma, removed by prostatectomy at New York Hospital, Cornell Medical Center. A modification of the Hedley technique was used to process the samples. This part of the study was conducted by Dr. James Amberson. The results obtained on 68 patients, with one exception stages B, C, and D, are shown in Table 9-6.

The results of the combined prospective and retrospective studies, shown in Table 9-7, clearly indicate that small, incidentally observed prostatic carcinomas are for the most part diploid. With the progression of the tumors to more advanced stages, the ploidy pattern shifts perceptibly to the aneuploid. In this study, all tetraploid tumors were considered to be "nondiploid."

These results of DNA distribution in stages of prostatic carcinoma are nearly identical to those reported by Tribukait and summarized in Table 9-3. Several conclusions appear to be permissible: aneuploid prostatic cancers are likely to progress beyond the prostate and become metastatic. Some diploid car-

cinomas may also progress, but the probability of progression appears to be much smaller than for the aneuploid tumors. Distinguishing between the diploid tumors that are not likely to progress and those that may progress cannot be achieved by flow cytometry or, most likely, by any other method of DNA measurements.

A number of papers from the Mayo Clinic confirmed the prognostic value of DNA ploidy measurements by flow cytometry (Winkler et al., 1988; Nativ et al., 1989; Nativ et al., 1990). Winkler and his colleagues documented that patients undergoing radical prostatectomy for tumors with diploid or tetraploid DNA patterns and receiving hormonal treatment have a much better survival rate than patients with aneuploid tumors. The data suggest that these observations are applicable even to patients with stage C and D tumors. Nativ et al. (1990) also noted that patients with operable diploid prostatic carcinoma tended to have lower PSA values in serum.

It must be stressed again that some diploid carcinomas do progress to invasive and metastatic disease. It is possible that by studying such tumors with fluorescent in situ hybridization (FISH), using DNA probes to various chromosomes, a pattern of chromosomal

TABLE 9-6

Prostate: Retrospective Study, Correlation of DNA Ploidy with Stages of Prostatic Carcinoma

	n	Intraprostatic		Disseminated	
		A	B	C	D
Diploid	17	1	6	1	9
Nondiploid	51	0	13	7	31
Total	68				

(Modified from Amberson, J.B., and Koss, L.G. Measurements of DNA as a prognostic factor in prostatic carcinoma. *In* Karr, J.P., Coffey, D.S., and Gardner, W., Jr. [Eds.]: Prognostic Cytometry and Cytopathology of Prostate Cancer. pp. 281–286. New York, Elsevier, 1988.)

TABLE 9-7
Prostatic Carcinoma: Combined DNA Ploidy Data
From the Prospective and Retrospective Studies

| | *n* | *Stage* | | | |
		A	B	C	D
Diploid	71	35	30	7	9
Nondiploid	69	0	18	13	38
Total	150	35	48	20	47

(Modified from Amberson, J.B., and Koss, L.G. Measurements of DNA as a prognostic factor in prostatic carcinoma. *In* Karr, J.P., Coffey, D.S., and Gardner, W., Jr. [Eds.]: Prognostic Cytometry and Cytopathology of Prostate Cancer. pp. 281–286. New York, Elsevier, 1988.)

abnormalities may emerge that will allow a subdivision of diploid tumors into those with stable behavior and those with aggressive behavior. Unfortunately, the conclusions of this work were not applied preoperatively in a prospective fashion, which could have very likely prevented some unnecessary prostatectomies.

It appears, though, that even the progression rate of metastatic diploid prostatic carcinomas is low and much slower than the progression rate of aneuploid prostatic cancers (Stephenson, 1987; Winkler, 1988). Major differences in behavior of prostatic carcinomas according to DNA ploidy pattern were observed in retrospective studies in 1976 by Zetterberg and Esposti. These authors used Feulgen-stained prostatic aspiration smears studied by image analysis. Only patients with "moderately" or "poorly" differentiated carcinomas were included in the study. There were 61 patients alive after 10 years of endocrine therapy and 82 patients who died of disease under similar circumstances. The survivors had, for the most part, diploid, diploid–tetraploid, or tetraploid tumors, whereas nearly all the patients who died of disease had aneuploid DNA values (Fig. 9-18). A follow-up study was presented by Auer and Zetterberg (1984) and another by Forsslund and Zetterberg in 1990. In a recent study, Zetterberg (1993) pointed out that patients with diploid and tetraploid ploidy patterns had stable karyotypes that became aneuploid in only 10% of the patients.

Thus, the DNA measurement in prostatic carcinoma, particularly when the tumor is still confined to the prostate, and, preferably, to one lobe, appears to be an important parameter that, taken together with other data, such as the level of prostate-specific antigen, may offer a triage technique for selecting treatment options, above and beyond clinical and ultrasound findings and histologic grading.

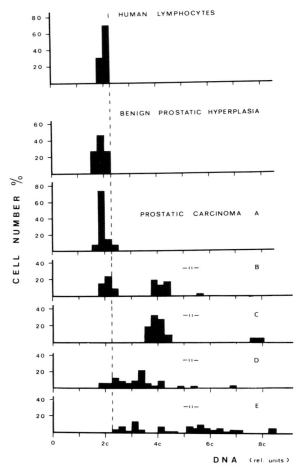

FIGURE 9-18. DNA distribution patterns in aspiration smears of prostatic carcinoma, observed in 143 patients, 61 of whom were alive after 10 years and 82 of whom were dead of disease, in spite of endocrine therapy. The patterns of DNA are diploid in control lymphocytes, benign prostatic hypertrophy and prostatic carcinomas (A). The pattern is diploid–tetraploid (B), tetraploid (C), and aneuploid (D,E). The survivors belonged almost without exception to patterns A, B, and C, whereas patients dying of disease had DNA patterns D or E. (From Auer, G., and Zetterberg, A. The prognostic significance of nuclear DNA content in malignant tumors of breast, prostate, and cartilage. *In* Koss, L. G., and Coleman, D. V. (Eds.): Advances in Clinical Cytology, Vol. 2. New York, Masson, 1984, pp. 123–134, with permission.)

Image Analysis Applied to Prostatic Adenocarcinoma

Image analysis techniques have also been applied to prostatic tumors. One of the observations that emerged from these studies was the "nuclear roundness factor" (Diamond et al., 1982; Epstein et al., 1984; Miller et al., 1988; Mohler et al., 1988). Significant survival differences were observed based on variance of roundness, with tumors with round nuclei showing a better survival pattern than tumors with non-round nuclei (Partin et al., 1992). Tosi et al. (1992) observed that nuclear shape changes could be observed in aspiration smears and in tissues. Helpap (1981) and Helpap and Otten (1982) also studied the morphology of nuclei and nucleoli and cell kinetic in prostatic carcinoma. These authors also concluded that abnormalities of nuclear and nuclear shape were of prognostic value. In a subsequent communication, Helpap (1988) concluded that the presence of two or more nucleoli in prostatic cells was a sure sign of carcinoma.

The observations are somewhat mysterious because the cause or causes of atypias of nuclear shape remain unknown. The possibility that DNA ploidy is somehow involved in the configuration of nuclei must be considered.

Leistenschneider and Nagel (1984) considered nuclear changes in aspiration biopsies of prostatic carcinoma undergoing hormonal treatment as an index of response to therapy. Nuclear pyknosis, reduction in nuclear and nucleolar sizes among other changes in tumor cells, were considered to be evidence of response to therapy. Unfortunately, these changes were based only on visual analysis of smears and were not subjected to an objective evaluation.

Chromosomal In Situ Hybridization

Because of significant difficulties in obtaining direct chromosomal spreads from prostatic carcinoma, the FISH technique has been applied (Poddighe et al., 1992; Breitkreutz et al., 1993; Henke et al., 1993; Macoska et al., 1993; Micale et al., 1993). Specific correlation between documented chromosomal abnormalities and prognosis of prostatic carcinoma have not yet emerged at the time of this writing (1994). However, the approach offers significant promise for the future, particularly with further developments in molecular genetics and availability of probes to individual genes (see Chap. 11).

Renal Tumors

Measurements of DNA

A number of retrospective studies of paraffin-embedded tumors of the kidney, using the method of Hedley or one of its modifications, have been published. Thus, renal carcinomas, oncocytomas, and Wilms' tumors have been studied.

FLOW CYTOMETRY OF RENAL CARCINOMAS

In reference to renal carcinomas, the published data appear to be controversial, inasmuch as the conclusions having to do with prognostic values of DNA ploidy vary from author to author. It was established by Ljungberg et al. (1985) that a significant proportion of renal carcinomas (44%) are heterogeneous, *i.e.*, show different DNA ploidy patterns in adjacent areas. This observation alone renders subsequent retrospective studies, based on single tissue blocks of tumors, of questionable value. Another problem may be with histograms based on nuclei prepared by the Hedley method. For this reason, Feitz et al. (1986) used antibodies to keratin and vimentin, two types of intermediate filaments commonly observed in cells of renal carcinoma, to identify cancer cells in flow cytometric studies.

Several observers reported that diploid tumors have a more favorable prognosis than aneuploid tumors (Rainwater et al., 1987; de Kernion et al., 1989; Grignon et al., 1989; Baisch et al., 1990). Ljungberg et al., 1989, who originally shared this view, subsequently attributed only a marginal value to DNA ploidy patterns (Ljungberg et al., 1991). Osterwijk et al. (1988) and Wolman et al. (1988) failed to observe any significant prognostic value in DNA measurements above tumor stage and grade.

Prospective studies of renal carcinomas are extremely difficult to conduct. Therefore, it is unlikely that in this anatomic area significant contributions can be expected from the flow cytometric studies.

IMAGE ANALYSIS OF RENAL CARCINOMAS

Tosi et al. (1986) proposed that nuclear area is of prognostic significance in stage I renal carcinomas. Using 32 μm^2 as a threshold, nearly all survivors had a smaller nuclear area, and nearly all patients with larger nuclear area died of disease within 5 years. Similar observations were reported by González-Cámpora et al. (1991), who also correlated survival with nuclear grading and other morphologic nuclear features. The information is obviously too scanty to warrant any conclusions at the time of this writing (1994).

OTHER RENAL TUMORS

Oncocytomas. The DNA content of 65 oncocytomas, 44 classified as grade 1 and 21 classified as grade 2 tumors, was reported by Rainwater et al. (1986). In keeping with the substantial nuclear abnormalities observed in these tumors (see p. 207) nearly half of them, regardless of grade, displayed aneuploid or aneuploid-tetraploid pattern of DNA. This observation justifies the classification of these tumors as tumors of uncertain behavior, with a minuscule chance of local recurrence and virtual absence of metastases.

Wilms' Tumors. Only one study of ploidy of Wilms' tumors is known to us. Rainwater (1987) observed that the tetraploid-aneuploid tumors had a lower survival rate than either diploid or non-tetraploid aneuploid tumors. A confirmation of this information would be desirable.

Renal Pelvic Carcinomas. These tumors are discussed on p. 267.

Adrenal Tumors

Pheochromocytoma

Flow cytometric DNA ploidy analysis of pheochromocytomas and related tumors, whether of adrenal origin or from other primary sites, was reported from several institutions, using archival tissue blocks (Hosaka et al., 1986; Nativ et al., 1992; Pang and Tsao, 1993; Lai et al., 1994). The results of all these studies were surprisingly similar: about $1/3$ of the tumors were diploid, $1/3$ aneuploid-tetraploid, and $1/3$ aneuploid-nontetraploid. With one exception, the tumors with malignant behavior (local recurrence, vascular invasion, and/or metastases) were either tetraploid or aneuploid-nontetraploid. The one exception was a diploid tumor with local extension reported by Nativ et al. On the other hand, only a relatively small fraction of aneuploid tumors (probably not more than 10–15%) showed malignant behavior. Hence, aneuploidy in pheochromocytomas does not necessarily constitute evidence of a malignant tumor.

On the other hand, ploidy studies based on image analysis of tissues (González-Cámpora et al., 1993) reported a much higher level of aneuploidy (15 of 16 cases). Similarly, Padberg et al. (1990) reported that only 5 of 43 adrenal pheochromocytomas were diploid.

As discussed in Chapter 8, the morphologic make-up of pheochromocytomas (and related tumors) is such that large cells and large nuclei (undoubtedly with a high DNA content) are extremely common and have no bearing on the behavior of the tumors. The data generated by flow cytometry are obviously quite different from the data generated by image analysis and clearly pertain to two different populations of cells. There is most likely a major loss of large nuclei during the tissue processing for flow cytometry, accounting for the higher proportion of diploid cases (see comments, p. 259).

Regardless of these considerations, the data clearly show that non-diploid pheochromocytomas are somewhat more likely to behave in an aggressive fashion than diploid tumors and probably deserve closer surveillance. The question of the true proportion of diploid tumors must await further studies.

In the Mayo Clinic study (Nativ et al., 1992), familial pheochromocytomas, although frequently bilateral, had variable DNA patterns. There was no correlation of tumor size with ploidy or behavior. Padberg et al. (1990) consider weight above 200 g as an ominous prognostic sign, regardless of ploidy.

OTHER ADRENAL TUMORS

I am not familiar with any substantial quantitative analytical studies of other adrenal tumors.

EPILOGUE

In the brief overview of established and experimental quantitative cytologic techniques in urology given in this chapter, the obvious emphasis was on the common malignant tumors of the bladder and prostate. It may be stated without equivocation that any urologist who deals with cancer of the urinary tract and who does not avail himself or herself of the diagnostic and prognostic modalities outlined in this chapter is not practicing state-of-the-art urology. Any pathologist who is not conversant with the accomplishments and pitfalls of quantitative techniques is not providing urologists with the help that their patients need and deserve.

Appendix: Essential Technical Methods in Flow Cytometry*

EQUIPMENT OF LABORATORY

Large Items

Flow cytometer

Refrigerated centrifuge with swinging bucket rotor

Coulter cell counter or equivalent instrument (may be replaced by a manual hemocytometer)

Micropipettor

Microcentrifuge

Small Items

Pasteur pipettes, various lengths. The most useful are 5$\frac{3}{4}$-inch-long (about 15 cm) pipettes.

Disposable serologic pipettes, various sizes

Disposable syringes, 1 ml, with fitting 21-caliber needles

Nylon mesh, 47 to 53 μm, cut into 1 × 1-inch (2.5 × 2.5 cm) squares

Disposable centrifuge tubes, conical, 15 ml

Microcentrifuge tubes, various sizes

*Protocols established by Robert P. Wersto, Ph.D., during his tenure at the Montefiore Medical Center, Albert Einstein College of Medicine, Bronx, N.Y. From Koss, L. G.: Diagnostic Cytology and Its Histopathologic Bases. Ed. 4. Philadelphia, J. B. Lippincott, 1992.

Note: The nylon mesh removes larger fragments of tissue from the nuclear suspension. The optimal way of processing, proposed by Wersto, is to aspirate the suspension into an *unarmed* syringe, place the nylon mesh on the tip of the syringe, and then fit the needle hub onto the syringe. The liquid expressed from the syringe is filtered across the nylon mesh, before entering the needle.

DNA ANALYSIS

Specimen Collection

The following options are available:

1. *Fresh material:* Fresh material, not otherwise preserved, must be processed within 30 to 60 minutes after removal.
2. *Fresh material, methods of preservation:*
   a. phosphate-buffered saline (PBS)
   b. bone marrow transport medium (RPMI 1640 with 10% calf serum and 14.3 U of sodium heparin/ml) (Gibco, Grand Island, N.Y. 14072)
   c. 70% ethanol or methanol

Processing should occur within 24 hours of collection.

3. *Fresh material,* snap frozen in liquid nitrogen, or at least frozen to −20°C, can be kept indefinitely before processing.

275

4. *Archival material:* Only tissue or fluids fixed in 10% buffered formalin for at least 24 hours are suitable for processing. If paraffin-embedded material is processed, the same principles of fixation apply. Smaller paraffin-embedded samples give better and cleaner histograms than large tissue blocks.

General Principles

With few exceptions, the measurements of DNA in human material are performed on nuclei stripped of cytoplasm. The cytoplasm is destroyed either by acid (citric acid–sodium citrate [CASC] procedure, Krishan's procedure) or by proteolytic enzymes (Vindelöv's procedures, see below). If an enzyme is used, the reaction must be timed and stopped. *All samples must be treated by RNAse, to avoid binding of the fluorochrome to RNA.*

If RNA measurements are desirable, DNAse must be used.

Control Cells

All flow cytometric measurements must be carefully controlled.

Peripheral blood lymphocytes, preferably from the same donor, must be prepared by the Ficoll-Hypaque method from heparinized blood. Samples can be stored at −70°C in a buffer composed of dimethyl sulfoxide (Sigma) with 10% calf serum. Aliquots of the stored lymphocytes can be diluted for use with the buffer used for the DNA procedure (*i.e.*, CASC, Vindelöv's buffer, Krishan's buffer—see below). The deep-frozen samples can be used for 6 to 12 months after preparation. There is a slightly lower DNA content in males than in females (a Y chromosome is somewhat smaller than an X chromosome), and matching the sex of the donor with the sex of the lymphocyte sample may be advisable.

Nucleated erythrocytes (chicken erythrocytes, Environmental Diagnostics, Burlington, N.C. 27215) or trout erythrocytes (no constant source of supply) may also be used and should be mixed with the unknown sample before use (see p. 278).

RNAse Solution and Use

REAGENTS

RNAse (ribonuclease A), type 1-A, bovine pancreas (Sigma). Phosphate buffered saline (PBS).

PREPARATION OF SOLUTION

Dissolve 100 mg of RNAse in 10 ml of PBS. Store at 4°C (lasts 1 week).

METHOD OF PROCEDURE

To the fluorochrome-stained sample in PBS, add 10 μl. of the RNAse solution and incubate for 30 minutes at 37°C in the dark. Store incubated samples at 4°C for at least 2 hours before DNA analysis (samples remain stable for 72 hours if stored in the dark).

METHODS OF SAMPLE PROCESSING

Citric Acid–Sodium Citrate Method (CASC)

The CASC method was initially developed to isolate nuclei from squamous epithelial cells, which often resist other methods of processing (Koss et al., 1977). The method is applicable to a number of cell-rich tissues, and it offers the advantage of simplicity.

Reagents

Preparation of 0.01M solution of citric acid: Dissolve 2.10 gm of citric acid monohydrate (formula weight 210.14) in 1 L of distilled water. Store at 4°C.

Preparation of 0.09M solution of sodium citrate: Dissolve 26.47 gm of sodium citrate (formula weight 294.10) in 1 L of distilled water. Store at 4°C.

Procedure

For use, mix in equal parts. Mince tissues in about 5 ml of the solution. Centrifuge for 10 minutes at 220 × g; discard supernatant. Add 50 ml of CASC and incubate for 30 minutes, using a magnetic stirrer. Filter through gauze or nylon mesh and syringe, as described above. Incubate with RNAse. The sample can be processed with any fluorochrome for DNA analysis.

For general comments on flow cytometric procedure, see below, p. 278.

Vindelöv's Procedure

Principle

DNA analysis is performed on nuclei stripped free of cytoplasm, using trypsin. Trypsin inhibitor is used to stop the reaction, and the nuclei are treated with RNAse before staining with propidium iodide. The reagents needed are listed in the following table.

Reagents Needed in Vindelövs Procedure

REAGENT/GRADE	SOURCE	CATALOG NO.
Citric acid, trisodium salt	Sigma*	C-7254
Propidium iodide	Calbiochem†	537059
Dimethyl sulfoxide, ACS reagent	Sigma	D-8779
Nonidet P-40 (NP-40)	Sigma	N-3516
RNAse (ribonuclease A), type 1-A, bovine pancreas	Sigma	R-4875
Spermine tetrahydrochloride	Sigma	S-2876
Sucrose, enzyme grade	Sigma	
Tris buffer, free base, reagent grade	Sigma	T1503
Trypsin, type IX, from porcine pancreas	Sigma	T-0134
Trypsin inhibitor, type II-O, from chicken egg white	Sigma	T-9253

*Sigma Chemical Company, P.O. Box 14508, St. Louis, Mo. 63178-9916
†Calbiochem Brand Biochemicals, Behring Diagnostics, PO Box 12087, San Diego, Calif. 92112-4180.

Reagent Preparation

1. Sample storage buffer:
   85.50 gm sucrose (250 mM)
   11.76 gm citric acid, trisodium salt (40 mM)
   50 ml dimethyl sulfoxide (DMSO)
   Dissolve the first two reagents in approximately 800 to 900 ml of distilled water and add the DMSO. Add additional distilled water to bring the volume to 1,000 ml. Adjust the pH to 7.60, and date and store at 4°C. (Normally, 250 ml of this solution is made up.)
   Label as Vindelöv Storage Buffer, with the date of preparation and an expiration date (90 days).

2. Staining buffer:
   2.0 gm citric acid, trisodium salt (3.4 mM)
   1.044 gm spermine tetrahydrochloride (1.5 mM)
   0.121 gm Tris buffer, free base (0.5 mM)
   2.0 ml Nonidet P40 (NP 40) (0.1%)
   Dissolve all reagents in 2,000 ml of distilled water and adjust the pH to 7.60. This solution becomes the buffer solution for the preparation of Vindelöv solutions A, B, and C and is used immediately. Excess is discarded.

3. Solution A:
   15 mg trypsin
   Dissolve in 500 ml of staining buffer (step 2), adjust pH to 7.60, and store aliquots in 15-ml centrifuge tubes. Usually aliquots of 3, 5, and 10 ml are useful. Label tubes on sides and on caps with A, date batch, and immediately store in a −70°C freezer. Make about 500 ml.

4. Solution B:
   250 mg trypsin inhibitor
   50 mg RNAse A
   Dissolve in 500 ml of staining buffer, adjust pH to 7.60. Usually aliquots of 3, 5, and 10 ml are useful. Label tubes on sides and on caps with B, date batch, and immediately store in a −70°C freezer. Make about 500 ml, and aliquot and freeze as described for Solution A.

5. Solution C:
   208 mg propidium iodide (PI)
   580 mg spermine tetrahydrochloride
   Dissolve in 500 ml of staining buffer, and adjust pH to 7.60. If the PI is purchased from Sigma Chemical Co., the purity is 95% to 97%, and some insoluble matter will be noted. Before freezing aliquots, filter Solution C through a 0.2 μl sterile filter unit. PI purchased from Calbiochem requires no filtering. Usually aliquots of 3, 5, and 10 ml are useful. Label tubes on sides and on caps with C, date batch, and immediately store in a −70°C freezer. Make about 500 ml, and aliquot and freeze as described for Solution A. Protect the PI solution from light at all times.

6. *General reagent notes.* The pH should be adjusted to 7.60 ± 0.5 units, although it appears to work better on the low side (7.53 to 7.58) than over pH 7.60. All solutions are stored frozen. If the freezer thaws, make new solutions. Usually when the enzyme solutions start to deteriorate, the G_1 coefficient of variation (CV) of control lymphocytes increases. Each batch *must* be tested with lymphocyte controls before use on clinical samples. Staining solutions that yield CVs above 4% on lymphocytes that had CVs of 2% to 3% with prior batches of stain indicate that an error was made and the solutions should be remade. Reagents with specific catalog numbers should not be substituted.

Procedure

1. Transport frozen aliquots of solutions A, B, and C on ice (and covered with aluminum foil) after removal from the −70°C freezer. Using warm water (≤37°C), rapidly thaw these frozen solutions by inverting the tubes under a constant stream of warm water. Solutions A and B can be placed in a rack at room temperature for up to 10 to 15 minutes before use. The thawed Solution C is stored *on ice* and covered.

2. To 200 μl (0.2 ml) of thawed sample, containing 5 × 10⁵ cells, add the following:

   a. 1.8 ml of Solution A. Set a timer for 10 minutes and start it immediately after the addition of Solution A to the first tube. *Incubate 10 minutes at room temperature, inverting several times during this period.*

   b. 1.5 ml of Solution B. Start timer as above, and *incubate for 10 minutes at room temperature, inverting several times during this period.*

   c. 1.5 ml of Solution C. Start timer as above, and *incubate for 15 minutes on ice in the dark (or covered), inverting several times during this period.*

3. Centrifuge samples at 500 × g (1,500) rpm at 4° to 10°C for 5 minutes to concentrate samples and transfer the centrifuged tubes with pellets, *undisturbed,* to an ice bucket, which is covered at all times or left uncovered in a totally darkened flow laboratory (or one with a background yellow or red darkroom light). Samples should be analyzed within 3 hours of preparation. For large numbers of samples, it is a good idea to prepare them in batches.

4. To analyze the sample, gently remove most of the clear supernatant using a clean Pasteur pipette so that approximately 0.5 ml of supernatant remains. This volume is dependent on the sample concentration and can be altered upward or downward to achieve an adequate concentration. This prevents an increase in sample pressure on the instrument. Resuspend the pellet in the remaining supernatant using the same Pasteur pipette, and transfer the solution to a 1.5-ml microcentrifuge tube. Using a 1-ml plastic syringe (with the needle removed), fill the syringe with the cell suspension and place a piece of 47 to 53 μm nylon mesh (approximately 1 to 2 cm square) between the barrel of the syringe and the hub of a 27-gauge needle. Tighten the needle and slowly filter the cell suspension through the mesh into a 0.5-ml microcentrifuge tube that has the cap removed (in order to fit in the flow cytometer's sample holder). Keep the filtered sample in the dark and on ice at all times before analysis.

General Notes and Comments

I. LONG-TERM STORAGE OF CELLS

Besides yielding DNA histograms with good resolution in terms of CVs, the other benefit of Vindelöv's procedure is the long term-storage of clinical specimens, which permits batch-type analysis. Generally, solid tissues are finely minced in a small Petri dish, flooded with some sample storage buffer (DMSO/sucrose/citrate), and filtered through a 350-μm mesh. The filtrate is then counted and adjusted so that the cell number is 2.5 × 10⁶ cells per ml. Counting minced tumor samples is often difficult, and the sample density can be estimated by eye or by comparison with that of the lymphocytes used as external DNA standards. The specimens at all times are kept on ice and immediately transferred to a −70°C freezer, where they may be kept for up to 6 months to 1 year before analysis. For thin-needle aspirates of the breast, colon, or prostate, generally no counting or mincing is necessary and the sample can be directly resuspended in 200 μl of the sample storage buffer and frozen. The same applies to touch or scrape preparations as well as bladder washings. The samples may be "snap" or quick frozen in liquid N₂ and then transferred to the −70°C freezer.

II. INTERNAL STANDARDS

For accurate DNA analysis, all clinical samples must have an internal standard admixed with the test specimen to control for stain and instrument variability. Nucleated chicken erythrocytes (CRBC) are useful (see above). Usually, 50 ml of CRBCs shipped in citrate will last for several years. On receipt, wash 10 to 15 ml of the solution two to three times with a large volume of the Vindelöv's sample storage buffer (DMSO/sucrose/citrate) or until the supernatant is clear. Decant the supernatant and resuspend the pellet in 10 ml of the sample storage buffer and count an aliquot of the CRBCs. Freeze 50 to 100 μl aliquots of the cells in 0.5-ml microcentrifuge tubes at −70°C. For use, thaw a frozen tube in your hand (about 15 seconds) and add an appropriate amount to the clinical specimen. Based on our experience, the CRBC concentration should be 5% to 10% of the total cell number. Therefore, 5 μl of the concentrated cells is placed in 4.5 ml of the sample storage buffer. Mix well and add 5 to 10 μl of the diluted CRBC to 200 μl of the clinical sample. It is best to check the dilutions by analyzing control lymphocytes with various dilutions of the CRBCs.

III. EXTERNAL STANDARDS

Peripheral blood lymphocytes from a "normal" donor are used as external standards for defining the channel position of the G_0/G_1 peak of the clinical sample. These are prepared by centrifugation of 10 ml of whole heparinized blood (or diluted 1 : 1 with RPMI 1640 tissue culture medium) onto a pad of 10 ml of Ficoll-Hypaque for 30 minutes at 300 × g at 22°C. The interface containing the cells is removed using a Pasteur pipette or a spinal tap needle, and washed three times (10 minutes, 1,100 rpm at 4° to 8°C; 200 × g) with a large volume of cold RPMI 1640 (at least 40 to 50 ml each time). After the final wash, the pellet is resuspended in 2 to 5 ml of the medium, counted, and recentrifuged. At this point, slowly pour off the supernatant, place the inverted tube on a clean paper towel for about a minute, invert to upright, and tap the pellet to dislodge it. Add the appropriate amount of sample storage buffer (DMSO/sucrose/citrate) so that the lymphocyte concentration is 2.5×10^6 cells per ml or 5×10^5 cells per 400 μl. Pour aliquots of 500-μl samples into 0.5-ml microcentrifuge tubes on ice and immediately freeze in a −70°C freezer. It is a good idea to test each batch against a previous batch with known good CV. If possible, lymphocytes from the same patient from whom the clinical sample was obtained should be used.

IV. FLOW CYTOMETRY: GENERAL COMMENTS

1. Try to use as few optical filters as possible to analyze the sample. The Coulter EPICS instruments require a 510-nm interference filter, 515-nm-long pass filter, and 590-nm-long pass filter (in this order toward the photomultiplier tube). If the 515-nm-long pass filter has no defects, the 590-nm one can be omitted. For other instruments, follow the manufacturer's directions.
2. For optimal resolution, sample flow rates should be 30 to 50 events per second (75 to 100 per second is acceptable).
3. The sample sheath fluid is distilled water. Since the sample is kept on ice before analysis, it is advantageous to configure the flow cytometer with temperature control of both the sheath and sample and run samples at 4°C.

4. Instrument optical alignment is accomplished with DNA check microspheres (10 μm, Fine Particle Division, Coulter Electronics, Hialeah, Fla.), which on linear fluorescence and forward-angle light scatter have a CV of less than 2%.
5. For practical purposes, the high voltage of the fluorescent signal required for the selected probe should be adjusted for the mean channel position of the G_0/G_1 peak of control lymphocytes to be near channel 70 (± 5 channels). In this case, the diploid (2N) peak is in channel 70, a tetraploid peak in channel 140, and an aneuploid (6N) peak in channel 210. This setup gives both good positioning of aneuploid peaks in the >2N and <5N range, which account for nearly all possible aneuploid combinations. If the 2N peak is in channel 70, the peak position of admixed CRBC should be in channel 25. Thus, the ratio of the diploid 2N peak position to that of the CRBCs is always 2.8 ± 0.05, and variation outside of this range indicates either poor staining or a nonlinear fluorescent signal. Notwithstanding, the position of the diploid (2N) peak is a trade-off. If one were to analyze cancer cells that may be in the 8N range, these would be off-scale with lymphocytes in channel 70 (4 × 70 = channel 280). However, positioning of the CRBCs in channels below 25 would prevent setting the discriminator high enough to gate out debris.

Krishan's Technique for Fresh/Frozen Tissue

Principle

DNA analysis is performed on nuclei stripped free of cytoplasm, using hypotonic lysis in dilute citric acid. The technique works best on nonfixed fresh or frozen tissue. The nuclei are treated with RNAse before staining with propidium iodide. The reagents needed are listed in the table below.

Regents Needed in Krishan's Technique

REAGENT/GRADE	SOURCE	CATALOG NO.
Citric acid, trisodium salt, Molecular Biology grade	Sigma*	C-8532
Propidium iodide (PI)	Calbiochem†	537059
Nonidet P-40 (NP-40)	Sigma	N-3516
RNAse (ribonuclease A), type 1-A, bovine pancreas	Sigma	R-4875

*Sigma Chemical Company, P.O. Box 14508, St. Louis, Mo. 63178-9916.
†Calbiochem Brand Biochemicals, Behring Diagnostics, P.O. Box 12087, San Diego, Calif. 92112-4180.

Reagent Preparation—Modified Krishan Buffer

To 250 ml of distilled water, add the following:

0.25 gm sodium citrate
(0.1% final concentration)
0.005 gm RNAse
(0.02 mg/ml final concentration)
0.75 ml NP-40
(0.3% final concentration)
0.0125 gm PI
(0.05 mg/ml final concentration)

Although pH is not critical, the pH of the buffer should be 7.4 before the addition of the PI. Cover the buffer with aluminum foil and store in the dark at 4°C. Label as Modified Krishan Buffer with the preparer's initials, the date of preparation, and an expiration date (3 weeks).

Procedure

1. With a pipette place 1-ml aliquots of the dissociated tumor tissue containing 1-2 $\times$ 10^6 cells into a 12 mm $\times$ 75 mm conical centrifuge tube and centrifuge at 250 $\times$ g (1,000 rpm) for 5 minutes at 4°C.
2. Remove the supernatant from the tubes, and add 1 ml of the Modified Krishan Buffer per 1 $\times$ 10^6 cells. Vortex each sample for 10 seconds.
3. Incubate samples for a minimum of 30 minutes to 1 hour at 4°C in an ice bucket, which is covered with aluminum foil to protect the samples from photobleaching.
4. Remove samples from ice bath and centrifuge at 250 $\times$ g (1,000 rpm) for 5 minutes at 4°C.
5. Remove the supernatant from the tubes, and add 1 ml of fresh Modified Krishan Buffer per 1 $\times$ 10^6 cells. Vortex each sample for 10 seconds and syringe each sample through a 47- to 53-μm nylon mesh, which is placed between the barrel of a 1-ml syringe and the hub of a 27-gauge needle, before analysis on the flow cytometer.

General Notes

1. Samples are stable for at least 3 hours on ice in the dark.
2. Distilled water is used as the instrument sample sheath.
3. See general comments on Vindelöv's procedure, above.

DNA Analysis of Paraffin-Embedded Samples (Hedley's Procedure Modified by Amberson and Wersto, Semiautomated)

Principle

DNA analysis is performed on nuclei, stripped free of cytoplasm using pronase, from deparaffinized tissue sections that have been fixed in formalin. The technique was originally designed by Hedley et al., specifically for single-parameter DNA analysis from archival material. The nuclei are treated with RNAse before staining with propidium iodide.

The reagents are listed in the table below.

Reagent Preparation

1. Pronase Solution: To 50 ml of PBS, add 50 mg of Pronase (Protease type XXI, Sigma). Make an aliquot of the solution and freeze at −70°C. Label as Pronase Solution with the date of preparation and an expiration date (6 months). Once thawed, the solution should be used immediately, and the remainder discarded.
2. PI stain, archival:
   To 100 ml of distilled water, add the following:

MgCl$_2$	0.102 gm
PI	0.5 mg
Sodium azide	0.100 gm
Tris	0.121 gm

   Dissolve well, and adjust the pH to 7.4. Store in

Reagents Needed in Modified Hedley's Procedure

REAGENT/GRADE	SOURCE	CATALOG NO.
MgCl$_2$, hexahydrate	Sigma*	
Pronase	Sigma	P-8038
Propidium iodide (PI)	Calbiochem[†]	537059
RNAse (ribonuclease A), type 1-A, bovine pancreas	Sigma	R-4875
Sodium azide	Sigma	
Tris hydrochloride		

*Sigma Chemical Company, P.O. Box 14508, St. Louis, Mo. 63178-9916.
[†]Calbiochem Brand Biochemicals, Behring Diagnostics, P.O. Box 12087, San Diego, Calif. 92112-4180.

an aluminum foil–wrapped bottle in the dark at 4°C. Label the date of preparation and an expiration date (1 week).

3. RNAse solution, archival:

To 10 ml of PBS, add 100 mg of RNAse (final concentration is 10 mg/ml). Store at 4°C for no more than 1 week, or make an aliquot and freeze for long-term storage of up to 3 months. Label with the date of preparation and an expiration date (1 week).

Procedure

1. Select tissue blocks showing the least amount of necrosis and the highest cellularity.
2. Cut two to three 50- to 100-μm sections, and place the sections from each patient sample into an embedding paper bag and then into a plastic tissue cassette.
3. Deparaffinize and hydrate the cut sections by running the samples through a tissue processor following this schedule, *usually overnight:*

a. Xylene	3 hours
b. Xylene	4 hours
c. 100% ethanol	3 hours
d. 100% ethanol	2 hours
e. 95% ethanol	2 hours
f. 70% ethanol	1 hour
g. 50% ethanol	1 hour
h. Distilled H$_2$O	1 hour
i. Distilled H$_2$O	1 hour
j. Distilled H$_2$O	Until removed

4. Remove the cassettes from the processor, and immediately place them in PBS. Change this solution after approximately 10 minutes.
5. Carefully transfer the dewaxed tissue sections to a 15-ml centrifuge tube, either manually or with forceps or by removing the specimen from the embedding bag with 3 to 5 ml of PBS. If the latter technique is used, centrifuge the specimen at 250 × g (1,100 rpm) for 5 minutes, before proceeding to the next step.
6. Add 1 to 2 ml of Pronase Solution to the deparaffinized sections in the centrifuge tube and incubate at 37°C for 30 minutes, vortexing every 5 to 10 minutes. A cloudy solution is indicative of a successful cellular digestion.
7. Filter each specimen through a piece of 47- to 53-μm nylon mesh into a clean 4.5-ml conical centrifuge tube.
8. Centrifuge the sample at 300 × g (1,300 to 1,500 rpm) for 5 minutes at 4°C.
9. Remove the supernatant and add 2 ml of PBS, vortexing gently. Repeat steps 8 and 9, with a final resuspension of the samples in PBS.

10. Samples can now either be stored in PBS at 4°C for up to 2 days or centrifuged as described in step 8 and, after decanting the supernatant, resuspended in 1 ml of the PI stain for immediate analysis.
11. Stain the sample for 30 minutes at 4°C in the dark.
12. Add 10 μl of the RNAse solution to each of the stained samples and incubate for 30 minutes at 37°C. Store the samples wrapped in aluminum foil in the dark at 4°C for at least 2 hours before analysis. Stained samples are stable for 72 hours at 4°C when stored in the dark. RNAse and PI can be added to the sample at the same time.

General Notes

1. Distilled water is used as the instrument sample sheath.
2. See general comments for Vindelöv's procedure.
3. *Diploid lymphocytes or chick red blood cells cannot be used as standards. In all instances, benign tissue from the same block* or *a fixed specimen of benign tissue from the same organ site and patient must be used for calculation of the tumor DNA index.*

IMMUNOFLUORESCENCE STAINING FOR THE SIMULTANEOUS MEASUREMENT OF INDIVIDUAL PROTEINS AND DNA CONTENT BY FLOW CYTOMETRY*

Stock Solutions

1. 0.01M phosphate-buffered saline solution (PBS, pH 7.4)
2. 0.5% paraformaldehyde in PBS
3. 100% methanol (−20°C)
4. 5% albumin in PBS
5. Primary antibody (specificity must be tested by Western blotting)
6. Fluorescein isothiocyanate (FITC)-conjugated secondary antibody
7. Propidium iodide (PI) solution (100 μg/ml in PBS).

Procedure

1. Dilute the primary and secondary antibodies in PBS containing 5% albumin. Working dilution

---

*Method developed by B. Czerniak, M.D., and F. Herz, Ph. D.

varies depending on the type of antibody and its source.

2. Fix the cells (in suspension) for 5 minutes at 4°C with 0.5% paraformaldehyde in PBS.
3. Wash the cells three times with PBS at 4°C and centrifuge.
4. Permeabilize the cells by resuspension in 100% methanol (5 minutes at −20°C).
5. Count the cells and transfer an aliquot containing 1×10^6 cells into a 5-ml conical test tube.
6. Centrifuge the cells and resuspend in 200 μl of the primary antibody solution.
7. Incubate at room temperature for 1 hour or at 4°C overnight.
8. Wash the cells three times with PBS and centrifugate.
9. Resuspend the cells in 200 μl of the secondary antibody solution.
10. Incubate the cells with the secondary antibody for 30 minutes at room temperature.
11. Wash the cell three times in PBS followed by centrifugation.
12. Resuspend the cells in 0.9 ml of PBS.
13. Immediately before the measurements, add 0.1 ml of stock (PI) solution (final concentration: 10 μl/ml) and keep at 4°C for 5 minutes.
14. Perform flow cytometric measurements of green (FITC) and red (PI) fluorescence.

Control samples are prepared following the same protocol, except that instead of being incubated with primary antibody (step 7), the cells are incubated with 5% albumin solution in PBS. For inhibition assays in step 7, the cells are exposed to the primary antibody, which was preincubated overnight at the working dilution with its corresponding immunogen at a molar antibody: immunogen ratio >2.

BIBLIOGRAPHY

Principles of Analytical Cytology
Bladder and other Urotheliel Tumors
Prostate
Renal Tumors
Adrenal Tumors

Principles of Analytical Cytology

Agarwal, V., Greenebaum, E., Wersto, R., and Koss, L. G.: DNA ploidy of spindle cell soft tissue tumors and its relationship to histology and clinical outcome. Arch. Pathol. Lab. Med., *115*, 558–562, 1991.

Amberson, J. B., and Wersto, R. P.: Semiautomated method of preparation of paraffin embedded tissue for flow cytometric analysis. *In* Koss, L. G.: Diagnostic Cytology and its Histopathologic Bases, 4th Ed. Philadelphia, J. B. Lippincott, 1992, pp. 1647–1648.

Auer, G. U., Caspersson, T. O., and Wallgren, A. S.: DNA content and survival in mammary carcinoma. Anal. Quant. Cytol., *2*, 161–165, 1980.

Baak, J. P. A.: Basic points in and practical aspects of application of diagnostic morphometry. Pathol. Res. Pract., *179*, 193–199, 1984.

Baak, J. P. A.: The principles and advances of quantitative pathology. Anal. Quant. Cytol. Histol., *9*, 89–95, 1987.

Baak, J. P. A., Noteboom, E., and Koevoets, J. J. M.: The influence of fixatives and other variations in tissue processing on nuclear morphometric features. Anal. Quant. Cytol. Histol., *11*, 219–224, 1989.

Baak, J. P. A., and Oort, J.: Morphometry in Diagnostic Pathology. Berlin, Springer Verlag, 1983.

Bacus, S. S., Bacus, J. W., Slamon, D. J., and Press, M. F.: HER-2/Neu oncogene expression and DNA ploidy analysis in breast cancer. Arch. Pathol. Lab. Med., *114*, 164–169, 1990.

Bacus, S., Flowers, J. L., Press, M. F., Bacus, J. W., and McCarty, K. S., Jr.: The evaluation of estrogen receptor in primary breast carcinoma by computer assisted image analysis. Am. J. Clin. Pathol., *90*, 233, 1988.

Bacus, S. S., Goldschmidt, R., Chin, D., Moran, G., Wienberg, D., and Bacus, J. W.: Biologic grading of breast cancer using antibodies to proliferating cells and other markers. Am. J. Pathol., *135*, 783–792, 1989.

Bagwell, C. B., Hudson, J. L., and Irvin, G. L.: Nonparametric flow cytometry analysis. J. Histochem. Cytochem., *27*, 293–296, 1979.

Bahr, G. F., Bartels, P. H., Dytch, H. E., Koss, L. G., and Wied, G. L.: Image analysis and its applications to cytology. *In* Koss, L. G.: Diagnostic Cytology and its Histopathologic Bases. 4th Ed. Philadelphia, J. B. Lippincott, 1992.

Bartels, P. H., Bahr, G. F., Bibbo, M., and Wièd, G. L.: Objective cell image analysis. J. Histochem. Cytochem., *20*, 239–254, 1972.

Bartels, P. H., Koss, L. G., and Wied, G. L.: Automated cell diagnosis in clinical cytology. *In* Koss, L. G., and Coleman, D. V. (Eds.): Advances in Clinical Cytology. London, Butterworth and Co., 1980, pp. 314–342.

Bauer, K. D., Duque, R. E., and Shankey, T. V. (Eds.): Clinical Flow Cytometry. Principles and Applications. Baltimore, Williams & Wilkins, 1993.

Bauer, T. W., Tubbs, R. R., Edinger, M. G., Suit, P. F., Gephart, G. N., and Levin, H. S.: A prospective comparison of DNA quantitation by image and flow cytometry. Am. J. Clin. Pathol., *93*, 322–326, 1990.

Bibbo, M., Bartels, P. H., Dytch, H. E., and Wied, G. L.: Ploidy measurements by high-resolution cytometry. Anal. Quant. Cytol. Histol., *7*, 81–88, 1985.

Brugal, G., and Adelh, D.: SAMBA 200: An industrial prototype for high resolution analysis of colored cells images. International Conference on High Resolution Cell Image Analysis, Los Angeles, 24–26, 1982.

Caspersson, T.: Cell Growth and Cell Function: A Cytochemical Study. New York, W.W. Norton, 1950.

Caspersson, T., and Santesson, L.: Studies on protein metabolism in cells of epithelial tumors. Acta Radiol. (Suppl.), *46*, 1–105, 1942.

Chieco, P., Jonker, A., Melchiorri, C., Vanni, G., and Van Norden, C. J. F.: A user's guide for avoiding errors in absorbance image cytometry: a review with original experimental observations. Histochem. J., *26,* 1–19, 1994.

Clark, G. M., Dressler, L. G., Owens, M. A., Pounds, G., Oldaker, T., and McGuire, W. L.: Predictions of relapse or survival in patients with node-negative breast cancer by DNA flow cytometry. N. Engl. J. Med., *320,* 627–633, 1989.

Clevenger, C. V., Bauer, K. D., and Epstein, A. L.: A method of simultaneous nuclear immunofluorescence and DNA content quantitation using monoclonal antibodies and flow cytometry. Cytometry, *6,* 208–214, 1985.

Cohen, J. H. M., Aubrey, J. P., Banchereau, J., and Revillard, J. P.: Identification of cell subpopulations by dual-color surface immunofluorescence using biotinylated and unlabeled monoclonal antibodies. Cytometry, *9,* 303–308, 1988.

Cohen, P. S., Seeger, R. C., Triche, T. J., and Israel, M. A.: Detection of N-*myc* gene expression in neuroblastoma tumors by in situ hybridization. Am. J. Pathol., *131,* 391–397, 1988.

Collan, Y., Torkkeli, T., Kosma, V. M., Pesonen, E., Kosunen, O., Jantunen, E., Mariuzzi, G. M., Montironi, R., Marinelli, F., and Collina, G.: Sampling in diagnostic morphometry. Pathol. Res. Pract., *182,* 401–406, 1987.

Coon, J. S., Landay, A. L., and Weinstein, R. S.: Advances in flow cytometry for diagnostic pathology. Lab. Invest., *57,* 453–479, 1987.

Cope, C., Rowe, D., Delbridge, L., and Friedlander, M.: Comparison of image analysis and flow cytometric determination of cellular DNA content. J. Clin. Path., *44,* 147–151, 1991.

Cornelisse, C. J., van de Velde, C. J. H., Caspers, R. J. C., Moolenaar, A. J., and Hermans, J.: DNA ploidy and survival in breast cancer patients. Cytometry, *8,* 225–234, 1987.

Cornelisse, C. J., and van Driel-Kulker, A. M.: DNA image cytometry on machine-selected breast cancer cells and a comparison between flow cytometry and scanning cytophotometry. Cytometry, *6,* 471–477, 1985.

Crissman, H. A., and Tobey, R. A.: Cell-cycle analysis in 20 minutes. Science, *184,* 1297–1298, 1974.

Czerniak, B., Chen, R., Tuziak, T., Markiewski, M., Kram, A., Gorczyca, W., Deitch, D., Herz, F., and Koss, L. G.: Expression of *ras* oncogene p21 protein in relation to regional spread of human breast carcinomas. Cancer, *63,* 2008–2013, 1989.

Czerniak, B., Darzynkiewicz, Z., Staiano-Coico, L., Herz, F., and Koss, L. G.: Expression of Ca antigen in relation to cycle in cultured human tumor cells. Cancer Res., *44,* 4342–4346, 1984.

Czerniak, B., Herz, F., and Koss, L. G.: DNA distribution patterns in early gastric carcinomas. A Feulgen cytometric study of gastric brush smears. Cancer, *59,* 113–117, 1987A.

Czerniak, B., Herz, F., Wersto, R. P., and Koss, L. G.: Asymmetric distribution of oncogene products at mitosis. Proc. Nat. Acad. Sci. (USA), *89,* 1199–1204, 1992.

Czerniak, B., Herz, F., Wersto, R. P., and Koss, L. G.: Expression of Ha-*ras* oncogene p21 protein in relation to the cell cycle of cultured human tumor cells. Am. J. Pathol., *126,* 411–416, 1987B.

Czerniak, B., Herz, F., Wersto, R. P., Alster, P., Puszkin, E., Schwarz, E., and Koss, L. G.: Quantitation of oncogene products by computer-assisted image analysis and flow cytometry. J. Histochem. Cytochem., *38,* 463–466, 1990.

Czerniak, B., Herz, F., Wersto, R. P., and Koss, L. G.: Modification of Ha-*ras* oncogene p21 expression and cell cycle progression in the human colonic cancer cell line HT-29. Cancer Res., *47,* 2826–2830, 1987C.

Czerniak, B., Papenhausen, P. R., Herz, F., and Koss, L. G.: Flow cytometric identification of cancer cells in effusions with Ca1 monoclonal antibody. Cancer, *55,* 2783–2788, 1985.

Darzynkiewicz, Z.: Cellular RNA content, a feature correlated with cell kinetics and tumor prognosis. Leukemia, *2,* 777–787, 1988.

Darzynkiewicz, Z.: Metabolic and kinetic compartments of the cell cycle distinguished by multiparameter flow cytometry. *In* Skehan, P., and Friedman, S. J. (Eds.): Growth, Cancer, and the Cell Cycle. Clifton, New Jersey, Humana Press, 1986, pp. 291–336.

Darzynkiewicz, Z.: Molecular interactions and cellular changes during the cell cycle. Pharmacol. Ther., *21,* 143–188, 1983.

Darzynkiewicz, Z., Andreeff, M., Traganos, R., Sharpless, T., and Melamed, M. R.: Discrimination of cycling and noncycling lymphocytes by BUdR-suppressed acridine orange fluorescence in a flow cytometric system. Exp. Cell Res., *115,* 1938–1942, 1978.

Darzynkiewicz, Z., Crissman, H., Traganos, F., and Steinkamp, J.: Cell heterogeneity during the cell cycle. J. Cell. Physiol., *113,* 465–474, 1982.

Darzynkiewicz, Z., Traganos, F., Kapuscinski, J., Staiano-Coico, L., and Melamed, M. R.: Accessibility of DNA in situ to various fluorochromes: relationship to chromatin changes during erythroid differentiation of Friend leukemia cells. Cytometry, *5,* 355–363, 1984.

Darzynkiewicz, Z., Traganos, F., and Melamed, M. R.: New cell cycle compartments identified by multiparameter flow cytometry. Cytometry, *1,* 95–108, 1980.

Dean, P. H., and Jett, J. H.: Mathematical analysis of DNA distributions derived from flow microfluorometry. J. Cell Biol., *60,* 523–527, 1974.

Dytch, H. E., and Wied, L. G.: Artificial neural networks and their use in quantitative pathology. Anal. Quant. Cytol. Histol., *12,* 379–393, 1990.

Ensley, J. F., Maciorowski, Z., Pietraszkiewicz, H., Hassan, M., Kish, J., AL-Sarraf, M., Jacobs, J., Weaver, A., Atkinson, D., and Crissman, J.: Solid tumor preparation for clinical application of flow cytometry. Cytometry, *8,* 488–493, 1987.

Fallenius, A. G., Askensten, U. G., Skoog, L. K., and Auer, G. U.: The reliability of microspectrophotometric and flow cytometric nuclear DNA measurements in adenocarcinomas of the breast. Cytometry, *8,* 260–266, 1987.

Fallenius, A. G., Auer, G. U., and Carstensen, J. M.: Prognostic significance of DNA measurements in 409 consecutive breast cancer patients. Cancer, *62,* 331–341, 1988.

Fallenius, A. G., Franzén, S. A., and Auer, G. U.: Predictive value of nuclear DNA content in breast cancer in relation to clinical and morphologic factors. Cancer, *62,* 521–530, 1988.

Fallenius, A., Svane, G., Auer, G., and Caspersson, T. O.: Cytochemical classification of nonpalpable breast carcinoma. Analyt. Quant. Cytol., *5,* 9–12, 1983.

Feitz, W. F. J., Beck, H. L. M., Smeets, A. W. G., Debruyne, F. M. J., Vooijs, G. P., Herman, C. J., and Ramaekers, F. C. S.: Tissue-specific markers in flow cytometry of urological cancers: Cytokeratins in bladder carcinoma. Int. J. Cancer, *36,* 349–356, 1985.

Feulgen, R., and Rossenbeck, H.: Mikroskopisch-chemischer Nachweis einer Nukleinsäure von Typus der Thymonukleinsaure Preparaten. Hoppe-Seylers Z Phys. Chem., *135,* 203–248, 1924.

Frankfurt, O. S., Arbuck, S. G., Chin, J. L., Greco, W. R., Pavelic, Z. P., Slocum, H. K., Mittelman, A., Piver, S. M., Pontes, E. J., and Rustum, Y. M.: Prognostic application of DNA flow cytometry for human solid tumors. Ann. N.Y. Acad. Sci., *468,* 276–290, 1986.

Friedlander, M. L., Hedley, D. W., and Taylor, I. W.: Clinical and biological significance of aneuploidy in human tumours. J. Clin. Pathol., *37,* 961–974, 1984.

Friedlander, M. L., Hedley, D. W., Taylor, I. W., Russell, P., Coates, A. S., and Tattersall, M. H.: Influence of cellular DNA content on survival in advanced ovarian cancer. Cancer Res., *44,* 397–400, 1984.

Fu, Y. S., and Hall, T. L.: DNA ploidy measurements in tissue sections. Analyt. Quant. Cytol., *7,* 90–95, 1985.

Gaub, J., Auer, G., and Zetterberg, A.: Quantitative cytochemical aspects of a combined Feulgen naphthol yellow S staining procedure for the simultaneous determination of nuclear and cytoplasmic proteins and DNA in mammalian cells. Exp. Cell Res., *92,* 323–332, 1975.

Gray, J. W., and Mayall, B. H. (Eds.): Monoclonal Antibodies Against Bromodeoxyuridine. New York, Allan R. Liss, 1985.

Greenebaum, E., Koss, L. G., Sherman, A. B., and Elequin, F.: Comparison of needle aspiration and solid biopsy technics in the flow cytometric study of DNA distributions of surgically resected tumors. Am. J. Clin. Pathol., *82,* 559–564, 1984.

Greenebaum, E., Koss, L. G., Elequin, F., and Silver, C. E.: The diagnostic value of flow cytometric DNA measurements in follicular tumors of the thyroid gland. Cancer, *56,* 2011–2018, 1985.

Haag, D., Feichter, G., Goerttler, K., and Kaufmann, M.: Influence of systematic errors on the evaluation of the S phase portions from DNA distributions of solid tumors as shown for 328 breast carcinomas. Cytometry, *8,* 377–385, 1987.

Hedley, D. W., Friedlander, M. L., and Taylor, I. W.: Application of DNA flow cytometry to paraffin-embedded archival material for the study of aneuploidy and its clinical significance. Cytometry, *6,* 327–333, 1985.

Hedley, D. W., Friedlander, M. L., Taylor, I. W., Rugg, C. A., and Musgrove, E. A.: DNA flow cytometry of paraffin-embedded tissue. Cytometry, *5,* 1660, 1984.

Hedley, D. W., Friedlander, M. L., Taylor, I. W., Rugg, C. A., and Musgrove, E. A.: Method for analysis of cellular DNA content of paraffin-embedded pathological material using flow cytometry. J. Histochem. Cytochem., *31,* 1333–1335, 1983.

Heiden, T., Strang, P., Stendahl, U., and Tribukait, B.: The reproducibility of flow cytometric analyses in human tumors. Methodological aspects. Anticancer Res., *10,* 49–54, 1990.

Hiddemann, W., Schumann, J., Andreeff, M., Barlogie, B., Herman, C. J., Leif, R. C., Mayall, B. M., Murphy, R. F., and Sandberg, A.: Convention on nomenclature for DNA cytometry. Cancer Genet. Cytogenet., *13,* 181–183, 1984.

Hopman, A. H. N., Ramaekers, F. C. S., Raap, A. K., Beck, J. L. M., Devilbe, P., van der Ploeg, M., and Vooijs, G. P.: In situ hybridization as a tool to study numerical chromosome aberrations in solid bladder tumors. Histochemistry, *89,* 307–316, 1988.

Horan, P. K., and Wheeless, L. L.: Quantitative single cell analysis and sorting. Science, *198,* 149–157, 1977.

Hunt, T., and Kirschner, M. W. (Eds.): Cell multiplication. Curr. Opinion Cell Biol., *5, issue 2,* 1993.

Hutchinson, M. L., Schultz, D. S., Stephenson, R. A., Wong, K. L., Harry, T., and Zahnizer, D. J.: Computerized microscopic analysis of prostate fine needle aspirates: Comparison with breast aspirates. Anal. Quant. Cytol. Histol., *11,* 105–110, 1989.

Jacobberger, J. W., Fogleman, D., and Lehman, J. M.: Analysis of intracellular antigens by flow cytometry. Cytometry, *7,* 356–364, 1986.

Jakobsen, A.: The use of trout erythrocytes and human lymphocytes for standardization in flow cytometry. Cytometry, *4,* 161–165, 1983.

Johnston, D. A., White, R. A., and Barlogie, B.: Automatic processing and interpretation of DNA distributions. Comparison of several techniques. Comput. Biomed. Res., *11,* 393–404, 1978.

Kallioniemi, O. P., Blanco, G., Alavaikko, M., et al.: Improving the prognostic value of DNA cytometry in breast cancer by combining DNA index and S-phase fraction. Cancer, *62,* 2183–2190, 1988.

Kallioniemi, O. P., Visakorpi, K., Holli, K., Heikkinen, A., Isola, J., and Koivula, T.: Improved prognostic impact of S-phase values from paraffin embedded breast and prostate carcinoma after correcting for nuclear slicing. Cytometry, *12,* 413–421, 1991.

Kamel, O. W., Franklin, W. A., Ringus, J. C., and Meyer, J. S.: Thymidine labeling index and Ki-67 growth fraction in lesions of the breast. Am. J. Pathol., *134,* 107–113, 1989.

Kamel, O. W., LeBrun, D. P., Davis, R. E., et al.: Growth fraction estimation of malignant lymphomas in formalin-fixed paraffin-embedded tissue using anti-PCNA/Cyclin 19A2. Am. J. Pathol., *138,* 1471–1477, 1991.

Kamentsky, L. A., Derman, H., and Melamed, M. R.: Ultraviolet absorption of epidermoid cancer cells. Science, *142,* 1580–1583, 1963.

Kamentsky, L. A., and Kamentsky, L. D.: Microscope-based multiparameter laser scanning cytometer yielding data comparable to flow cytometry data. Cytometry, *12,* 381–387, 1991.

Kamentsky, L. A., Melamed, M. R., and Derman, H.: Spectrophotometer: New instrument for ultrarapid cell analysis. Science, *150,* 630–631, 1965.

Koss, L. G.: Analytical and quantitative cytology: A historical perspective. Anal. Quant. Cytol. Histol., *4,* 251–256, 1982.

Koss, L. G.: The application of computerized high resolution scanning techniques to the identification of human cells and tissues. *In* Sklansky, J., Bisconte, J-C. (Eds.): Biomedical Images and Computers. New York, Springer-Verlag, 1982, pp. 1–10.

Koss, L. G.: Automated cytology and histology: A historical perspective. Anal. Quant. Cytol. Histol., *9,* 369–374, 1987.

Koss, L. G.: Diagnostic Cytology and Its Histopathologic Bases. 4th Ed. Philadelphia, J. B. Lippincott, 1992.

Koss, L. G.: Flow Cytometry. *In* Koss, L. G.: Diagnostic Cytology and its Histopathologic Bases. 4th Ed. Philadelphia, J. B. Lippincott, 1992.

Koss, L. G.: The future of cytology. The Wachtel lecture for 1988. Acta Cytol., *34,* 1–9, 1990.

Koss, L. G.: Image cytophotometry and flow cytometry. *In* Coon, J. S., and Weinstein, R. S. (Eds.): Diagnostic Flow Cytometry. Baltimore, Williams & Wilkins, 1992, pp. 147–163.

Koss, L. G., Czerniak, B. H., Herz, F., and Wersto, R. P.: Flow cytometric measurements of DNA and other cell components in human tumors: A critical appraisal. Hum. Pathol., *20,* 528–548, 1989.

Koss, L. G., Dembitzer, H. M., Herz, F., Herzig, N., Schreiber, K., and Wolley, R. C.: The monodisperse cell sample. I. Problems and possible solutions. *In* Wied, G. L., and Bahr, G. (Eds.): Proc. Int. Conf. on Automation of Uterine Cervix Cytology. Chicago, Chicago University Press, 1976.

Koss, L. G., and Greenebaum, E.: Measuring DNA in human cancer (Editorial). J.A.M.A., *255,* 3158–3159, 1986.

Koss, L. G., Lin, E., Schreiber, K., Elgert, P., and Mango, L.: Evaluation of the PAPNET cytologic screening system for quality control of cervical smears. Am. J. Clin. Pathol., *101,* 220–229, 1994.

Koss, L. G., Wolley, R. C., Schreiber, K., and Mendecki, J.: Flow microfluorometric analysis of nuclei isolated from various normal and malignant human epithelial cells. J. Histochem. Cytochem., *25,* 565–572, 1977.

Krishan, A.: Rapid flow cytofluorometric analysis of mammalian cell cycle by propidium iodide staining. J. Cell Biol., *66,* 188–193, 1975.

Lacombe, F., Belloc, F., Bernard, P., and Boisseau, M. R.: Evaluation of four methods of DNA distribution data analysis based on bromodeoxyuridine/DNA bivariate data. Cytometry, *9,* 245–253, 1988.

Latt, S. A.: Fluorescent probes of chromosome structure and replication. Canadian Journal of Genetics and Cytology, *19,* 603–623, 1977.

Mayall, B. H., Carrano, A. V., Moore, D. H., II, Ashworth, L. K., Bennett, D. E., and Mendelsohn, M. L.: The DNA-based karyotype. Cytometry, *5,* 376–385, 1984.

McDivitt, R. W., Stone, K. R., and Meyer, J. S.: A method for dissociation of viable human breast cancer cells that produce flow cytometric kinetic information similar to that obtained by thymidine labeling. Cancer Res., *44,* 2628–2633, 1984.

Melamed, M. R., and Kamentsky, L. A.: Automated cytology. Int. Rev. Exp. Pathol., *14,* 205–295, 1975.

Melamed, M. R., Lidmo, T., and Mendelsohn, M. L. (Eds.): Flow Cytometry and Sorting. 2nd Ed. New York, Wiley-Liss, 1990.

Mellors, R. C., Glassman, A., and Papanicolaou, G. N.: A microfluorometric scanning method for the detection of cancer cells in smears of exfoliated cells. Cancer, *5,* 458–468, 1954.

Mendecki, J., Dillmann, W. H., Wolley, R. C., Oppenheimer, J. H., and Koss, L. G.: Effect of thyroid hormone on the ploidy of rat liver nuclei as determined by flow cytometry. Proc. Soc. Exp. Biol. Med., *158,* 63–67, 1978.

Mendelsohn, M. L., Mayall, B. H., Prewitt, J. M. S., Bostrom, R. S., and Holcomb, W. G.: Digital transformation and computer analysis of microscopic images. *In* Barer, R., and Cosslett, V. E. (Eds.): Advances in Optical and Electron Microscopy. New York, Academic Press, 1968.

Merkel, D. E., Dressler, L. G., and McGuire, W. L.: Flow cytometry, cellular DNA content, and prognosis in human malignancy. J. Clin. Oncol., *5,* 1690–1703, 1987.

Meyer, J. S.: Cell kinetic measurements of human tumors. Hum. Pathol., *13,* 874–877, 1982.

Meyer, J. S., Bauer, W. C., and Rao, B. R.: Subpopulation of breast carcinoma defined by S-phase fraction, morphology, and estrogen receptor content. Lab. Invest., *39,* 225–235, 1978.

Meyer, J. S., and Coplin, M. D.: Thymidine labeling index, flow cytometric S-phase measurement, and DNA index in human tumors. Comparisons and correlations. Am. J. Clin. Pathol., *89,* 586–595, 1988.

Mikel, U. V., Fishbein, W. N., and Bahr, G. F.: Some practical consideration in quantitative absorbance microspectrophotometry: Preparation techniques in DNA cytophotometry. Anal. Quant. Cytol. Histol., *7,* 107–118, 1985.

Murray, A., and Hunt, T.: The Cell Cycle. New York, W. H. Freeman, 1993.

Ohtsubo, M., and Roberts, J. M.: Cyclin-dependent regulation of G1 in mammalian fibroblasts. Science, *259,* 1908–1912, 1993.

Oud, P. S., Hanselaar, T. G. J., Reubsaet-Veldhuizen, J. A. M., Meijer, J. W. R., Gemmink, A. H., Pahlplatz, M. M. M., Beck, H. L. M., and Vooijs, G. P.: Extraction of nuclei from selected regions in paraffin-embedded tissue. Cytometry, *7,* 595–600, 1986.

Poddighe, P. J., Ramaekers, F. C. S., and Hopman, A. H. N.: Interphase cytogenetics of tumours. J. Pathol., *166*, 215–224, 1992.

Preston, K. J.: Automation of the analysis of cell images. Anal. Quant. Cytol., *2*, 1–14, 1980.

Prewitt, J. M. S., and Mendelsohn, M. L.: The analysis of cell images. Ann. N.Y. Acad. Sci., *128*, 1035–1043, 1966.

Rabinovitch, P. S., Kubbies, M., Chen, Y. C., Schindler, D., and Hoehn, H.: BrdU-Hoechst Flow Cytometry: A unique tool for quantitative cell cycle analysis. Exper. Cell Res., *174*, 309–318, 1988.

Riley, R. S., Mahin, E. J., and Ross, W.: Clinical Applications of Flow Cytometry. New York, Igaku-Shoin, 1993.

Ryan, D. H., Fallon, M. A., and Horan, P. K.: Flow cytometry in the clinical laboratory. Clin. Chim. Acta, *171*, 125–197, 1988.

Sahni, K., Tribukait, B., and Einhorn, N.: Flow cytometric measurement of ploidy and proliferation in effusions of ovarian carcinoma and their possible prognostic significance. Gynecol. Oncol., *35*, 240–245, 1989.

Schneller, J., Eppich, E., Greenebaum, E., Elequin, F., Sherman, A., Wersto, R., and Koss, L. G.: Flow cytometry and Feulgen cytophotometry in evaluation of effusions. Cancer, *59*, 1307–1313, 1987.

Schutte, B., Reynders, M. M. J., van Assche, C. L. M. V. J., Hupperets, P. S. G. J., Bosman, F. T., and Blijham, G. H.: An improved method for the immunocytochemical detection of bromodeoxyuridine labeled nuclei using flow cytometry. Cytometry, *8*, 372–376, 1987.

Shackney, S. E., Erickson, B. W., and Skramstad, K. S.: The T-lymphocyte as a diploid reference standard for flow cytometry. Cancer Res., *39*, 4418–4427, 1979.

Shapiro, H. M.: Multistation multi-parameter flow cytometry: a critical review and rationale. Cytometry, *3*, 227–243, 1983.

Shapiro, H. M.: Practical Flow Cytometry. New York, Alan R. Liss, 1985.

Shapiro, H. M.: Technical developments in flow cytometry. Hum. Pathol., *17*, 649–651, 1986.

Sharpless, T. K., and Melamed, M. R.: Estimation of cell size from pulse shape in flow cytofluorometry. J. Histochem. Cytochem., *24*, 257–264, 1976.

Sivestrini, R., and the SICCAB Group for Quality Control of Cell Kinetic Determination: Quality control for evaluation of S-phase fraction by flow cytometry: a multicentric study. Cytometry, *18*, 11–16, 1994.

Smeets, A. W. G., Pauwels, R. P. E., Beck, H. L. M., Feitz, W. F. J., Geraedts, J. P. M., Debruyne, F. M. J., Laarakkers, L., Vooijs, G. P., and Ramaekers, F. C. S.: Comparison of tissue disaggregation techniques of transitional cell bladder carcinomas for flow cytometry and chromosomal analysis. Cytometry, *8*, 14–19, 1987.

Smeets, A. W. G., Pauwels, R. P. E., Beck, J. P. M., Geraedts, J. P. M., Debruyne, F. M. J., Laarakkers, L., Feitz, W. F. J., Vooijs, G. P., and Ramaekers, F. C. S.: Tissue specific markers in flow cytometry of urological cancers. III. Comparing chromosomal and flow cytometric DNA analysis of bladder tumors. Int. J. Cancer, *39*, 304–310, 1987.

Steinkamp, J. A., Hansen, K. M., and Crissman, H. A.: Flow microfluorometric and light-scatter measurement of nuclear and cytoplasmic size in mammalian cells. J. Histochem. Cytochem., *24*, 292–297, 1976.

Thornwaite, J. F., Seckinger, D., Sugarbaker, E. V., Rosenthal, P. K., and Vazquez, D. A.: Dual immunofluorescent analysis of human peripheral blood lymphocytes. Am. J. Clin. Pathol., *82*, 48–56, 1984.

Thronwaite, J. T., Sugarbaker, E. V., and Temple, W. J.: Preparation of tissues for DNA flow cytometric analysis. Cytometry, *1*, 229–237, 1980.

Traganos, F.: Flow cytometry. Principles and applications. II. Cancer Invest., *2*, 239–258, 1984.

van Dierendonck, J. H., Wijdman, J. H., Keijzer, R., et al.: Cell-cycle related staining patterns of anti-proliferating cell nuclear antigen monoclonal antibodies: comparison with BrdU labelling and Ki-67 staining. Am. J. Pathol., *138*, 1165–1172, 1991.

van Diest, P. J., Smeulders, A. W. M., Thunnissen, F. B. J., and Baak, J. P. A.: Cytomorphometry. A Methodologic study of preparation techniques, selection methods and sample sizes. Anal. Quant. Cytol. Histol., *11*, 225–231, 1989.

Van Dilla, M. A., Trujillo, T. T., Mullaney, P. F., and Coulter, J. R.: Cell microfluorometry: A method for rapid fluorescence measurement. Science, *163*, 1213–1214, 1969.

Vindeløv, L. L., Christensen, I. J., and Nissen, N. I.: A detergent-trypsin method for the preparation of nuclei for flow cytometric DNA analysis. Cytometry, *3*, 323–327, 1983.

Vindeløv, L. L., Christensen, I. J., and Nissen, N. J.: Standardization of high-resolution flow cytometric DNA analysis by the simultaneous use of chicken and trout red blood cells as internal reference standards. Cytometry, *3*, 328–331, 1983.

Watson, J. V.: Quantitation of molecular and cellular probes in populations of single cells using fluorescence. Mol. Cell. Probes, *1*, 121–136, 1987.

Watson, J. V., Stewart, J., Cox, H., Sikora, K., and Even, G. I.: Flow cytometric quantitation of the c-*myc* oncoprotein in archival neoplastic biopsies of the colon. Mol. Cell Probes, *1*, 151–157, 1987.

Wersto, R. P., Greenebaum, E., Deitch, D., Kerstenberger, K., and Koss, L. G.: Deoxyribonucleic acid ploidy and cell cycle events in benign colonic epithelium peripheral to carcinoma. Lab. Invest., *58*, 218–225, 1988.

Wersto, R. P., Herz, F., Gallagher, R. E., and Koss, L. G.: Cell cycle-dependent reactivity with the monoclonal antibody Ki-67 during myeloid cell differentiation. Exp. Cell Res., *179*, 79–88, 1988.

Wersto, R. P., Liblit, R. L., Deitch, D., and Koss, L. G.: Variability in DNA measurements in multiple samples of human colonic carcinoma. Cancer, *67*, 106–115, 1991.

Wersto, R. P., Liblit, R. L., and Koss, L. G.: Flow cytometric analysis of human solid tumors: a review of the interpretation of DNA histograms. Hum. Pathol., *22*, 1085–1098, 1991.

Wheeless, L. L., Coon, J. S., Cox, C., Deitch, A. D.,

deVere White, R. W., Koss, L. G., Melamed, R. M., O'Connell, M. J., Reeder, J. E., Weinstein, R. S., and Wersto, R. P.: Measurement variability in DNA flow cytometry of replicate samples. Cytometry, *10*, 731–738, 1989.

Wheeless, L. L., Coon, J. S., Cox, C., Deitch, A. D., deVere White, R. W., Fradet, Y., Koss, L. G., Melamed, M. R., O'Connell, M. J., Reeder, J. E., Weinstein, R. S., and Wersto, R. P.: Precision of DNA flow cytometry in inter-institutional analysis. Cytometry, *12*, 405–412, 1991.

Wied, G. L., Bartels, P. H., Bibbo, M., and Dytch, H. E.: Image analysis and quantitative cyto- and histopathology. Hum. Pathol., *20*, 549–571, 1989.

Wied, G. L., Bartels, P. H., Bahr, G. F., and Oldfield, D. G.: Taxonomic intracellular analytic system (TICAS) for cell identification. Acta Cytol., *12*, 180–204, 1968.

Wolley, R. C., Herz, F., Dembitzer, H. M., Schreiber, K., and Koss, L. G.: The monodisperse cervical smear. Quantitative analysis of cell dispersion and loss with enzymatic and chemical agents. Anal. Quant. Cytol., *1*, 43–49, 1979.

Wolley, R. C., Herz, F., and Koss, L. G.: Caution on the use of lymphocytes as standards in the flow cytometric analysis of cultured cells. Cytometry, *2*, 370–372, 1982.

Wolley, R. C., Schreiber, K., Koss, L. G., Karas, M., and Sherman, A.: DNA distribution in human colon carcinomas and its relationship to clinical behavior. J. Natl. Cancer Inst., *69*, 15–22, 1982.

Bladder and Other Urothelial Tumors

Aamodt, R. L., Coon, J. S., Deitch, A., deVere White, R. W., Koss, L. G., Melamed, M. R., Weinstein, R. S., and Wheeless, L. L.: Flow cytometric evaluation of bladder cancer: recommendations of the NCI flow cytometry network for bladder cancer. World J. Urol., *10*, 63–67, 1992.

Amberson, J. B., and Laino, J.: Image cytometric deoxyribonucleic acid analysis of urine specimens as an adjunct to visual cytology in the detection of urothelial cell carcinoma. J. Urol., *149*, 42–45, 1993.

Baak, J. P. A., and Oort, J.: Morphometry in Diagnostic Pathology. Berlin, Springer Verlag, 1983.

Badalament, R. A., Fair, W. R., Whitmore, W. F., Jr., and Melamed, M. R.: The relative value of cytometry and cytology in the management of bladder cancer: The Memorial Sloan-Kettering Cancer Center experience. Semin. Urol., *6*, 22–30, 1988.

Badalament, R. A., Gary, H., Whitmore, W. F., Jr., et al.: Monitoring intravesical bacillus Calmette-Guerin treatment of superficial bladder carcinoma by serial flow cytometry. Cancer, *58*, 2751–2757, 1986.

Badalament, R. A., Hermansen, D. K., Kimmel, M., et al.: The sensitivity of bladder wash flow cytometry, bladder wash cytology, and voided cytology in the detection of bladder carcinoma. Cancer, *60*, 1423–1427, 1987.

Blomjous, C. E., Schipper, N. W., Baak, J. P., van Galen, E. M., de Voogt, H. J., and Meyer, C. J.: Retrospective study of prognostic importance of DNA flow cytometry of urinary bladder carcinoma. J. Clin. Pathol., *41*, 21–25, 1988.

Blomjous, E. C., Schipper, N. W., Baak, J. P., Vos, W., De Voogt, H. J., and Meijer, C. J.: The value of morphometry and DNA flow cytometry in addition to classic prognosticators in superficial urinary bladder carcinoma. Am. J. Clin. Pathol., *91*, 243–248, 1989.

Blute, M. L., Tsushima, K., Farrow, G. M., Therneau, T. M., and Lieber, M. M.: Transitional cell carcinoma of the renal pelvis: nuclear deoxyribonucleic acid ploidy studied by flow cytometry. J. Urol., *140*, 944–949, 1988.

Bretton, P. R., Herr, H. W., Kimmel, M., Fair, W. R., Whitmore, W. F., and Melamed, M. R.: Flow cytometry as a predictor of response and progression in patients with superficial bladder cancer treated with Bacillus Calmette-Guerin. J. Urol., *141*, 1332–1336, 1989.

Chin, J. L., Huben, R. P., Nava, E., Rustum, Y. M., Greco, J. M., Pontes, E., and Frankfurt, O. S.: Flow cytometric analysis of DNA content in human bladder tumors and irrigation specimens. Cancer, *56*, 1677–1681, 1985.

Collste, L. G., Devonec, M., Darzynkiewicz, Z., Traganos, F., Sharpless, T. K., Whitmore, W. F., Jr., and Melamed, M. R.: Bladder cancer diagnosis by flow cytometry. Correlation between cell samples from biopsy and bladder irrigation fluid. Cancer, *45*, 2389–2394, 1980.

Coon, J. S., Deitch, A. D., DeVere White, R. W., Koss, L. G., Melamed, M. R., Reeder, J. E., Weinstein, R. S., Wersto, R. P., and Wheeless, L. L.: Interinstitutional variability in DNA flow cytometric analysis of tumors. The National Cancer Institutes flow cytometry network experience. Cancer, *61*, 126–130, 1988.

Coon, J. S., Schwartz, D., Summers, J. L., Miller, A. W., and Weinstein, R. S.: Flow cytometric analysis of deparaffinized nuclei in urinary bladder carcinomas. Comparison with cytogenetic analysis. Cancer, *57*, 1594–1601, 1986.

Corrado, F., Ferri, C., Mannini, D., Corrado, G., Bertoni, F., Bachini, P., Lelli, G., Lieber, M. M., and Song, J. M.: Transitional cell carcinoma of the upper urinary tract: evaluation of prognostic factors by histopathology and flow cytometric analysis. J. Urol., *145*, 1159–1163, 1991.

Czerniak, B., Cohen, G. L., Etkin, P., Deitch, D., Simmons, H., Herz, F., and Koss, L. G.: Concurrent mutations of coding and regulatory sequences of the Ha-*ras* gene in urinary bladder carcinoma. Hum. Pathol., *23*, 1199–1204, 1992.

Czerniak, B., Deitch, D., Simmons, H., Etkind, P., Herz, F., and Koss, L. G.: Ha-*ras* gene codon 12 mutation and ploidy in urinary bladder cancer. Br. J. Cancer, *62*, 762–763, 1990.

Czerniak, B., and Koss, L. G.: Expression of Ca antigen on human urinary bladder tumors. Cancer, *55*, 2380–2383, 1985.

Czerniak, B., Koss, L. G., and Sherman, A.: Nuclear pores and DNA ploidy in human bladder carcinomas. Cancer Res., *44*, 3752–3756, 1984.

Dean, P. J., and Murphy, W. M.: Importance of urinary cytology and future role of flow cytometry. Urology, *26* (*Suppl.*), 11–15, 1985.

deVere White, R. W., Deitch, A. D., Baker, W. C., Jr., and Strand, M. A.: Urine: A suitable sample for deoxyribonucleic acid flow cytometry studies in patients with bladder cancer. J. Urol., *139*, 926–928, 1988.

deVere White, R. W., Olsson, C. A., and Deitch, A. D.: Flow cytometry: Role in monitoring transitional cell carcinoma of bladder. Urology, *8*, 15–20, 1986.

Devonec, M., Darzynkiewicz, Z., Kostyrka-Claps, M. L., Collste, L., Whitmore, W. F., and Melamed, M. R.: Flow cytometry of low stage bladder tumors: correlation with cytologic and cytoscopic diagnosis. Cancer, *49*, 109–118, 1982.

Devonec, M., Darzynkiewicz, Z., Whitmore, W. F., and Melamed, M. R.: Flow cytometry for follow-up examinations of conservatively treated low stage bladder tumors. J. Urol., *126*, 166–170, 1981.

Esrig, D., Elmajian, D., Groshen, S., Freeman, J. A., Stein, J. P., Chen, S. C., Nichols, P. W., Skinner, D. G., Jones, P. A., and Cote, R. J.: Accumulation of nuclear p53 and tumor progression in bladder cancer. New Engl. J. Med., *331*, 1259–1264, 1994.

Farsund, T.: Preparation of bladder mucosa for micro-flow fluorometry. Virch. Arch. B (Cell Path), *16*, 35–42, 1974.

Farsund, T.: Selective sampling of cells for morphological and quantitative cytology of bladder epithelium. J. Urol., *128*, 267–271, 1982.

Feitz, W. F. J., Beck, H. L. M., Smeets, A. W. G., Debruyne, F. M. J., Vooijs, G. P., Herman, C. J., and Ramaekers, F. C. S.: Tissue-specific markers in flow cytometry of urological cancers: Cytokeratins in bladder carcinoma. Int. J. Cancer, *36*, 349–356, 1985.

Giella, J. G., Ring, K., Olsson, C. A., Karp, F. S., and Benson, M. C.: The predictive value of flow cytometry and urinary cytology in the follow-up of patients with transitional cell carcinoma of bladder. J. Urol., *148*, 293–296, 1992.

Gustafson, H., Tribukait, B., and Esposti, L.: DNA profile and tumor progression in patients with superficial bladder tumors. Urol. Res., *10*, 13–18, 1982.

Hopman, A. H. N., Ramaekers, F. C. S., Raap, A. K., Beck, J. L. M., Devilbe, P., van der Ploeg, M., and Vooijs, G. P.: In situ hybridization as a tool to study numerical chromosome aberrations in solid bladder tumors. Histochemistry, *89*, 307–316, 1988.

Kirkhus, B., Clausen, O. P. F., Fjordvang, H., Helander, K., Iversen, O. H., Reitan, J. B., and Vaage, S.: Characterisation of bladder tumors by multiparameter flow cytometry with special reference to grade II tumors. APMIS, *96*, 783–792, 1988.

Klein, F. A., Herr, H. W., Sogani, P. C., Whitmore, W. F., Jr., and Melamed, M. R.: Detection and follow-up of carcinoma of the urinary bladder by flow cytometry. Cancer, *50*, 389–395, 1982.

Klein, F. A., Herr, H. W., Whitmore, W. F., Pinsky, C. M., Oettgen, H., and Melamed, M. R.: Automated flow cytometry to monitor intravesical therapy for superficial bladder cancer. Urology, *17*, 310–314, 1981.

Klein, F. A., Herr, H. W., Whitmore, W. F., Sogani, P. C., and Melamed, M. R.: An evaluation of automated flow cytometry (FCM) in detection of carcinoma in situ of the urinary bladder. Cancer, *50*, 1003–1008, 1982.

Koss, L. G., Bartels, P. H., Bibbo, M., Freed, S. Z., Sychra, J. J., Taylor, J., and Wied, G. L.: Computer analysis of atypical urothelial cells. I. Classification by supervised learning algorithms. Acta Cytol., *21*, 247–260, 1977.

Koss, L. G., Bartels, P. H., Bibbo, M., Freed, S. Z., Taylor, J., and Wied, G. L.: Computer discrimination between benign and malignant urothelial cells. Acta Cytol., *19*, 378–391, 1975.

Koss, L. G., Bartels, P. H., Sychra, J. J., and Wied, G. L.: Computer analysis of atypical urothelial cells. II. Classification by unsupervised learning algorithms. Acta Cytol., *21*, 261–265, 1977.

Koss, L. G., Bartels, P. H., Bibbo, M., Freed, S. Z., Sychra, J. J., Taylor, J., and Wied, G. L.: Computer analysis of atypical urothelial cells. I. Classification by supervised learning algorithms. Acta Cytol., *21*, 247–260, 1977.

Koss, L. G., Bartels, P. H., Sherman, A., Sychra, J. J., Schreiber, K., Moussouris, H. S., and Wied, G. L.: Computer identification of degenerated urothelial cells. Anal. Quant. Cytol., *2*, 107–111, 1980.

Koss, L. G., Bartels, P. H., Sychra, J. J., and Wied, G. L.: Diagnostic cytologic sample profiles in patients with bladder cancer using TICAS system. Acta Cytol., *22*, 392–397, 1978.

Koss, L. G., Bartels, P., and Wied, G. L.: Computer-based diagnostic analysis of cells in the urinary sediment. J. Urol., *123*, 846–849, 1980.

Koss, L. G., and Czerniak, B.: Image analysis and flow cytometry of tumors of prostate and bladder. With a comment on molecular biology of urothelial tumors. *In:* Weinstein, R. and Gardner, W. A., Jr. (Eds.) Pathology and Pathobiology of the Urinary Bladder and Prostate. Baltimore, Williams & Wilkins, 1992.

Koss, L. G., Eppich, E. M., Medler, K. H., and Wersto, R. P.: DNA cytophotometry of voided urine sediment: Comparison with results of cytologic diagnosis and image analysis. Anal. Quant. Cytol. Hist., *9*, 398–404, 1987.

Koss, L. G., Sherman, A. B., and Eppich, E.: Image analysis and DNA content of urothelial cells infected with human polyomavirus. Anal. Quant. Cytol., *6*, 89–94, 1984.

Koss, L. G., Sherman, A. B., and Adams, S. E.: The use of hierarchic classification in the image analysis of a complex cell population. Experience with the sediment of voided urine. Anal. Quant. Cytol., *5*, 159–166, 1983.

Koss, L. G., Wersto, R. P., Simmons, D. A., Deitch, D., Herz, F., and Freed, S. Z.: Predictive value of DNA measurements in bladder washings. Comparison of flow cytometry, image cytophotometry, and cytology in patients with a past history of urothelial tumors. Cancer, *64*, 916–924, 1989.

Lederer, B., Mikuz, G., Gutter, W., and zur Neiden, G.: Zytophotometrische Untersuchungen von Tumoren des Ubergangsepithels der Harnblase. Vergleich zytophotometrischer Untersuchungsergebnisse mit dem histologischen Grading. Beitr. Pathol., *147,* 379–389, 1972.

Melamed, M. R.: Flow cytometry of the urinary bladder. Urol. Clin. North Am., *11,* 599–608, 1984.

Melamed, M. R., and Klein, F. A.: Flow cytometry of urinary bladder irrigation specimens. Hum. Pathol., *15,* 302–302, 1984.

Melamed, M. R., Traganos, F., Sharpless, T., and Darzynkiewicz, Z.: Urinary cytology automation. Preliminary studies with Acridine Orange stain and flow-through cytofluorometry. Invest. Urol., *13,* 331–338, 1976.

Murphy, W. M., Emerson, L. D., Chandler, R. W., Moinuddin, S. M., and Soloway, M. S.: Flow cytometry versus urinary cytology in the evaluation of patients with bladder cancer. J. Urol., *136,* 815–819, 1986.

Nativ, O., Winkler, H. Z., Reiman, H. M., and Lieber, M. M.: Squamous cell carcinoma of the renal pelvis: nuclear deoxyribonucleic acid ploidy studied by flow cytometry. J. Urol., *144,* 23–26, 1990.

Norming, U., Nyman, C. R., and Tribukait, B.: Comparative flow cytometric deoxyribonucleic acid studies on exophytic tumors and random mucosal biopsies in untreated carcinoma of the bladder. J. Urol., *142,* 1442–1447, 1989.

Norming, U., Tribukait, B., Gustafson, H., Nyman, C. R., Wang, N., and Wijkstrom, H.: Deoxyribonucleic acid profile and tumor progression in primary carcinoma in situ of the bladder: A study of 63 patients with grade 3 lesions. J. Urol., *147,* 11–15, 1992.

Oldbring, J., Hellsten, S., Lindholm, K., Mikulowski, P., and Tribukait, B.: Flow DNA analysis in the characterisation of carcinoma of the renal pelvis and ureter. Cancer, *64,* 2141–2145, 1989.

Orihuela, E., Varadachay, S., Herr, H. W., Melamed, M. R., and Whitmore, W. F.: The practical use of tumor marker determination in bladder washing specimens. Assessing the urothelium of patients with superficial bladder cancer. Cancer, *60,* 1009–1016, 1987.

Poddighe, P. J., Ramaekers, F. C. S., Smeets, A. W. G., Vooijs, G. P., and Hopman, A. H. N.: Structural chromosome 1 aberrations in transitional cell carcinoma of the bladder: interphase cytogenetics combining a centromeric, telomeric, and library DNA probe. Cancer Res., *52,* 4929–4934, 1992.

Shaaban, A. A., Tribukait, B., Abdel-Fattah, A. E.-B., and Ghoneim, M. A.: Characterisation of squamous cell bladder tumors by flow cytometric deoxyribonucleic acid analysis: a report of 100 cases. J. Urol., *144,* 879–883, 1990.

Shabaik, A. S., Pow-Sang, J. M., Lockhard, J., and Nicosia, S. V.: Role of DNA image cytometry in the follow-up of patients with urinary tract transitional cell carcinoma. Anal. Quant. Cytol. Histol., *15,* 115–123, 1993.

Shankey, T. V.: Urologic cancers. *In* Bauer, K. D., Duque, R. E., Shankey, T. V. (Eds.): Clinical Flow Cytometry. Principles and Applications. Baltimore, Williams & Wilkins, 1993, pp. 271–305.

Sherman, A., Koss, L. G., Adams, S., Schreiber, K.,

Moussouris, H. F., Fred, S. Z., Bartels, P. H., and Wied, G. L.: Bladder cancer diagnosis by image analysis of cells in voided urine using a small computer. Anal. Quant. Cytol., *3,* 239–249, 1981.

Sherman, A. B., Koss, L. G., Wyschogrod, D., Melder, K. H., Eppich, E. M., and Bales, C. E.: Bladder cancer diagnosis by computer image analysis of cells in the sediment of voided urine using a video scanning system. Anal. Quant. Cytol. Histol., *8,* 177–186, 1986.

Sherman, A. B., Koss, L. G., and Adams, S. E.: Interobserver and intraobserver differences in the diagnosis of urothelial cells. Comparison with classification by computer. Anal. Quant. Cytol., *6,* 112–120, 1984.

Smeets, A. W. G., Pauwels, R. P. E., Beck, H. L. M., Feitz, W. F. J., Geraedts, J. P. M., Debruyne, F. M. J., Laarakkers, L., Vooijs, G. P., and Ramaekers, F. C. S.: Comparison of tissue disaggregation techniques of transitional cell bladder carcinomas for flow cytometry and chromosomal analysis. Cytometry, *8,* 14–19, 1987.

Smeets, A. W. G., Pauwels, R. P. E., Beck, J. P. M., Geraedts, J. P. M., Debruyne, F. M. J., Laarakers, L., Feitz, W. F. J., Vooijs, G. P., and Ramaekers, F. C. S.: Tissue specific markers in flow cytometry of urological cancers. III. Comparing chromosomal and flow cytometric DNA analysis of bladder tumors. Int. J. Cancer, *39,* 304–310, 1987.

Stockle, M., Steinbach, F., Voges, G., and Hohenfeller, R.: Image analysis DNA cytometry of bladder cancer. Rec. Res. Cancer Res., *126,* 151–163, 1993.

Stoiano-Coico, L., Huffman, J., Wolf, R., Pinsky, C. M., Herr, H. W., Whitmore, W. F., Jr., Oettgen, H. F., Darzynkiewicz, Z., and Melamed, M. R.: Monitoring intravesical Bacillus Calmette-Guerin treatment of bladder carcinoma by flow cytometry. J. Urol., *133,* 786–788, 1985.

Tribukait, B.: Flow cytometry in surgical pathology and cytology of tumors of the genito-urinary tract. *In* Koss, L. G., and Coleman, D. V. (Eds.). Advances in Clinical Cytology. Vol. 2. New York, Masson, 1984, pp. 163–189.

Tribukait, B.: Flow cytometry in assessing the clinical aggressiveness of genito-urinary neoplasms. World J. Urol., *5,* 108–122, 1987.

Tribukait, B., Gustafson, H., and Esposti, P. L.: Ploidy and proliferation of human bladder tumors as measured by flow-cytofluorometric DNA-analysis and its relations to histopathology and cytology. Cancer, *43,* 1742–1751, 1979.

Tribukait, B., Gustafson, H., and Esposti, P. L.: The significance of ploidy and proliferation in the clinical and biological evaluation of human tumors: A study of 100 untreated bladder carcinomas. Br. J. Urol., *54,* 130–135, 1982.

Wheeless, L. L., Badalament, R. A., deVere White, R. W., Fradet, Y., and Tribukait, B.: Consensus review of the clinical utility of DNA cytometry in bladder cancer. Cytometry, *14,* 478–481, 1993.

Wheeless, L. L., Coon, J. S., Cox, C., Deitch, A. D., deVere White, R. W., Fradet, Y., Koss, L. G., Melamed, M. R., O'Connell, M. J., Reeder, J. E., Weinstein, R. S., and Wersto, R. P.: Precision of DNA flow cytometry in inter-institutional analysis. Cytometry, *12*, 405–412, 1991.

Wheeless, L. L., Coon, J. S., Deitch, A. D., deVere White, R. W., Koss, L. G., Melamed, M. R., Reeder, J. E., Robinson, R. D., Weinstein, R. S., and Wersto, R. W.: Comparison of automated and manual techniques for analysis of DNA frequency distributions in bladder washings. Cytometry, *9*, 600–604, 1988.

Wijkstrom, H., Granberg-Ohman, I., and Tribukait, B.: Chromosomal and DNA patterns in transitional cell bladder carcinoma. A comparative cytogenetic and flow-cytofluorometric DNA study. Cancer, *53*, 1718–1723, 1984.

Wong, E. K., Liang, E. H., Lin, E. K., Simmons, D. A., and Koss, L. G.: A selective mapping algorithm for computer analysis of voided urine cell images. Anal. Quant. Cytol. Histol., *11*, 203–210, 1989.

Prostate

Adolfsson, J., Ronstrom, L., Herlund, P., Löwhagen, T., Carstensen, J., and Tribukait, B.: The prognostic value of modal deoxyribonucleic acid in low grade, low stage untreated prostate cancer. J. Urol., *144*, 1404–1407, 1990.

Adolfsson, J., and Tribukait, B.: Evaluation of tumor progression by repeated fine needle biopsies in prostate adenocarcinoma: modal deoxyribonucleic acid value and cytological differentiation. J. Urol., *144*, 1408–1410, 1990.

Amberson, J. B., and Koss, L. G.: Measurements of DNA as a prognostic factor in prostatic carcinoma. *In* Karr, J. P., Coffey, D. S., Gardner, W., Jr. (Eds.): Prognostic Cytometry and Cytopathology of Prostate Cancer. New York, Elsevier, 1988, pp. 281–286.

Auer, G., and Zetterberg, A.: The prognostic significance of nuclear DNA content in malignant tumors of breast, prostate, and cartilage. *In* Koss, L. G., and Coleman, D. V. (Eds.): Advances in Clinical Cytology. Vol. 2. New York, Masson Publishing USA, 1984, pp. 123–134.

Black, W. C., and Welch, H. G.: Advances in diagnostic imaging and overestimation of disease prevalence and the benefits of therapy. N. Engl. J. Med., *328*, 1237–1243, 1993.

Böcking, A., Aufferman, W., Jochman, D., et al.: DNA grading of malignancy and tumor regression in prostatic carcinoma under hormone therapy. Applied Pathology, *3*, 206–214, 1985.

Breitkreutz, T., Romanakis, K., Lutz, S., Seitz, G., Bonkoff, H., Unteregger, G., Zwergel, T., Zang, K. D., and Wullich, B.: Genotypic characterization of prostatic carcinoma: a combined cytogenetic, flow cytometry, and in situ hybridization study. Cancer Res., *53*, 4035–4040, 1993.

Deitch, A. D., Strand, M. A., and deVere White, R. W.: Deoxyribonucleic acid flow cytometry of benign prostatic disease. J. Urol., *142*, 759–762, 1989.

deVere White, R. W., Deitch, A. D., Tesluk, H., Lamborn, K. R., and Meyers, F. J.: Prognosis in disseminated prostate cancer as related to tumor ploidy and differentiation. World J. Urol., *8*, 47–50, 1990.

Diamond, D. A., Berry, S. J., Umbricht, C., Jewett, H. J., and Coffey, D. S.: Computerized image analysis of nuclear shape as a prognostic factor for prostatic cancer. Prostate, *3*, 351–355, 1982.

Epstein, J. I., Berry, S. J., and Egglestone, J. C.: Nuclear roundness factor: A predictor of prognosis in untreated stage A2 prostate cancer. Cancer, *54*, 1666–1671, 1984.

Fordham, M. V. P., Burge, A. H., Matthews, J., Williams, G., and Cooke, T.: Prostatic carcinoma cell DNA content measured by flow cytometry and its relation to clinical outcome. Br. J. Surg., *73*, 400–403, 1986.

Forsslund, G., and Zetterberg, A.: Ploidy level determination in high-grade and low-grade malignant variants of prostatic carcinoma. Cancer Res., *50*, 4281–4285, 1990.

Greene, D. R., Taylor, S. R., Wheeler, T. M., and Scardino, P. T.: DNA ploidy by image analysis of individual foci of prostate cancer: a preliminary report. Cancer Res., *51*, 4084–4089, 1991.

Henke, R. P., Kruger, E., Ayhan, N., Hubner, D., and Hammerer, P.: Numerical chromosomal aberrations in prostate cancer: correlation with morphology and cell kinetics. Virchow's Arch. (A), *422*, 61–66, 1993.

Helpap, B.: Cell kinetics and cytological grading of prostatic carcinoma. Virchows Arch (Pathol. Anat.), *393*, 205–214, 1981.

Helpap, B.: Observations on the number, size, and localization of nucleoli in hyperplastic and neoplastic prostatic disease. Histopathol., *13*, 203–211, 1988.

Helpap, B., and Otten, J.: Histologisch-cytologisches Grading von uniformen und pluriform Prostatacarcinomen. Pathologe, *3*, 216–222, 1982.

Jones, E. C., McNeal, J., Bruchovsky, N., and de Jong, G.: DNA content in prostatic adenocarcinoma. A flow cytometry study of the predictive value of aneuploidy for tumor volume, percentage Gleason grade 4 and 5, and lymph node metastases. Cancer, *66*, 752–757, 1990.

Kallioniemi, O. P., Visakorpi, K., Holli, K., Heikkinen, A., Isola, J., and Koivula, T.: Improved prognostic impact of S-phase values from paraffin embedded breast and prostate carcinoma after correcting for nuclear slicing. Cytometry, *12*, 413–421, 1991.

Koss, L. G.: The puzzle of prostatic carcinoma (Editorial). Mayo Clin. Proc., *63*, 193–197, 1988.

Koss, L. G., and Czerniak, B.: Image analysis and flow cytometry of tumors of prostate and bladder. With a comment on molecular biology of urothelial tumors. *In* Weinstein, R., and Gardner, W. A., Jr. (Eds.) Pathology and Pathobiology of the Urinary Bladder and Prostate. Baltimore, Williams & Wilkins, 1992.

Leistenschneider, W., and Nagel, R.: Atlas of Prostatic Cytology. Berlin and New York, Springer, 1984.

Lieber, M. M.: Prostatic dysplasia: Significance in relation to nuclear DNA ploidy studies of prostate adenocarcinoma. Urology, *34 (Suppl.)*, 43–48, 1989.

Lu-Yao, G. L., McLerran, D., Wasson, J., and Wennberg, J. E.: An assessment of radical prostatectomy. Time trends, geographic variation, and outcomes. J.A.M.A., *269*, 2633–2636, 1993.

Macoska, J. A., Micale, M. A., Sakr, W. A., Benson, P. D., and Wolman, S. R.: Extensive genetic alterations in prostate cancer revealed by dual PCR and FISH analysis. Genes, Chromosom. Cancer, 8, 88–97, 1993.

Micale, M. A., Sanford, J. S., Powell, I. J., Sakr, W. A., and Wolman, S. R.: Defining the nature of cytogenetic events in prostatic adenocarcinoma: paraffin FISH vs. Metaphase analysis. Cancer Genet. Cytogenet., 69, 7–12, 1993.

Miller, G. J., and Shikes, J. L.: Nuclear roundness as a predictor of response to hormonal therapy of patients with stage D2 prostatic carcinoma. In Karr, J. P., Coffey, D. S., and Gardner, W. (Eds.): Prognostic Cytometry and Cytopathology of Prostate Cancer. New York, Elsevier, 1988, pp. 349–354.

Miller, J., Horsfall, D. J., Marshall, V. R., Rao, D. M., and Leong, A. S-Y.: The prognostic value of deoxyribonucleic acid flow cytometric analysis in stage D2 prostatic carcinoma. J. Urol., 145, 1192–1196, 1991.

Mohler, J. L., Partin, A. W., Lohr, D. W., and Coffey, D. S.: Nuclear roundness factor measurement for assessment of prognosis of patients with prostatic carcinoma. I. Testing of digitization system. J. Urol., 139, 1080–1084, 1988.

Montgomery, B. T., Nativ, O., Blute, M. L., Farrow, G. M., Myers, R. P., Zincke, H., Therneau, T. M., and Lieber, M. M.: Stage B Prostate adenocarcinoma. Flow cytometric nuclear DNA ploidy analysis. Arch. Surg., 125, 327–331, 1990.

Nativ, O., and Lieber, M. M.: Prostatic carcinoma: Prognostic importance of static and flow cytometric nuclear DNA ploidy measurements. J. Urol., 178–183, 1991.

Nativ, O., Myers, R. P., Farrow, G. M., Therneau, T. M., Zincke, H., and Lieber, M.: Nuclear deoxyribonucleic acid ploidy and serum prostate specific antigen in operable prostatic carcinoma. J. Urol., 144, 303–306, 1990.

Nativ, O., Winkler, H. Z., Raz, Y., Therneau, T., Farrow, G. M., Myers, R. P., Zincke, H., and Lieber, M. M.: Stage C prostatic adenocarcinoma: flow cytometric nuclear DNA ploidy analysis. Mayo Clin. Proc., 64, 911–919, 1989.

Nemoto, R., Kawamura, H., Miyakawa, I., Uchida, K., Hattori, K., Koiso, K., and Harada, M.: Immunohistochemical detection of proliferating cell nuclear antigen (PCNA/cyclin) in human prostate adenocarcinoma. J. Urol., 149, 165–169, 1993.

Palazzo, J. P., Ellison, D., and Petersen, R. O.: DNA content in prostate adenocarcinoma. Correlation with Gleason score, nuclear grade and histologic subtypes. J. Urol. Path., 1, 283–292, 1993.

Partin, A. W., Carter, H. B., Epstein, J. I., and Coffey, D. S.: The biology of prostate cancer: new and future directions in predicting tumor behavior. In Weinstein, R. S., and Gardner, W. A. (Eds.): Pathology and Pathobiology of the Urinary Bladder and Prostate. Baltimore, Williams & Wilkins, 1992. pp. 198–218.

Partin, A. W., Walsh, A. C., Pitcock, R. V., Mohler, J. L., Epstein, J. I., and Coffey, D. S.: A comparison of nuclear morphometry and Gleason grade as a predictor of prognosis in stage A2 prostate cancer. A critical analysis. J. Urol., 142, 1254–1258, 1989.

Petersen, R. O.: Urologic Pathology. 2nd Ed. Philadelphia, J. B. Lippincott, 1992.

Rönström, L., Tribukait, B., and Esposti, P. L.: DNA pattern and cytological findings in fine-needle aspirates of untreated prostatic tumors. A flow-cytofluorometric study. Prostate, 2, 79–88, 1981.

Shankey, T. V.: Urologic cancers. In Bauer, K. D., Duque, R. E., Shankey, T. V. (Eds.): Clinical Flow Cytometry. Principles and Applications. Baltimore, Williams & Wilkins, 1993, pp. 271–305.

Sprenger, E., Volk, L., and Michaelis, W. E.: The significance of nuclear DNA measurements in the diagnosis of prostatic carcinomas. Beitr. Pathol., 153, 370–378, 1974.

Stephenson, R. A., James, B. C., Gay, H., Fair, W. R., Whitmore, W. F., Jr., and Melamed, M. R.: Flow cytometry of prostate cancer: relationship of DNA content to survival. Cancer Res., 47, 2504–2507, 1987.

Tardif, C. P., Partin, A. W., Qaqish, B., Epstein, J. P., and Mohler, J. L.: Comparison of nuclear shape in aspirated and histologic specimens of prostatic carcinoma. Anal. Quant. Cytol. Histol., 14, 474–482, 1992.

Tribukait, B.: DNA flow cytometry in carcinoma of the prostate for diagnosis, prognosis and study of tumor biology. Acta Oncologica, 30, 187–192, 1991.

Tribukait, B.: Flow cytometry in surgical pathology and cytology of tumors of the genito-urinary tract. In Koss, L. G., and Coleman, D. V. (Eds.). Advances in Clinical Cytology, Vol. 2, New York, Masson, 1984, pp. 163–189.

Tribukait, B.: Flow cytometry in assessing the clinical aggressiveness of genito-urinary neoplasms. World J. Urol., 5, 108–122, 1987.

Wasson, J. H., Cushman, C. C., Bruskewitz, R. C., Littenberg, B., Mulley, A. G. J., and Wennberg, J. E.: A structured literature review of treatment for localized prostate cancer. Arch. Fam. Med., 487–493, 1993.

Winkler, H. Z., Rainwater, L. M., Myers, R. P., Farrow, G. M., Therneau, J. M., Zincke, H., and Lieber, M. M.: Stage D1 prostatic adenocarcinoma: significance of nuclear DNA ploidy patterns studied by flow cytometry. Mayo Clin. Proc., 63, 103–112, 1988.

Zetterberg, A.: Stability of diploid genome in carcinoma of the prostate with long follow up. WHO Consensus Meeting on Prostatic Carcinoma. Stockholm, 1993.

Zetterberg, A., and Esposti, P. L.: Cytophotometric DNA-analysis of aspirated cells from prostatic carcinoma. Acta Cytol., 20, 46–57, 1976.

Zetterberg, A., and Esposti, P. L.: Prognostic significance of nuclear DNA levels in prostatic carcinoma. Scand. J. Urol. Nephrol. (Suppl.), 55, 53–58, 1980.

Renal Tumors

Baish, H., Koppel, G., and Otto, U.: DNA analysis in renal neoplasia. In Eble, J. N. (Ed.). Tumors and Tumor-like Conditions of the Kidney and Ureter. New York, Churchill Livingstone, 1990, pp. 250–251.

Banner, B. F., Erstoff, M. S., Bahnson, R. R., Titus-Erstoff, L., and Taylor, S. R.: Quantitative DNA analysis of small renal cortical neoplasms. Hum. Pathol., 22, 247–253, 1991.

Bibbo, M., Galera-Davidson, H., Dytch, H. E., González de Chaves, J., Lopez-Garrido, J., Bartels, P. H., and

Wied, G. L.: Karyometry and histometry of renal-cell carcinoma. Anal. Quant. Cytol. Histol., 9, 182–187, 1987.

Chin, J. L., Pontes, J. E., and Frankfurt, O. S.: Flow cytometric deoxyribonucleic acid analysis of primary and metastatic human renal cell carcinoma. J. Urol., 133, 582–585, 1985.

Currin, S. M., Lee, S. E., and Walther, P. J.: Flow cytometric assessment of deoxyribonucleic acid content in renal adenocarcinoma. Does ploidy status enhance prognostic stratification? J. Urol., 143, 458–463, 1990.

deKernion, J. B., Mukamel, E., Ritchie, A. W. S., Blyth, B., Hannah, J., and Bohman, R.: Prognostic significance of the DNA content of renal carcinoma. Cancer, 64, 1669–1673, 1989.

deKernion, J. B., Ramming, K. P., and Smith, R. B.: The natural history of metastatic renal cell carcinoma: a computer analysis. J. Urol., 120, 148–152, 1978.

Ekfors, T. O., Lipasti, J., Nurmi, M. J., and Eerola, B.: Flow cytometric analysis of the DNA profile of renal cell carcinoma. Pathol. Res. Pract., 182, 58–62, 1987.

Farnsworth, W. V., Cohen, C., McCue, P. A., and DeRose, P. B.: DNA analysis of small renal cortical neoplasms. J. Urol. Path., 2, 65–79, 1994.

Feitz, W. F. J., Karthaus, H. F. M., Beck, H. L. M., et al.: Tissue-specific markers in flow cytometry of urological cancers. II. Cytokeratin and vimentin in renal cell tumors. Int. J. Cancer, 37, 201–207, 1986.

González-Cámpora, R., González-de Chaves, F. J., Mora-Marin, J., Rodriguez-González, R., Rubi-Uria, J., and Galera-Davidson, H.: Nuclear planimetry in renal-cell tumors. Anal. Quant. Cytol. Histol., 13, 54–60, 1991.

Grignon, D. J., Ayala, A. G., El-Naggar, A., Wishnow, K. I., Ro, J. Y., Swanson, D. A., McLemore, D., Giacco, G. G., and Guinee, V. F.: Renal cell carcinoma. A clinicopathologic and DNA flow cytometric analysis of 103 cases. Cancer, 64, 2133–2140, 1989.

Grignon, D. J., el-Naggar, A., Green, L. K., Ayala, A. G., Ro, J. Y., Swanson, D. A., Troncoso, P., McLemore, D., Giaccio, G. G., and Guinee, V. F.: DNA flow cytometry as a predictor of outcome in stage I renal cell carcinoma. Cancer, 63, 1161–1165, 1989.

Kloeppel, G., Knoefel, W. T., Baisch, H., and Otto, U.: Prognosis of renal cell carcinoma related to nuclear grade, DNA content, and Robson stage. Europ. Urol., 12, 426–431, 1986.

Ljungberg, B., Forsslund, G., Stenling, R., and Zetterberg, A.: Prognostic significance of the DNA content in renal cell carcinoma. J. Urol., 135, 422–426, 1986.

Ljungberg, B., Larsson, P., Stenling, R., and Roos, G.: Flow cytometric deoxyribonucleic acid analysis in stage I renal cell carcinoma. J. Urol., 146, 697–699, 1991.

Ljungberg, B., Stenling, R., and Roos, G.: DNA content in renal cell carcinoma with reference to tumor heterogeneity. Cancer, 56, 503–508, 1985.

Ljungberg, B., Stenling, R., and Roos, G.: Prognostic value of deoxyribonucleic acid content in metastatic renal cell carcinoma. J. Urol., 136, 801–804, 1986.

Nativ, O., Winkler, H. Z., Reiman, H. M., and Lieber, M. M.: Squamous cell carcinoma of the renal pelvis: nuclear deoxyribonucleic acid ploidy studied by flow cytometry. J. Urol., 144, 23–26, 1990.

Oosterwij, E., Warnaar, S. O., Zwartenduk, J., van der Velde, E. A., Fleuren, G. J., and Cornelisse, C. J.: Relationship between DNA ploidy, antigen expression and survival in renal cell carcinoma. Int. J. Cancer, 42, 703–708, 1988.

Rainwater, L. M., Farrow, G. M., Hay, I. D., and Lieber, M. M.: Oncocytic tumours of the salivary gland, kidney, and thyroid: Nuclear DNA patterns studied by flow cytometry. Br. J. Cancer, 53, 799–804, 1986.

Rainwater, L. M., Farrow, G. M., and Lieber, M. M.: Flow cytometry of renal oncocytoma: common occurrence of deoxyribonucleic acid polyploidy and aneuploidy. J. Urol., 135, 1167–1171, 1986.

Rainwater, L. M., Hosaka, Y., Farrow, G. M., and Lieber, M. M.: Well differentiated clear cell carcinoma: significance of nuclear deoxyribonucleic acid patterns studied by flow cytometry. J. Urol., 137, 15–20, 1987.

Rainwater, L. M., Hosaka, Y., Farrow, G. M., Kramer, S. A., Kelalis, P. P., and Lieber, M. M.: Wilms tumors: relationship of nuclear deoxyribonucleic acid ploidy to patient survival. J. Urol., 138, 974–977, 1987.

Shankey, T. V.: Urologic cancers. In Bauer, K. D., Duque, R. E., and Shankey, T. V. (Eds.): Clinical Flow Cytometry. Principles and Applications. Baltimore, Williams & Wilkins, 1993, pp. 271–305.

Tosi, P., Luzi, P., Baak, J. P. A., Mirraco, C., Santopietra, R., Vindigni, C., Mattei, F. M., Acconcia, A., and Massai, M. R.: Nuclear morphometry as an important prognostic factor in stage I renal cell carcinoma. Cancer, 58, 2512–2518, 1986.

Von Willebrand, E.: Fine needle aspiration cytology of renal transplants: Background and present applications. Transplant Proc., 17, 2071–2074, 1985.

Wolman, S. R., Catmuto, P. M., Golimbu, M., and Schinella, R.: Cytogenetic, flow cytometric and ultrastructural studies of twenty-nine nonfamilial human renal carcinomas. Cancer Res., 48, 2890–2897, 1988.

Adrenal Tumors

González-Cámpora, R., Diaz-Cano, S., Lerma-Puertas, E., Rios-Martin, J. J., Salguero-Villadiego, M., Villar-Rodriguez, J. L., Bibbo, M., and Davidson, H. G.: Paragangliomas. Static cytometric studies of nuclear DNA patterns. Cancer, 71, 820–824, 1993.

Hosaka, Y., Aso, Y., Rainwater, L. M., Grant, C. S., Farrow, G. M., van Heerden, J. A., and Lieber, M. M.: Flow cytometric DNA histograms of paraffin-embedded pheochromocytomas. Urologia Internat., 47, 100–103, 1991.

Hosaka, Y., Rainwater, L. M., Grant, C. S., Farrow, G. M., Heerden, J. A., and Lieber, M. M.: Pheochromocytoma: nuclear deoxyribonucleic acid pattern studied by flow cytometry. Surgery, 100, 1003–1009, 1986.

Lai, M. K., Sun, C. F., Chen, C. S., Huang, C. C., Chu, S. H., and Chuang, C. K.: Deoxyribonucleic acid flow cytometric study in pheochromocytomas and its correlation with clinical parameters. Urology, *44*, 185–188, 1994.

Nativ, O., Grant, C. S., Sheps, S. G., O'Fallon, J. R., Farrow, G. M., van Herden, J. A., and Lieber, M. M.: The clinical significance of nuclear DNA ploidy pattern in 184 patients with pheochromocytoma. Cancer, *69*, 2683–2687, 1992A.

Nativ, O., Grant, C. S., Sheps, S. G., O'Fallon, J. R., Farrow, G. M., van Herden, J. A., and Lieber, M. M.: Prognostic profile for patients with pheochromocytoma derived from clinical and pathological factors and DNA ploidy pattern. J. Surg. Oncol., *50*, 258–262, 1992B.

Padberg, B. C., Achilles, E., Garbe, E., Dralle, H., Kloppel, G., and Schroder, S.: Histology, immunocytochemistry and DNA cytophotometry of adrenal gland pheochromocytoma (PCC)—a morphologic clinical study of 64 tumors (in German). Verh. Deutsch. Ges. Path., *74*, 289–294, 1990.

Pang, L. C., and Tsao, K. C.: Flow cytometric DNA analysis for the determination of malignant potential in adrenal and extra-adrenal pheochromocytomas or paragangliomas. Arch. Path. Lab. Med., *117*, 1142–1147, 1993.

CHAPTER 10

Immunohistology and Immunocytology of the Urinary Tract

Walter Nathrath, M.D.

Immunochemical methods have become well established in the diagnostic examination of cells and tissues since the 1980s. The identification of specific poly- or monoclonal antibodies, reacting with biochemically characterized cell epitopes (antigens), adds a molecular aspect to microscopic analysis and is often of diagnostic value.

Most markers currently used for diagnostic purposes define components of the cell membrane or the cytoplasm, and are associated with events in cell or tissue differentiation (Table 10-1). Lymphocytic antigens and intermediate filament proteins are examples of such markers. Other markers identify extracellular products of normal or pathologic origin, such as collagens or amyloids. Another group of markers, expressed either in the nucleus, the cytoplasm or the cell membrane, is linked to normal or neoplastic growth. Examples include proliferation markers, tumor suppressor antigens, or growth factor receptors. Finally, some markers are used for the identification of infectious agents (*e.g.,* hepatitis B antigens).

The practical aspects of routine microscopic diagnosis require careful selection of markers in specific categories, particularly for a precise classification of poorly differentiated tumors (for review see Bander, 1987; Domagala and Osborn, 1992; Listrom and Fenoglio-Preiser, 1992). A core panel of about five to ten antibodies is generally used for initial classification of such tumors, followed, if necessary, by a second series of antibodies.

Using appropriate antibodies, virtually all antigens can now be detected equally well on either frozen or formalin fixed, paraffin-embedded tissue sections, and on cytologic preparations. Antigen unmasking, by either enzymatic methods or the recently developed microwave oven system, has significantly increased the range of antibodies that can be successfully used in routinely processed material (Shi et al., 1991; Cattoretti et al., 1993; Taylor et al., 1994; von Wasielewsky et al., 1994). It is still important, however, to identify the optimal tissue treatment for each antibody, because the results may vary widely according to the method of processing (see also the section on Methods, p. 327).

Although these general principles of immunopathology are valid in reference to the urinary tract, a large number of antibodies has been developed that deal specifically with the unique normal and neoplastic aspects of this system. These antibodies are the primary target of this chapter.

There are three main groups of markers of particular importance for the urinary tract:

1. Markers that characterize normal urothelium and form a basis for the analysis of urothelial tumors

2. Markers that are related to carcinomas and may either
   a. Help to distinguish normal from neoplastic cells
   b. Be of predictive value of tumor behavior

3. Markers that can be helpful in distinguishing between urothelial and non-urothelial tumors.

TABLE 10-1
Selected Markers in Routine Diagnostic Immunomorphology

Antigens	*Antibodies*
Differentiation Markers	
Epithelial	
All epithelia	
Broad-spectrum keratins	Iu 5 (van Overbeck et al. 1985)
	AE1/AE3 (Cooper et al. 1985)
	LP34 (Lane, Alexander 1990)
	TS8 (Sundström et al. 1988)
Restricted epithelial spectrum	
Non-epidermal epithelia	
Epithelial membrane antigen (EMA)	E 29 (Heyderman et al. 1985)
Ber EP4-antigen	BerEP4 (Latza et al. 1990)
Human epithelial antigen (HEA)	HEA 1
Simple epithelia	
Tissue polypeptide antigen (TPA)	anti-TPA (Björklund 1979;
	Nathrath et al. 1985)
Keratin 19	KS19.1; LP2k (Osborn et al.
	1985; Lane et al. 1985)
Keratin 18	LE 61 (Lane 1982)
Keratin 8	TS1 (Sundström et al. 1989)
Keratin 7	CK7 (Tölle et al. 1985)
Keratin 20	CK20 (Moll et al. 1992)
Squamous epithelia	
Keratin 4	6B10 (van Muijen et al. 1986)
Keratin 13	KS13.1 (Moll et al. 1988)
Keratin 10	
Keratin 14	LLoo1 (Purkis et al. 1990)
Oncofetal epithelia	
Carcinoembryonic antigen (CEA)	(Hammarström et al. 1989)
Alpha-fetoprotein (AFP)	(Abelev 1974)
Cell Type Specific	
Prostate-specific antigen (PSA)	(Oesterling 1991)
Prostate-specific and phosphatase (PSAP)	(Oesterling 1991)
Beta HCG	(Braunstein et al. 1973)
Endocrine	
Broad Spectrum	
Chromogranin	(Wilson and Lloyd 1984)
gamma neuron-specific enolase (NSE)	(Schmechel 1985)
pHe 5	(Riddell et al. 1987)
Synaptophysin	(Gould et al. 1987)
Hormone receptors	
Estrogen receptor	(Greene et al. 1980)
Progesterone receptor	(Logeat et al. 1983)
Hormone specific	
Gastrin	(Larsson et al. 1974)
Bombesin	(Polak et al. 1978)
5-hydroxytryptamine	(Facer et al. 1979)
Neuroglial	
Neural	
Neuron-specific enolase	(Tapia et al. 1981)
Neurofilament	(Debus et al. 1983a)
Glial	
Glial fibrillary acidic protein (GFAP)	(Debus et al. 1983a)
Neurocrest	
S–100 protein	(Nakajima et al. 1982)
Melanoma antigen	AMB-45 (Gown et al. 1986)

TABLE 10-1 *(Continued)*

Antigens	*Antibodies*
Mesenchymal	
Broad spectrum	
Vimentin	(Osborn et al. 1984)
Cell type specific	
Macrophage antigen	MAC 387
Muscle	
Desmin	DE-A-7 (Debus et al. 1983b)
Smooth muscle antigen (sMA)	HHF35 (Tsukada et al. 1987)
Vascular	
Endothelin	CD31
Factor VIII–related antigen	(Mukai et al. 1980)
Lymphoid	
Broad spectrum	
CD45	T200 (Warnke et al. 1983)
Restricted spectrum	
CD20 (B cells)	LE26 (Cartun et al. 1987)
CD 3 (T cells)	CD3
Cell type specific	
Ig kappa/lambda	
Growth-Associated Markers	
Proliferation Markers	
Ki 67	MiB–1 (Key et al. 1993)
PCNA	PC10 (Waseem, Lane 1990)
Growth Factor Receptors	
Epidermal growth factor receptor (EGFR)	528 (Kawamoto et al. 1983)
Oncogenes	
c–erb B 2	NCL CB11 (Corbett et al. 1990)
Tumor suppressor antigens	
p 53 antigen	CM1 (Midgley et al. 1992)
Intercellular Substance	
Normal	
Collagens	
Laminin	
Pathological	
Amyloids	
Infectious Organisms	
Viral Antigens	
Hepatitis B antigens	
Bacterial Antigens	
Fungal Antigens	

MARKERS ASSOCIATED WITH UROTHELIAL DIFFERENTIATION

Epithelial Markers

Epithelial markers have been described as a result of three different pathways of investigation: the search for tumor-specific antigens (Björklund, 1958; Gold and Freedman, 1965; Nathrath et al., 1983); the search for organ-specific antigens (Ceriani et al., 1977; Nathrath, 1978; Nathrath et al., 1979; Heydermann et al., 1979) and the study of cytoplasmic structural components, mainly the intermediate filaments. The latter approach led to the identification of keratins (Franke et al., 1978; Sun and Green, 1978).

Keratins

Keratins are the most important group of intermediate filaments representative of epithelial antigens. They comprise at least 20 different polypeptides and belong to two genetically closely related intermediate filament protein families: type I (acidic) and type II (basic). At least one member of each family is expressed in any epithelium, resulting in various combinations depending on the epithelial type and on the state of epithelial differentiation (Moll et al., 1982; Sun et al., 1984; Moll et al., 1992). For example, keratins 8 and 18 are found in all simple, non-stratifying epithelia; many simple epithelia also express keratin 19 (for example, intestinal epithelium) and 7 (for example, ducts of glands). The recently identified keratin 20 is almost entirely restricted to the gastric foveolar cells and to the intestinal epithelium, the urothelium, and Merkel cells of the epidermis (Moll et al., 1992). Keratins 5 and 14 are characteristic of all stratified squamous epithelia, which also express another pair of keratins, depending on their level of differentiation: thus, keratins 1 and 10 are expressed in cornifying epithelium, keratins 4 and 13 in non-cornifying stratified epithelium, and keratins 6 and 16 in abnormally proliferating squamous epithelium (Moll et al., 1982; Sun et al., 1984; van Muijen et al., 1986).

KERATINS IN NORMAL UROTHELIUM

Keratins 7, 8, 18, 19 and 20, corresponding to simple epithelia, and keratins 4, 5, 13 and 17, common to stratified epithelia, have been identified in normal human urothelium (Moll et al., 1982; Achtstätter et al., 1985; Cooper et al., 1985; Quinlan et al., 1985; Table 10-2). Keratins 7 and 19 can be demonstrated throughout the entire urothelium. Different antibodies to keratins 8 and 18 show different staining patterns in normal urothelium, *i.e.*, either an extensive immunostaining in all cell layers or a more restricted, umbrella cell-related pattern, thus reflecting quantitative differences of their respective epitopes (Ramaekers et al., 1985; Schaafsma et al.,

1990). Keratin 20 is found almost exclusively in the umbrella cells (Moll et al., 1992) (Fig. 10-1). Keratins 13 and 4 (the latter in only trace amounts) are expressed in all urothelial cells, except in the umbrella cells (Fig. 10-2) (Achtstätter et al., 1985; Ramaekers et al., 1985; Rheinwald and O'Connell, 1985; Moll et al., 1988; Moll, 1989; Schaafsma et al., 1990; Moll, 1991). This pattern is unique: the keratins of the umbrella cells are entirely of the simple epithelial type (keratins 7, 8, 18, 19, and 20), comparable to the pattern of gastric epithelial cells lining gastric pits. On the other hand, the cells from the deeper urothelial layers combine the features of non-cornifying stratified epithelium (keratins 4, 13) and of simple intestinal tract epithelium, such as the biliary and pancreatic ducts (keratins 7, 8, 18, 19).

It should be emphasized that the expression of keratins in normal urothelium differs from other stratified epithelia. Keratin 14, characteristic of all (or sometimes only the basal cells) of the stratified squamous epithelium, is not detected (Moll et al., 1988; Schaafsma et al., 1990). The expression pattern of keratin 4 is not related to that of keratin 13, as is customary in non-cornifying squamous epithelia (Moll et al., 1988; Schaafsma et al., 1990). The expression of keratin 13 in the urothelium does not follow the patterns observed in other stratified epithelia such as the esophagus (Moll et al., 1982; Sun et al., 1984; Cooper et al., 1985; Lane et al., 1985; van Muijen et al., 1986). Conversely, in the urothelium the deeper cell layers express keratin 13 (see Fig. 10-2) as an indication of squamous cell differentiation. Moll et al. (1988) have pointed out that this feature may be related to the ability of the urothelium

TABLE 10-2
Keratins (K) and Uroplakin III in Normal and Neoplastic Urothelium

Antigens	Normal urothelium		Urothelial carcinoma					
	UMBRELLA CELLS	DEEPER LAYERS	PAPILLARY			NON-PAPILLARY		SQUAMOUS CELL
			pTa	*pT1*	*pT2/3*	*CIS*	*invasive*	
K4	−	−/+	−/+	−/+	−	−/+	−	+/−
K7	++	++	++	++	+/−	+	−/+	−/+
K 8/18	++	+	++	++	+	+	−/+	−/+
K 10	−	−	−	−	−	−	−	+/−
K 13	−	++	−/+	−/+	−/+	−/+	−/+	+
K 14	−	−	−	−	−/+	−	−/+	+
K 19	++	++	++	+	+	+	−/+	−/+
K 20	++	−	++	++	−/+	+/−	−/+	−
Uroplakin III	++	−	+	+	−/+	n.d.	n.d.	n.d.

Abbreviations: pTa, pT1, pT2/3, papillary tumors according to stage; *CIS*, carcinoma in situ; Level of expression indicated by none (−), slight (+/−), moderate (+), and high (++); n.d. not done.

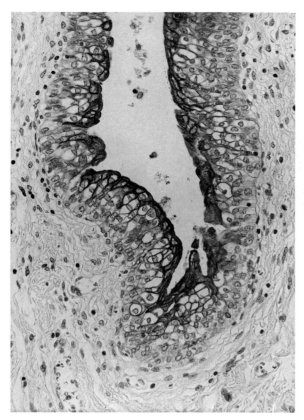

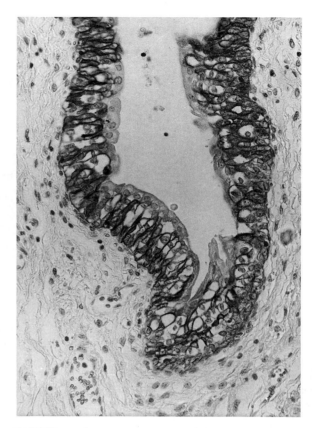

FIGURE 10-1. Keratin 18. Normal urothelium. The staining is confined almost exclusively to umbrella cells. This staining pattern is the same as that for keratin 20.

FIGURE 10-2. Keratin 13. Normal urothelium. The staining is confined exclusively to the lower cell layers.

to develop squamous metaplasia (Hicks, 1975; Koss, 1975a; Koss, 1975b; Hicks and Chowaniec, 1978).

KERATINS IN UROTHELIAL CARCINOMAS

Non-invasive papillary carcinomas, carcinomas in situ, and invasive carcinomas, including poorly differentiated carcinomas, are reactive with all the broad spectrum keratin antibodies, usually in a diffuse pattern (Nathrath et al., 1982b; Ramaekers et al., 1985; Sanchez-Fernandes de Sevilla et al., 1992). By gel electrophoresis all carcinomas contain the simple epithelium-type keratins 7, 8, 18, 19, and 20. Stratified epithelium-type keratins, such as keratins 17 and 13, are found in variable amounts or only occasionally. Keratins 4, 5, 6, 10, 14, and 16 are found only in trace amounts (Achtstätter et al., 1985; Moll et al., 1988; Moll, 1991).

In non-invasive papillary tumors, keratins 8, 18, and 20 tend to be expressed more strongly in super-

ficial cells (obviously, an equivalent of the normal umbrella cells). Such keratins are also expressed in deeper cells of less–well-differentiated, non-invasive papillary carcinomas, and by all cells of *in situ* and frankly invasive carcinomas (Fig. 10-3) (Achtstätter et al., 1985; Ramaekers et al., 1985; Moll et al., 1988; Cintorino et al., 1988; Schaafsma et al., 1990; Moll, 1991). On the other hand, keratin 13 is expressed only by rare cells in high grade carcinomas or in their metastases (Fig. 10-4) (Moll et al., 1988; Nathrath, 1988; Schaafsma et al., 1989; Schaafsma et al., 1990; Moll, 1991). An increasing level of expression of keratin 14 was reported in higher grade and stage urothelial carcinomas (Schaafsma et al., 1990).

Rare high grade carcinomas express only the simple epithelium-type keratins. Such tumors cannot be distinguished immunologically from some adenocarcinomas of other organs, such as the breast and pancreas (Moll et al., 1988; Schaafsma et al., 1990).

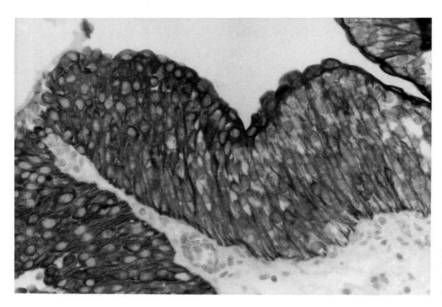

FIGURE 10-3. Keratin 18. Urothelial carcinoma in situ of the bladder. There is staining of all carcinoma cells.

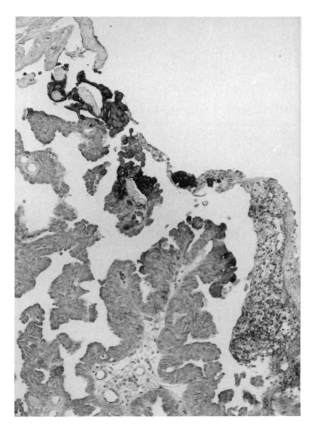

FIGURE 10-4. Keratin 13. Papillary carcinoma of the bladder. The staining is focal and confined to isolated cell clusters.

Surprisingly, with increasing level of malignancy, some urothelial carcinomas show a decrease of keratin 13 expression (see Fig. 10-4), and an appearance of keratin 14 with a simultaneous increase in the number of cells expressing keratins 18 and 20 (see Fig. 10-3). Such tumors are immunologically comparable to the normal umbrella cells. These findings suggest that these carcinomas either originate from well-differentiated neoplastic cells or express a disorderly umbrella cell–type differentiation, as hypothesized by Ramaekers et al. (1985) and Moll et al. (1988).

Urothelial carcinomas with foci of squamous metaplasia and pure squamous cell carcinomas of the urinary tract express an increased amount of the keratins 4, 6, 16, and 17 of the stratified epithelial type (see Table 10-2). In single cells of these tumors even the epidermal differentiation keratins 1, 2, 10, 11, and 14 can be seen. These tumors also maintain keratin 13 expression and focally express the simple epithelial keratins 7, 8, 18, and 19, and are thus different from squamous carcinomas of many other organs (Achtstätter et al., 1985; Fukushima et al., 1987; Moll et al., 1988; Nathrath, 1988; Schaafsma et al., 1990; Moll, 1991).

These observations suggest that urothelial carcinoma may differentiate in the direction of either squamous carcinoma (keratin 13) or umbrella cells (keratin 20).

Diagnostic Application of Keratin Antibodies in Urinary Tract Tumors

The dual nature of urothelial carcinomas with respect to keratin molecules may be helpful in the differential diagnosis of metastasis. The expression of keratin 20 and (although in small amounts) of keratin 13 suggests urothelial origin of poorly differentiated metastatic tumors (Moll et al., 1988). Within the urinary tract, the urothelium-specific keratin 20 allows the distinction between urothelial carcinoma and prostatic or renal carcinomas that do not express it (see Table 10-9). Immunostaining may also be helpful in distinguishing a squamous carcinoma of urothelial origin from other similar tumors (Moll et al., 1988).

Analogously, in urinary immunocytology, the demonstration of keratins 8, 18, and particularly keratins 13, 14, and 20 in tumor cells could be used to distinguish between urothelial and non-urothelial neoplasms. Quantitative changes of these keratins in urothelial cancer cells may conceivably be of prognostic value, using the quantitative immunocytological (QUIC) approach, as proposed by Huland and coworkers for the antibody 486 p3/12 (Huland et al., 1990; Klän et al., 1991). Another quantitative approach is with image analysis of cell products, which was discussed in Chapter 9.

It is also possible that the studies of keratin expression may identify early neoplastic changes in mapping biopsies of the bladder. For example, demonstration of keratins 8, 18, and 20 in deeper urothelial layers may indicate a malignant transformation. Careful analyses of keratin staining patterns are still needed with regard to urothelial carcinoma differentiation (grading), growth patterns (papillary versus non-papillary), and behavior (invasive versus non-invasive). Differences in keratin expression also may be of prognostic value in urothelial carcinomas.

Keratin Antibodies Useful In Urinary Tract Tumor Analysis

More than 120 monoclonal keratin-antibodies are now being used for typing of epithelial cells (Lane and Alexander, 1990). Antibodies that are either mono- or polyspecific, i.e., reactive with one or more than one keratin type, are available. Most monoclonal antibodies recognize a definable type or subtype of epithelial tissues. The most important distinction is between antibodies that react with simple epithelia but not with stratified squamous epithelia, as these usually contain non-overlapping sets of keratins. There are only a few antibodies that are "pan-epithelial." We have found that the antibodies discussed in this section work well on formalin-fixed, paraffin-embedded material and on urine cytology specimens (see Table 10-1).

PAN-EPITHELIAL ANTIBODIES

AE1 (against keratins 10, 14, 15, 16, and 19), AE3 (against keratins 1–8), keratin cocktail (Cooper et al., 1985), Lu5 (Von Overbeck et al., 1985), and LP34 (Lane et al., 1985) recognize keratins common to all epithelial cells. LP34 requires microwave oven treatment (Lane and Alexander, 1990). All these antibodies recognize all cell layers of normal urothelium and are also reactive with virtually all urothelial carcinomas. They can be used to identify epithelial cells in normal tissues and in tumors and can distinguish a carcinoma from a non-epithelial tumor (Osborn and Weber, 1986).

MONOSPECIFIC KERATIN ANTIBODIES

The following monoclonal antibodies identify individual keratin markers (see Table 10-2): TS1 for keratin 8 (Sundström et al., 1989), RGE 53 for keratin 18 (Herman et al., 1983), Ks 7.18 for keratin 7 (Bartek et al., 1991b), Ks 19.1 for keratin 19 (Karsten et al., 1985), Ks 13.1 for keratin 13 (Moll et al., 1988), and Ks 20.8 for keratin 20 (Moll et al., 1992).

Other Epithelial Markers

In addition to keratins, several other epithelial markers have been discovered (Nathrath, 1978; Heyderman et al., 1979; Nathrath et al., 1979; Wilson et al., 1982). Most of them show a broad spectrum of staining distribution patterns (Nathrath et al., 1982a; Nathrath et al., 1985).

TISSUE POLYPEPTIDE ANTIGEN

Tissue polypeptide antigen (TPA) was the first tumor marker described (Björklund et al., 1958) that has been extensively used for clinical serologic monitoring of tumor patients. Immunohistochemically, TPA was shown to be an epithelium-specific differentiation antigen present in almost all simple and stratified epithelia with the notable exception of epidermis and hepatocytes. Thus, its distribution is comparable to that of other broad spectrum epithelial antibodies, including those that react with keratins characterizing simple epithelia, such as keratin 19 (Nathrath et al., 1982a; Nathrath et al., 1983; Nathrath et al., 1985). TPA is also expressed in all cell layers of the normal urothelium and in all grades of urothelial carcinomas (Nathrath et al., 1983; Senatore et al., 1987). Biochemically, TPA represents keratins 8, 18, and 19 (Weber et al., 1984) or fragments of keratins 8 and 18 (Leube et al., 1986).

EPITHELIAL MEMBRANE ANTIGEN

Epithelial membrane antigen (EMA) is a glycoprotein (Mw 265–400 kd) originally purified from the membrane of human milk fat globules (Ceriani et al., 1977). Poly- and monoclonal antibodies show a widely distributed, epithelium-specific reactivity that includes the urothelium (Heyderman et al., 1979;

Heyderman et al., 1984; Heyderman et al., 1985). These antibodies do not stain hepatocytes and show only irregular staining in squamous epithelia. Staining for EMA is typically cell membrane–associated. Staining also has been observed in plasma cells, other lymphocytes, and macrophages. EMA has been found in most carcinomas but also in some mesenchymal tumors, including sarcomas and lymphomas. Thus, the EMA is of limited value in the differential diagnosis of tumors, although it gives a characteristic staining pattern in mesothelioma (Leong et al., 1990). Poorly differentiated and invasive urothelial carcinomas express EMA in the cell membrane and also show strong cytoplasmic staining (Takashi et al., 1987; Sanchez-Fernandez de Sevilla et al., 1992).

HEA 125 AND BER-EP4 ANTIGENS

The two monoclonal antibodies HEA 125, raised against the colon carcinoma cell line HT29 (Momburg et al., 1987), and Ber-EP4, raised against the breast carcinoma cell line MCF-7 (Latza et al., 1990), apparently recognize a neighboring or identical epitope of the same antigen within the protein moiety of two 34- and 39-kd glycopeptide chains (Latza et al., 1990). The antigen is different from carcinoembryonic antigen (CEA), EMA, and keratins. Immunohistologically, it is present on the cell surface of almost all normal epithelia, including the urothelium, but it is not found in the epidermis, mesothelium, hepatocytes, or parietal gastric epithelial cells. Antibody reactivity has been seen with most epithelial neoplasms, but not with malignant mesotheliomas (Momburg et al., 1987; Latza et al., 1990).

In the diagnosis of urinary tract lesions, the antibodies described above recognize virtually all cells of normal and neoplastic urothelium and therefore play essentially the same role as the panepithelial keratin antibodies.

Urothelium-Specific Markers

Urothelium-Specific and Urothelial Membrane Antigen

The existence of a urothelium-specific antigen in the human was first demonstrated immunohistochemically by absorption studies of a polyclonal antiserum raised against calf bladder urothelium (Nathrath, 1978; Nathrath et al., 1979; Nathrath et al., 1982). Urothelium-specific staining was found on the surface of umbrella cells of the normal fetal and adult human urothelium, suggestive of localization in the glycocalix of the asymmetric unit membrane (AUM)

(Hicks, 1965; Hicks and Ketterer, 1969; Hicks, 1975). Bovine, mouse, rat, and hamster (but not guinea pig) urothelium, human bladder biopsy specimens, and cell lines of human urothelial carcinomas (Nathrath et al., 1979; Nathrath and Franks, 1981), also showed staining.

Subsequently, a *urothelial membrane antigen* has been identified by a polyclonal antibody raised against a preparation of the AUM of calf urothelium (Trejdosiewicz et al., 1984). The antigen was found to be a predominantly membrane-associated peptide of cross-species reactivity. This peptide is approximately 54 kd in size and is localized by light and electron microscopy in normal luminal urothelial cells and in human bladder carcinoma cell lines (Trejdosiewicz et al., 1984).

Uroplakins I–III (see Table 10-2)

Uroplakin I, II, and III, three distinct proteins of 15, 27, and 47 kd, respectively, were isolated from the asymmetrical unit membrane (AUM) of bovine urothelium using gradient centrifugation (Wu et al., 1990; see Table 10-2). Monospecific polyclonal antibodies to these three proteins found that all of them are AUM-associated. Uroplakins I and II were detected exclusively on the luminal side of the mature apical AUM. Uroplakin III is a transmembrane glycoprotein with a core-protein (28.9 kilodaltons) and sugar molecules attached to it (Wu et al., 1990; Yu et al., 1990; Surya et al., 1990; Moll et al., 1993; see also Chapter 2).

Using a polyclonal antiserum against uroplakin III, Moll and coworkers found that this protein was urothelium-specific and that the apical membrane staining pattern seen in normal urothelial umbrella cells was partially maintained in cell clusters of metastatic urothelial carcinoma. The membranes of cytoplasmic vesicles (which are also lined by AUM; see Chapter 2) also showed staining (Moll et al., 1993). Positive reaction (sometimes focal) was found in routine histologic sections in 16 of 18 papillary noninvasive urothelial carcinomas (89%), in 21 of 37 invasive carcinomas (57%), and in 12 of 15 metastases (80%). Only two out of 70 urothelial carcinomas did not show any reaction. All non-urothelial carcinomas were consistently negative (Moll et al., 1993).

Although it is of intermediate sensitivity, mainly because of its overall weak but very specific staining pattern, uroplakin III can be expected to serve as a marker of urothelial differentiation.

The application of this antibody to diagnostic urine cytology should yield favorable results. An expression of uroplakin III is comparable to keratin 20 and to the 486 P3/12-antigen (Huland et al., 1990).

MARKERS CHARACTERIZING UROTHELIAL TRANSFORMATION

Blood Group–Related Antigens

ABO-Related Antigens

The blood group antigens A, B, and H(O) are either glycoproteins or glycolipids, their fundamental constituent being a backbone precursor carbohydrate chain of type 1 or type 2 (Table 10-3). This carbohydrate backbone is converted into type 1 or type 2 H-substance, an important intermediate structure, and then into A or B determinants, by sequential specific transferase-mediated addition of fucose and N-acetyl galactosamine or D-galactose, respectively (Sheinfeld et al., 1992). These antigens are present on erythrocytes, endothelial cells, and the cells of many epithelial tissues (Szulman, 1962). The expression in the latter, as in serum, urine and secretions, depends on the secretory-gene–controlled fucosylation of the precursor chain into H-substance. Therefore, this antigen is absent on the urothelium of non-secretors (Cordon-Cardo et al., 1988; Sheinfeld et al., 1992). Most individuals (80%) are secretors and express H-, A-, or B-antigens on their urothelium. These antigens have been demonstrated immunohistochemically in the luminal zone of the umbrella cells and in nearly all basal and intermediate cells (Szulman, 1962; Juhl, 1985; Cordon-Cardo et al., 1986) (see Table 10-3).

In 1961, Kay and Wallace reported a correlation between the absence of ABO antigens and anaplasia in biopsies of bladder, suggesting that the test was of prognostic value. Using human anti A and B serum, and Ulex europaeus 1 agglutinin (UEA-1) for H-antigen with a red cell adherence (RCA) or peroxidase visualization technique, some observers reported that tumors expressing blood group antigens were less likely to become invasive than negative tumors (DeCenzo et al., 1975; Weinstein et al., 1979; Newman et al., 1980; Limas and Lange, 1980; Weinstein et al., 1981; Coon and Weinstein, 1981; Orihuela et al., 1987).

Applying the RCA test to bladder washing specimens from patients with recurrent multifocal superficial bladder carcinomas, Orihuela and coworkers found a correlation of ABO negativity with aneuploidy. ABO negativity also correlated with the potential of the urothelium to form new tumors and with the likelihood of invasion. BCG-treatment induced a prognostically favorable conversion of marker expression. Lack of such conversion was predictive of persistent disease, regardless of type or stage of the initial tumor (Orihuela et al., 1987).

Other investigators, however, have failed to confirm that these markers have any clinical relevance (Kovarik et al., 1968; Davidsohn, 1979; Gynter et al., 1983). Studies with monoclonal antibodies to ABO antigens have demonstrated a variable relationship between antigen expression and histologic grade of urothelial carcinomas. The prognostic value was either partial (Summers et al., 1983; Juhl et al., 1986; Cordon-Cardo et al., 1988; Limas, 1993) or none (Pauwels et al., 1988; Aprikian et al., 1993). These conflicting results may be explained in part by methodologic factors, including differences in tissue preparation technique, in visualization and quantification of antigen expression (Coon and Weinstein, 1981; Yamase et al., 1981; Juhl, 1985; Juhl et al., 1986; Sheinfeld et al., 1992). Secretor status obviously determines the expression of the major blood group antigens on both normal and neoplastic epithelial cells, necessitating the separation of patients into different ABO secretor groups (Juhl et al., 1986; Cordon-Cardo et al., 1986; Cordon-Cardo et al., 1988).

Recent studies have emphasized the complexity of

TABLE 10-3
Blood Group–Related Antigens

	Normal Urothelium		Urothelial Carcinoma Stages				
	UMBRELLA CELLS	BASAL CELLS	pTA	pT1	pT2	pT3/4	CIS
ABO	++	+	+	+	−	−	−/+
Lewis X	+	−	+	+/−	+/−	+/−	+
Thomsen-Friedenreich							
Tcr +	+	−	+	+/−	−	−	+/−
T +	−	−	−	−/+	+	+/−	−/+

++, strong reaction; +, moderate/minimal reaction; −, no reaction; pTa, pT1, pT2, pT3/4, papillary tumors according to stage; CIS, carcinoma in situ.

the ABO phenotypes and the interdependence among the various blood groups. Part of this complexity is based on either suppression of active or activation of quiescent glycosyltransferases, resulting in deletion of ABO antigens in secretors. Such events may also result in accumulation of precursor structures that are not normally present, or aberrant synthesis of Lewis X-antigen, or, in non-secretors, of H-, Lewis b-, or Lewis y-antigens (Cordon-Cardo et al., 1986; Cordon-Cardo et al., 1988; Limas, 1993; Sheinfeld, 1993). Furthermore, other cell markers have been found to be altered in synchrony with changes in the blood group antigens. Thus, a strong expression of epidermal growth factor receptor and elevated proliferation indices have been found to be associated with blood group antigen depression and severe atypia of cancer cells (Limas, 1993). A study of blood group antigen expression and of other markers may be useful, particularly in secretor individuals with the ABO antigens deletion (Summers et al., 1983; Coon and Weinstein, 1986; Orihuela et al., 1987; Cordon-Cardo et al., 1988; Limas, 1993).

Lewis X-Related Antigen

Lewis X-related antigen (LeX), an oncodevelopmental antigen also known as the X-hapten or stage-specific mouse embryonic antigen (SSEA-1) (Solter and Knowles, 1978; Hakomori, 1985), is formed by the 1-3 fucosylation of a type 2 blood group backbone chain. This antigen is expressed on human granulocytes (but not on erythrocytes) independently from the secretor status, and on some normal epithelial cells, including renal tubules (Magnani, 1984; Cordon-Cardo et al., 1986).

Normal urothelium is negative for the LeX, with the exception of occasional umbrella cells (see Table 10-3) (Cordon-Cardo et al., 1986; Cordon-Cardo et al., 1988; Sheinfeld, 1993). LeX is associated with a variety of human adenocarcinomas and urothelial carcinomas (Hakomori, 1985; Taki et al., 1988; Hoff et al., 1989; Shirahama et al., 1992). Using a monoclonal antibody against SSEA-1, a correlation was found between the expression of this antigen with stage, grade, and lymph node metastases of urothelial carcinomas (see Table 10-3) (Shirahama et al., 1992). Similar observations were made with the fucose-binding proteins (FBP) of *Lotus tetragonolobus*-lectin (Shirahama et al., 1991). LeX antigen is expressed in over 90% of bladder tumors regardless of histologic grade, stage, secretory status, or clinical behavior (Cordon-Cardo et al., 1988).

In a cytologic study, using the monoclonal LeX antibody P-12 as a cancer detection system on cells in bladder lavage specimens from about 300 bladder

carcinoma patients, Sheinfeld et al. found a high level of diagnostic sensitivity when the two methods were combined. The LeX immunocytologic expression was a predictor of tumor recurrences in disease-free, high-risk patients with prior superficial bladder carcinoma (Sheinfeld et al., 1990; Sheinfeld, 1992).

These results suggest that LeX immunostaining may be useful in cytopathology of the urinary sediment, and may assist in the detection of low grade urothelial tumors that are difficult to identify in routine cytology (Aprikian et al., 1993; see also Chapter 5). The observations are comparable to similar findings, with antibodies G4 (Chopin et al., 1985), M344 (Fradet et al., 1987), or 486 P3/12 (Huland et al., 1987), which apparently recognize either the LeX or a related antigen (Fradet, 1990; Fradet et al., 1990b). These antibodies are discussed in more detail later in this chapter (see Tumor-Associated Antigens, p. 305).

Thomsen-Friedenreich–Related Antigen (T-antigen)

Thomsen-Friedenreich–related antigen (T antigen) is a neuraminic-acid–shielded disaccharide (galactose/N-acetylgalactosamine) that was originally found on pathologically agglutinating erythrocytes, wherein it is carried on the major intrinsic membrane protein, glycophorin. This peptide is shared with the MN blood group antigens; it provides the hapten for the T-epitope, represented by three distinctly antigenic glycoproteins of 39, 42, and 46 kd, recognized by the T-specific monoclonal antibody HH8 (Langkilde et al., 1992). There appears to be slight staining differences among the different T-antibodies (Springer, 1983; Longenecker et al., 1984; Clausen et al., 1988; Langkilde et al., 1992). Strong differences, however, are recognized with the peanut agglutinin, which reacts in part with the same epitopes as the HH8 antibody, but also with several other high molecular weight molecules (Langkilde et al., 1992).

Neuraminidase treatment of tissue sections uncovers the shielded form of the T-antigen (Rauvala and Finne, 1979). There are three possible expressions of the T-antigen: reactivity only after neuraminidase treatment (the cryptic T-antigen, Tcr+), reactivity without pretreatment (the overt T-antigen, T+), and no reactivity, regardless of pretreatment (negative T, Tcr−) (Coon and Weinstein, 1986). The T+ phenotype is expressed in only some normal cells, such as some lymphocytes and macrophages, whereas the Tcr+ is much more common in normal cells and tissues, and is expressed on erythrocytes, endothelial cells, and many mesenchymal and epithelial tissues, including normal urothelium (Coon and Weinstein, 1986).

In normal urothelium, the Tcr+ can be demonstrated in the umbrella and intermediate cells, but not in the basal cells (Juhl et al., 1987; Langkilde et al., 1992). Many human carcinoma cells express the unmasked phenotype (T+), suggesting that T-antigen expression may be an adjunct to conventional histology in assessing borderline lesions of the bladder as either benign or malignant (Summers et al., 1983). Similar observations were made on breast tissue (Springer et al., 1975; Springer, 1983). There is agreement that T staining of urothelial carcinomas correlates with stage and grade: Tcr+ antigen expression is predominant in low-grade tumors, whereas T+ and Tcr− phenotypes increase with increasing grade of tumors. T expression may be deleted (Tcr−) from areas of high grade and invasive carcinomas (Summers et al., 1983; Lehmann et al., 1984; Coon and Weinstein, 1986; Juhl et al., 1987; Langkilde et al., 1992). Measurements of T antigen expression were found to be of value in predicting subsequent recurrence in patients with low grade and stage urothelial carcinomas, particularly when associated with negative blood group expression and chromosomal abnormalities (Summers et al., 1983; Coon and Weinstein, 1986). In other hands, T staining was not significantly correlated with the clinical course of urothelial carcinomas (Longenecker et al., 1984; Lehman et al., 1984; Juhl et al., 1987). Thus, the molecular specificity and clinical value of the T-reagents is not clear (Langkilde et al., 1992). Further investigation in combination with other markers may be of interest (Summers et al., 1983).

UROTHELIAL TUMOR–ASSOCIATED ANTIGENS

The antibodies of the urothelial tumor–associated antigens were raised against urinary bladder carcinomas and carcinoma cell lines in the search for tumor specific markers (Nathrath et al., 1979). Although the immunohistochemical staining products of most of these antibodies are strongly expressed in urothelial carcinomas, the corresponding antigens also occur in normal urothelium.

A large number of such monoclonal antibodies have been described by different investigators. However, the extent to which the relevant epitopes have been characterized differs widely from one group to the other. Some of these antibodies may be related to the Lewis X-blood group antigen (Fradet et al., 1990).

Well-Characterized Antigens

M344 and 19A211 Antigens as Markers of Early Malignant Transformation

The markers M344 and 19A211 appear to be restricted to early stages of urothelial carcinoma. Both are sialoglycoproteins, of approximately 300 and 200 kd molecular weight, respectively, that were identified using monoclonal antibodies raised by simultaneous active immunization against intact grade 1 papillary carcinoma cells and passive immunization with normal urothelium (Fradet et al., 1987; Fradet et al., 1990b). Both antigens have been found to be distinct from other high-molecular-weight and mucin-like antigens, such as the major blood group antigens, EMA, or CEA (Cordon-Cardo et al., 1992). Immunohistologically, both antigens are stable and well preserved on deparaffinized tissue sections (Cordon-Cardo et al., 1992). Normal urothelium does not stain except for rare umbrella cells (Huland et al., 1991; Cordon-Cardo et al., 1992; Fradet, 1993). Both antibodies display a patchy reactivity in squamous metaplasia of the urothelium (Cordon-Cardo et al., 1992). M344 shows no or only weak reactivity, and 19A211 shows consistent staining of renal tubules (Huland et al., 1991; Cordon-Cardo et al., 1992). Both antibodies react with a few cells of occasional low-grade carcinomas of colon and breast. M344 also reacts with some prostatic and endometrial carcinomas (Cordon-Cardo et al., 1992). The expression of the 19A211 antigen on cervical condylomas and carcinomas suggests an association with a viral etiology for some bladder cancers. Human papillomavirus (HPV) 16 DNA sequences have been detected in a significant proportion of bladder tumors (Fradet et al., 1992), although this issue is a subject of a considerable debate.

In urothelial carcinomas, both markers are expressed mainly by low-grade superficial papillary tumors (Table 10-4). They are expressed on approximately 80% of Ta and T1 tumors but on only 15% of muscle-invading carcinomas. The frequency of antigen expression also decreases with increasing tumor grade (Fradet et al., 1987). The staining behavior of the two antibodies is not always identical. For example, only 2% of carcinoma in situ lesions coexpress both antigens, whereas 17% express M344 and 50% express 19A211 (Cordon-Cardo et al., 1992). The presence of M344 and 19A211 antigens on exfoliated cells from previously treated but currently tumor-free patients appears to be predictive of tumor recurrence (Fradet et al., 1993). It has also been suggested that these antigenic changes may provide tools to monitor the effects of chemotherapy (Fradet et al., 1992).

TABLE 10-4
Urothelial Tumor–Associated Antigens

Antibody	Immunogen	Antigen	Normal Urothelium		Urothelial Carcinoma					Other Tissues		Reference
			UMBRELLA CELLS	DEEPER LAYERS	pTA	pT1	pT2	pT3/4	CIS	NORMAL	NEOPLASTIC	
M344	Papillary carcinoma	300-kd sialoglycoprotein	-/+	-	+/-	+	-/+	-	-/+	-	Different carcinomas	Cordon-Cardo et al., 1992a
19A211	Papillary carcinoma	200-kd sialoglycoprotein	-/+	-	+/-	+	-/+	-/+	+/-	Renal tubules	Different carcinomas	Cordon-Cardo et al., 1992a Huland et al., 1991a
BL2-10D1	Papillary carcinoma	Non-protein	-/+	-	+	+/-	-/+	-	+	Squamous cells		Longin et al. 1989
486 P3/12	486P	200-kd glycoprotein	-/+	-	+/-	+	-/+	-	+/-	Renal tubules, granulocytes		Huland et al. 1991a
Due ABC3	SW1710	Glycolipid	-/+	-/+						Renal tubules, granulocytes	Renal cell carcinoma	Decken et al. 1992
T43	Papillary carcinoma	85-kd glycoprotein	-	-	-/+	-/+	+	+	-/+	Renal tubules	Different carcinomas	Fradet 1993
T138	Papillary carcinoma	25-kd sialoglycoprotein	-	-	-/+	-/+	+	+	-/+	Endothelial	Different carcinomas	Fradet 1993

Symbols represent the reaction most often reported: + +, considerable reaction; +, moderate/minimal reaction; -, no reaction; -/+ and +/-, degrees of slight reaction. For other abbreviations, see Table 10–3.

M344 expression on superficial papillary tumors may also be predictive of recurrence (Fradet et al., 1993). The predictive value of M344 staining was further increased when it was combined with the identification of the oncogene Ha-*ras* point mutations, found in 40% of the tumors in Fradet's 1993 report. In this group, recurrences were observed in 75% of the M344-positive and in only 14% of the M344-negative cases. On the other hand, in the tumors containing the wild type (non-mutated) Ha-*ras* gene, M344 staining had no predictive value (Fradet et al., 1993). When combined with DNA ploidy measurements and cytology, the M344 sensitivity for low-grade tumors was 88%, and for high grade tumors 95% (Bonner et al., 1993).

BL2-10D1 Antigen

The monoclonal antibody BL2-10D1 is another marker of early malignant transformation. This antigen, raised against human bladder carcinoma, reacts with 5% to 10% of umbrella cells (see Table 10-4) and in a variable fashion with normal squamous cells (Longin et al., 1990). Preliminary data suggest that the antigenic determinant is not a protein. This marker is expressed mainly by low-grade papillary tumors and carcinomas in situ of the urothelium. High-grade papillary and invasive non-papillary urothelial carcinomas show only poor reactivity (Longin et al., 1989).

BL2-10D1 is of great interest in immunocytology, because specific immunostaining has been reported on exfoliated urinary cells in all patients with a grade 1 papillary carcinoma, carcinoma in situ, or dysplastic lesions, whereas a variable or no reactivity has been found in urinary sediment from patients with grade 2 and 3 carcinomas (Longin et al., 1990). Similar results have been obtained in a flow cytometric study (Hijazi et al., 1989). Furthermore, a combination of the BL2-10D1 antibody and standard cytology has been reported to be more accurate than either method alone, determining the presence of tumor cells before and after immunotherapy (Chicheportiche et al., 1993). The staining distribution of this antigen is similar to that of the LeX, M344, and 486 P3/12 antigens (Chicheportiche et al., 1993).

T43 and T138 Antigens

T43 and T138 have been classified as cancer-progression markers (Fradet et al., 1990; Fradet et al., 1992; see Table 10-4). Both show a reactivity in 15% to 20% of superficial tumors and in 60% of invasive urothelial carcinomas. The antigens are also DNA-ploidy–dependent and are expressed in 15% of diploid and 60% of aneuploid tumors (Fradet et al., 1993). Some important points must be considered separately for each of these antigens:

T43 antigen is an 85-kd surface glycoprotein that can be detected on fresh or frozen cells, but not on formalin-fixed tissues. Most normal tissues and benign epithelia are negative, but the antigen is found in metabolically active cells of the proximal tubules of the kidney and in the basal cell layer of stratified squamous epithelia. Carcinomas of various origins express T43 antigen.

T138 antigen is a 25-kd surface glycoprotein, which is restricted in normal tissues to endothelial cells. It is also expressed on a few primary non-urothelial tumors. In urothelial carcinomas, it is particularly valuable in dividing invasive bladder cancers into progressor and non-progressor groups. Moreover, 4 of 5 patients with Ta- or T1-tumors that later progressed to invasive or metastatic stage were T138-positive when initially analyzed (Fradet et al., 1990; Bretton et al., 1990; Fradet et al., 1992; Fradet and Cordon-Cardo, 1993). A correlation has been suggested between the rapidity of cancer progression and the increased proportion of T138 positive cells within the initial sample. The value of T138 antigen as a clinical cancer progression marker in primary tumors was documented in a prospective study of 38 patients with more than 2 years of follow-up (Fradet et al., 1990). Fifty-six percent of the patients with T138-positive tumor samples developed metastases or died of bladder cancer, in contrast with only 5% of those whose samples were T138-negative. T138 antigen is also expressed in most non-urothelial metastatic carcinomas of different types, suggesting that it may be involved in the metastatic process (Fradet et al., 1992). Although it has been found to be a better prognostic indicator than the DNA-ploidy status, the combination of ploidy and T138 expression was also predictive of survival. Death rate of bladder cancer at 2 years ranged from 0% for patients with diploid, T138-negative tumors to 63% for aneuploid, T138-positive tumor samples. For further comments on DNA ploidy in bladder tumors, see Chapter 9.

486 P3/12 Antigen

486 P3/12 antigen, identified by a mouse monoclonal antibody raised against the urothelial carcinoma cell line 486p, is a 200-kd glycoprotein, related to, but not identical to, CEA and NCA-1 (Arndt et al., 1987; see Table 10-4). It has been suggested that the 486 P3/12 antibody recognizes an LeX-related antigen (Fradet, 1990; Chicheportiche et al., 1993). The antigen can be demonstrated in single umbrella cells of the normal urothelium, in granulocytes, and in epithelium of normal kidney, stomach, and breast.

The antigen is also found in renal, gastric, and mammary carcinomas (Arndt et al., 1987). Furthermore, tumor cells in about 90% (17 of 19) of urothelial carcinomas expressed the 486 P3/12-antigen (Arndt et al., 1987). An increased 486 P3/12 antigen expression was shown to be associated with decreased expression of ABO(H)-antigen and with deletion of T-antigen not only in urothelial carcinomas but also in adjacent epithelium that appeared histologically benign. This observation suggested that patterns of abnormal antigen expression may identify cells with potential for tumor development or recurrence (Heinzer et al., 1992).

The diagnostic value of this antigen was evaluated by Huland et al. with a "quantitative immunocytology" (QUIC)-approach (Huland et al., 1987; Arndt et al., 1987). In each urinary sediment, 100 urothelial cells were counted and the percentage of cells reactive with the 486 P3/12 antibody was noted. With an arbitrary threshold established at 30% positive cells, it was possible to discriminate between cancer and non-cancer groups (Huland et al., 1990).

To document that this approach was also effective with low-grade tumors, Huland et al. (1990) studied 241 unselected patients with urothelial tumors. In this group standard cytology was positive in 59.2%, 63.8%, and 84.7% for grade 1, 2, and 3 tumors, respectively. The corresponding DNA flow cytometry in the first 69 patients of this population showed abnormalities in only 27.7%, 48.6%, and 57.1%, respectively. The QUIC test, however, was positive in 91.8%, 98.4%, and 92.9% for the three tumor grades (Huland et al., 1990; Klän et al., 1991).

Huland et al. (1990) also used the QUIC approach to identify patients who were not at risk of recurrence. Voided urinary specimens were examined at 4-weekly intervals after transurethral resection of Ta- and T1 bladder tumors. In 22 of 55 patients who remained negative with the QUIC procedure, only 2 developed recurrent tumors, which were also negative for 486 P3/12. Of the 33 patients who had positive results at least once during the 2 years of monitoring, 14 developed a recurrent tumor within 2 to 5 months after the initial positive immunocytologic test.

False-positive QUIC tests were observed in patients with renal stones (Huland et al., 1991a). The QUIC method shows high sensitivity but low specificity and is not likely to be of prognostic value, because it is equally sensitive in all tumor grades. Further developments in the application of the 486 P3/12 antigen may be of interest and may prove to be of clinical value (Huland et al., 1991b; Droller, 1990; Oyasu, 1990). The QUIC method may be applicable to other antibodies, such as antibodies against keratin 20 and uroplakins.

Other Markers Identifying Urothelial Tumors

A number of other monoclonal antibodies directed against bladder tumor–associated antigens has been described during the last decade, but none of them has been characterized as extensively as the antibodies just described. Among antibodies raised against bladder carcinoma cell lines or tumor cells, the antibodies RBS-31, RBS-85, RBA-1, and HBP-1 reacted more strongly with urine samples from bladder cancer patients than with those from normal subjects, as estimated by ELISA (Grossman, 1983; Masuko et al., 1984; Masuko et al., 1989; Trejdosiewicz et al., 1985; Montgomerie et al., 1992; Masuko et al., 1989).

It has been suggested that some of these antibodies (but also 486 P3/12, A7, G4, and BL2-10D1), recognize the LeX blood group antigen (Fradet, 1990; Chicheportiche et al., 1993). The following sections describe some of these antibodies.

G4 and A7 Antigens

The G4 and A7 antigens were identified by the G4 and A7 antibodies raised against bladder carcinoma and were found to recognize occasional umbrella cells in the normal urothelium (Hijazi et al., 1993). In view of the suggestion that both antibodies recognize LeX-antigen (Fradet, 1990), they may have similar properties to the BL2-10D1 antibody (Longin et al., 1989; Longin et al., 1990; Hijazi et al., 1993). Both antibodies were shown to detect malignant urothelial cells in bladder washings in 78% of patients with bladder carcinomas, whereas bladder washings of non-tumor patients and from those without evidence of a tumor recurrence did not show any specific staining (Chopin et al., 1985). In a flow-cytometric analysis, these antibodies preferentially labeled cells from high-grade urothelial carcinomas (Hijazi et al., 1993).

LBS Antigens

Eleven monoclonal antibodies were raised in mice against the human urothelial carcinoma cell line RT112 and divided into three groups according to their reactivity with a panel of cell lines. Two antibodies were "panepithelial" (group I), four antibodies were restricted to human urothelial cells (group II), and five reacted with human and murine urothelial cell lines (group III) (Trejdosiewicz et al., 1985). The group II antibodies reacted predominantly with well-differentiated urothelial carcinoma cell lines, whereas the group III antibodies failed to react. These data suggest that the LBS series may be of value in characterizing normal and neoplastic urothelial cells (Trejdosiewicz et al., 1985). Huland et al. (1991a) compared some of the LBS antibodies with the 486

P3/12 antibody (discussed earlier in this chapter) on urine samples from patients with bladder carcinoma, prostatic hypertrophy, and renal stones and found a similarity between some of the LBS antibodies and the 486 P3/12 antibody.

28K Antigen

An antigen of 28-kd molecular weight was identified by a monoclonal antibody within the umbrella cells of normal urothelium, in squamous metaplasia, in squamous cell carcinomas of the bladder, and in basal cells of the epidermis (Montgomerie et al., 1992). This distribution differs from that of another 28-kd protein, which was derived from Mano cells and localized in the basal layer, but not in the umbrella cells of normal urothelium (Arndt et al., 1987).

Leu-M1 Antigen

Leu-M1 antigen was originally recognized by the monoclonal antibody Leu-M1 directed against a human histiocytic cell line (Hanjan et al., 1982; Hsu and Jaffe, 1984), and subsequently has been identified as the 3-fucosyl N-acetyllactamine (CD15) antigen. It is used as a marker of myeloid differentiation and is also found in non-hematopoietic neoplasms, including urinary bladder carcinomas (Pinkus and Said, 1986; Sanders et al., 1988). However, there is no significant correlation with the grade or stage of urothelial carcinomas (Hoshi et al., 1986). Recent studies suggest that the CD15 antigen is identical with the LeX antigen (Sheinfeld et al., 1992).

Due ABC 3 Antigen

The Due ABC 3-antigen was identified by a mouse monoclonal antibody, raised against the human bladder carcinoma cell line SW 1710 (see Table 10-4). Preliminary results disclosed that the antigen is a neutral glycolipid of the cell membrane, stable after formaldehyde fixation and paraffin embedding and different from the CD15 or LeX antigens (Decken et al., 1992).

The Due ABC 3-antigen was present in normal urothelium in 7 of 25 samples, only in the umbrella cells in some of those. It also has been found in proximal tubular epithelium of the kidney, and in some gastrointestinal epithelia, in normal granulocytes, in ovarian and breast carcinomas, and in 7 out of 12 renal cell carcinomas examined (Decken et al., 1992).

Using this antibody in a quantitative evaluation of voided urinary specimens with a cutoff value of 20% antigen positive urothelial cells, 49 of 74 specimens (66%) from patients with urothelial carcinomas were classified correctly, whereas conventional cytology was positive in only 35 of these specimens (47%). However, the results were impaired by purulent exu-

date, because of staining of granulocytes (Schmitz-Dräger et al., 1991; Decken et al., 1992). Specificity of conventional cytology (92%) was higher when compared to immunocytology (58%). The sensitivity of the combined analysis of conventional cytology and Due ABC 3 immunocytology was higher than conventional cytology alone, but specificity remained the same. The clinical evaluation of this antibody awaits further work, particularly in the recognition of low-grade urothelial tumors (Schmitz-Dräger et al., 1991).

CELL ADHESION MARKERS

E-cadherin

E-cadherin is the epithelial member of the cadherin molecule family, each member of which displays a unique tissue distribution, *e.g.*, E-cadherin (epithelial), P-cadherin (placental), N-cadherin (neural), and L-CAM (liver cell adhesion molecule) (Table 10-5). The cadherins belong to the group of adhesion molecules together with integrin, selectin, and immunoglobulins (Takeichi, 1991). Cadherins are glycoproteins of cell membrane, of between 80 and 120 kd molecular weight and between 723 and 748 aminoacids, with an extracellular, a membranous, and a cytoplasmic domain. The extracellular domain contains the binding site for calcium, which protects the molecule from proteolysis. The cytoplasmic domain forms complexes with caterins and cytoskeletal elements. The proper anchorage to these molecules is a prerequisite for the cell-binding function of the extracellular domain of cadherin (Takeichi, 1991). Several lines of evidence indicate that the cell-adhesiveness, mediated by cadherins, is critically important for morphogenesis and integrity of the normal structure and function of adult tissues. A relationship between suppressed cadherin function and the invasive capacity of tumors has recently received strong support (Behrens et al., 1989; Eidelman et al., 1989; Shiozaki et al., 1991; Vleminckx et al., 1991; Becker et al., 1993; Becker et al., 1994).

Using monoclonal and polyclonal antibodies (*e.g.*, HECD-1: Shiozaki et al., 1991; anti GP-80: Eidelman et al., 1989) on frozen sections, E-cadherin (CAM 120/80) was found in all normal epithelial tissues, and two distinct staining patterns were noted. A nonpolarized staining along the cell circumference was seen in squamous epithelia and the urothelium, while a polarized lateral cell border expression was found in ductal and glandular epithelia (Eidelman et al., 1989). E-cadherin expression in many carcinomas was reduced and heterogeneous, the polarization was less

TABLE 10-5
Distribution of Adhesion Molecules and CEA

		Normal Urothelium	Low Stage: pTa/pT1	High Stage: pT2–4
E-Cadherin		Membranous expression at all cell borders, except umbrella surface, basal aspect of basal cells[*]	Disturbed expression (decreased/heterogeneous/cytoplasmic/negative) 21% (5/24)[*,†]	76% (19/25)[*,†]
			Disturbed expression also correlates with increased tumor grade and shortened survival	
Integrin beta 1	alpha 1	No expression		7% (2/28)
	alpha 2	Mainly membranous; basal cells more than luminal cells	46% (6/13)[*,‡]	24% (8/34)[*,‡]
	alpha 3		77% (10/13)[*,‡]	68% (19/28)[*,‡]
	alpha 4	No expression		No expression
	alpha 5			10% (3/31)[*,‡]
	alpha 6 (α6β4)	Co-localization polarized at the basal and lateral junction side of basal cells	α6β4 { Nonpolarized overexpression on basal and suprabasal cells; 5/6[*,§]	Severe disturbance of co-localization of integrin (often increased) and collagen VII (often lost)
Collagen VII (C VII)			C VII { Unchanged expression: polarized on basal cells only	83% (25/30)[*,§]
Carcinoembryonic antigen (CEA)		Rarely expressed (luminal)	Expression increases with grade and stage	

[†] Reactive cases; percentage and/or absolute figures: first number = tumors reactive; second number = tumors investigated
[*] Bringuier et al., 1993
[§] Liebert et al., 1994a
[‡] Liebert et al., 1994b

pronounced, and in some tumors the staining was located in the cytoplasm. These observations suggested a reduced cell adhesiveness in cancer (Eidelman et al., 1989; Shiozaki et al., 1991).

In urothelial carcinomas, the RT4 and RT112 cell lines express E-cadherin and are not invasive, whereas the EJ24 cell line does not express E-cadherin and is invasive (Frixen et al., 1991). Immunohistologically, normal human urothelium shows a homogeneous expression of E-cadherin with a typical membranous staining at cell-cell borders. The luminal membranes of the umbrella cells are devoid of staining, as is the part of cells in contact with the basement membrane (Eidelman et al., 1989; Bringuier et al., 1993). Abnormal staining patterns (negative, cytoplasmic, or heterogeneous) were found in 5 of 24 (21%) of low-stage tumors, and in 19 of 25 (76%) of invasive tumors. This strong correlation with tumor stage seems to indicate that a disturbance of E-cadherin expression may play a role in bladder tumor invasiveness. Most invasive tumors were composed of positive and negative areas (Bringuier et al., 1993; see Table 10-5).

A strong correlation between decreased E-cadherin staining and survival in bladder cancer has been noted, and thus may be of prognostic value. Conversely, conservation of normal E-cadherin staining pattern appears to indicate a relatively good prognosis, even if the tumor is at an advanced stage. Given the low rate of progression of superficial papillary bladder tumors (about 4%) to invasive cancer, a large scale prospective study is needed to accurately evaluate the clinical application of E-cadherin immunostaining in bladder tumor biopsies and urine samples (Bringuier et al., 1993).

Integrins

The integrins, another of the families of adhesion molecules, are transmembrane heterodimers of noncovalently associated alpha and beta subunits (see Table 10-5). There are at least eight different subfamilies of integrins, each with a common beta subunit capable of combining with various alpha subunits (Hynes, 1992). They function as receptors for extracellular molecules and can be segregated broadly into those that bind primarily to major constituents of the basement membrane (collagens, laminin), those that bind primarily to extracellular matrix proteins (fibrinogen, fibronectin, thrombospodin), and those that function as cell–cell adhesion molecules (found primarily on leukocytes). Because of these functions, integrins have been suspected of participating in progression of tumors (Albelda, 1993).

Following the development of monoclonal antibodies to specific alpha and beta subunits (Albelda, 1993; Liebert et al., 1993), the distribution of integrins has been investigated immunohistochemically in normal and neoplastic tissues. The cells of most tissues express the beta 1 integrins and alpha 1, alpha 2, alpha 3, and alpha 6, involved in adhesion to basement membrane proteins. In a number of studies of tumors, the integrin expression was heterogeneous but showed a general down-regulation (particularly of the basement-membrane protein-binding integrins) in the more aggressive neoplasms (Falcioni et al., 1988; Wolf et al., 1990; Van Waes et al., 1991; Sollberg et al., 1992; Albelda, 1993). Decreased adhesion to basement membrane or matrix molecules may be of importance in the early stages of tumor invasion. Enhanced expression of integrins on invasive and circulating tumor cells may conceivably promote metastases and aid implantation (Albelda, 1993).

Liebert and her colleagues have recently presented two studies on the expression of integrins in human urothelial carcinomas (Liebert et al., 1994a; Liebert et al., 1994b). Using monoclonal antibodies to members of the beta 1 integrin family on frozen sections of normal and malignant urothelium, they found that normal urothelium did not express alpha 1, alpha 4, and alpha 5, but showed cell membrane staining for alpha 2 and alpha 3, more strongly in the basal cell layers than in the luminal cells. This staining distribution suggested that these two integrins function as cell-to-basement membrane and as cell-to-cell adhesion molecules (Liebert et al., 1994a). The striking finding was the progressive loss of alpha 2 beta 1 expression, and less so of alpha 3 beta 1 expression, comparing Ta/T1 to T2/T3 carcinomas. Only a few high-stage carcinomas showed new expression of alpha 1 (7%) and alpha 5 (10%). The loss of alpha 2 expression may be an indication of reduced cell-to-cell adherence and of invasive potential (see Table 10-5). This altered integrin composition may play a role in the development of invasion and metastases (Liebert et al., 1994a).

The second study was concerned with the relationship between the expression of collagen VII and the alpha 6 beta 4 integrin in the hemidesmosome cell–anchoring structures in normal urothelium and in bladder carcinomas. Appropriate monoclonal antibodies were used in frozen sections (Liebert et al., 1993; Liebert et al., 1994b). Previously, the alpha 6 beta 4 integrin had been demonstrated in the hemidesmosomal anchoring complexes on the basal surface of the basal cells of normal epithelia; it was overexpressed in human carcinomas (Falcioni et al., 1988; Carter et al., 1990; Wolf et al., 1990; Sonnenberg et al., 1991; Van Waes et al., 1991). Integrin disruption combined with a disturbance of collagen VII has been suggested as a possible mechanism implicated in invasion and metastases (Sollberg et al., 1992).

In normal urothelium, the alpha 6 beta 4 integrin co-localizes with collagen VII at the junction of the basal cells and the lamina propria (Sollberg et al., 1992; Liebert et al., 1994b). In 5 of 6 non-invasive bladder tumors integrin expression was found on suprabasal and basal cells, whereas the collagen VII expression had remained unchanged at the hemidesmosomal anchoring complexes. This finding was consistent with published results on collagen VII expression in urothelial carcinomas (Wetzels et al., 1991) and suggested that the anchoring complex in low-stage tumors is normal or nearly normal (Liebert et al., 1994b). By contrast, 25 of 30 invasive bladder cancers showed either loss of integrin and/or collagen VII expression or a lack of co-localization of the two molecules (Liebert et al., 1994b; see Table 10-5). Thus, disturbance in the co-localization of these two antigens appears to be a fairly consistent event in bladder carcinomas. These changes may also explain why tumor cells may migrate (invade) and may predispose them to metastases (Wetzels et al., 1991; Liebert et al., 1994a,b). The value of these markers in diagnostic urologic immunohistology and immunocytology has yet to be evaluated.

Carcinoembryonic Antigen

Carcinoembryonic antigen (CEA), an important marker of carcinomas, originally was thought to be specifically associated with embryonic and neoplastic colon epithelium (Gold and Freedman, 1965). The antigen is a high-molecular-weight glycoprotein (180 kd), consisting of a single polypeptide chain with approximately 40 N-linked oligosaccharide chains. It shares several epitopes with other genetically related macromolecules, including the nonspecific cross-reacting antigen (NCA), the biliary glycoprotein I (BGP), and the meconium antigen (MA) (Yachi and Shively, 1989). These molecules comprise the CEA-related family with well-established cell adhesion properties (Thompson et al., 1991) and have been found to be members of the immunoglobulin superfamily. Unlike many members of the superfamily, the CEA lacks a true cytoplasmic domain (Benchimol et al., 1989). It has been suggested that the presence of excess CEA on tumor cells could interfere with the function of the normal cell-to-cell adhesion molecules (Benchimol et al., 1989; Albelda, 1993).

In a competitive inhibition assay study, the reactivities of 52 monoclonal CEA antibodies could be grouped into five essentially non–cross-reacting CEA epitope groups (GOLD 1–5), of which the GOLD 1 and GOLD 3 groups recognize the most specific CEA epitopes (Hammarström et al., 1989). Therefore, the results obtained with absorbed or unabsorbed polyclonal and monoclonal antibodies of different specificities cannot be compared. However, unabsorbed polyclonal anti-CEA antiserum is still a valuable tool in immunohistochemistry, because it indicates the total CEA-related reactivity within a tissue. Immunostaining of carcinomas with poly- and monoclonal CEA-antibodies has given essentially comparable staining patterns, confirming the initial observations about CEA distribution in tumors (Goldenberg et al., 1976; Sanders et al., 1993).

In general, CEA is expressed by nearly all adenocarcinomas, squamous cell carcinomas, and urothelial carcinomas (Goldenberg et al., 1976; Jautzke and Altenaehr, 1982; Nathrath et al., 1982; Sanchez-Fernandez de Sevilla et al., 1992; Sanders et al., 1993). CEA has been found to be absent or weak in normal urothelium and progressively more strongly expressed in dysplasia and carcinoma in situ (see Table 10-5). CEA is also associated with an increase in the degree of malignancy of papillary and invasive carcinomas: more CEA-positive cells have been observed in invasive than in superficial carcinomas. Luminal cell-membrane staining is found in areas of urothelial carcinomas showing glandular differentiation (Goldenberg and Wahren, 1978; Jautzke and Altenaehr, 1982; Nathrath et al., 1982b; Fujioka et al., 1986; Sanchez-Fernandez de Sevilla et al., 1992). Still, some investigators have found variable staining results in carcinomas of higher grade and stage (Heyderman et al., 1984) or more CEA staining in lower than in higher grade carcinomas (Wahren et al., 1977; Nathrath et al., 1982a).

Although CEA was demonstrated in the urine of patients with urothelial carcinoma (Hall, 1973), there is—to our knowledge—only one immunocytologic study of CEA in urinary sediment. Wahren and co-workers (1977) reported that in 40 patients with either a primary tumor or a recurrence 1 to 6 years after radiation treatment, bladder washings of 18 contained a variable percentage of CEA-stained tumor cells. Most of the positive cases (14 of 23) were well- and moderately differentiated tumors, compared to only 4 of the 17 poorly differentiated carcinomas.

Clearly, additional histologic and cytologic studies of urothelial carcinomas are needed with well-defined antibodies, to elucidate the role of the CEA-related antigens with regard to their diagnostic value.

PROLIFERATION MARKERS

Ki-67 Antigen

Ki-67 antigen was identified by a monoclonal antibody exclusively in the nucleus of cycling cells (G1, S, G2, M), referred to as the "growth fraction," (Gerdes et al., 1983; Gerdes et al., 1984). It is a nuclear bimolecular protein complex of molecular weight 354 and 395 kd (Gerdes et al., 1991). The Ki-67 antigen is related to an alpha polymerase, which is involved in the duplication of DNA for messenger RNA synthesis and for replicase activity (Wersto et al., 1988) and is encoded by the Ki-67 gene (MK167), which has been assigned to chromosome 10 (10q25) (Fonatsch et al., 1991).

The original Ki-67 antibody had to be used on unfixed material (Gerdes et al., 1983). The recently developed antibody MIB1, raised against a fixation resistant epitope of the Ki-67 antigen, recognizes the same epitope as the original Ki-67 antibody, and can be used on formalin-fixed, paraffin-embedded sections (Key et al., 1993) after suitable microwave oven heating for antigen retrieval (Shi et al., 1991; Cattoretti et al., 1993; Schwarting, 1993; Taylor et al., 1994). However, most studies published on urothelial tumors have used the Ki-67 antibody on frozen sections. This antibody has been employed in the studies of a large number of human cancers, in most of which the growth fraction correlated well with the tumor grade and the number of mitoses (Brown and Gatter, 1990).

Immunohistochemical Ki-67 expression on frozen sections of normal urothelium was very low; it increased somewhat in benign conditions such as inflammation and metaplasia (Limas, 1993) (Table 10-6). Moderately atypical urothelium varied widely in the expression of Ki-67, but severe atypia and carcinoma in situ consistently showed marked elevation in the numbers of stained tumor nuclei (Limas, 1993). Frozen sections of 101 bladder carcinomas of all grades and stages showed a significant correlation between the percentage of Ki-67 staining tumor cells and histologic grade, even though within each grade tumors with different proliferation indexes were observed. This may explain why bladder carcinomas of an equal histologic grade may have different levels of biologic aggressiveness. However, there was no significant correlation between proliferation and staging (Fontana et al., 1992). Furthermore, two distribution patterns of Ki-67 staining were distinguished: one in which most of the stained cells were seen in the superficial portion of the tumor, and one in which the stained cells were widely distributed and mainly localized in the basal portion of a tumor (Figs. 10-5 and

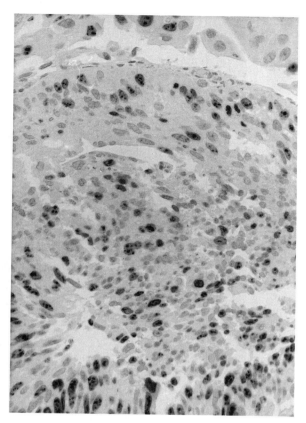

FIGURE 10-5. Ki-67 (antibody MiB1). Invasive carcinoma. Nuclear staining of carcinoma cells is seen in the area of invasion.

10-6). In invasive tumors (stages T1 to T4), the latter pattern was always present, with most of the stained cells in the area of invasive carcinoma. Of the noninvasive tumors (stage Ta), 57% showed the superficial staining pattern, and there were no recurrences at follow-up. Forty-three percent of the tumors exhibited the second pattern of staining distribution, and 94% of these cases developed a carcinoma recurrence (Fontana et al., 1992). An association between Ki-67 labeling index and p53 staining (CM1-antibody, see below) has been described in precancerous urothelium (Wagner et al., 1994). Ki-67 staining may be demonstrated in cancer cells in the urinary sediment (see Fig. 10-6). The diagnostic and prognostic value of this observation must still be established.

Proliferating Cell Nuclear Antigen

Proliferating cell nuclear antigen (PCNA) was originally identified in proliferating cells by auto-

TABLE 10-6
Frequency and Prognostic Value of Tumor Suppressor Antigens and Proliferation Markers

Nuclear Staining		Normal Urothelium	Urothelial Carcinoma					
			pTA	Carcinoma in situ		pT1		pT2–4
			Reactive Tumors	Annual Rate		Reactive Tumors	Annual Rate of Progression	
				Progression	Death			
p53-reactive tumor cells	<20%	No expression	54%* (18/33)	16.7%*	0*	42% (18/43)†	2.5%†	
	>20%		45%* (15/33)	86.7%	8.4%	58%† (25/43)	20.5%†	
		Percentage of reactive cells correlates strongly with stage, grade, and prognosis						
pRb		Suprabasal layers more than basal cells	Most cells	Heterogeneous or absent staining in approximately 30–37%‡,§ correlated with clinically aggressive tumors and with decreased long-term survival of patients				
Ki-67		Rare single cells	57%‡ staining in superficial tumor compartment‖	No recurrence‖		100%‡ staining, mainly in the basal tumor compartment‖		
			43% basal compartment‖	94% recurrence‖				
		Percentage of reactive cells correlates with grade but not with stage‖						
PCNA		Rare single cells	Percentage of reactive cells correlates with grade but not with stage¶					

* Sarkis et al. 1994
† Sarkis et al. 1993
‡ Tumors reactive
§ Cordon-Cardo et al. 1992b; Logothetis et al. 1992
‖ Fontana et al. 1992
¶ Cohen et al. 1993; Krüger et al. 1993; Lipponen et al. 1993

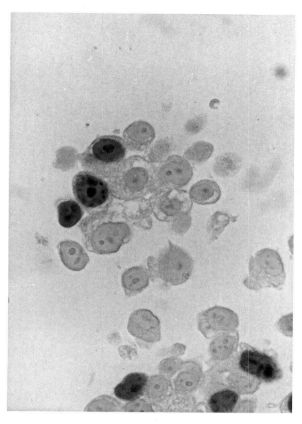

FIGURE 10-6. Ki-67 (antibody MiB1). Exfoliated cells of a high-grade papillary carcinoma. Nuclear staining of some of the malignant cells is shown.

antibodies from patients with systemic lupus erythematosus (Miyachi et al., 1978). It is an evolutionary, highly conserved, 36-kd acidic nuclear protein associated with polymerase-delta in the cell cycle during DNA synthesis (Suzuka et al., 1989; Bravo et al., 1987; Prelich et al., 1987; Hall et al., 1990; McCormick et al., 1992). The distribution of PCNA increases through G1, is predominantly expressed during the G1/S-phase interface, and decreases during G2. It is lowest in the M-phase and is virtually undetectable in G0 cells (Morris and Mathews, 1989; Coltrera and Gown, 1991). Accumulation of the PCNA mRNA and the deregulated synthesis of high levels of the protein is stimulated by growth factors (Jaskulski et al., 1988). This and the relatively long half-life of approximately 20 hours may explain why PCNA is immunologically detectable in cells that have recently left the cell cycle (Bravo and MacDonald-Bravo, 1987; McCormick and Hall, 1992).

Using monoclonal antibodies against the formalin resistant epitope of PCNA, such as 19A2 (Garcia et al., 1989) or PC10 (Waseem and Lane, 1990), a linear relationship has been found between the nuclear immunoreactivity for PCNA (or that of Ki-67) and the S-phase fraction in some tumors (Woods et al., 1990; Kamel et al., 1991) but not in others (Leonardi et al., 1992). Conflicting results have also been reported with regard to the correlation between the level of PCNA-immunostaining and prognosis or prognostic variables in tumors (Bianchi et al., 1993; Schmitt et al., 1994). Such divergent results have been explained by different degrees of disturbance of DNA synthesis, different cycle times, different growth factor susceptibility, and different immunohistochemical approaches (Hall et al., 1990; McCormick and Hall, 1992; Sabattini et al., 1993; Schmitt et al., 1994; Thiele et al., 1994).

In 26 carcinomas of the bladder, Cohen and coworkers (1993) used BrdU (see Chap. 9) as a standard of DNA synthesis for comparison with mitotic counts, AgNOR,* Ki-67, and PCNA immunohistochemistry. Krüger and associates (1993) assessed nuclear area, AgNOR, Ki-67, and PCNA in 69, and Lipponen (1993) investigated PCNA, p53, and c-erbB-2, in 104 bladder carcinomas. All three studies showed a significant correlation between PCNA and tumor grade, but no useful correlation was found with tumor stage (see Table 10-6). The proliferation markers correlated with each other (Cohen et al., 1993; Krüger et al., 1993), with the exception of AgNOR in the Cohen study. Lipponen found that the expression of PCNA was correlated with that of both p53 and c-erbB-2 (see following discussion). All three proteins were simultaneously expressed in 15% of the papillary carcinomas, in about 10% of the Ta–T1 tumors, and in 20% of invasive T2–T4 tumors. In reference to grade, the simultaneous expression of the three antigens was rare in grade 1 tumors, whereas up to 35% of the grade 2 and 3 tumors were reactive (Lipponen, 1993).

TUMOR SUPPRESSOR GENES

p53 Protein

p53 is a DNA-binding phosphoprotein (53 kd; 393 amino acids) and is coded for by the p53 tumor suppressor gene, which is located on the short arm of chromosome 17 in the region 17p13.1 (Isobe et al., 1986; Foord et al., 1991). p53 is a transcription factor that regulates cell growth and inhibits cells from entering the S phase (Lane, 1992). Lane has recently

---

*Estimation of nucleolar numbers and sizes by silver staining, as an index of cell proliferation.

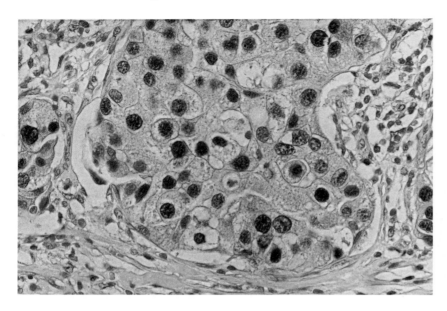

FIGURE 10-7. p53 (antibody CM1). Invasive urothelial carcinoma. There is nuclear staining of most carcinoma cells.

suggested that p53 functions as a cell cycle checkpoint, on which appropriate cell replication and division depend (Lane, 1992). p53 mutations (Bartek et al., 1990; Marks et al., 1991), or functional inactivations with intact p53 genes (Momand et al., 1992; Helland et al., 1993) have been found in a wide range of human cancers, reflecting a loss of the normal growth regulatory response (Lohmann et al., 1993; Vojtesek and Lane, 1993). p53 mutations result in prolonged half-life and accumulation of the p53 protein to a level that makes it detectable immunohistochemically in tumor cell nuclei. Overexpression of p53 protein has been shown to be associated with poor prognosis in a variety of tumors (Bartek et al., 1991a; Marks et al., 1991; Scott et al., 1991; Thor et al., 1992).

Most p53 specific antibodies can be used on deparaffinized formalin sections (Bartek et al., 1993; Baas et al., 1994). However, staining results may vary due to differences in fixation, specimen pretreatment, and differences in antibodies (Baas et al., 1994; Hall and Lane, 1994; Lambkin et al., 1994). The binding sites on the large p53 molecule have been reported to be different for a number of these antibodies. For example, the monoclonal antibody PAb1801 recognizes an epitope between amino acid residues 32 and 79 (Banks et al., 1986), the monoclonal antibody PAb 240 is specific for an epitope in an altered-mutated conformation (Gannon et al., 1990) but has been judged unreliable for immunochemistry (Baas et al., 1994), and the rabbit antibody CM1 is directed against a full length of the p53 protein (Midgley et al., 1992).

In urothelial carcinomas, nuclear p53 protein immunostaining (Fig. 10-7) correlates strongly with high grade and stage, with tumor progression, and also with p53 mutations including 17p deletion and chromosome 17 polysomy (Sidransky et al., 1991; Wright et al., 1991; Dalbagni et al., 1993; Esrig et al., 1993; Sarkis et al., 1993; Cordon-Cardo et al., 1994; Sauter et al., 1994). In particular, p53 immunoreactivity and 17p deletion have been found to be closely, although not exclusively, associated with each other and with p53 gene mutation in bladder carcinoma (Sidransky et al., 1991; Dalbagni et al., 1993; Esrig et al., 1993; Sauter et al., 1994) (see Table 10-6). For example, Sauter and associates found a strong correlation between 17p alteration (deletion or polysomy) and p53 immunostaining in a group of 106 urothelial carcinomas. Within a subgroup of 25 T1 tumors, there were 18 with a 17p deletion. Furthermore, in two retrospective studies of 43 T1 and 33 in situ (TIS) cases with a median follow-up of 119 and 124 months, respectively, Sarkis and coworkers strikingly demonstrated the prognostic significance of p53 immunostaining in urothelial carcinomas, using the PAb1801 antibody (Sarkis et al., 1993; Sarkis et al., 1994). A Cox proportional hazards model of 20% or more cells stained was the most significant factor affecting outcome and allowed a stratification into two groups. In the T1 bladder carcinoma group, 25 patients (58%) with more than 20% staining had a progression rate of 20.5% per year; 18 patients (42%) with less than 20% tumor cells staining had progression rates of 2.5% per year (Sarkis et al., 1993). In the TIS group, 15 carcinomas showed more than 20%

immunostaining, with annual progression rates of 86.7% and a death rate of 8.4%. In the TIS with values below 20%, the progression rate was 16.7% and the death rate 0 (Sarkis et al., 1994). In both studies, p53 reactivity was the only independent predictor of tumor progression and was not associated with age, sex, grade, or vascular invasion, suggesting that p53 overexpression can be employed as a stratification variable for treatment. Furthermore, in the T1 group, the authors found significantly more reactive tumor cells in areas with lamina propria invasion than in superficial, non-invasive tumor fields (Sarkis et al., 1993). Esrig et al. (1994b) again confirmed the ominous prognostic significance of p53 staining as a factor independent of stage and grade of bladder tumors (see Table 10-6). The significance of p53 staining in T1 carcinomas was corroborated by the finding of Sauter and coworkers that differences in 17p deletions and polysomy are much greater between pTa and pT1 tumors than between pT1 and pT2–T4 tumors, suggesting that the pT1 tumors are biologically closer to pT2–T4 than to pTa tumors (Sauter et al., 1994).

The data from Sarkis' studies are also in agreement with those of Spruck et al. (1994), who emphasized the importance of p53 gene mutations for progression of urothelial carcinoma. The very high rate of tumor progression and death in the carcinoma in situ cases with p53 overexpression (Sarkis et al., 1994a) is in line with the hypothesis of Spruck et al. (1994), that p53 alterations—either because of mutations or viral activation (as suggested by Reznikoff et al., 1993)—are the principal genetic events in the progression of the urothelial carcinoma in situ. In contrast, p53 mutations were almost nonexistent in Ta carcinomas, which also showed a significant predominance of a chromosome 9 allelic loss (see Chap. 11). It has been suggested that chromosome 9 defect may be less destabilizing as an early event than p53 gene inactivation (Spruck et al., 1994). These data support a relevant biologic distinction between two pathways of urothelial carcinogenesis (Koss, 1979; Reznikoff et al., 1993; Kroft and Oyasu, 1994; Spruck et al., 1994; also see Chaps. 5 and 11). p53 gene alterations and p53 protein overexpression also are associated with higher stages of invasive urothelial carcinoma and metastases, but not necessarily with each other (Sidransky et al., 1991; Fujimoto et al., 1992; Moch et al., 1993; Sauter et al., 1994). It is also quite possible that another tumor suppressor gene is located on 17p, as has recently been proposed for breast and brain tumors (Coles et al., 1990; Cogen et al., 1992).

p53 mutations have been identified in between 1% and 7% of cells within the urine sediment of three patients tested, using the polymerase chain reaction and oligomere specific hybridization (Sidransky et

al., 1991). Thus, there is a clear link of immunocytology with genetic analysis of cells in urine sediment (see also Chapter 11 for comments on detecting *ras* gene mutations in urinary sediment).

Retinoblastoma Protein

Retinoblastoma protein (pRb) is an approximately 105-kd phosphoprotein, coded for by the Rb gene that has been mapped to chromosome regions 13q14 (Lee et al., 1987), and is believed to function as cell cycle and general transcription regulator (Nevins, 1992). The phosphorylation of pRb is cell-cycle–dependent, with a highly phosphorylated state in late G1 and early S, but an underphosphorylated form in early G1. The latter form seems to represent the functionally active state of pRb (Mittnacht and Weinberg, 1991; Xu et al., 1991). pRb is expressed in all human tissues; the percentage of immunohistochemically staining nuclei has been found to be higher in maturing than in progenitor cells. This has been observed in stratified epithelia, including the urothelium, and in simple epithelia, suggesting a regulatory function in the differentiation of certain cell lineages (Cordon-Cardo and Richon, 1994).

Rb is considered the prototype tumor suppressor gene. Mutational inactivation of the Rb gene as well as reduction of pRb expression was detected originally in retinoblastomas (Knudson, 1971; Lee et al., 1987; Weinberg, 1991) and also in other human cancers (Cance et al., 1990; Horowitz et al., 1990; Shimizu et al., 1994). pRb can be inactivated by the protein corresponding to the open reading frame E6 of HPV type 16 without mutation of the Rb gene (Dyson et al., 1989). Similar observations have been reported with p53 protein. Inactivation of pRb may be an important event in tumorigenesis (Lee et al., 1987).

In urothelial carcinomas, mutations of the Rb gene have been reported (Horowitz et al., 1989; Ishikawa et al., 1991). Employing polyclonal (Horowitz et al., 1990; Logothetis et al., 1992) or monoclonal (Presti et al., 1991; Cordon-Cardo et al., 1992b) antibodies, an "altered" (*i.e.*, undetectable or heterogeneous) expression of pRb has been described in clinically aggressive tumors and tumors with poor prognosis (see Table 10-6). Benign urothelial lesions and noninvasive urothelial carcinomas show pRb immunohistochemical staining in most cells (Ishikawa et al., 1991; Presti et al., 1991; Cordon-Cardo et al., 1992b; Logothetis et al., 1992). Variations in reported frequencies of altered pRb expression—from about 75% (Presti et al., 1991) to 7% (Ishikawa et al., 1991)—may be explained by the use of different antibodies, different modes of preparation of tumor tissue (frozen versus paraffin-embedded), scoring methods, and size of study populations. In spite of such methodologic differences, the results of the two more recent immunohistochemical pRb studies were comparable with each other (Cordon-Cardo et al., 1992b; Logothetis et al., 1992). Also, long-term survival was decreased in patients with altered pRb expression (Cordon-Cardo et al., 1992b; Logothetis et al., 1992; see Table 10-6). It is possible that altered pRb expression is a late event in the pathogenesis of human urothelial carcinomas (Presti et al., 1991; Logothetis et al., 1992) and may serve as an important marker of tumor progression (Presti et al., 1991; Logothetis et al., 1992). For further comments on Rb gene in bladder tumors, see Chapter 11.

ONCOGENES

C-erbB-2 Gene Product (neu; Her-2; p185)

The c-erbB proto-oncogene, present as a single copy gene in normal cells, has been mapped to human chromosome 17q12-21.32 (Popescu et al., 1989), and encodes a protein that is located in the cytoplasmic membrane. This protein has an external (c-erbB-1/Her-1) component, a transmembrane, and an internal, 185-kd cytoplasmic (c-erbB-2/Her-2) component. The latter portion is similar to the oncogene product of the avian erythroblastosis virus (v-erb B), has ty-

rosine kinase activity, and shares 85% homology with the epidermal growth factor receptor protein [EGFr] (Akiyama et al., 1986). The transmembrane segment is not closely related to EGFr, while the extracellular domain shares 40% homology with EGFr (Coussens et al., 1985; Yamamoto et al., 1986). In spite of the similarities between c-erbB-2 and EGFr, the two recently identified ligands for c-erbB-2 are distinct from the ligands for EGFr (Tarakhovsky et al., 1991; Yarden and Peles, 1991).

Using immunohistochemistry, the c-erbB-2 antigen is commonly expressed in normal and precancerous urothelium (Wagner et al., 1994), in urothelial tumors (Coombs et al., 1993), but rarely in disease-free adult tissues (Mori et al., 1989; Slamon et al., 1989; Coombs et al., 1993) (Table 10-7). Overexpression of erbB-2 protein has been found to be prognostically relevant in a variety of human tumors (McCann et al., 1991; Yonemura et al., 1991). However, conflicting reports have been published concerning the frequency of c-erbB-2 expression—for example between 2% (Porter et al., 1991) and approximately 50% (Bacus et al., 1990) in breast carcinomas. The prognostic significance of immunohistochemical expression of c-erbB-2 protein in tumors is uncertain. Discrepancies among reports seem to be related to differences in tumor classes, patients investigated, and the variation in the antibodies and fixation methods employed (Coombs et al., 1993; Penault-Llorca et al., 1994). The characteristic cellular localization of c-erbB-2 staining in urothelial carcinomas is on the

TABLE 10-7
Growth Factors/Receptor and c-erbB-2

	Normal Urothelium	*pTa*	*CIS*	*pT1*	*pT2–4*
EGFR	Mainly membranous, basal cells	5% (1/22)[*]		14% (3/21)[*]	71% (24/34)[*,†]
		Increased expression also correlates with grade,[*] subsequent muscle invasion, and recurrence rate[†]		Prominent staining at invasion front (independent of grade or stage)[*]	
aFGF	Umbrella cells	Correlation of staining intensity with grade and stage[‡]			
c-erbB-2	Occasional, membranous	49% (23/47)[§]		74% (23/31)[§]	56% (55/100)[§] 89% (8/9)[‖]
		Increased expression correlates with high grade,[‖,¶] recurrences,[¶] and metastases[§]			

pTa, pT1, pT2–4, papillary tumors according to stage. CIS, carcinoma in situ.
[*]Sauter et al. 1994
[†]Neal et al. 1990
[‡]Ravery et al. 1992; Chopin et al. 1993
[§]Moch et al. 1993
[‖]Moriyama et al. 1991
[¶]Ding-Wei et al. 1993

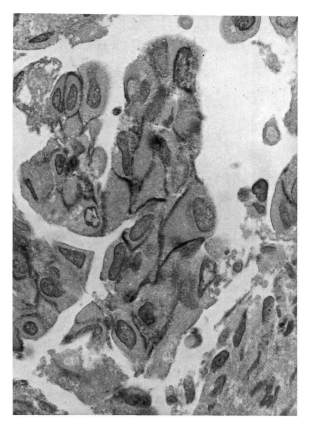

FIGURE 10-8. c-erbB-2 (antibody NCL CB11). Invasive urothelial carcinoma. There is cell membrane staining of many cancer cells.

cell membrane (Fig. 10-8). Cytoplasmic reactivity has also been reported (Wright et al., 1991; Coombs et al., 1993). In general, the stained cells are distributed diffusely within the urothelial carcinoma, with no preference for the luminal or the basal aspect of the tumor (Moriyama et al., 1991).

Variable frequency of c-erbB-2 protein expression have been found in urothelial carcinomas, ranging from 2% to 65% (Coombs et al., 1993; see Table 10-7). With regard to grade and stage, Moch et al. (1993) reported erbB-2 immunostaining in 74% (23 of 31) of pT1 and in 49% (23 of 47) of pTa carcinomas, whereas Moriyama et al. (1991) reported erbB-2 expression in 20% (9 of 45) of Tis–T1b carcinomas and 89% (8 of 9) in pT2–4 carcinomas. These and other observers correlated c-erbB-2 expression with recurrent and metastatic tumors of high grade and stage (Moriyama et al., 1991; Ding-Wei et al., 1993; Moch et al., 1993). Other investigators failed to observe a significant correlation between c-erbB-2 staining and the biologic behavior of urothelial carcinomas

(Wright et al., 1991; Swanson et al., 1992). c-erbB-2 protein expression was also described in normal urothelium (Coombs et al., 1993; Moch et al., 1993; Wagner et al., 1994), in 4 of 21 mild or moderate dysplasias, and in 5 of 7 carcinomas in situ (Wagner et al., 1994).

Thus, c-erbB-2 immunohistochemistry requires careful standardization of methods and antibodies. Studies comparing Southern, northern, and immunoblotting with immunohistochemistry of the same tumor have shown concordance between immunohistochemistry and molecular biology in only 74% (Coombs et al., 1993; Penault-Llorca et al., 1994). The selection of appropriate antibodies is essential (Corbett et al., 1990; Singleton et al., 1992; Penault-Llorca et al., 1994).

High c-erbB-2 protein expression may prove to be an important early event in urothelial carcinogenesis (Coombs et al., 1993; Moch et al., 1993). The expression of the protein in non-neoplastic conditions, such as inflammation, may limit its use as an indicator of malignancy, particularly in cytology (Wagner et al., 1994). Further studies are needed to evaluate the potential of the c-erbB-2 gene product as a diagnostic or prognostic marker for bladder carcinoma. For further comments on Ha-*ras* and other oncogenes in bladder tumors, see Chapter 11.

GROWTH FACTORS/RECEPTORS

Epidermal Growth Factor Receptor

The epidermal growth factor receptor (EGFR), encoded by a proto-oncogene located on chromosome 7p13, is a transmembrane, growth-regulating 170-kd glycoprotein (Downward et al., 1984a). Its extracellular domain (in its mature form), carries about 11 to 12 oligosaccharide residues with sequences shared by blood group antigens, particularly the A determinant (Cummings et al., 1985). The extracellular domain represents the ligand binding site and is a receptor for the cytokine's epidermal growth factor (EGF) and transforming growth factor alpha (TGF-α) (Atlas et al., 1992). Epidermal growth factor is a 53-amino acid peptide of 6 kd, widely distributed in human tissues and is a potent mitogen (Cohen, 1983; Matilla, 1986). EGF is excreted in urine in high concentrations, probably as a result of renal tubular function (Matilla, 1986), thus gaining access to receptors (EGFR) on normal and neoplastic urothelium (Messing and Reznikoff, 1987). The actions of EGF are mediated by binding to the external domain of the EGFR, whose cytoplasmic internal domain has a close similarity with the oncogene product of the avian erythroblastosis virus (v-erbB-2). Binding of EGF to its receptor results in down-regulation of the receptor and stimulation of a tyrosine kinase (Cohen, 1983; Downward, 1984b).

EGFRs have been identified on many different cell types, including the basal layers of normal urothelium. The staining pattern is predominantly membranous, although cytoplasmic staining may be observed (Messing et al., 1987; Messing, 1990; Neal et al., 1990; Limas, 1991; Sauter et al., 1994). The distribution of specific immunostaining was found to be comparable in frozen and deparaffinized, formalin-fixed sections of urothelial carcinomas (Messing, 1990; Neal et al., 1990; Wright et al., 1991; Sauter et al., 1994; see Table 10-7). Because the intensity of EGFR-immunostaining in bladder tumors is variable, EGFR-positivity has been defined as equal to specific immunostaining of a normal placenta (Neal et al., 1990; Sauter et al., 1994). Variable EGFR staining may be attributable in part to different states of glycosylation of the external domain, which apparently increases during the maturation process (Limas, 1991). Concomitantly, the availability of the core peptide sites appears to decrease, resulting in loss of peptide-specific EGFR immunoreactivity and in a declining response to EGF. The unglycosylated core peptide of the EGFR, however, is characteristic of normal immature and of malignant urothelial cells. This is well in line with the reported combination of strong EGFR and absence of blood group immunostaining in normal basal and malignant urothelial cells (Limas, 1991).

An overall staining has been found in approximately 50% of bladder carcinomas, increasing to 71% in pT2–4 tumors (Neal et al., 1990; Sauter et al., 1994). Staining frequently is most prominent at the line of invasion of tumors (Sauter et al., 1994). A general relationship has been found between EGFR positivity and bladder carcinoma aggressiveness (Berger et al., 1987; Messing, 1990; Neal et al., 1990; Wright et al., 1991; Sauter et al., 1994) and death from bladder cancer (Neal et al., 1990; see Table 10-7). A prospective study on newly diagnosed bladder carcinomas disclosed an increased immunochemical expression of EGFR in those superficial tumors that later developed muscle invasion. The level of EGFR expression in superficial tumors also correlated with time to recurrence and with recurrence rates (Neal et al., 1990). The cumulative prognostic impact of EGFR positivity is statistically independent of T-category, grade, and tumor size (Neal et al., 1990). Histologically normal peripheral urothelium in patients with bladder carcinomas may show a "malignant" staining pattern of EGFR, including a positive reaction in the superficial and deeper epithelial layers.

This is thought to reflect the potential tumorigenic effects of EGF (Messing, 1990). The strong association found between EGFR staining and the proliferation index (using BUdr) in bladder carcinomas suggests that EGFR expression may be involved in promoting urothelial carcinoma proliferation (Gullick et al., 1991; Sauter et al., 1994). Furthermore, the combination of increased EGFR immunostaining with "loss" of blood group antigen and the spontaneous expression of the T antigen (see earlier discussion) suggests that defective glycosylation is involved in urothelial carcinogenesis and is associated with invasive growth (Limas and Lange, 1980; Limas and Lange, 1986; Limas 1991).

Clearly, these findings indicate the potential of immunohistochemical or immunocytologic determination of EGFR as a prognostic marker. However, before the value of the marker is firmly established, further careful follow-up studies are necessary, preferably together with other markers of possible prognostic value, *e.g.*, blood group antigens and proliferation markers.

Acidic Fibroblast Growth Factor

Acidic fibroblast growth factor (aFGF) is a monomeric 16-kd protein that was purified from normal brain and is widely distributed in normal tissues (Schweigerer, 1990). It belongs to a family of structurally related mitogens that stimulates proliferation of fibroblasts, angiogenesis, cell differentiation, and cell motility (Schweigerer, 1990; Valles et al., 1990). Valles (1990) and her colleagues reported that both the acidic and the related basic fibroblast growth factor were mitogenic for cells derived from a rat bladder carcinoma (cell line NBT-II). Only the acidic FGF, however, induced the epithelial cells to pass from a stationary state to a dissociated, highly mobile state. Two distinct populations of receptors for acidic FGF and basic FGF were distinguished by their ligand-binding characteristics.

Using polyclonal rabbit antisera, Chopin et al. (1993) found specific immunostaining for aFGF restricted to umbrella cells of normal urothelium, and in the epithelial tumor cells of 49 out of 50 urothelial carcinoma samples. Similarly, Ravery et al. (1992) reported aFGF staining in all urothelial carcinomas investigated, but weak staining or none in normal urothelium (see Table 10-7). The intensity of immunostaining and the frequency of aFGF detection were correlated with the stage of the urothelial carcinoma (Chopin et al., 1993). A correlation has also been seen between aFGF-staining intensity and the grade of urothelial carcinomas (Ravery et al., 1992). By con-

TABLE 10-8
Drug Resistance Markers

		Carcinoma		
	Normal	TREATED[*]	UNTREATED[*] BLADDER	UPPER URINARY TRACT
Pgp	No expression	all (4/4)[†]	cytoplasmic staining of: 31% (6/19)[†] 75%[‡]	72% (13/18)[†]
		No correlation with grade, stage, tumor morphology. No predictive value for treatment success/failure[†,‡]		
Metallothionein	No expression	Cytoplasmic staining weak in invasive compartment, strong in CIS. No correlation of staining pattern and clinical outcome.[§]		

[*] Chemotherapy
[†] Naito et al. 1992
[‡] Park et al. 1994
[§] Bahnson et al. 1991

trast, a polyclonal antibody against the basic fibro-blast growth factor reacted immunohistologically with vessels and basal membranes, but did not react with urothelium (Ravery et al., 1992).

A competitive enzyme immunoassay on urine samples from 579 individuals showed a significant difference in the frequency of urinary aFGF detection between patients with invasive urothelial carcinoma and those of a control group, which included patients with benign prostatic disease and prostatic carcinoma (Chopin et al., 1993).

The acidic growth factor is another potential marker for bladder tumors that is worthy of further study in large patient populations.

DRUG RESISTANCE MARKERS

P-glycoprotein

P-glycoprotein (Pgp) is a 170-kd plasma membrane glycoprotein (P170; Pgp) of 1280 amino acids, and is coded for by the multidrug resistance (MDR) gene-1, which has been localized to chromosome 7q36 (Bell et al., 1986). The gene is overexpressed during the development of drug resistance (Bradley et al., 1988). Pgp acts as an energy-dependent drug reflux pump involved as a major mechanism in the phenomenon of multidrug resistance (Juranka et al., 1989). Pgp has been demonstrated immunohistochemically on the apical membrane of excretory epithelial cells, including those of the gastrointestinal tract, lung, kidney, and various glands (Thiebaut et al., 1987; Volm et al., 1989; Cordon-Cardo et al., 1990). Cancers that arise from these organs normally express a high level of Pgp and are resistant to chemo-

therapy (Goldstein et al., 1989). Normal urothelium of the ureter and urinary bladder has no detectable Pgp immunostaining (Cordon-Cardo et al., 1990; Naito et al., 1992).

The monoclonal Pgp-antibody MRK16 (Thiebaut et al., 1987) was used on frozen sections of biopsies of urinary bladder carcinoma, adjacent normal urothelium, and carcinomas of the upper urothelial tract. A specific cytoplasmic reaction was seen in only 6 of the 19 (31%) untreated bladder tumors, compared to 13 of 18 (72%) untreated carcinomas of the upper urinary tract (Naito et al., 1992). Four carcinomas previously treated with chemotherapy had positive immunostaining (Naito et al., 1992). The difference between tumors of the bladder and of the upper urinary tract was confirmed in a chemosensitivity test (Naito et al., 1992). This observation, suggesting a biologic difference between these two urothelial tract locations, needs to be confirmed. However, Pgp expression in 75% of bladder carcinomas without any prior chemotherapy was reported in another immunohistochemical study, using a polyclonal rabbit anti–human-Pgp antibody on formalin-fixed, paraffin-embedded cancer tissue sections (Park et al., 1994). The presence of Pgp on carcinoma cells before chemotherapy did not correlate with success or failure of the treatment, *i.e.*, it did not predict tumor recurrence (see Table 10-8). In neither study was there a correlation between Pgp expression and the grade, stage, or morphology of the carcinoma (Naito et al., 1992; Park et al., 1994). This is at variance with the results of a flow cytometric study using the monoclonal antibody 219 (Kartner et al., 1985). In this study deeply invasive bladder carcinomas showed an increase of Pgp expression in comparison with non-invasive carcinomas (Benson et al., 1991). Differences in detection systems and antibodies used in different studies may explain the inconsistent results (Volm et al., 1989; Benson et al., 1991; Naito et al., 1992; Park et al., 1994; Toth et al., 1994).

It is clearly desirable to establish a reliable method with which the success of chemotherapy for urothelial carcinomas could be predicted and monitored at the molecular level. In spite of the present controversy, immunocytology and immunohistology, with appropriate specific antibodies, may prove to be of clinical value after suitable controlled clinical trials.

Metallothioneins

Metallothioneins belong to a family of low-molecular-weight cytosolic proteins, which are involved in binding, absorption, transport, and metabolism of heavy metals and seem to affect the sensitivity of cells to heavy metal anti-cancer agents, particularly cisplatin (Kelley et al., 1988). Metallothioneins are widely distributed among vertebrate species and are also found in some lower species. They have also been found in human carcinomas (Nartey et al., 1987; Schmidt and Hamer, 1986).

Using a rabbit anti-metallothionein antibody, Bahnson et al. (1991) retrospectively found specific cytoplasmic immunostaining of primary bladder tumors from eight patients who subsequently received cisplatin-based chemotherapy. Staining was weak and variable in the invasive portion of the carcinomas, but intense in areas of carcinoma in situ (see Table 10-8). These findings are of interest with respect to the observation that cisplatin combination chemotherapy of invasive urothelial carcinomas often is ineffective against carcinoma in situ (Scher et al., 1988). No correlation has been found between the staining pattern of tumors and the clinical outcome. However, intense staining of normal urothelium was found in three patients who developed progression of their carcinoma and died of it, but in only 1 of the 5 patients who have remained disease-free for 2 years (Bahnson et al., 1991).

MARKERS USEFUL IN DIFFERENTIAL DIAGNOSIS OF URINARY TRACT TUMORS

Whereas the preceding sections have focused on markers of normal and neoplastic urothelial differentiation with emphasis on markers of potentially prognostic value, the following section describes markers that are helpful in distinguishing between urothelial and non-urothelial neoplasms. Such markers are useful when a definitive diagnosis cannot be made by routine microscopy and are applicable to histologic and cytologic specimens from the urinary tract and adjacent organs.

Markers Characteristic of Urothelial, Prostatic, and Renal Epithelium

Normal Epithelia of the Urinary Tract

Immunochemistry is rarely, if ever, required in the identification of normal epithelia. Some of the same markers, however, can be used in the identification of tumors.

As can be seen from Table 10-9 (and also Tables 10-1 and 10-2), the antigenic distinction among the urothelium, prostatic epithelium, and renal epithelium is based on differences in staining distribution of the prostate-specific antigens, keratins, vimentin, and villin. The most important markers are the prostate-specific antigen (PSA) and the prostate-specific acid phosphatase (PSAP). Both are expressed strongly in the luminal secretory cells lining the acini, ducts, and adjacent urethra of the normal and hyperplastic prostates, while basal prostatic cells, the urothelium (except for some areas lining the trigone of the bladder—see Chap. 3), and the epithelium of seminal vesicles do not express either (Mostofi et al., 1992). In spite of occasionally observed "non-specific" cross-reactivities with epitopes in other glandular tissues, one can consider these antigens as highly prostate specific (van Krieken, 1993; Poller, 1994; Allhoff et al., 1983; Allsbrook and Simms, 1992). The expression of the simple epithelial type keratins 7, 8, 18, and 19 in the luminal cells of the adult prostate is not specific and is shared by the urothelium and the renal tubular epithelium. The prostatic basal cells combine keratin 7 and 19 with squamous cell type keratins 13 and 14. These two keratins are expressed in basal cell hyperplasia, but not in prostatic carcinomas (Wernert et al., 1987) and can therefore be helpful in the distinction between these two entities. For further comments on the use of anti-keratin antibodies in prostatic disease, see Chapter 7.

The expression of keratin 20 in the umbrella cells of the urothelium is specific within the urinary tract and therefore exploitable for diagnostic purposes (Moll et al., 1992). Keratin 14, a widely distributed basal cell marker, is not found in adult urothelium (Purkis et al., 1990). Instead, the keratins 4, 5, and particularly 13 are present in the basal and intermediate urothelial cells, but not in the umbrella cells (Achtstätter et al., 1985; Wernert et al., 1987; Schaafsma et al., 1990; Moll et al., 1988) and together with keratin 20 provide a typical urothelial staining pattern (see also Figs. 10-1 and 10-2).

Some other markers are also expressed specifically in the umbrella cells, but are not as specific as keratin 20. These are the urothelial tumor-associated antigens, recognized by the monoclonal antibodies 486 P3/12 (Arndt et al., 1987), M344, and 19A211 (Fradet et al., 1990b; Huland et al., 1991; Cordon-Cardo et al., 1992a), which also show a distinct staining pattern in the normal renal tubules (Huland et al., 1991a). Other umbrella cell–reactive antibodies, such as the BL2-10D1 (Longin et al., 1990), the LeX (Cordon-Cardo et al., 1986), and Tcr+ antibodies (Juhl et al., 1987; Langkilde et al., 1992), or the URO antibodies (Cordon-Cardo et al., 1984) may perhaps be of some value in distinguishing epithelial cells of different sites of origin in the urinary tract. In general these markers still have to be tested for their wider diagnostic applicability. Such an evaluation has been carried out for the umbrella cell specific uroplakin III (Moll et al., 1993).

Villin is expressed along the apical surface of the cells of the proximal tubules of the kidney but no-where else within the urinary tract (Moll et al., 1987). It is an actin-associated protein typical of brush border microvilli of intestinal epithelial cells (Moll et al., 1987). Vimentin is of some value in renal carcinoma diagnosis (see discussion later in this chapter and Chapter 8) (Osborn and Weber, 1986) but it is also found in single prostatic glandular cells (Wernert et al., 1987). Vimentin has been demonstrated in single epithelial cells of proximal and collecting tubules of the normal kidney (Moll, 1989; Störkel and Jacobi, 1989).

Malignant Tumors

The immunochemical identification of a carcinoma of urothelial, prostatic, or renal origin can be based on the demonstration of the respective histogenic pattern of differentiation markers described above: PSA, PSAP, keratin 20, 13, vimentin, and villin (see Table 10-9). Thus, urothelial carcinomas tend to express keratin 20 in most of their cells and show loss of keratin 13 expression with increasing dedifferentiation. However, the combination of single keratin 13

TABLE 10-9
Markers Characteristic of Renal, Urothelial, and Prostatic Epithelium

	Villin Vimentin	Prostate antigens PSA, PSAP	Keratin types				
			SIMPLE EPITHELIUM			SQUAMOUS EPITHELIUM	
			7/19	8/18	20	13	14
Urothelium							
Umbrella cells	−	−	+	+	+	−	−
Basal cells	−	−	+	+ or −*	−	+	−
Urothelial carcinoma grade							
Low	−	−	+	+	+	−/+	−
High	−	−	+/−	+	−/+	−/+	−/+
Prostate glands							
Basal cells	−	−	+	−	−	−/+	+
Luminal cells	−†	+	+	+	−	−	−
Carcinoma	−†	+	+‡	+	−	−	−
Kidney							
Proximal tubules	+	−	−	+	−	−	−
Henle's loop	−	−	+	+	−	−	−
Distal tubules	−	−	−	+	−	−	−
Collecting ducts	−	−	+/−	+	−	−	−
Renal carcinoma type							
Clear cell	+	−	+/−	+	−	−	−
Chromophilic	+	−	+/−	+	−	−	−
Chromophobe	−	−	−/+	+	−	−	−
Oncocytic	−	−	+/−	+	−	−	−
Bellini Duct	−	−	+	+	−	−	−

*Two different patterns, antibody-type dependent
†Expressed focally
‡Negative segments and cases possible

reactive cells with keratin 20 (see also Figs. 10-3 and 10-4) and absence of prostate-specific antigens in a carcinoma within the urinary tract can be considered as urothelium specific (Moll et al., 1988).

Keratins 4 and 13 are expressed strongly in foci of urothelial carcinomas with squamous metaplasia, together with focal expression of the squamous differentiation (keratins 1, 2, 10, or 14). These carcinomas can still be recognized as urothelial because of the expression of keratin 20 (Moll et al., 1988; Schaafsma et al., 1990). This pattern is not seen either in prostatic or in renal cell carcinomas (Moll et al., 1988; Störkel and Jacobi, 1989). However, when the squamous carcinomas of the urothelial tract lack keratin 20 expression, they cannot be distinguished from squamous cell cancers of other primary origin.

Glandular differentiation of urothelial carcinomas is characterized by the expression of keratins 8, 18, 19, and 20, with or without the expression of keratin 7. These staining patterns are indistinguishable from those of some carcinomas of the gastrointestinal tract, including stomach and large intestine (Alroy et al., 1981; Nathrath et al., 1982b) (also see discussion of epithelial tumors later in this chapter).

The simple epithelial keratins 7, 8, 18, and 19 are also found in prostatic carcinomas, for which PSA and PSAP are the markers of choice (Wernert et al., 1987; Mostofi et al., 1992; Brawer, 1993). In spite of occasionally observed "nonspecific" cross-reactivities with epitopes in other glandular tissues (van Krieken, 1993; Poller, 1994), they are particularly helpful in the diagnosis of lymph node metastases of unknown origin (Nadji et al., 1980; Nadji et al., 1981; Henttu et al., 1992).

For the identification of renal cell carcinomas, the expression of the simple epithelial keratin profile, although shared by urothelial and prostatic carcinomas, is helpful in combination with vimentin (Pitz et al., 1987; Wernert et al., 1987; Moll et al., 1988; Schaafsma et al., 1990; Herman et al., 1983; Holthöfer et al., 1984; Waldherr and Schwechheimer, 1985; Pitz et al., 1987; Medeiros et al., 1988; Donhuijsen and Schulz, 1989; Schaafsma et al., 1990) and villin (Moll et al., 1987; Störkel and Jacobi, 1989). Thoenes and coworkers have shown that this pattern is typical only for the clear and chromophilic renal cell carcinomas and that neither vimentin nor villin is expressed in chromophobe cell carcinomas or in oncocytomas of the kidney (Thoenes et al., 1988; Störkel and Jacobi, 1989). Based on macroscopic and microscopic differences and on their different antigenic patterns, the clear and chromophilic renal cell carcinomas have been related histogenetically to the proximal tubules, the chromophobe cell carcinomas and the oncocytomas to different segments of the col-

lecting ducts, and the Bellini duct carcinomas to the medullary area of the collecting ducts of the kidney (Pitz et al., 1987; Thoenes et al., 1988; Störkel and Jacobi, 1989; see also Chap. 8).

The different antigenic patterns of the urothelial, prostatic, and renal area have been established by immunohistology, but they are also recognizable in cytologic preparations (Hart et al., 1994). For example, the dual staining pattern (keratin and vimentin) is particularly helpful in the identification of metastatic renal carcinoma in aspirates (Domagala et al., 1988). Such a distinctive immunocytochemistry not only helps in the differential diagnosis among the principal carcinoma types of the urinary tract but also among renal subtypes. One should be aware, however, that poorly differentiated carcinomas may be negative for one or all of the characteristic markers (Ellis et al., 1984; Wernert et al., 1987; Brawer, 1993).

MARKERS OF OTHER PRIMARY OR SECONDARY TUMORS OF THE URINARY TRACT

Besides urothelial carcinomas, a number of rare epithelial and non-epithelial tumors can occur in the urothelial tract (Koss, 1975a; Koss, 1985). In less well differentiated tumors, the stepwise marker characterization (see Table 10-1) helps to narrow the differential diagnostic possibilities or even to pinpoint the diagnosis of a given tumor. Because all these tumors may shed malignant cells into the urinary sediment, immunocytology may be helpful in tumor identification. A definitive immunologic distinction between a primary tumor and a metastatic tumor is sometimes possible.

Epithelial Tumors

Adenocarcinomas

The infrequent pure adenocarcinomas of the urinary tract express the typical markers shared by adenocarcinomas of other organ systems. These include keratins 7, 8, 18, 19, and 20, general epithelial markers, and CEA. Thus, a primary adenocarcinoma of the urinary bladder cannot be distinguished immunologically from a metastasis from the gastrointestinal tract or from the ovary. Keratins may be of some help, in that bile duct and pancreatic duct carcinomas express keratins 7, 8, 18, and 19, whereas gastrointestinal and mucinous ovary carcinomas tend to express keratin 20 and keratin 19, but not keratin 7 (Moll et al., 1992). Signet ring cell carcinomas of the bladder (Koss, 1985) and metastatic signet ring cell carcinomas, particularly from the stomach, again cannot be distinguished because both express the same markers, mucin and keratins 7, 8, and 19.

Carcinoid Tumors

Carcinoid tumors (Colby, 1980; Cramer et al., 1981; Koss, 1985) can be recognized by the expression of neuroendocrine markers, particularly chromogranin (Wilson and Lloyd, 1984), and neuron-specific enolase (NSE) (Tapia et al., 1981), in addition to simple epithelial markers, particularly keratins 8 and 18.

Small Cell Carcinomas

Small cell carcinomas of the urinary tract are rare (Koss, 1975a; Cramer et al., 1981). Lopez et al. (1994) found six cases (1%) among 552 bladder carcinomas. Both oat cell and intermediate types have been described, identical to the small cell carcinomas of the lung. They are also characterized by the variable double expression of epithelial and neuroendocrine markers, particularly keratin 8, 18, NSE and—less often—chromogranin (Lopez et al., 1994). The keratins may sometimes show a typical paranuclear spot staining pattern characteristic of cells of neuroendocrine tumors including Merkel cell tumors (Domagala et al., 1987). Thus, these tumors are histologically and immunomorphologically analogous to small cell carcinomas of other sites, particularly the lung, and cannot be distinguished from their metastases (Grignon et al., 1992).

Squamous Cell Carcinomas

The squamous cell carcinoma of urothelial origin is rare in its pure form (except in Africa; see Chap. 5), while foci of squamous differentiation are relatively frequent in urothelial carcinomas (Pugh, 1959; Koss, 1975a). Immunohistochemically squamous cancer is characterized by the expression of non-keratinizing and keratinizing squamous epithelial markers, particularly keratins 4, 5, and 13, and 1, 2, and 10, of which the latter three are not found in normal urothelium (Moll et al., 1988; Schaafsma et al., 1990).

Spindle Cell Carcinomas

The keratins and other epithelial markers are of help in the differential diagnosis between spindle cell sarcomas and the rare squamous carcinomas with atypical morphologic growth patterns, such as the spindle and giant cell carcinomas (Koss, 1975a). The spindle cell carcinomas, also described as carcinosarcomas or sarcomatoid carcinomas, are characterized by a carcinomatous and a spindle cell component

(Mahadevia et al., 1989). Broad spectrum keratin or other epithelial specific antibodies (see Table 10-1) have been used to identify the epithelial nature of these tumors, which always co-express vimentin (Cross et al., 1989; Torenbeek et al., 1994). However, keratin or EMA reactivity may occur in normal and neoplastic smooth muscle and in macrophages (Miettinen, 1988; Knapp and Franke, 1989). To avoid an erroneous diagnosis of a carcinoma in a case of a sarcoma or, particularly, an inflammatory pseudotumor (Jones et al., 1993; Torenbeek et al., 1994), a panel of antibodies to different epithelial markers, including keratins, and non-epithelial intermediate filament proteins should be employed (see Table 10-1). In smooth muscle tumors, keratin expression is never seen in the absence of desmin and vimentin (Torenbeek et al., 1994). These markers may also be helpful in the distinction between the epithelial and non-epithelial component of squamous carcinomas with pseudosarcomatous stroma (Anderson et al., 1977; Koss 1985).

Lymphoepithelioma-like Carcinomas

The very rare lymphoepithelioma-like carcinoma of the urinary bladder (Zukerberg et al., 1991; Amin et al., 1994) must be distinguished from malignant lymphoma, chronic cystitis, small cell carcinoma of the bladder, and urothelial carcinoma with a strong inflammatory reaction. Broad spectrum markers for epithelial, lymphoid, and endocrine differentiation can be used (Siegelbaum et al., 1986; see Table 10-1).

Mesodermal Mixed Tumors

Mesodermal mixed tumors can be difficult to distinguish from spindle cell carcinomas and pure sarcomas, depending on their carcinomatous and sarcomatous make-up (Koss, 1975a). The former is often represented by urothelial carcinoma, whereas the latter can be an undifferentiated or a differentiated mesenchymal component, e.g., osteo-, chondro-, or leiomyosarcoma (Holtz et al., 1972; Kunze et al., 1994). Assessment of the different components can be achieved by different specific epithelial markers, including broad spectrum keratins, in parallel with a panel of antibodies to non-epithelial intermediate filament proteins (see Table 10-1).

Non-epithelial Tumors

Tumors of Muscle

Leiomyomatous and rhabdomyomatous tumors, both benign and malignant, represent about half of the rare mesenchymal tumors of the urinary bladder (Koss, 1975a; Mills et al., 1989; Teran et al., 1989;

Kunze et al., 1994). Muscle-specific actin (*e.g.*, monoclonal antibody HHF35) was found in virtually all tumors of smooth and striated muscle origin, while desmin was negative in a number of cases (Mills et al., 1989; Miettinen, 1990; Kunze et al., 1994). Kunze et al. (1994) also identified specific staining for S-100 protein (Mills et al., 1989), and focal staining for NSE and alpha-1-antichymotrypsin. Rhabdomyosarcomas may also co-express myoglobin and myosin (Altmannsberger et al., 1982; de Jong et al., 1987; Pettinato et al., 1989). The distinction between differentiated leiomyosarcoma and rhabdomyosarcoma may be difficult not only by conventional histology but also by immunomorphology. Undifferentiated leiomyosarcomas may lack expression of any of the myogenic markers (Spiro and Koss, 1965; Domagala and Osborn, 1992).

Fibrohistiocytic Tumors

Fibrohistiocytic tumors represent about one third of the mesenchymal urinary tract tumors, the majority of which are malignant fibrous histiocytomas (Rew et al., 1988; Kunze et al., 1994). Alpha-1-antichymotrypsin was most consistently expressed, analogous to malignant fibrous histiocytomas at other sites (Meister and Nathrath, 1981), while the histiocytic marker CD 68 was found only focally in a few tumor cells (Kunze et al., 1994).

An important differential diagnosis within this group is the *inflammatory pseudotumor,* also called pseudomalignant spindle cell proliferation or pseudosarcomatous fibromyxoid tumor of the urinary bladder (Jones et al., 1993; Lundgren et al., 1994; Ro et al., 1994). They were all immunoreactive for vimentin and muscle-specific actin, but occasionally showed only focal staining for keratins, EMA, smooth muscle actin, and desmin. There was no staining for S-100 protein or a range of histiocytic, vascular, and myogenic markers (Ro et al., 1994; Jones et al., 1993; Lundgren et al., 1994).

Angiosarcomas

Angiosarcomas are rare in the urothelial tract (Koss, 1975a). They usually express endothelial markers, particularly the factor VIII–associated antigen (Ordonez and Batsakis, 1984; Little et al., 1986).

Neurogenic Tumors

Neurogenic tumors are also rare in the urothelial tract (Koss, 1975a). S-100 protein is a neurocrest marker and is found in peripheral neurogenic tumors with Schwann cell differentiation, particularly in neurofibromas and schwannomas. Other tumors that express S-100 protein include chondrosarcomas, liposarcomas, clear cell sarcomas, malignant melanomas, hemangiopericytomas, and glomus tumors (Nakajima et al., 1982; Kahn et al., 1983; Weiss et al., 1983; Porter et al., 1991a). In some of them, additional expression of NSE, neurofilament, and muscle antigens may be helpful in the differential diagnostic identification of soft tissue tumors and tumor subtypes (Shimada et al., 1985; Porter et al., 1991a).

Pheochromocytoma

Pheochromocytomas, benign or malignant (Zimmerman et al., 1953), can be identified by morphology and by neuroendocrine broad spectrum markers reactive with the normal adrenal medulla, *i.e.*, chromogranin and NSE. The epithelial markers are negative (Tapia et al., 1981; Wilson and Lloyd, 1984).

Malignant Melanomas

Malignant melanomas usually, but not always, lack epithelial antigens and express S-100 protein (Nakajima et al., 1982) and react with antibody HMB-45 (Gown et al., 1986).

Malignant Lymphoma

Malignant lymphomas are fairly common in the urothelial tract, rarely as primary tumor (Koss, 1975a; Aigen and Phillips, 1986; Siegelbaum et al., 1986; Simpson et al., 1991; see also Chap. 5). CD 45 is the marker of choice for the differential diagnostic separation from other small cell blue tumors (Warnke et al., 1983; Kurtin and Pinkus, 1985), although plasmocytomas and large cell lymphomas may present a problem in immunolabeling (Kurtin and Pinkus, 1985; Cartun et al., 1987). For such lymphomas and for further subclassification, particularly according to B- and T-cell differentiation, additional antibodies of the CD series must be employed (Cartun et al., 1987; Chan et al., 1988). (For detailed analysis, see Domagala and Osborn, 1992; Listrom and Fenoglio-Preiser, 1992).

CONCLUSIONS

The purpose of this chapter is to review the diagnostic and prognostic markers of urothelial tumors. An increasing number of well-defined antibodies that can be used equally well on unfixed and formalin-fixed tissue sections and on cytologic preparations from the urinary tract to complement routine microscopy has become available. It is important to recognize that histologic and clinical features are an essential background for the immunologic approach and provide the framework for the interpretation of the results. Some of the markers discussed in this chapter may help in predicting the biologic behavior of a tumor. Some antigens, such as keratins 20, 13, or uroplakin III, may be used simultaneously for diagnostic and prognostic purposes. However, large-scale prospective studies with well-defined antibodies are still needed for these and some other markers discussed above (*e.g.*, blood group–related antigens, the adhesion markers c-erbB2 or EGFR) to accurately evaluate their clinical relevance. Antibody characterization should include a definition of their reactivity pattern on differently fixed and masked or unmasked normal and neoplastic tissues and cells.

The unique antigenic pattern of the normal urothelium and tumors derived therefrom constitutes an exceptional opportunity for such studies. A significant and valuable addition to the immunologic studies is the quantitation of antigen expressions. The technology currently available includes flow cytometry and image analysis, both discussed in Chapter 9. Flow cytometry may provide information on antigen expression and other markers (*e.g.*, proliferation markers) in a population of cells. The technique has been extensively used in separating cell types in mixed populations—for example, subgroups of lymphocytes. Using fluorescent keratin antibodies, it is now possible to measure different epitopes (or DNA ploidy) separately in epithelial cells and compare them to other cells in the mixture (see Chap. 9). Image analysis allows the quantitation of individual cell components. It has been shown by this approach that quantitation of DNA and of gene expression in a population of cells is possible and may yield valuable information on changes of this expression in cell cycle (Czerniak et al., 1987, 1990, 1992; Bacus, 1990). Application of these techniques to the many antibodies discussed in this chapter may provide a new way to evaluate their diagnostic and prognostic value.

APPENDIX
IMMUNOLOGIC METHODS

Although the preparation of cytologic and histologic specimens is different, the antibodies and the detection methods used are identical for both approaches.

Preparation of Cytologic Smears from Urine

A negative control preparation is always needed. *Cytocentrifugation* is carried out at room temperature (about 20°C ± 5°), using voided urine or bladder washings. The urine is centrifuged for 10 minutes at 2000 revolutions per minute. The supernatant is drained off and the sediment, after stirring with phosphate-buffered saline (PBS), centrifuged again for 10 minutes at 2000 revolutions per minute. One ml of sodium chloride is added to prepare from 10 to 50 cytocentrifuge preparations (700 revolutions per minute for 5 minutes) from each half urine sample (the other half is to be used for standard cytologic examination). Air-drying of cytocentrifugation samples takes about 2 hours. The samples are either processed immediately after air-drying, or put into airtight boxes and stored at −70°C until used. (Storage at −20° to −30°C for shorter time periods gives acceptable results.) Alternatively, the cytocentrifugation specimens can be lyophilized, wrapped in aluminum foil, and kept in airtight plastic bags until used.

It must be stressed that the cells in the cytocentrifugation preparations should form a monolayer (see discussion of Bales' method in Chapter 1).

When they are ready to use, the cytocentrifugation specimens are fixed in acetone for 5 minutes at room temperature to permeabilize the cells, air-dried, and then rehydrated by rinsing in PBS for 10 minutes.

The following steps are the same for immunocytology using cytocentrifugation slides and for immunohistology on unfixed frozen or deparaffinized, permeabilized, formalin-fixed histologic sections.

Staining Procedures

Avidin-Biotin-Complex-Peroxidase

After the slides have been rehydrated in PBS for 5 minutes, endogenous peroxidase is blocked by overlaying a 3% H_2O_2 in PBS for 30 minutes at room temperature. The slides are then covered with 5% normal serum from the same animal species as that of the linking antibody and incubated for 10 minutes. The excess of normal serum is carefully removed, using an Eppendorf pipette. Slides are covered by 100 μl of primary, appropriately diluted antibody and incubated in a humidity chamber for 30 minutes at room temperature.

After washing in PBS for 5 minutes, the slides are incubated with the biotinylated linking antibody in a humidity chamber for 30 minutes at room temperature. After another wash in PBS for 5 minutes, the streptavidin-biotin-peroxidase complex is added for one half hour at room temperature. After washing in PBS, the slides are incubated with 0.125 mg of diaminobenzidine dissolved in 20 ml of PBS with 40 μl of 30% H_2O_2 for 5 minutes at room temperature. The slides are then washed with distilled water for 5 minutes, counterstained with Mayer's hematoxylin, washed in tap water, dehydrated, mounted in Permount, and slipcovered.

Alkaline Phosphatase Anti-Alkaline Phosphatase Complex Staining

All steps are the same as for the avidin-biotin-peroxidase method, including the PBS-washing after application of the primary antibody.

The slides are incubated with the linking antibody (*i.e.,* rabbit anti-mouse, in case of a mouse monoclonal primary antibody), and appropriately diluted in PBS/normal human serum (v/v 5:1) for 30 minutes at room temperature. After two washes in PBS, 5 minutes each, the slides are incubated with the alkaline phosphatase–anti-alkaline phosphatase (mouse) complex, appropriately diluted in PBS for 30 minutes at room temperature, followed by two PBS washes for 5 minutes.

PREPARATION OF THE CHROMOGEN

15 mg of naphthol-AS-MX-phosphate is dissolved in 750 ml dimethylformamide, which is then mixed with veronal acetate buffer (pH 9.2). Fifty (50) mg Fast Red salt and 10 mg levamisole are then added to this solution. After filtration and pH control, 1 ml is put onto each slide and left at room temperature for 30 minutes. After a brief rinse in distilled water, sections or smears are counterstained with Mayer's hematoxylin and blued in saturated lithium carbonate solution for 5 minutes. After a brief rinse in distilled water, the slides are mounted in glycerine jelly.

BIBLIOGRAPHY

Abelev, G. I.: Alpha-fetoprotein as a marker of embryo-specific differentiations in normal and tumor tissues. Transplant. Rev., *20:* 3–37, 1974.

Achtstätter, T., Moll, R., Moore, B., and Franke, W. W.: Cytokeratin polypeptide patterns of different epithelia of the human male urogenital tract. J. Histochem. Cytochem., *33:* 415–426, 1985.

Adolphs, H. D., and Oehr, P.: Significance of plasma tissue polypeptide antigen determination for diagnosis and follow-up of urothelial bladder cancer. Urol. Res., *12:* 125–128, 1984.

Aigen, A. B., and Phillips, M.: Primary malignant lymphoma of the urinary bladder. Urology, *28:* 235–237, 1986.

Akiyama, T., Sudo, C., Ogawara, H., Toyoshima, K., and Yamamoto, T.: The product of the human c-erbB-2 gene: A 185-kilodalton glycoprotein with tyrosine kinase activity. Science, *232:* 1644–1646, 1986.

Albelda, S. M.: Role of integrins and other cell adhesion molecules in tumor progression and metastasis. Lab. Invest., *68:* 4–17, 1993.

Allhoff, E. P., Proppe, K. H., Chapman, C. M., Lin, C. -W., and Prout, G. R.: Evaluation of prostate specific acid phosphatase and prostate specific antigen in identification of prostatic cancer. J. Urol., *129:* 315–318, 1983.

Allsbrook, W. C., and Simms, W. W.: Histochemistry of the prostate. Hum. Pathol., *23:* 297–305, 1992.

Alroy, J., Roganovic, D., Banner, B. F., Jacobs, J. B., Merk, F. B., Ucci, A. A., Kwan, P. W. L., Coon, J. S., and Miller, A.W.: Primary adenocarcinomas of the human urinary bladder: Histochemical, immunological and ultrastructural studies. Virchows Arch., *393:* 165–181, 1981.

Altmannsberger, M., Osborn, M., Treuner, J., Hölscher, A., Weber, K., and Schauer, A.: Diagnosis of human childhood rhabdomyosarcoma by antibodies to desmin, the structural protein of muscle specific intermediate antibodies. Virchows Arch., *B 39:* 203–215, 1982.

Altmannsberger, M., Osborn, M., Droese, M., Weber, K., and Schauer, A.: Diagnostic value of intermediate filament antibodies in clinical cytology. Klin. Wochenschr., *62:* 114–123, 1984.

Altmannsberger, M., Alles, J. U., Fitz, H., Jundt, G., and Osborn, M.: Mesenchymale Tumormarker. Verh. Dtsch. Ges. Path., *70:* 51–63, 1986.

Amin, M. B., Ro, J. Y., Lee, K. M., Ordonez, N. G., Dinney, C. P., Gulley, M. L., and Ayala, A. G.: Lymphoepithelioma-like carcinoma of the urinary bladder. Am. J. Surg. Pathol., *18:* 466–473, 1994.

Anderson, J. D., Scardino, P., and Smith, R. B.: Inflammatory fibrous histiocytoma presenting as a renal pelvic and bladder mass. J. Urol., *118:* 470–471, 1977.

Anwar, K., Naiki, H., Nakakuki, K., and Inuzuka, M.: High frequency of human papillomavirus infection in carcinoma of the urinary bladder. Cancer Res., *70:* 1967–1973, 1992.

Aprikian, A. G., Sarkis, A. S., Reuter, V. F., Cordon-Cardo, C., and Sheinfeld, J.: Biological markers of prognosis in transitional cell carcinoma of the bladder: current concepts. Sem. Urol., *11:* 137–144, 1993.

Arndt, R., Dürkopf, H., Huland, H., Donn, F., Loening, Th., and Kalthoff, H.: Monoclonal antibodies for characterization of the heterogeneity of normal and malignant transitional cells. J. Urol., *137:* 758–763, 1987.

Asamoto, M., Fukushima, S., Oosumi, H., Tatemoto, Y., and Mori, M.: Immunohistochemical distribution of epithelial membrane antigen in bladder carcinomas as detected with a monoclonal antibody. Urol. Res., *17:* 273–277, 1989.

Atlas, I., Mendelsohn, J., Baselga, J., Fair, W. R., Masui, H., and Kumar, R.: Growth regulation of human renal-cells: role of transforming growth factor alpha. Cancer Res., *52:* 3335–3339, 1992.

Baas, I. O., Mulder, J. -W. R., Offerhaus, G. J. A., Vogelstein, B., and Hamilton, S. R.: An evaluation of six antibodies for immunohistochemistry of mutant p53 gene product in archival colorectal neoplasms. J. Pathol., *172:* 5–12, 1994.

Bacus, S. S., Bacus, J. W., Slamon, D. J., and Press,

M. F.: HER-2/neu oncogene expression and DNA ploidy analysis in breast cancer. Arch. Pathol. Lab. Med., *114;* 164, 1990.

Bahnson, R. R., Banner, B., Ernstoff, M. S., Lazo, J. S., Cherian, M. G., Banerjee, D., and Chin, J. L.: Immunohistochemical localization of metallothionein in transitional cell carcinoma of the bladder. J. Urol., *146:* 1518–1520, 1991.

Bander, N. H.: Monoclonal antibodies: State of the art. J. Urol., *137:* 603–612, 1987.

Banks, S. J., Matlashewiski, G., and Crawford, L.: Isolation of human p53 specific monoclonal antibodies and their use in the studies of human p53 expression. Eur. J. Biochem., *159:* 529–534, 1986.

Bartek, J., Iggo, R., Gannon, J., and Lane, D. P.: Genetic and immunochemical analysis of mutant p53 in human breast cancer cell lines. Oncogene, *5:* 893–899, 1990.

Bartek, J., Bartkova, J., Vojtesek, B., Staskova, Z., Lukas, J., Rejthar, A., Kovarik, J., Midgley, C. A., Gannon, J. V., and Lane, D. P.: Aberrant expression of the p53 oncoprotein is a common feature of a wide spectrum of human malignancies. Oncogene, *6:* 1699–1703, 1991a.

Bartek, J., Vojtesek, B., Staskova, Z., Bartkova, J., Kerekes, Z., Rejthar, A., and Kovarik, J.: A series of 14 new monoclonal antibodies to keratins: characterization and value in diagnostic histopathology. J. Pathol., *164:* 215–224, 1991b.

Bartek, J., Bartkova, J., Lukas, J., Staskova, Z., Vojtesek, B., and Lane, D. P.: Immunohistochemical analysis of the p53 oncoprotein on paraffin sections using a series of novel monoclonal antibodies. J. Pathol., *169:* 27–34, 1993.

Bashar, H., Urano, T., Fukuta, K., Pietraszek, M. H., Suzuki, K., Kawabe, K., Takada, Y., and Takada, A.: Plasminogen activators and plasminogen activator inhibitor 1 in urinary tract cancer. Urol. Int., *52:* 4–8, 1994.

Becker, K. -F., Atkinson, M. J., Reich, U., Huang, H. -H., Nekarda, H., Siewert, J. R., and Höfler, H.: Exon skipping in the E-cadherin gene transcript in metastatic human gastric carcinomas. Hum. Mol. Gen., *2:* 803–804, 1993.

Becker, K. -F., Atkinson, M. J., Reich, U., Becker, I., Nekarda, H., Siewert, J. R., and Höfler, H.: E-cadherin gene mutations provide clues to diffuse type gastric carcinomas. Cancer Res., *54:* 3845–3852, 1994.

Behrens, J., Marcel, M. M., Van Roy, F. M., and Birchmeier, W.: Dissecting tumor cell invasion: epithelial cells acquire invasive properties after the loss of uvomorulin-mediated cell-cell adhesion. J. Cell. Biol., *108:* 2435–2447, 1989.

Bell, D. R., Trent, J. M., Willard, H. F., Riorden, J. R., and Ling, V.: Chromosomal location of human P-glycoprotein sequences. Cancer Genet. Cytol., *45:* 12–15, 1986.

Benchimol, S., Fuks, A., Jothy, S., Beauchemin, N., Shirota, K., and Stanners, C. P.: Carcinoembryonic antigen, a human tumor marker, functions as an intercellular adhesion molecule. Cell, *57:* 327–334, 1989.

Benson, M. C., Giella, J., Whang, I. S., Buttyan, R.,

Hensle, T. W., Karp, F., and Olsson, C. A.: Flow cytometric determination of the multidrug resistant phenotype in transitional cell cancer of the bladder: Implications and applications. J. Urol., *146:* 982–986, 1991.

Berger, M. S., Greenfield, C., Gullick, W. J., Haley, J., Downward, J., Neal, D. E., Harris, A. L., and Waterfield, M. D.: Evaluation of epidermal-growth-factor receptors in bladder tumours. Brit. J. Cancer, *56:* 533–537, 1987.

Bianchi, S., Paglierani, M., Zampi, G., Cardona, G., Cataliotti, L., Bonardi, R., Zappa, M., and Ciatto, S.: Prognostic value of proliferating cell nuclear antigen in lymph node negative breast cancer. Cancer, *72:* 120–125, 1993.

Björklund, B., Lundblad, G., and Björklund, V.: Antigenicity of pooled human malignant and normal tissues by cyto-immunological technique. II. Nature of tumor antigen. Int. Arch. Allergy, *12:* 241, 1958.

Björklund, V., and Björklund, B.: Localisation of synthesis of TPA in normal and malignant human tissues by immunohistochemical techniques. *In* Peters, H. (Ed.): Protides of the Biological Fluids. Oxford, Pergamon Press, 1979, pp. 229–232.

Bonner, R. B., Hemstreet, G. P., Fradet, Y., Rao, J. Y., Min, K. W., and Hurst, R. E.: Bladder cancer risk assessment with quantitative fluorescence image analysis of tumor markers in exfoliated bladder cells. Cancer, *72:* 2461–2469, 1993.

Bradley, G., Juranka, P. F., and Ling, V.: Mechanism of multidrug-resistance. Biochim. Biophys. Acta, *948:* 87–128, 1988.

Braunstein, G. D., Vaitukaitis, J. L., Carbone, P. P., and Ross, G. T.: Ectopic production of human chorionic gonadotrophin by neoplasms. Ann. Int. Med., *78:* 39–45, 1973.

Bravo, R., Frank, R., Blundell, P. A., and Mac-Donald-Bravo, H.: Cyclin/PCNA in the auxiliary protein of DNA polymerase-delta. Nature, *326:* 515–520, 1987.

Bravo, R., and MacDonald-Bravo, H.: Existence of two populations of cyclin/proliferation cell nuclear antigen during the cell cycle: association with DNA replication sites. J. Cell Biol., *105:* 1549–1554, 1987.

Brawer, M. K.: The diagnosis of prostatic carcinoma. Cancer, *71:* 899–905, 1993.

Bringuier, P. P., Umbas, R., Schaafsma, H. E., Karthaus, H. F., Debruyne, F. M., and Schalken, J. A.: Decreased E-cadherin immunoreactivity correlates with poor survival in patients with bladder tumors. Cancer Res., *53:* 3241–3245, 1993.

Brown, D. C., and Gatter, K. C.: Monoclonal antibody Ki-67: Its use in histopathology. Histopathology, *17:* 489–503, 1990.

Cance, W. G., Brennan, M. F., Dudas, M. E., Huang, C. M., and Cordon-Cardo, C.: Altered expression of the retinoblastoma gene product in human sarcomas. N. Engl. J. Med., *323:* 1457–1462, 1990.

Carter, W. G., Kaur, P., Gil, S. G., Gahr, P. J., and Wayner, E. A.: Distinct functions for integrins alpha 3 beta 1 in focal adhesions and alpha 6 beta 4/bullous pemphigoid antigen in a new stable anchoring contact (SAC) of keratinocytes: relation to hemidesmosomes. J. Cell. Biol., *111:* 3141–3154, 1990.

Cartun, R. W., Coles, F. B., and Pastuszak, W. T.: Utilization of monoclonal antibody L26 in the identification and confirmation of B-cell lymphomas. A sensitive and specific marker applicable to formalin- and B5-fixed, paraffin-embedded tissues. Am. J. Pathol., *129:* 415–421, 1987.

Cattoretti, G., Pileri, S., Parravicini, C., Becker, M. H. G., Poggi, S., Bifulco, C., Key, G., D'Amato, L., Sabattini, E., Feudale, E., Reynolds, F., Gerdes, J., and Rilke, F.: Antigen unmasking on formalin-fixed, paraffin-embedded tissue sections. J. Pathol., *171:* 83–98, 1993.

Ceriani, R. L., Thompson, K., Peterson, J. A., and Abraham, S.: Surface differentiation antigens of human mammary epithelial cells carried on the human milk fat globule. Proc. Natl. Acad. Sci., *74:* 582–586, 1977.

Chan, J. K. C., Ng, C. S., and Hui, P. K.: A simple guide to the terminology and application of leucocyte monoclonal antibodies. Histopathology, *12:* 461–480, 1988.

Chicheportiche, C., Gazarossian, E., Longin, A., Lebreuil, G., Hermanowicz, M., Richaud, C., Beley, S., Kaphan, S., Fontaniere, B., Cotte, G., and Laurent, J. -C.: Combination of standard cytology and immunocytology with BL2-10D1 monoclonal antibody for monitoring treated bladder cancer patients. Eur. Urol., *23:* 405–408, 1993.

Chopin, D. K., Bubbers, J. E., De Kernion, J. B., and Fahey, J. L.: Monoclonal antibodies against tumor associated antigens on human transitional cell carcinoma of the bladder. J. Urol., *131:* 107 A, 1982.

Chopin, D. K., De Kernion, J. B., Rosenthal, D. L., and Fahey, J. L.: Monoclonal antibodies against transitional cell carcinoma for detection of malignant urothelial cells in bladder washing. J. Urol., *134:* 260–265, 1985.

Chopin, D. K., and DeKernion, J. B.: Detection of transitional cell carcinoma in bladder by intravesical injection of monoclonal antibodies. Urol. Res., *14:* 145–148, 1986.

Chopin, D. K., Caruelle, J. -P., Colombel, M., Palcy, S., Ravery, V., Caruelle, D., Abbou, C. C., and Barritault, D.: Increased immunodetection of acidic fibroblast growth factor in bladder cancer, detectable in urine. J. Urol., *150:* 1126–1130, 1993.

Cintorino, M., Del Vecchio, M. T., Bugnoli, M., Petracca, R., and Leoncini, P.: Cytokeratin pattern in normal and pathological bladder urothelium: immunohistochemical investigation using monoclonal antibodies. J. Urol., *139:* 428–432, 1988.

Clausen, H., Stroud, M. R., Parker, J., Springer, G., and Hakomori, S.: Monoclonal antibodies directed to the blood group A associated structure, galactosyl-A: Specificity and relation to the Thomsen-Friedenreich antigen. Mol. Immunol., *25:* 199–204, 1988.

Cline, M. J.: Biology of disease. Molecular diagnosis of human cancer. Lab. Invest., *61:* 368, 1989.

Cogen, P. H., Daneshvar, L., Metzger, A. K., Duyk, G., Edwards, M. S., and Sheffield, V. C.: Involvement of multiple chromosome 17p loci in medulloblastoma tumorigenesis. Am. J. Hum. Genet., *50:* 584–589, 1992.

Cohen, M. B., Waldman, F. M., Carroll, P. R., Kerschmann, R., Chew, K., and Mayall, B. H.: Comparison of five histopathologic methods to assess cellular proliferation in transitional cell carcinoma of the urinary bladder. Hum. Pathol., *24:* 772–778, 1993.

Cohen, S.: The epidermal growth factor. Cancer, *51:* 1787–1791, 1983.

Colby, T. V.: Carcinoid tumor of the bladder. Arch. Pathol. Lab. Med., *104:* 199–200, 1980.

Coles, C., Thompson, A., Elder, P., Cohen, B., and Mackenzie, I.: Evidence implicating at least two genes on chromosome 17a in breast carcinogenesis. Lancet, *336:* 761–763, 1990.

Coltrera, M. C., and Gown, A. M.: PCNA/Cyclin expression and BrdUrd uptake define different subpopulations in different cell lines. J. Histochem. Cytochem., *39:* 23–30, 1991.

Coombes, G. B., Hall, R. R., Laurence, D. J. R., and Neville, A. M.: Urinary carcinoembryonic antigen (CEA)-like molecules and urothelial malignancy. A clinical appraisal. Br. J. Cancer, *31:* 35–142, 1975.

Coombs, L. M., Oliver, S., Sweeney, E., and Knowles, M.: Immunocytochemical localization of c-erbB-2 protein in transitional cell carcinoma of the urinary bladder. J. Pathol., *169:* 35–42, 1993.

Coon, J. S., and Weinstein, R. S.: Detection of ABH tissue isoantigens by immunoperoxidase methods in normal and neoplastic urothelium. Comparison with the erythrocyte adherence method. Am. J. Clin. Pathol., *76:* 163–171, 1981.

Coon, J. S., and Weinstein, R. S.: Blood group related antigens as markers of malignant potential and heterogeneity in human carcinomas. Hum. Pathol., *17:* 1089–1106, 1986.

Cooper, D., Schermer, A., and Sun, R. -T.: Classification of human epithelia and their neoplasms using monoclonal antibodies for keratins: Strategies, applications and limitations. Lab. Invest., *32:* 243–256, 1985.

Corbett, I. P., Henry, J. A., Brian, A., Watchorn, C. J., Wilkinson, L., Hennessy, C., Gullick, W. J., Tuzi, N. L., May, F. E. B., Westley, B. R., and Horne, C. H. W.: NCL-CB11, a new monoclonal antibody recognizing the internal domain of the c-erbB-2 oncogene protein effective for use on formalin-fixed, paraffin-embedded tissue. J. Pathol., *161:* 15–25, 1990.

Cordon-Cardo, C., Bander, N. H., Fradet, Y., Finstad, C. F., Whitmore, W. F., Lloyd, K. O., Oettgen, H. F., Melamed, M. R., and Old, L. J.: Immunoanatomic dissection of the human urinary tract by monoclonal antibodies. J. Histochem. Cytochem., *32:* 1035–1040, 1984.

Cordon-Cardo, C., Lloyd, K. O., Finstad, C. F., McGroarty, M. E., Reuter, V. E., Bander, N. H., Old, L. J., and Melamed, M. R.: Immunoanatomic distribution of blood group antigens in the human urinary tract: Influence of secretor status. Lab. Invest., *55:* 444–454, 1986.

Cordon-Cardo, C., Reuter, V. E., and Lloyd, K. O.: Blood

group-related antigens in human urothelium: Enhanced expression of precursor, Le(x), and Le(y) determinants in urothelial carcinoma. Cancer Res., 48: 4113–4120, 1988.

Cordon-Cardo, C., O'Brien, J. P., Boccia, J., Casals, D., Bertino, J. R., and Melamed, M. R.: Expression of the multidrug resistance gene product (P-glycoprotein) in human normal and tumor tissues. J. Histochem. Cytochem., 38: 1277–1287, 1990.

Cordon-Cardo, C., Wartinger, D. D., Melamed, M. R., Fair, W., and Fradet, Y.: Immunopathologic analysis of human urinary bladder cancer. Characterization of two new antigens associated with low-grade superficial bladder tumors. Am. J. Pathol., 140: 375–385, 1992a.

Cordon-Cardo, C., Wartinger, D. D., Petrylak, D., Dalbagni, G., Fair, W. R., Fuks, Z., and Reuter, V. E.: Altered expression of the retinoblastoma gene product: prognostic indicator in bladder cancer. J. Natl. Cancer Inst., 84: 1251–1256, 1992b.

Cordon-Cardo, C., Dalbagni, G., Saez, G. T., Oliva, M. R., Zhang, Z. -F., Rosai, J., Reuter, V. E., and Pellicer, A.: p53 mutations in human bladder cancer: genotypic versus phenotypic patterns. Int. J. Cancer, 56: 347–353, 1994.

Cordon-Cardo, C., and Richon, V. M.: Expression of the retinoblastoma protein is regulated in normal tissues. Am. J. Pathol., 144: 500–510, 1994.

Coussens, L., Yang-Feng, T. L., Liao, Y. -C., Chen, E., Gray, A., McGrath, J., Seeburg, P. H., Libermann, T. A., Schlessinger, J., Franke, U., Levinson, A., and Ullrich, A.: Tyrosine kinase receptor with extensive homology to EGF receptor shares chromosomal location with neu oncogene. Science, 230: 1132–1139, 1985.

Cramer, S. F., Aikawa, M., and Cebelin, M.: Neurosecretory granules in small cell invasive carcinoma of the urinary bladder. Cancer, 47: 724–730, 1981.

Cross, P. A., Eyden, B. P., and Joglekar, V. M.: Carcinosarcoma of the urinary bladder. A light, immunohistochemical and electron microscopical case report. Virchows Arch. A Pathol. Anat., 415: 91–95, 1989.

Cummings, R. D., Soderquist, A. M., and Carpenter, G.: The oligosaccharide moieties on the epidermal growth factor receptor in A-431 cells. J. Biol. Chem., 260: 11944–11952, 1985.

Czerniak, B., Herz, F., Wersto, R. P., and Koss, L. G.: Asymmetric distribution of oncogene products at mitosis. Proc. Nat. Acad. Sci. USA, 89: 1199–1204, 1992.

Czerniak, B., Herz, F., Wersto, R. P., and Koss, L. G.: Expression of Ha-ras oncogene p21 protein in relation to the cell cycle of cultured human tumor cells. Am. J. Pathol., 126: 411–416, 1987.

Czerniak, B., Herz, F., Wersto, R. P., Alster, P., Puszkin, E., Schwarz, E., and Koss, L. G.: Quantitation of oncogene products by computer-assisted image analysis and flow cytometry. J. Histochem. Cytochem., 38: 463–466, 1990.

Dalbagni, G., Presti, J. C., Jr., Reuter, V. E., Zhang, Z. -F., Sarkis, A. S., Fair, W. R., and Cordon-Cardo, C.: Molecular genetic alterations of chromosome 17 and

p53 nuclear overexpression in human bladder cancer. Diagn. Mol. Pathol., 2: 4–13, 1993.

Davidsohn, I.: The loss of blood group antigens A, B and H from cancer cells. In Herberman, R. B., and McIntire, K. R. (Eds.): Immunodiagnosis of cancer. New York, Marcel Dekker, 1979, pp. 644–664.

Debus, E., Weber, K., and Osborn, M.: Monoclonal antibodies specific for each of the neuro triplet filament proteins. Differentiation, 25: 193–203, 1983a.

Debus, E., Weber, K., and Osborn, M.: Monoclonal antibodies to desmin, the muscle-specific intermediate filament protein. EMBO J., 2: 2305–2312, 1983b.

DeCenzo, J. M., Howard, P., and Irish, C. E.: Antigenic deletion and prognosis of patients with stage A transitional cell bladder carcinoma. J. Urol., 114: 874–878, 1975.

Decken, K., Schmitz-Dräger, B. J., Rohde, D., Nakamura, S., Ebert, T., and Ackermann, R.: Monoclonal antibody Due ABC 3 directed against transitional cell carcinoma. I. Production, specificity analysis, and preliminary characterization of the antigen. J. Urol., 147: 235–241, 1992.

DeJong, A. S. H., van Kessel-van Vark, M., and van Heerde, P.: Fine needle aspiration biopsy diagnosis of rhabdomyosarcoma. An immunohistochemical study. Acta Cytol., 31: 573–577, 1987.

Ding-Wei, Y., Jia-Fu, Z., and Yong-Jiang, M.: Correlation between the expression of oncogenes ras and c-erb B-2 and the biological behavior of bladder tumors. Urol. Res., 21: 39–43, 1993.

Domagala, W., Lubinski, J., Lasota, J., Giryn, I., Weber, K., and Osborn, M.: Neuroendocrine (Merkel-cell) skin carcinoma: Cytology, intermediate filament typing, and ultrastructure of tumor cells in fine needle aspirates. Acta Cytol., 31: 267–275, 1987.

Domagala, W., Lasota, J., Wolska, H., Lubinski, J., Weber, K., and Osborn, H.: Diagnosis of metastatic renal cell and thyroid carcinomas by intermediate filament typing and cytology of tumor cell in fine needle aspirates. Acta Cytol., 32: 415–421, 1988.

Domagala, W., and Osborn, M.: Immunocytochemistry. In Koss, L. G., Woyke, S., and Olszewski, W. (Eds.): Aspiration Biopsy: Cytologic Interpretatory and Histopathologic Bases, 2nd ed. New York, Igaku Shoin, 1992.

Donhuijsen, K., and Schulz, S.: Prognostic significance of vimentin positivity in formalin-fixed renal cell carcinoma. Pathol. Res. Pract., 184: 287–291, 1989.

Downward, J., Parker, P., and Waterfield, M. D.: Autophosphorylation sites on the epidermal growth factor receptor. Nature, 311: 483–485, 1984a.

Downward, J., Yarden, Y., Mayes, E., Scrace, G., Totty, N., Stockwell, P., Ullrich, A., Schlessinger, J., and Waterfield, M. D. Close similarity of epidermal growth factor receptor and v-erb-B oncogene protein sequences. Nature, 307: 521–527, 1984b.

Droller, M. J.: Editorial comments. J. Urol., 144: 6, 1990.

Dyson, N., Howley, P. M., Munger, K., and Harlow, E.: The human papillomavirus-16 E7 oncoprotein is able to bind to the retinoblastoma gene product. Science, 243: 934–937, 1989.

Eidelman, S., Damsky, C. H., Wheelock, M. J., and Damjanov, I.: Expression of the cell–cell adhesion glycoprotein cell-CAM 120/80 in normal human tissues and tumors. Am. J. Pathol., *135:* 101–110, 1989.

Ellis, D. W., Leffers, S., Davies, J. S., and Ng, A. B. P.: Multiple immunoperoxidase markers in benign hyperplasia and adenocarcinoma of the prostate. Am. J. Clin. Pathol., *81:* 279–284, 1984.

Esrig, D., Spruck III, C. H., Nichols, P. W., Chaiwun, B., Steven, K., Groshen, S., Chen, S. -C., Skinner, D. G., Jones, P. A., and Cote, R. J.: p53 nuclear protein accumulation correlates with mutations in the p53 gene, tumor grade, and stage in bladder cancer. Am. J. Pathol., *143:* 1389–1397, 1993.

Esrig, D., Elmajian, D., Groshen, S., Freeman, J. A., Stein, J. P., Chen, S. C., Nichols, P. W., Skinner, D. G., Jones, P. A., and Cote, R. J.: Accumulation of nuclear p53 and tumor progression in bladder cancer. N. Engl. J. Med., *331:* 1259–1264, 1994.

Facer, P., Polak, J. M., Jaffe, B. M., and Pearse, A. G.: Immunocytochemical demonstration of 5-hydroxytryptamine in gastrointestinal endocrine cells. Histochem. J., *11:* 117–121, 1979.

Falcioni, R., Sacchi, A., Resau, J., and Kennel, S. J.: Monoclonal antibody to human carcinoma-associated protein complex: quantitation in normal and tumor tissue. Cancer Res., *48:* 816–821, 1988.

Farha, K. M. M. A., Menheere, P. P. C. A., Nieman, F. H. M., Janknegt, R. A., and Arends, J. W.: Urine laminin P1 assessment discriminates between invasive and noninvasive urothelial cell carcinoma of the bladder. Urol. Int., *51:* 204–208, 1993.

Feitz, W. F., Ramaekers, F. C., Beck, H. L. M., Vooijs, G. P., Debryune, F. M. J., and Hermann, C. J.: Flow cytometric analysis of bladder tumors using cytokeratin as a tissue marker. J. Urol., *133:* 295A, 1985.

Fonatsch, C., Duchrow, M., Rieder, H., Schlüter, C., and Gerdes, J.: Assignment of the human Ki-67 gene (MK 167) to 10q25-qter. Genomics, *11:* 476–477, 1991.

Fontana, D., Bellina, M., Gubetta, L., Fasolis, G., Rolle, L., Scoffone, C., Porpiglia, F., Colombo, M., Tarabuzzi, R., and Leonardo, E.: Monoclonal antibody Ki-67 in the study of the proliferative activity of bladder carcinoma. J. Urol., *148:* 1149–1151, 1992.

Foord, O., Bhattacharya, P., Reich, Z., and Rotter, V.: A DNA binding domain is contained in the C-terminus of wild type p53 protein. Nucleic Acids Res., *19:* 5191–5198, 1991.

Fradet, Y.: Biological markers of prognosis in invasive bladder cancer. Sem. Oncol., *17:* 533–543, 1990.

Fradet, Y., Cordon-Cardo, C., Thomson, T., Daly, M. E., Whitmore, W. F., Lloyd, K. O., Melamed, M. R., and Old, L. J.: Cell surface antigens of human bladder cancer defined by mouse monoclonal antibodies. Proc. Natl. Acad. Sci. USA, *81:* 224–228, 1984.

Fradet, Y., Cordon-Cardo, C., Whitmore, W. F. Jr., Melamed, M. R., and Old, L. R.: Cell surface antigens of human bladder tumors: Definition of tumor subsets by monoclonal antibodies and correlation with growth characteristics. Cancer Res., *46:* 5183–5188, 1986.

Fradet, Y., Islam, N., and Boucher, L., Parent-Vaugeois, C., and Tardif, M.: Polymorphic expression of a human superficial bladder tumor antigen defined by mouse monoclonal antibodies. Proc. Natl. Acad. Sci. USA, *84:* 7227–7231, 1987.

Fradet, Y., Tardif, M., Bourget, L., Robert, J.: Clinical cancer progression in urinary bladder tumors evaluated by multiparameter flow cytometry with monoclonal antibodies. Cancer Res., *50:* 432–437, 1990a.

Fradet, Y., LaRue, H., Parent-Vaugeois, C., Bergeron, A., Dufour, C., Boucher, L., and Bernier, L.: Monoclonal antibody against a tumor-associated sialoglycoprotein of superficial papillary bladder tumors and cervical condylomas. Int. J. Cancer, *46:* 990–997, 1990b.

Fradet, Y., Tardif, M., Bourget, L., and the Laval University Urology Group: Clinical cancer progression in urinary bladder tumors evaluated by multiparameter flow cytometry with monoclonal antibodies. Cancer Res., *50:* 432–437, 1990c.

Fradet, Y., Lafleur, L., and LaRue, H.: Strategies of chemoprevention based on antigenic and molecular markers of early and premalignant lesions of the bladder. J. Cell Biochem., Suppl. 161: 85–92, 1992.

Fradet, Y., and Cordon-Cardo, C.: Critical appraisal of tumor markers in bladder cancer. Semin. Urol., *11:* 145–153, 1993.

Franke, W. W., Weber, K., Osborn, M., Schmid, E., and Freudenstein, C.: Antibody to prekeratin: Decoration of tonofilament-like arrays in various cells of epithelial character. Exp. Cell Res., *116:* 429–445, 1978.

Franke, W. W., Winter, S., von Overbeck, J., Gudat, F., Heitz, P. U., and Stahli, C.: Identification of the conserved, confirmation-dependent cytokeratin epitope recognized by monoclonal antibody (lu-5). Virchows Arch. A, *411:* 137–147, 1987.

Frixen, U. H., Behrens, J., Sachs, M., Eberle, G., Voss, B., Warda, A., Lochner, D., and Birchmeier, W.: E-cadherin-mediated cell-cell adhesion prevents invasiveness of human carcinoma cells. J. Cell. Biol., *113:* 173–185, 1991.

Fujimoto, K., Yamada, Y., Okajima, E., Kakizoe, T., Sasaki, H., Sugimura, T., and Terada, M.: Frequent association of p53 gene mutation in invasive bladder cancer. Cancer Res., *52:* 1393–1398, 1992.

Fujioka, R., Ohhori, T., Lovrekovich, L. et al.: Investigation of blood group antigens and carcinoembryonic antigen in urinary bladder carcinoma. Urol. Int., *41:* 397–402, 1986.

Fukushima, S., Ito, N., El-Bolkaing, M. N., Tawfik, H. N., Tatemoto, Y., and Mori, M.: Immunohistochemical observations of keratins, involucrin, and epithelial membrane antigen in urinary bladder carcinomas from patients infected with schistosoma haematobium. Virchows Arch., A 411, 103–115, 1987.

Gannon, J. V., Greaves, R., Iggo, R., Lane, D. P.: Activating mutations in p53 produce a common conformational effect. A monoclonal antibody specific for the mutant form. EMBO J., *9:* 1559–1602, 1990.

Garcia, R. L., Coltresa, M. D., and Gown, A. M.: Analysis of proliferative grade using anti-PCNA/cyclin antibodies in fixed, embedded tissues. Comparison with flow cytometry analysis. Am. J. Pathol., *134:* 733–739, 1989.

Gauthier, J., and Fradet, Y.: Growth-regulated surface glycoproteins of human bladder cancer. Cancer Res., *50:* 293–298, 1990.

Gerdes, J., Schwab, U., Lemke, H., and Stein, H.: Production of a mouse monoclonal antibody reactive with a human nuclear antigen associated with cell proliferation. Int. J. Cancer, *31:* 13–20, 1983.

Gerdes, J., Lemke, H., Baisch, H., Wacker, H. H., Schwab, U., and Stein, H.: Cell cycle analysis of a cell proliferation-associated human nuclear antigen defined by the monoclonal antibody Ki-67. J. Immunol., *133:* 1710–1715, 1984.

Gerdes, J., Li, L., Schlueter, C., Duchrow, M., Wohlenberg, C., Gerlach, C., Stahmer, I., Kloth, S., Brandt, E., and Flad, H. -D.: Immunobiochemical and molecular biological characterisation of the cell proliferation-associated nuclear antigen that is defined by monoclonal antibody Ki-67. Am. J. Pathol., *138:* 867–873, 1991.

Gold, P., and Freedman, S.: Demonstration of tumor-specific antigens in human colon carcinomata by immunological tolerance and absorption techniques. J. Exp. Med., *121:* 439–462, 1965.

Goldenberg, D. M., Sharkey, R. M., and Primus, F. J.: Carcinoembryonic antigen in histopathology: Immunoperoxidase staining of conventional tissue sections. J. Natl. Cancer Inst., *57:* 11–22, 1976.

Goldenberg, D. M., and Wahren, B.: Immunoperoxidase staining of carcinoembryonic antigen in urinary bladder cancer. Urol. Res., *6:* 211–214, 1978.

Goldstein, L. J., Galski, H., Fojo, A., Willingham, M., Lai, S. -L., Gazdar, A., Pirker, R., Green, A., Crist, W., Brodeur, G. M., Lieber, M., Cossman, J., Gottesman, M. M., and Pastan, I.: Expression of multidrug resistance gene in human tumors. J. Natl. Cancer Inst., *81:* 116–124, 1989.

Gould, V. E., Wiedenmann, B., Lee, I., Schwechheimer, K., Dockhorn-Dworniczak, B., Radosevich, J. A., Moll, R., and Franke, W. W.: Synaptophysin expression in neuroendocrine neoplasms as determined by immunocytochemistry. Am. J. Pathol., *126:* 243–257, 1987.

Gown, A. M., Vogel, A. M., Hoak, D., Gough, F., and McNutt, M. A.: Monoclonal antibodies specific for melanocytic tumors distinguish subpopulations of melanocytes. Am. J. Pathol., *123:* 195–203, 1986.

Greene, G. L., Nolan, C., Engler, J. P., and Jensen, E. V.: Monoclonal antibodies to human estrogen receptors. Proc. Natl. Acad. Sci. USA, *77:* 5115–5119, 1980.

Grignon, D. J., Ro, J. Y., and Ayala, A. G.: Small cell carcinoma of the urinary bladder. A clinicopathologic analysis of 22 cases. Cancer, *69:* 527–536, 1992.

Gross, J. L., Krupp, M. N., Rifkin, D. B., and Lane, D. M.: Down–regulation of epidermal growth factor receptor correlates with plasminogen activator activity in human A431 epidermoid carcinoma cells. Proc. Natl. Acad. Sci. USA, *80:* 2276–2280, 1983.

Grossman, H. B.: Hybridoma antibodies reactive with human bladder carcinoma cell surface antigens. J. Urol., *130:* 610–614, 1983.

Guirguis, R., Schiffmann, E., Liu, B., Birkbeck, D., Engel, J., and Liotta, L.: Detection of autocrine motility factor in urine as a marker of bladder cancer. J. Natl. Cancer Inst., *80:* 1203–1211, 1988.

Gullick, W. J., Hughes, C. M., Mellon, K., Neal, D. E., and Lemoine, N. R.: Immunohistochemical detection of the epidermal-growth-factor receptor in paraffin-embedded human tissues. J. Pathol., *164:* 285–289, 1991.

Gynter, P. A., De Abela-Borg, J., Pugh, R. C. B.: Urothelium and the specific red cell adherence test. Br. J. Urol., *55:* 10–16, 1983.

Hakomori, S.: Aberrant glycosylation in cancer cell membranes as focused on glycolipids: overview and perspectives. Cancer Res., *45:* 2405–2414, 1985.

Hall, P. A., and Lane, D. P.: p53 in tumour pathology: can we trust immunohistochemistry?—Revisited! J. Pathol., *172:* 1–4, 1994.

Hall, P. A., Levison, D. A., Woods, A. L., Yu, C. C., Kellock, D. B., Watkins, J. A., Barnes, D. M., Gillett, C. E., Camplejohn, R., Dover, R., et al.: Proliferating cell nuclear antigen (PCNA) immunolocalization in paraffin sections: an index of cell proliferation with evidence of deregulated expression in some neoplasms. J. Path., *162,* 285–294, 1990.

Hall, R.: Carcinoembryonic antigen in the urine of patients with urothelial carcinoma. Br. J. Urol., *45:* 88–92, 1973.

Hammarström, S., Shively, J. E., and Paxton, R. J.: Antigenic sites in carcinoembryonic antigen. Cancer Res., *49:* 4852–4858, 1989.

Hanjan, S. N. S., Kearney, J. F., and Cooper, M. D.: A monoclonal antibody (MMA) that identifies a differentiation antigen on human myelomonocytic cells. Clin. Immunol. Immunopathol., *23:* 172–188, 1982.

Hart, A. P., Brown, R., Lechago, J., and Truong, L. D.: Collision of transitional cell carcinoma and renal cell carcinoma. Cancer, *73:* 154–159, 1994.

Hasul, Y., Marutsuka, K., Nishi, S., Kitada, S., Osada, Y., and Sumiyoshi, A.: The content of urokinase-type plasminogen activator and tumor recurrence in superficial bladder cancer. J. Urol., *151:* 16–20, 1994.

Heinzer, H., Huland, E., Mönk, M., and Huland, H.: Distribution of 486 P3/12 antigen, ABO(H) blood group antigen and T antigen in cystectomy specimens from patients with stage T2 transitional cell carcinoma of the bladder. J. Urol., *148:* 802–805, 1992.

Helland, A., Holm, R., Kristensen, G., Kaern, J., Karlsen, F., Trope, C., Nesland, J. M., and Börresen, A. -L.: Genetic alterations of the TP53 gene, p53 protein expression and HPV infection in primary cervical carcinomas. J. Pathol., *171:* 105–114, 1993.

Henttu, P., Liao, S., and Vihko, P.: Androgens up-regulate the human prostate-specific antigen messenger ribonucleic acid (mRNA), but down-regulate the prostatic acid phosphatase mRNA in the LNCaP cell line. Endocrinol., *130:* 766–772, 1992.

Herman, C. J., Moesker, O., Kant, A., Huysmans, A.,

Vooijs, G. P., and Ramaekers, F. C. S.: Is renal cell (Grawitz) tumor a carcinosarcoma? Virchows Arch. A (Path. Anat.), *44:* 73–83, 1983.

Heyderman, E., Steele, K., and Ormerod, M. G.: A new antigen on the epithelial membrane: its immunoperoxidase localisation in normal and neoplastic tissue. J. Clin. Pathol., *32:* 35–39, 1979.

Heyderman, E., Brown, B. H., and Richardson, T. C.: Epithelial markers in prostatic, bladder and colorectal cancer: An immunoperoxidase study of epithelial membrane antigen, carcinoembryonic antigen and prostatic acid phosphatase. J. Clin. Pathol., *37:* 1363–1369, 1984.

Heyderman, E., Strudley, I., Powell, G., Richardson, T. C., Cordell, J. L., and Mason, D. Y.: A new monoclonal antibody to epithelial membrane antigen (EMA)-E29. A comparison of its immunocytochemical reactivity with polyclonal anti-EMA antibodies and with another monoclonal antibody, HMFG-2. Br. J. Cancer, *52:* 355–361, 1985.

Hicks, R. M.: The fine structure of the transitional epithelium of rat ureter. J. Cell. Biol., *26:* 25–48, 1965.

Hicks, R.M.: The mammalian urinary bladder: An accommodating organ. Biol. Rev., *50:* 215–246, 1975.

Hicks, R. M., and Ketterer, B.: Hexagonal lattice of subunits in the thick luminal membrane of the rat urinary bladder. Nature, *224:* 1304–1305, 1969.

Hicks, R. M., and Chowaniec, J.: Experimental induction, histology, and ultrastructure of hyperplasia and neoplasia of the urinary bladder epithelium. Int. Rev. Exp. Pathol., *18:* 199–280, 1978.

Hijazi, A., Devonec, M., Bouvier, R., Escourro, G., Longin, A., Perrin, P., and Revillard, J. P.: Phenotyping of 76 human bladder tumors with a panel of monoclonal antibodies correlation between pathology, surface immunofluorescence and DNA content. Eur. J. Cancer Clin. Oncol., *25:* 777–783, 1989.

Hijazi, A., Devonec, M., Bouvier, R., Revillard, J. P.: Flow cytometry study of cytokeratin 18 expression according to tumor grade and deoxyribonucleic acid content in human bladder tumors. J. Urol., *141:* 522–526, 1989.

Hijazi, A., Caratero, A., Rischmann, P., Bes, J. -C., Chopin, D., Laurent, J. C., Mazerolles, C., Kassar, G., Sarramon, J. -P., and Caratero, C.: Antibodies to bladder-tumor-associated antigens as prognosis probes in the flow-cytometric analysis. Eur. Urol., *23:* 469–474, 1993.

Hoff, S. D., Matsushita, Y., Ota, D. M., Cleary, K. R., Yamori, T., Hakomori, S., and Irimura, T.: Increased expression of sialylidimeric Le(x) antigen in liver metastases of human colorectal carcinoma. Cancer Res., *49:* 6883–6888, 1989.

Holthöfer, H., Mietinen, A., Letho, V. P., Lehtonen, E., and Virtanen, I.: Expression of vimentin and cytokeratin types of intermediate filament proteins in developing and adult human kidneys. Lab. Invest., *50:* 552–559, 1984.

Holtz, F., Fox, J. E., Abell, M. R.: Carcinosarcoma of the urinary bladder. Cancer, *29:* 294–304, 1972.

Horowitz, J. M., Park, S. -H., Bogenmann, E., Cheng, J. C., Yandell, D. W., Kaye, F. J., Minna, J. D., Dryja, T. P., and Weinberg, R. A.: Frequent inactivation of the retinoblasoma anti-oncogene is restricted to a subset of human tumor cells. Proc. Natl. Acad. Sci. USA, *87:* 2775–2779, 1990.

Horowitz, J. M., Yandell, D. W., Park, S. -H., Canning, S., Whyte, P., Buchkovich, K., Harlow, E., Weinberg, R. A., and Dryja, T. P.: Point mutational inactivation of the retinoblastoma antioncogene. Science, *243:* 937–940, 1989.

Hoshi, S., Orikasa, S., Numata, I., and Nose, M.: Expression of Leu-M1 antigens in carcinoma of the urinary bladder. J. Urol., *135:* 1075–1077, 1986.

Hsu, S. M., and Jaffe, E. S.: Leu-M1 and peanut agglutinin stain the neoplastic cells of Hodgkin's disease. Am. J. Clin. Pathol., *82:* 29–32, 1984.

Huland, H., Arndt, R., Huland, E., Loening, Th., and Steffens, M.: Monoclonal antibody 486 P3/12: A valuable bladder carcinoma marker for immunocytology. J. Urol., *137:* 654–659, 1987.

Huland, E., Huland, H., and Schneider, A. W.: Quantitative immunocytology in the management of patients with superficial bladder carcinoma. I. A marker to identify patients who do not require prophylaxis. J. Urol., *144:* 637–640, 1990.

Huland, E., Huland, H., Meier, Th., Baricordi, O., Fradet, Y., Grossman, H. B., Hodges, G. M., Messing, E. M., and Schmitz-Dräger, B. J.: Comparison of 15 monoclonal antibodies against tumor-associated antigens of transitional cell carcinoma of the human bladder. J. Urol., *146:* 1631–1636, 1991a.

Huland, E., Huland, H., Meier, T., Baricordi, O., Fradet, Y., Grossman, H. B., Hodges, G. M., Messing, E. M., and Schmitz-Dräger, B. J.: The significance of immune cytological diagnostics for bladder carcinoma. Onkologie, *14:* 385–390, 1991b.

Hynes, R. O.: Integrins: Versatility, modulation, and signaling in cell adhesion. Cell, *69:* 11–25, 1992.

Ikemoto, S., Iimori, H., Nishimoto, K., Hayahara, N., and Okamoto, S.: Two cases of urothelial tumor with high serum level of carcinoembryonic antigen and TA-4. Urol. Int., *51:* 105–107, 1993.

Ishikawa, J., Xu, H. -J., Hu, S. -X., Yandell, D. W., Maeda, S., Kamidono, S., Benedict, W. F., and Takahashi, R.: Inactivation of the retinoblastoma gene in human bladder and renal cell carcinomas. Cancer Res., *51:* 5736–5740, 1991.

Isobe, M., Emanuel, B., Givol, D., Oren, M., and Croce, C.: Localization of gene for human p53 tumour antigen to band 17p13. Nature, *320:* 84–85, 1986.

Jaskulski, D., Gatti, G., Travalli, S., Calabretta, B., Baserga, R.: Regulation of the proliferating cell nuclear antigen cyclin and thymidine kinase mRNA levels by growth factors. J. Biol. Chem., *263:* 10175–10179, 1988.

Jautzke, G., and Altenaehr, E.: Immunohistochemical demonstration of carcinoembryonic antigen (CEA) and its correlation with grading and staging on tissue sections of urinary bladder carcinomas. Cancer, *50:* 2052–2056, 1982.

Jones, E. C., Clement, P. B., and Young, R. H.: Inflammatory pseudotumor of the urinary bladder. A clinicopathological, immunohistochemical, ultrastructural, and flow cytometric study of 13 cases. Am. J. Surg. Pathol., *17:* 264–274, 1993.

Juhl, B. R.: Methodologic and genetic influence on immunohistochemical demonstration and semiquantitation of blood group antigen A in human ureter urothelium. J. Histochem. Cytochem., *33:* 21–26, 1985.

Juhl, B. R., Hartzen, S. H., and Hainau, B.: A, B, H antigen expression in transitional cell carcinomas of the urinary bladder. Cancer, *57:* 1768–1775, 1986.

Juhl, B. R., Hartvig-Hartzen, S., and Hainau, B.: Thomsen-Friedenreich-related antigen in non-neoplastic ureter urothelium and transitional cell tumours of the urinary bladder. An immunohistochemical study employing the monoclonal antibody 49H.8. Acta Path. Microbiol. Immunol. Scand. Sect. A., *95:* 83–91, 1987.

Juranka, P. F., Zastawny, R. L., and Ling, V.: P-glycoprotein: multidrug-resistance and a superfamily of membrane-associated transport proteins. FASEB J., *3:* 2583–2592, 1989.

Kahn, H. J., Marks, A., Thom, H., and Baumal, R.: Role of antibody to S100 protein in diagnostic pathology. Am. J. Clin. Pathol., *79:* 341–347, 1983.

Kamel, O. W., Le Brun, D. B., Davis, R. E., Berry, G. J., and Warnke, R. A.: Growth fraction estimation of malignant lymphomas in formalin-fixed paraffin embedded tissue using anti-PCNA/Cyclin 19A2. Correlation with Ki-67 labeling. Am. J. Pathol., *138:* 1471–1477, 1991.

Karsten, U., Papsdorf, G., Roloff, G., Stolley, P., Abel, H., Walther, I., and Weiss, H.: Monoclonal anti-cytokeratin antibody from a hybridoma clone generated by electrofusion. Eur. J. Cancer Clin. Oncol., *21:* 733–740, 1985.

Kartner, N., Evernden-Porelle, D., Bradley, G., and Ling, V.: Detection of P-glycoprotein in multidrug-resistant cell lines by monoclonal antibodies. Nature, *316:* 820–823, 1985.

Kawamoto, T., Sato, J. D., Le, A., Polikoff, J., Sato, G. H., and Mendelsohn, J.: Growth stimulation of A431 cells by epidermal growth factor: identification of high-affinity receptors for epidermal growth factor by an anti-receptor monoclonal antibody. Proc. Natl. Acad. Sci. USA, *80:* 1337–1341, 1983.

Kay, H. E. M., and Wallace, D. M.: A and B antigens of tumors arising from urinary epithelium. J. Natl. Cancer Inst., *26:* 1349–1365, 1961.

Kelley, S. L., Basu, A., Teicher, B. A., Hacker, M. P., Hamer, D. H., and Lazo, J. S.: Overexpression of metallothionein confers resistance to anticancer drugs. Science, *241:* 1813–1815, 1988.

Keshgegian, A., and Kline, T. S.: Immunoperoxidase demonstration of prostatic acid phosphatase in aspiration biopsy cytology (ABC). Am. J. Clin. Pathol., *82:* 586–589, 1984.

Key, G., Becker, M. H. G., Baron, B., Duchrow, M., Schlüter, C., Flad, H. -D., and Gerdes, J.: New Ki-67-equivalent murine monoclonal antibodies (MIB 1-3) generated against bacterially expressed parts of the Ki-67 cDNA containing three 62 base pair repetitive elements encoding for the Ki-67 epitope. Lab. Invest., *68:* 629–636, 1993.

Klän, R., Huland, E., Baisch, H., and Huland, H.: Sensitivity of urinary quantitative immunocytology with monoclonal antibody 486 P3/12 in 241 unselected patients with bladder carcinoma. J. Urol., *145:* 495–497, 1991.

Knapp, A. C., and Franke, W. W.: Spontaneous losses of control of cytokeratin gene expression in transformed, non-epithelial human cells occurring at different levels of regulation. Cell, *59:* 67–79, 1989.

Knudson, A. G., Jr.: Mutation and cancer: Statistical study of retinoblastoma. Proc. Natl. Acad. Sci. USA, *68:* 820–823, 1971.

Koss, L. G.: Tumors of the urinary bladder. Atlas of tumor pathology, 2nd series, fasc. 11. Washington, D.C., Armed Forces Institute of Pathology, 1975a.

Koss, L. G.: Cytology in the diagnosis of bladder cancer. *In* Cooper, E. H., and Williams, R. E. (Eds.): The Biology and Clinical Management of Bladder Cancer. Oxford, Blackwell Scientific Publ., 1975b, pp. 111–139.

Koss, L. G.: Mapping of the urinary bladder: Its impact on the concepts of bladder cancer. Human Pathol., *10:* 533–548, 1979.

Koss, L. G.: Tumors of the urinary bladder. Supplement. Washington, D.C., Armed Forces Institute of Pathology, 1985.

Kovarik, S., Davidsohn, I., and Stejskal, R.: ABO antigens in cancer. Arch. Pathol., *86:* 12–21, 1968.

Kroft, S. H., and Oyasu, R.: Urinary bladder cancer: mechanisms of development and progression. Lab. Invest., *71:* 158–174, 1994.

Krüger, S., Kahl, Fabian, T., Hörlin, A., Herrmann, G., Müller, H., and Schneider, M.: Morphometrical, cytochemical and immunohistochemical studies on the proliferative activity of urinary bladder carcinomas. Verh. Dtsch. Ges. Path., *77:* 231–235, 1993.

Kumar, S., Costello, C. B., Glashan, R. W., and Björklund, B.: The clinical significance of tissue polypeptide antigen (TPA) in the urine of bladder cancer patients. Br. J. Urol., *53:* 578–581, 1981.

Kunze, E., Theuring, F., and Krüger, G.: Primary mesenchymal tumors of the urinary bladder. A histological and immunohistochemical study of 30 cases. Path. Res. Pract., *190:* 311–332, 1994.

Kurtin, P. J., and Pinkus, G. S.: Leukocyte common antigen—A diagnostic discriminant between hematopoietic and nonhematopoietic neoplasms in paraffin sections using monoclonal antibodies: Correlation with immunologic studies and ultrastructural localization. Hum. Path., *16:* 353–365, 1985.

Lafuente, A., Giralt, M., Cervello, I., Pujol, F., and Mallol, J.: Glutathione-S-Transferase activity in human superficial transitional cell. Carcinoma of the bladder. Cancer, *65:* 2064–2068, 1990.

Lambkin, H. A., Mothersill, C. M., and Kelehan, P.: Variations in immunohistochemical detection of p53 protein overexpression in cervical carcinomas with different antibodies and methods of detection. J. Pathol., *172:* 13–18, 1994.

Lane, D. P.: p53, guardian of the genome. Nature, *358:* 15–16, 1992.

Lane, E. B.: Monoclonal antibodies provide specific intra-molecular markers for the study of epithelial tonofilament organization. J. Cell. Biol., *92:* 665–673, 1982.

Lane, E. B., Bartek, J., Purkis, P. E., and Leigh, I. M.: Keratin antigens in differentiating skin. Ann. N.Y. Acad. Sci., *455:* 241–258, 1985.

Lane, E. B., and Alexander, C. M.: Use of keratin antibodies in tumor diagnosis. Semin. Cancer Biol., *1:* 165–179, 1990.

Langkilde, N. C., Wolf, H., Clausen, H., and Örntoft, T. B.: Localization and identification of T-(Galβ1-3GalNAcal-O-R) and T-like antigens in experimental rat bladder cancer. J. Urol., *148:* 1279–1284, 1992.

Larsson, L. I., Rehfeld, J. F., Sundler, F., Hakanson, R., and Stadil, F.: Concomitant development of gastrin immunoreactivity and formaldehyde-ozone-induced fluorescence in gastrin cells of rabbit antropyloric mucosa. Cell Tissue Res., *149:* 329–332, 1974.

Latza, U., Niedobitek, G., Schwarting, R., Nekarda, H., and Stein, H.: Ber-EP4: a new monoclonal antibody which distinguishes epithelia from mesothelia. Clin. Pathol., *43:* 213–219, 1990.

Lee, W. -H., Bookstein, R., Hong, F., Young, L. -J., Shew, J. -Y., Lee, E. Y. -H. P.: Human retinoblastoma susceptibility gene. Cloning, identification, and sequence. Science, *235:* 1394–1399, 1987.

Lehman, T. P., Cooper, H. S., Mulholland, G.: Peanut lectin binding sites in transitional cell carcinoma of the urinary bladder. Cancer, *53:* 272–277, 1984.

Leonardi, E., Girlando, S., Serio, G., Mauri, F. A., Perrone, G., Scampini, S., Dalla Palma, P., and Barbareschi, M.: PCNA and Ki-67 expression in breast carcinoma: correlations with clinical and biological variables. J. Clin. Pathol., *45:* 416–419, 1992.

Leong, A. S. -Y., Parkinson, R., and Milios, J.: Thick cell membranes revealed by immunocytochemical staining: A clue to the diagnosis of mesothelioma. Cytopathol., *6:* 9–13, 1990.

Leube, R. E., Bosch, F. X., Romano, V., Zimbelmann, R., Höfler, H., and Franke, W. W.: Cytokeratin expression in simple epithelia. III. Detection of mRNAs encoding human cytokeratin nos. 8 and 18 in normal and tumor cells by hybridization with cDNA sequences in vitro and in situ. Differentiation, *33:* 69–85, 1986.

Levison, D. A., Woods, A. L., Yu, C. C. W., Kellock, D. B., Watkins, J. A., Barnes, D. M., Gillet, C. E., Camplejohn, R., Dover, R., Waseen, N. H., Lane, D. P.: Proliferating cell nuclear antigen (PCNA) immunolocalization in paraffin sections: an index of cell proliferation with evidence of deregulated expression in some neoplasms. J. Pathol., *162:* 289–294, 1990.

Liebert, M., Wedemeyer, G. A., Stein, J. A., Washington, R. W., Jr., Ren, L. Q., and Grossman, H. B.: Identification by monoclonal antibodies of an antigen shed by human bladder cancer cells. Cancer Res., *49:* 6720–6726, 1989.

Liebert, M., Wedemeyer, G., Stein, J. A., Washington, R. W., Jr., Van Waes, C., Carey, T. E., and Grossman, H. B.: The monoclonal antibody BQ16 identifies the alpha 6 beta 4 integrin on bladder cancer. Hybridoma, *12:* 67–80, 1993.

Liebert, M., Washington, R., Wedemeyer, G., Carey, Th.E., and Grossman, H. B.: Loss of co-localization of alpha 6 beta 4 integrin and collagen VII in bladder cancer. Am. J. Pathol., *144:* 787–795, 1994a.

Liebert, M., Washington, R., Stein, J., Wedemeyer, G., and Grossman, H. B.: Expression of the VLA β1 integrin family in bladder cancer. Am. J. Pathol., *144:* 1016–1022, 1994b.

Limas, C.: A, B blood group antigens in tissues of AB heterozygotes. Emphasis on normal and neoplastic urothelium. Am. J. Pathol., *137:* 1157–1162, 1990.

Limas, C.: Relationship of epidermal growth factor receptor detectability with the A, B, H blood group antigens. Emphasis on normal and neoplastic urothelium. Am. J. Pathol., *139:* 131–137, 1991.

Limas, C.: Proliferative state of the urothelium with benign and atypical changes. Correlation with transferrin and epidermal growth factor receptors and blood group antigens. J. Pathol., *171:* 39–41, 1993.

Limas, C., and Lange, P.: Altered reactivity for A, B, H antigens in transitional cell carcinomas of the urinary bladder. A study of the mechanisms involved. Cancer, *46:* 1366–1373, 1980.

Limas, C., and Lange, P. H.: T-antigen in normal and neoplastic urothelium. Cancer, *58:* 1236–1245, 1986.

Lipponen, P. K.: Review of cytometric methods in the assessment of prognosis in transitional cell bladder cancer. Eur. Urol., *21:* 177–183, 1992.

Lipponen, P. K.: Interrelationship between expression of p53, proliferating cell nuclear antigen and c-erbB-2 in bladder cancer. Pathobiol., *61:* 178–182, 1993.

Listrom, M. B., and Fenoglio-Preiser, C. M.: Immunochemistry in Cytology. *In* Koss, L. G. (Ed.): Diagnostic Cytology 4th ed. Philadelphia, J. B. Lippincott, 1992, pp. 1532–1560.

Little, D., Said, J. W., Siegel, R. J., Fealy, M., and Fishbein, M. C.: Endothelial cell markers in vascular neoplasms: an immunohistochemical study comparing factor VIII-related antigen, blood group specific antigens, 6-keto-PGF1 alpha, and ulex europaeus 1 lectin. J. Pathol., *149:* 89–95, 1986.

Logeat, F., Hai, M. T. V., Fournier, A., Legrain, P., Buttin, G., and Milgrom, E.: Monoclonal antibodies to rabbit progesterone receptor: cross reaction with other mammalian progesterone receptors. Proc. Natl. Acad. Sci. USA, *80:* 6456–6459, 1983.

Logothetis, C. J., Xu, H. -J., Ro, J. Y., Hu, S. -X., Sahin, A., Ordonez, N., and Benedict, W. F.: Altered expression of retinoblastoma protein and known prognostic variables in locally advanced cancer. J. Natl. Cancer Inst., *84:* 1256–1261, 1992.

Lohmann, D., Ruhri, C., Schmitt, M., Gräff, H., and Höfler, H.: Accumulation of p53 protein as an indicator for p53 gene mutation in breast cancer. Diagn. Mol. Pathol., *2:* 36–41, 1993.

Longenecker, B. M., Rahman, A. F. R., Leigh, J. B., Purser, R. A., Grenberg, A. H., Williams, D. J., Keller, O., Petrik, P. K., Thay, T. Y., Suresh, M. R., and

Noujaim, A. A.: Monoclonal antibody against a cryptic carbohydrate antigen of murine and human lymphocytes. I. Antigen expression in non-cryptic or unsubstituted form on certain murine lymphomas, and on several human adenocarcinomas. Int. J. Cancer, *33:* 123–129, 1984.

Longin, A., Hijazi, A., Berger-Dutrieux, N., Escourrou, G., Bouvier, R., Richer, G., Mironnean, I., Fontaniere, B., Devonec, M., and Laurent, J. S.: A monoclonal antibody (BL2-10D1) reacting with a bladder cancer associated antigen. Int. J. Cancer, *43:* 183–189, 1989.

Longin, A., Fontaniere, B., Berger-Dutrieux, N., Devonec, M., Laurent, J. C.: A useful monoclonal antibody (BL2-10D1) to identify tumor cells in urine cytology. Cancer, *65:* 1412–1417, 1990.

Lopez, J. I., Angulo, J. C., Flores, N., and Toledo, J. D.: Small cell carcinoma of the urinary bladder. A clinicopathological study of six cases. Br. J. Urol., *73:* 43–49, 1994.

Lundgren, L., Aldenborg, F., Angervall, L., and Kindblom, L. G.: Pseudomalignant spindle cell proliferation of the urinary bladder. Hum. Pathol., *25:* 181–191, 1994.

Magnani, J. L.: Carbohydrate differentiation and cancer-associated antigens detected by monoclonal antibodies. Biochem. Soc. Trans., *12:* 543–545, 1984.

Mahadevia, P. S., Alexander, J. E., Rojas-Corona, R., and Koss, L. G.: Pseudosarcomatous stromal reaction in primary and metastatic urothelial carcinoma. Am. J. Surg. Pathol., *13:* 782–790, 1989.

Marks, J. R., Davidoff, A. M., Kerns, B. J., Humphrey, P. A., Pence, J. C., Dodge, R. K., Clarke-Pearson, D. C., Inglehart, J. D., Bast, A. R. C., Jr., and Berchuck, A.: Overexpression and mutation of p53 in epithelial ovarian cancer. Cancer Res., *51:* 2979–2984, 1991.

Masuko, T., Yagita, H., and Hashimoto, Y.: Monoclonal antibodies against cell surface antigens present on human urinary bladder cancer cells. J. Natl. Cancer Inst., *72:* 523–530, 1984.

Masuko, T., Sugahara, K., Kamiya, T., and Hashimoto, Y.: Increase in murine monoclonal-antibody-defined urinary antigens in patients with bladder cancer and benign urogenital disease. Int. J. Cancer, *44:* 582–588, 1989.

Matilla, A. -L.: Human urinary epidermal growth factor: effects of age, sex and female endocrine status. Life Sci., *39:* 1879–1884, 1986.

McCann, A. H., Dervan, P. A., O'Regan, M., Codd, M. B., Gullick, W. J., Tobin, B. M., and Carney, D. N.: Prognostic significance of c-erbB-2 and estrogen receptor status in human breast cancer. Cancer Res., *51:* 3296–3303, 1991.

McCormick, D., and Hall, P. A.: The complexities of proliferating cell nuclear antigen. Histopathology, *21:* 591–594, 1992.

Medeiros, L. J., Michie, S. A., Johnson, D. E., Warnke, R. A., and Weiss, L. M.: An immunoperoxidase study of renal cell carcinomas: Correlation with nuclear grade, cell type, and histologic pattern. Hum. Path., *19:* 980–987, 1988.

Meister, P., and Nathrath, W. B. J.: Immunohistochemical characterisation of histiocytic tumours. Diagn. Histopathol., *4:* 79–87, 1981.

Melamed, M. R.: Flow cytometry of the urinary bladder cancer. Urol. Clin. North Am., *11:* 599–608, 1984.

Messing, E. M.: Clinical implications of the expression of epidermal growth factor receptors in human transitional cell carcinoma. Cancer Res., *50:* 2530–2537, 1990.

Messing, E. M., and Reznikoff, C. A.: Normal and malignant human urothelium: in vitro effects of epidermal growth factor. Cancer Res., *47:* 2230–2235, 1987.

Messing, E. M., Hanson, P., Ulrich, P., and Erturk, E.: Epidermal growth factor-interactions with normal and malignant urothelium: In vivo and in situ studies. J. Urol., *138:* 1329–1335, 1987.

Midgley, C. A., Fisher, C. J., Bartek, J., Vojtesek, B., Lane, D., and Barnes, D. M.: Analysis of p53 expression in human tumours: an antibody raised against human p53 expressed in *Escherichia coli*. J. Cell Sci., *101:* 183–189, 1992.

Miettinen, M.: Immunocytochemistry of soft-tissue tumors: Possibilities and limitations in surgical pathology. Pathol. Ann., *25:* 1–36, 1990.

Miettinen, M.: Immunoreactivity for cytokeratin and epithelial membrane antigen in leiomyosarcoma. Arch. Pathol. Lab. Med., *112:* 637–640, 1988.

Mills, S. E., Bova, G. S., Wick, M. R., and Young, R. H.: Leiomyosarcoma of the urinary bladder. A clinicopathological and immunohistochemical study of 15 cases. Am. J. Surg. Pathol., *13:* 480–489, 1989.

Mittnacht, S., and Weinberg, R. A.: G1/S phosphorylation of the retinoblastoma protein is associated with an altered affinity for the nuclear compartment. Cell, *65:* 381–393, 1991.

Miyachi, K., Fritzler, M. J., and Tan, E. M.: Autoantibodies to a nuclear antigen in proliferating cells. J. Immunol., *121:* 2228–2234, 1978.

Moch, H., Sauter, G., Moore, D., Mihatsch, M. J., Gudat, F., and Waldman, F.: p53 and erbB-2 protein overexpression are associated with early invasion and metastasis in bladder cancer. Virchows Arch., *423:* 329–334, 1993.

Moll, R.: Intermediärfilamentmuster des Nephrons und des Urothels. Verh. Dtsch. Ges. Path., *73:* 314–320, 1989.

Moll, R.: Differenzierung und Entdifferenzierung im Spiegel der Intermediärfilament-Expression: Untersuchungen an normalen, alterierten und malignen Epithelien mit Betonung der Cytokeratine. Verh. Dtsch. Ges. Path., *75:* 446–459, 1991.

Moll, R., Franke, W. W., Schiller, D. L., Geiger, B., and Krepler, R.: The catalog of human cytokeratins: patterns of expression in normal epithelia, tumors and cultured cells. Cell, *31:* 11–24, 1982.

Moll, R., Robine, S., Dudouet, B., and Louvard, D.: Villin: a cytoskeletal protein and a differentiation marker expressed in some human adenocarcinomas. Virchows Arch. B, *54:* 155–169, 1987.

Moll, R., Achtstätter, Th., Becht, E., Balcarova-Ständer, J., Ittensohn, M., and Franke, W. W.: Maintenance of expression of urothelial differentiation features in transitional cell carcinomas and bladder carcinoma cell culture lines. Am. J. Pathol., *132:* 123–144, 1988.

Moll, R., Löwe, A., Laufer, J., and Franke, W. W.: Cytokeratin 20 in human carcinomas. Am. J. Pathol., *140:* 427–447, 1992.

Moll, R., Laufer, J., Wu, X. R., and Sun, T. -T.: Uroplakin III, ein spezifisches Membranprotein von urothelialen Deckzellen, als histologischer Marker für metastatische Urothelkarzinome. Verh. Dtsch. Ges. Path., *77:* 260–265, 1993.

Momand, J., Zambetti, G. P., Olson, D. C., George, D., and Levine, A. J.: The mdm-2 oncogene product forms a complex with the p53 protein and inhibits p53-mediated transactivation. Cell, *69:* 1237–1245, 1992.

Momburg, F., Moldenhauer, G., Hämmerling, G. J., and Möller, P.: Immunohistochemical study of the expression of a Mr 34,000 human epithelium-specific surface glycoprotein in normal and malignant tissues. Cancer Res., *47:* 2883–2891, 1987.

Montgomerie, J. Z., Keyser, A. J., Holshuh, H. J., and Schick, D. G.: 28K antigen in the urothelium. J. Urol., *147:* 1388–1390, 1992.

Mori, S., Akiyama, T., Morishita, Y., Shimizu, S. -I., Sakai, K., Sudoh, K., Toyoshima, K., and Yamamoto, T.: Light and electron microscopical demonstration of c-erbB2-gene product-like immunoreactivity in human malignant tumors. Virchows Arch. B, *54:* 8–15, 1987.

Mori, S., Akiyama, T., Yamada, Y., Morishita, Y., Sugawara, I., Toyoshima, K., and Yamamoto, T.: C-erbB-2 gene product, a membrane protein commonly expressed on human fetal epithelial cells. Lab. Invest., *61:* 93–97, 1989.

Moriyama, M., Akiyama, T., Yamamoto, T., Kawamoto, T., Kato, T., Sato, K., Watanuki, T., Hikage, T., Katsuta, N., and Mori, S.: Expression of C-ErbB-2 gene product in urinary bladder cancer. J. Urol., *145:* 423–427, 1991.

Morris, G. F., and Mathews, M. B.: Regulation of proliferating cell nuclear antigen during the cell cycle. J. Cell. Biol., *264:* 13856–13864, 1989.

Mostofi, F. K., Sesterhenn, I. A., and Davies, C. C. J.: Prostatic carcinoma: Problems in the interpretation of prostatic biopsies. Hum. Pathol., *23:* 223–241, 1992.

Mukai, K., Rosai, J., and Burgdorf, W. H. C.: Localization of factor VIII-related antigen in vascular endothelial cells using an immunoperoxidase method. Am. J. Clin. Pathol., *4:* 273–276, 1980.

Mulder, A. H., Van Hootegem, J. C. S. P., Sylvester, R., Ten Kate, F. J. W., Kurth, K. H., Ooms, E. C. M., and Van der Kwast, Th. H.: Prognostic factors in bladder carcinoma: histologic parameters and expression of a cell cycle related nuclear antigen (Ki-67). J. Pathol., *166:* 37–43, 1992.

Nadji, M.: The potential value of immunoperoxidase techniques in diagnostic cytology. Acta Cytol., *24:* 442–447, 1980.

Nadji, M., Tabei, S. Z., Castro, A., Chu, T. M., and Morales, A. R.: Prostatic origin of tumors. An immunohistochemical study. Am. J. Clin. Pathol., *73:* 735–739, 1980.

Nadji, M., Tabei, S. Z., Castro, A., Chu, T. M., Murphy, G. P., Wang, M. C., and Morales, A. R.: Prostatic-specific antigen: An immunohistological marker for prostatic neoplasms. Cancer, *48:* 1229–1232, 1981.

Naito, S., Sakamoto, N., Kotoh, S., Goto, K., Matsumoto, T., and Kumazawa, J.: Correlation between the expression of P-glycoprotein and multidrug-resistant phenotype in transitional cell carcinoma of the urinary tract. Eur. Urol., *22:* 158–162, 1992.

Nakajima, T., Watanabe, S., Sato, Y., Kameya, T., Hirota, T., and Shimosato, Y.: An immunoperoxidase study of S-100 protein distribution in normal and neoplastic tissues. Am. J. Surg. Pathol., *6:* 715–727, 1982.

Nartey, N., Cherian, M. G., and Banerjee, D.: Immunohistochemical localization of metallothionein in human thyroid tumors. Am. J. Pathol., *129:* 177–182, 1987.

Nathrath, W. B. J.: Organ and tumour antigens in malignant disease: a review. J. Royal Soc. Med., *71:* 755–761, 1978.

Nathrath, W. B. J.: Morphologische und immunhistologische Untersuchungen von Mammakarzinomen unter besonderer Berücksichtigung von Cytokeratinen, im Vergleich zu anderen neoplastisch veränderten und den normalen Epithel-Geweben des Menschen. University of Munich, Habilitationsschrift, 1988.

Nathrath, W. B. J., Detheridge, F., and Franks, L. M.: Species cross-reacting epithelial and urothelial specific antigens in human fetal, adult, and neoplastic bladder epithelium. J. Natl. Cancer Inst., *63:* 1322–1330, 1979.

Nathrath, W. B. J., and Franks, L. M.: Localization of species cross-reactive epithelium and urothelium specific antigens in the urinary tract of the rat, mouse, hamster and guinea pig. J. Urol., *126:* 77–80, 1981.

Nathrath, W. B. J., Wilson, P. D., and Trejdosiewicz, L. K.: Immunohistochemical demonstration of epithelial and urothelial antigens at the light- and electron microscope levels. Acta Histochem., *Suppl. 25,* 73–82, 1982a.

Nathrath, W. B. J., Arnholdt, H., and Wilson, P. D.: Keratin, luminal epithelial antigen and carcinoembryonic antigen in human urinary bladder carcinomas. Pathol. Res. Pract. *175:* 299–307, 1982b.

Nathrath, W. B. J., and Heidenkummer, P.: Lokalisation von "Tissue Polypeptide Antigen" (TPA) in normalen und neoplastischen Geweben des Menschen. Verh. Dtsch. Ges. Path., *67:* 701, 1983.

Nathrath, W. B. J., Heidenkummer, P., Arnholdt, H., Bassermann, R., Löhrs, U., Permanetter, W., Remberger, K., and Wiebecke, B.: Distribution of tissue polypeptide antigen in normal and neoplastic human tissues. *In* Peters, H. (Ed.): Protides of the Biological Fluids. Oxford, Pergamon Press, 1983, pp. 437–440.

Nathrath, W. B. J., Heidenkummer, P., Björklund, V., and Björklund, B.: Distribution of tissue polypeptide antigen (TPA) in normal human tissues. J. Histochem. Cytochem., *33:* 99–109, 1985.

Neal, D. E., Marsh, C., Bennett, M. K., Abel, P. D., Hall, R. R., Sainsbury, J. R., and Harris, A. L.: Epidermal growth-factor receptors in human bladder cancer: comparison of invasive and superficial tumors. Lancet, *1:* 366–367, 1985.

Neal, D. E., Sharples, L., Smith, K., Fennelly, J., Hall, R., and Harris, A. L.: The epidermal growth factor receptor and the prognosis of bladder cancer. Cancer, *65:* 1619–1625, 1990.

Nevins, J. R.: E2F: A link between the Rb tumor suppressor protein and viral oncoproteins. Science, *258:* 424–429, 1992.

Newman, A. J., Carlton, C. E., Jr., Johnson, S.: Cell surface A, B, or O(H) blood group antigens as an indicator of malignant potential in stage A bladder carcinomas. J. Urol., *124:* 27–29, 1980.

Oesterling, J. E.: Prostate specific antigen: A critical assessment of the most useful tumor marker for adenocarcinoma of the prostate. J. Urol., *145:* 907–923, 1991.

Oljans, P. J., and Tanke, H. J.: Flow cytometric analysis of DNA content in bladder cancer: prognostic value of the DNA-index with respect to early tumor recurrence in G2 tumors. World J. Urol., *4:* 205–210, 1986.

Olumi, A. F., Tsai, Y. C., Nichols, P. W., Skinner, D. G., Cain, D. R., Bender, L. I., and Jones, P. A.: Allelic loss of chromosome 17p distinguishes high grade from low grade transitional cell carcinomas of the bladder. Cancer Res., *50:* 7081–7083, 1990.

Ordonez, N. G., and Batsakis; J. G.: Comparison of Ulex europaeus 1 lectin and factor VIII-related antigen in vascular lesions. Arch. Pathol. Lab. Med., *108:* 129–132, 1984.

Orihuela, E., Varadachay, S., Herr, H. W., Melamed, M. R., and Whitmore, W. F.: The practical use of tumor marker determination in bladder washing specimens. Assessing the urothelium of patients with superficial bladder cancer. Cancer, *60:* 1009–1016, 1987.

Osborn, M., Altmannsberger, M., Debus, E., and Weber, K.: Differentiation of the major human tumor groups using conventional and monoclonal antibodies specific for individual intermediate filament proteins. Ann. NY Acad. Sci., *455:* 649–668, 1985.

Osborn, M., Debus, E., and Weber, K.: Monoclonal antibodies specific for vimentin. Eur. J. Cell Biol., *34:* 137–143, 1984.

Osborn, M., and Weber, K.: Intermediate filament proteins: A multigene family distinguishing major cell lineages. Trans. Int. Biochem. Soc. 2, 469–472, 1986.

O'Toole, C., Price, Z. H., Ohnuki, Y., and Unsgaard, B.: Ultrastructure, karyology and immunology of a cell line originated from a human transitional cell carcinoma. Br. J. Cancer, *38:* 64, 1978.

Oyasu, R.: Editorial comments. J. Urol., *144:* 639–640, 1990.

Park, J., Shinohara, N., Liebert, M., Noto, L., Flint, A., and Grossman, H. B.: P-glycoprotein expression in bladder cancer. J. Urol., *151:* 43–46, 1994.

Pauwels, R. P. E., Shapers, R.F.M., Smeets, A. W. G. P., Jansen, L. E. G., Debruyne, F. M. F., and Geraedts, J. P. M.: Blood group isoantigen deletion and chromosomal abnormalities in bladder cancer. J. Urol., *140:* 959–963, 1988.

Penault-Llorca, F., Adelaide, J., Houvenaeghel, G., Hassoun, J., Birnbaum, D., and Jacquemier, J.: Optimiza-tion of immunohistochemical detection of ErbB-2 in human breast cancer: impact of fixation. J. Pathol., *173:* 65–75, 1994.

Pettinato, G., Swanson, P. E., Insabato, L., DeChiara, A., and Wick, M. R.: Undifferentiated small round-cell tumors of childhood: The immunocytochemical demonstration of myogenic differentiation in fine-needle aspirates. Diagn. Cytopathol., *5:* 194–199, 1989.

Pinkus, G. S., and Kurtin, P. J.: Epithelial membrane antigen: A diagnostic discriminant in surgical pathology: Immunohistochemical profile in epithelial, mesenchymal and hematopoietic neoplasms using paraffin sections and monoclonal antibodies. Hum. Pathol., *16:* 929–940, 1985.

Pinkus, G. S., and Said, J. W.: Leu-M1 immunoreactivity in nonhematopoietic neoplasms and myeloproliferative disorders. Am. J. Clin. Pathol., *85:* 278–282, 1986.

Pitz, S., Moll, R., Störkel, S., and Thoenes, W.: Expression of intermediate filament proteins in subtypes of renal cell carcinomas and in renal oncocytomas: Distinction of two classes of renal cell tumors. Lab. Invest., *56:* 642–653, 1987.

Polak, J. M.: Brain and gut peptides. J. Clin. Path., *Supp. 8,* 68–75, 1978.

Poller, D.: Prostate marker immunoreactivity in salivary gland neoplasms. Am. J. Surg. Pathol., *18:* 214, 1994.

Popescu, N. C., King, C. R., and Kraus, M. H.: Localisation of the human erbB-2 gene on normal and rearranged chromosomes 17 to bands q 12-21.32. Genomics, *4:* 362–366, 1989.

Porter, P. L., Bigler, S. A., McNutt, M., and Gown, A. M.: The immunophenotype of hemangiopericytomas and glomus tumors, with special reference to muscle protein expression: an immunohistochemical study and review of the literature. Mod. Pathol., *4:* 46–52, 1991a.

Porter, P. L., Garcia, R., Moe, R., Corwin, D. J., and Gown, A. M.: c-erbB-2 oncogene protein in in situ and invasive lobular breast neoplasia. Cancer, *68:* 331–334, 1991b.

Prelich, G., Tan, C. -K., Kostura, M., Mathews, M. B., So, A. G., Downy, K. M., and Stilman, B.: Functional identity of proliferating cell nuclear antigen and a DNA polymerase-delta auxiliary protein. Nature, *326:* 517–520, 1987.

Presti, J. C., Reuter, V. E., Galan, T., Fair, W. R., and Cordon-Cardo, C.: Molecular genetic alteration in superficial and locally advanced human bladder cancer. Cancer Res., *51:* 5405–5409, 1991.

Pugh, R. C. B.: The pathology of bladder tumours. *In:* Wallace, D. M. (Ed.): Tumours of the Bladder: Neoplastic Disease at Various Sites. Vol. 2. Edinburgh, E. & S. Livingstone; Baltimore, Williams & Wilkins, 1959, pp. 116–156.

Purkis, P. E., Steel, J. B., Mackenzie, I. C., Nathrath, W. B. J., Leigh, I. M., and Lane, E. B.: Antibody markers of basal cells in complex epithelia. J. Cell Sci., *97:* 30–50, 1990.

Quinlan, R. A., Schiller, D. L., Hatzfeld, M., Achstätter, Th., Moll, R., Jorcano, J. L., Magin, Th. M., and Franke, W. W.: Patterns of expression and organization of cytokeratin intermediate filaments. Ann. N.Y. Acad. Sci., *455:* 282–306, 1985.

Ramaekers, F. C. S., Moesker, O., Huysmans, A., Schaart, G., Westerhof, G., Wagenaar, Sj. Sc., Herman, C. J., and Vooijs, G. P.: Intermediate filament proteins in the study of tumor heterogeneity: An in-depth study of tumors of the urinary and respiratory tracts. Ann. N.Y. Acad. Sci., *455:* 614–634, 1985.

Rauvala, H., and Finne, J.: Structural similarity of the terminal carbohydrate sequences of glycoproteins and glycolipids. Febs. Letter, *97:* 1–8, 1979.

Ravery, V., Jouanneau, J., Gil-Diez, S., Abbou, C. C., Caruelle, J. P., Barritault, D., and Chopin, D. K.: Immunohistochemical detection of acidic fibroblast growth factor in bladder transitional cell carcinoma. Urol. Res., *20:* 211–214, 1992.

Rew, D. A., Woodhouse, C. R., Shearer, R. J., and Corbishley, C. M.: Malignant fibrous histiocytomas associated with the urinary tract. Br. J. Urol., *62:* 488–489, 1988.

Reznikoff, C. A., Kao, C., Messing, E. M., Newton, M., and Swaminathan, S.: A molecular genetic model of human bladder carcinogenesis. Semin. Cancer Biol., *4:* 143–152, 1993.

Rheinwald, J. G., and O'Connell, Th. M.: Intermediate filament proteins as distinguishing markers of cell type and differentiated state in cultured human urinary tract epithelia. Ann. N.Y. Acad. Sci., *455:* 259–268, 1985.

Riddell, K., Tippens, D., and Gown, A. M.: Phe5, a new monoclonal antibody to a unique neuro-endocrine granule protein. Lab. Invest., *56:* 64A, 1987.

Ro, J. Y., El-Naggar, A. K., Amin, M. B., Sahin, A. A., Ordonez, N. G., and Ayala, A. G.: Pseudosarcomatous fibromyxoid tumor of the urinary bladder and prostate. Immunohistochemical, ultrastructural, and DNA flow cytometric analyses of nine cases. Hum. Pathol., *25:* 181–191, 1994.

Sabattini, E., Gerdes, J., Gherlinzoni, P., Poggi, S., Zucchini, L., Melilli, G., Grigioni, F., Del Vecchio, M. T., Leoncini, L., Falini, B., and Pileri, S. A.: Comparison between the monoclonal antibodies Ki-67 and PC10 in 125 malignant lymphomas. J. Pathol., *169:* 397–403, 1993.

Sanchez-Fernandez de Sevilla, M. C., Morell-Quadreny, L., Gil-Salom, M., Fenollosa-Entrena, B., and Llombart-Bosch, A.: Behavior of epithelial differentiation antigens (carcinoembryonic antigen, epithelial membrane antigen, keratin and cytokeratin) in transitional cell carcinomas of the bladder. Urol. Int., *48:* 14–19, 1992.

Sanders, D. S. A., Kerr, M. A., Hopwood, D., Coghill, G., and Milne, A.: Expression of the 3-fucosyl N-acetyllactosamine (CD 15) antigen in normal, metaplastic, dysplastic, and neoplastic squamous epithelia. J. Pathol., *154:* 255–262, 1988.

Sanders, D. S. A., Ferryman, S. R., Bryant, F. J., and Rollason, T. P.: Patterns of CEA-related antigen expression in invasive squamous carcinoma of the cervix. J. Pathol., *171:* 21–26, 1993.

Sarkis, A. S., Dalbagni, G., Cordon-Cardo, C., Zhang, Z. F., Sheinfeld, J., Fair, W. R., Herr, H. W., and

Reuter, V. E.: Nuclear overexpression of p53 protein in transitional cell bladder carcinoma: a marker of disease progression. J. Natl. Cancer Inst., *85:* 53–59, 1993.

Sarkis, A. S., Dalbagni, G., Cordon-Cardo, C., Melamed, J., Zhang, Z. F., Sheinfeld, J., Fair, W. R., Herr, H. W., and Reuter, V. E.: Association of p53 nuclear overexpression and tumor progression in carcinoma in situ of the bladder. J. Urol., *152:* 388–392, 1994.

Sasaki, K., Murakami, T., Kawasaki, M., and Takahashi, M.: The cell cycle associated change of Ki-67 reactive nuclear antigen expression. J. Cell. Physiol., *133:* 579, 1987.

Sauter, G., Deng, G., Moch, H., Kerschmann, R., Matsumura, K., De Vries, S., George, T., Fuentes, J., Carroll, P., Mihatsch, M. J., and Waldman, F. M.: Physical deletion of the p53 gene in bladder cancer. Detection by fluorescence in situ hybridization. Am. J. Pathol. *144:* 756–766, 1994a.

Sauter, G., Haley, J., Chew, K., Kerschmann, R., Moore, D., Carroll, P., Moch, H., Gudat, F., Mihatsch, M. J., and Waldman, F. M.: Epidermal-growth-factor-receptor expression is associated with rapid tumor proliferation in bladder cancer. Int. J. Cancer, *57:* 508–514, 1994.

Schaafsma, H. E., Ramaekers, F. C. S., van Muijen, G. N. P., Ooms, E. C. M., and Ruiter, D. J.: Distribution of cytokeratin polypeptides in epithelia of the adult human urinary tract. Histochemistry, *91:* 151–159, 1989.

Schaafsma, H. E., Ramaekers, F. C. S., van Muijen, G. N. P., Lane, E. B., Leigh, I. M., Robben, H., Huijsmans, A., Ooms, E. C. M., and Ruiter, D. J.: Distribution of cytokeratin polypeptides in human transitional cell carcinomas, with special emphasis on changing expression patterns during tumor progression. Am. J. Pathol., *136:* 329–343, 1990.

Scher, H. I., Yagoda, A., Herr, H. W., Sternberg, C. N., Bosl, G., Morse, M. J., Sogani, P. C., Watson, R. C., Dershaw, D. D., Reuter, V., Geller, N., Hollander, P. S., Vaughan, E. D., Jr., Whitmore, W. F., Jr., and Fair, W. R.: Neoadjuvant M-VAC (methotrexate, vinblastine, doxorubicin and cisplatin) effect on the primary bladder lesion. J. Urol., *139:* 470–476, 1988.

Schmechel, D. E.: Gamma-subunit of the glycolytic enzyme enolase: nonspecific or neuron specific? Lab. Invest., *52:* 239–242, 1985.

Schmidt, C. J., and Hamer, D. H.: Cell specificity and an effect of *ras* on human metallothionein gene expression. Proc. Natl. Acad. Sci., *83:* 3346–3350, 1986.

Schmitt, F. C., Pereira, E. M., Andrade, L. M., Torresan, M., and de Lucca, L.: The proliferating cell nuclear antigen index in breast carcinomas does not correlate with mitotic index and estrogen receptor immunoreactivity. Pathol. Res. Pract., *190:* 786–791, 1994.

Schmitt, M. F., and Waldherr, R.: Epidermal-Growth-Factor-Rezeptor (EGFR 1) in Urothelkarzinomen. Verh. Dtsch. Ges. Path., *73:* 535, 1989.

Schmitz-Dräger, B. J., Nakamura, S., Decken, K., Pfitzer, P., Rottmann-Ickler, C., Ebert, Th., and Ackermann, R.: Monoclonal antibody Due ABC 3 directed against transitional cell carcinoma. II. Prospective trial on the diagnostic value of immunocytology using monoclonal antibody Due ABC 3. J. Urol., *146:* 1521–1524, 1991.

Schwarting, R.: Little missed markers and Ki-67. Lab. Invest., *68:* 597–599, 1993.

Schweigerer, L.: Basic fibroblast growth factor: properties and clinical applications. *In* Habenicht, A. (Ed.): Growth factors, differentiation factors, and cytokines. New York, Springer Verlag, 1990, pp. 42–55.

Scott, N., Sagar, P., Stewart, J., Blair, G. E., Dixon, M. F., and Quirke, P.: p53 in colorectal cancer: clinicopathological correlation and prognostic significance. Br. J. Cancer, *63:* 317–319, 1991.

Senatore, S., Attolini, A., Luccarelli, S., Candita, F., Trabucco, M.: Tissue polypeptide antigen in normal and neoplastic urinary bladder. Oncology, *123:* 118–123, 1987.

Sheibani, K., Shin, S. S., Kezirian, J., and Weiss, L. M.: Ber-EP4 antibody as a discriminant in the differential diagnosis of malignant mesothelioma versus adenocarcinoma. Am. J. Surg. Pathol., *15:* 779–784, 1991.

Sheinfeld, J., Reuter, V. E., Melamed, M. R., Fair, W. M., Morse, M., Sognani, P. C., Herr, H. W., Whitmore, W. F., and Cordon-Cardo, C.: Enhanced bladder cancer detection with the Lewis X antigen as a marker of neoplastic transformation. J. Urol., *143:* 285–288, 1990.

Sheinfeld, J., Reuter, V. E., Sarkis, A. S., and Cordon-Cardo, C.: Blood group antigens in normal and neoplastic urothelium. J. Cell. Biochem., *161:* 50–55, 1992a.

Sheinfeld, J., Reuter, V. E., Fair, W. R., and Cordon-Cardo, C.: Expression of blood group antigens in bladder cancer: current concepts. Review. Seminars Surg. Oncol., *8:* 308–315, 1992b.

Shevchuk, M. M., Fenoglio, C. M., and Richart, R. M.: Carcinoembryonic antigen localization in benign and malignant transitional epithelium. Cancer, *47:* 899–905, 1981.

Shi, S. R., Key, M. E., and Kalra, K. L.: Antigen retrieval in formalin-fixed, paraffin-embedded tissues: an enhancement method for immunohistochemical staining based on microwave oven heating of tissue sections. J. Histochem. Cytochem., *39:* 741–748, 1991.

Shimada, H., Aoyama, C., Chiba, T., and Newton, W. A.: Prognostic subgroups for undifferentiated neuroblastoma: Immunohistochemical study with anti-S-100 protein antibody. Hum. Pathol., *16:* 471–476, 1985.

Shimizu, E., Coxon, A., Otterson, G. A., Steinberg, S. M., Kratzke, R. A., Kim, Y. W., Fedorko, J., Oie, H., Johnson, B. E., Mulshine, J. L., Minna, J. D., Gazdar, A. F., and Kaye, F. J.: RB protein status and clinical correlation from 171 cell lines representing lung cancer, extrapulmonary small cell carcinoma, and mesothelioma. Oncogene, *9:* 2441–2448, 1994.

Shiozaki, H., Tahara, H., Oka, H., Miyata, M., Kobayashi, K., Tamura, S., Iihara, K., Doki, Y., Hirano, S., Takeichi, M., and Mori, T.: Expression of immunoreactive E-cadherin adhesion molecules in human cancers. Am. J. Pathol., *139:* 17–23, 1991.

Shirahama, T., Ikoma, M., Muramatsu, H., Muramatsu, T., and Ohi, Y.: Reactivity of fucose-binding proteins of Lotus tetragonolobus correlates with metastatic phenotype of transitional cell carcinoma of the bladder. J. Urol., *147:* 1659–1664, 1991.

Shirahama, T., Ikoma, M., Muramatsu, T., and Ohi, Y.: Expression of SSEA-1 Carbohydrate antigen correlates with stage, grade and metastatic potential of transitional cell carcinoma of the bladder. J. Urol., *148:* 1319–1322, 1992.

Sidransky, D., von Eschenbach, A., Tsai, Y. C., Jones, P., Summerhayes, I., Marshall, F., Paul, M., Green, P., Hamilton, S. R., Frost, P., and Vogelstein, B.: Identification of p53 gene mutations in bladder cancers and urine samples. Science, *252:* 706–709, 1991.

Siegelbaum, M. H., Edmonds, P., and Seidman, E. J.: Use of immunohistochemistry for identification of primary lymphoma of the bladder. J. Urol., *136:* 1074–1076, 1986.

Simpson, R. H. W., Bridger, J. E., and Anthony, P. P.: Malignant lymphoma of the lower urinary tract: a clinicopathologic study with review of literature. Br. J. Urol., *65:* 254–260, 1991.

Singleton, T. P., Niehans, G. A., Gu, F., Litz, C. E., Hagen, K., Qiu, Q., Kiang, D. T., and Strickler, J. G.: Detection of c-erbB-2 activation in paraffin-embedded tissue by immunochemistry. Hum. Pathol., *23:* 1141–1150, 1992.

Slamon, D. J., Godolphin, W., Jones, L. A., Holt, J. A., Wong, S. G., Keith, D. E., Levin, W. J., Stuart, S. G., Udove, J., Ullrich, A., and Press, M. F.: Studies of the HER-2/neu proto-oncogene in human breast and ovarian cancer. Science, *244:* 707–712, 1989.

Sloane, J. P., Macpath, B. S., and Ormerod, M. G.: Distribution of epithelial membrane antigen in normal and neoplastic tissues and its value in diagnostic tumor pathology. Cancer, *47:* 1786–1795, 1981.

Sollberg, S., Peltonen, J., and Uitto, J.: Differential expression of laminin isoforms and beta 4 integrin epitopes in the basement membrane zone of normal human skin and basal cell carcinomas. J. Invest. Dermatol., *98:* 864–870, 1992.

Solter, D., and Knowles, B. B.: Monoclonal antibody defining a stage-specific mouse embryonic antigen (SSEA-1). Proc. Natl. Acad. Sci. USA, *75:* 5565–5569, 1978.

Sonnenberg, A., Calafat, J., Janssen, H., Daams, H., van der Raaij-Helmer, L. M., Falcioni, R., Kennel, S. J., Aplin, J. D., Baker, J., Loizidou, M., and Garrod, D.: Integrin alpha 6 beta 4 complex is located in hemidesmosomes, suggesting a major role in epidermal cell-basement membrane adhesion. J. Cell. Biol., *113:* 907–917, 1991.

Spiro, R. H., and Koss, L. G.: Myosarcoma of the uterus. A clinicopathological study. Cancer, *18:* 571–588, 1965.

Springer, G. F., Desai, P. R., and Banatwala, I.: Blood group MN antigens in normal and malignant human breast glandular tissue. J. Natl. Cancer Inst., *54:* 335–339, 1975.

Springer, G. F.: Tn and T blood group precursor antigens are universal, clonal, epithelial cell-adhesive, autoimmunogenic carcinoma (CA) markers. Naturwissenschaften, *70:* 369–371, 1983.

Spruck III, C. H., Ohneseit, P. F., Gonzalez-Zulueta, M., Esrig, D., Miyao, N., Tsai, Y. C., Lerner, S. P., Schmütte, C., Yang, A. S., Cote, R., Dubeau, L., Nichols, P. W., Hermann, G. G., Steven, K., Horn, T., Skinner, D. G., and Jones, P. A.: Two molecular pathways to transitional cell carcinoma of the bladder. Cancer Res., *54:* 784–788, 1994.

Steeg, P. S., Bevilacqua, G., Kopper, L., et al.: Evidence for a novel gene associated with low tumor metastatic potential. J. Natl. Cancer Inst., *80:* 200–204, 1988.

Störkel, S., and Jacobi, G. H.: Systematik, Histogenese and Prognose der Nierenzellkarzinome und des renalen Onkozytoms. Verh. Dtsch. Ges. Path., *73:* 321–338, 1989.

Summerhayes, J. C., Mellhinney, R. A. J., Ponder, B. A. J., Shearer, R. J., and Poock, R. D.: Monoclonal antibodies raised against cell membrane component of human bladder tumor tissue recognizing subpopulations in normal urothelium. J. Natl. Cancer Inst., *75:* 1025–1038, 1985.

Summers, J. L., Coon, J. S., Ward, R. M., Falor, W. H., Miller, A. W., III, and Weinstein, R. S.: Prognosis in carcinoma of the urinary bladder based upon tissue blood group ABH and Thomsen-Friedenreich antigen status and karyotype of the initial tumor. Cancer Res., *43:* 934–939, 1983.

Sun, T. -T., and Green, H.: Immunofluorescent staining of keratin fibers in cultured cells. Cell, *14:* 469–476, 1978.

Sun, T. T., Eichner, R., Schermer, A., Cooper, D., Nelson, W. G., and Weiss, R. A.: Classification, expression and possible mechanisms of evolution of mammalian epithelial keratins: a unifying model. *In* Levine, A., Topp, W., Van Woode, G., Watson, J. D. (Eds.): The Cancer Cell (The Transformed Phenotype). Cold Spring Harbor, New York, Cold Spring Harbor Laboratory, 1984, pp. 169–176.

Sundström, B. E., Nathrath, W. B. J., and Stigbrand, T. I.: Diversity in immunoreactivity of tumor-derived cytokeratin monoclonal antibodies. J. Histochem. Cytochem., *37:* 1845–1854, 1989.

Surya, B., Yu, J., Manabe, M., and Sun, T. -T.: Assessing the differentiation state of cultured bovine urothelial cells: elevated synthesis of stratification-related K5 and K6 keratins and persistent expression of uroplakin I. J. Cell Sci., *97:* 419–432, 1990.

Suzuka, I., Daidoji, H., Matsuoka, M., Kadowaki, K., Takasaki, Y., Nakane, P. K., Moriuchi, T.: Gene for proliferating cell nuclear antigen (DNA polymerase-delta auxiliary protein) is present in both mammalian and higher plant genomes. Proc. Nat. Acad. Sci. (USA), *86:* 3189–3193, 1989.

Swanson, P. E., Frierson, H. F., and Wick, M. R.: c-erbB-2 (HER-2/neu) oncopeptide immunoreactivity in localized, high grade transitional cell carcinoma of the bladder. Mod. Pathol., *5:* 531–536, 1992.

Szulman, A. E.: The histological distribution of the blood group substances in man as disclosed by immunofluorescence. II. The H antigen and its relation to A and B antigens. J. Exp. Med., *115:* 977–996, 1962.

Takashi, M., Murase, T., Kinjo, T., et al.: Epithelial membrane antigen as an immunohistochemical marker for transitional cell carcinoma of the urinary bladder. Urol. Int., *42:* 170–175, 1987.

Takeichi, M.: Cadherin cell adhesion receptors as a morphogenetic regulator. Science, *251:* 1451–1455, 1991.

Taki, T., Takamatsu, M., Myoga, A., Tanaka, K., Ando, S., and Matsumoto, M.: Glycolipids of metastatic tissue in liver from colon cancer: Appearance of sialylated Le(x) and Le(y) lipids. J. Biochem., *103:* 998–1003, 1988.

Tapia, F. J., Barbosa, A. J. A., Marangos, P. J., Polak, J. M., Bloom, S. R., Dermody, C., and Pearse, A. G. E.: Neuron-specific enolase is produced by neuroendocrine tumours. Lancet, *1:* 808–811, 1981.

Tarakhovsky, A., Zaichuk, T., Prassolov, V., and Butenko, Z. A.: A 25 kDa polypeptide is the ligand for p185neu and is secreted by activated macrophages. Oncogene, *6:* 2187–2196, 1991.

Taylor, C. R., Shi, S. -R., Chaiwun, B., Young, L., Imam, S. A., Cote, R. J.: Strategies for improving the immunohistochemical staining of various intranuclear prognostic markers in formalin-paraffin sections: androgen receptor, estrogen receptor, progesterone receptor, p53 protein, proliferating cell nuclear antigen, and Ki-67 antigen revealed by antigen retrieval techniques. Hum. Pathol., *25:* 263–270, 1994.

Teran, A. Z., and Don Gambrell, R.: Leiomyoma of the bladder: case report and review of the literature. Int. J. Fertil., *34:* 289–292, 1989.

Thiebaut, T., Tsuruo, T., Hamada, H., Gottesman, M. M., Pastan, I., and Willingham, M. C.: Cellular localization of the multidrug-resistance gene product P-glycoprotein in normal human tissues. Proc. Natl. Acad. Sci., *84:* 7735–7738, 1987.

Thiele, J., Bertsch, H. P., Kracht, L. W., Anwander, T., Zimmer, J. D., Kreipe, H., and Fischer, R.: Ki-S1 and PCNA expression in erythroid precursors and megakaryocytes—A comparative study on proliferative and endoreduplicative activity in reactive and neoplastic bone marrow lesions. J. Pathol., *173:* 5–12, 1994.

Thoenes, W., Störkel, St., Rumpelt, H. -J., Moll, R., Baum, H. P., and Werner, S.: Chromophobe cell renal carcinoma and its variants—a report on 32 cases. J. Pathol., *155:* 277–287, 1988.

Thompson, J. A., Grunert, F., and Zimmermann, W.: Carcinoembryonic gene family: molecule biology and clinical perspectives. J. Clin. Lab. Anal., *5:* 344–366, 1991.

Thor, A. D., Moore II, D. H., Egerton, S. M., Kawasaki, E. S., Reihsaus, E., Lynch, H. T., Marcus, J. N., Schwartz, L., Chen, L. -C., and Mayall, B. H., and Smith, H. S.: Accumulation of p53 tumor suppressor gene protein: an independent marker of prognosis in breast cancer. J. Natl. Cancer Inst., *84:* 845–855, 1992.

Tölle, H. G., Weber, K., and Osborn, M.: Microinjection of monoclonal antibodies specific for one intermediate filament protein in cells containing multiple keratins allow insight into the composition of particular 10 nm filaments. Eur. J. Cell Biol., *38:* 234–244, 1985.

Torenbeek, R., Blomjous, C. E. M., de Bruin, P. C., Newling, D. W. W., and Meijer, C. J. L. M.: Sarcomatoid carcinoma of the urinary bladder. Clinicopathological analysis of 18 cases with immunohistochemical and electron microscopic findings. Am. J. Surg. Pathol., *18:* 241–249, 1994.

Toth, K., Vaughan, M. M., Slocum, H. K., Arredondo, M. A., Takita, H., Baker, R. M., and Rustum, Y. M.: New immunohistochemical "sandwich" staining method for mdr1 P-glycoprotein detection with JSB-1 monoclonal antibody in formalin-fixed, paraffin-embedded human tissues. Am. J. Pathol., *144:* 227–236, 1994.

Trejdosiewicz, L. K., Wilson, P. D., and Hodges, G. M.: Species cross-reactive membrane-associated urothelial differentiation antigen. J. Natl. Cancer Inst., *72:* 355–366, 1984.

Trejdosiewicz, L. K., Southgate, J., Donald, J. A., Masters, J. R. W., Hepburn, P. J., and Hodges, G. M.: Monoclonal antibodies to human urothelial cell lines and hybrids: Production and characterization. J. Urol., *133:* 533–538, 1985.

Tsai, Y. C., Nichols, P. W., Hiti, A. L., Williams, Z., Skinner, D. G., and Jones, P. A.: Allelic loss of chromosomes 9, 11, and 17 in human bladder cancer. Cancer Res., *50:* 44–47, 1990.

Tsukada, T., Tippens, D., Gordon, D., Ross, R., and Gown, A. M.: HHF35, a muscle-actin-specific monoclonal antibody. I. Immunocytochemical and biochemical characterization. Am. J. Pathol., *126:* 51–60, 1987.

Ueda, R., Ogata, S. -I., Morissey, D. M., Finstad, C. L., Szkudlarek, J., Whitmore, W. F., Oettgen, H. F., Lloyd, K. O., and Old, L. J.: Cell surface antigens of human renal cancer defined by mouse monoclonal antibodies: identification of tissue-specific kidney glycoproteins. Proc. Natl. Acad. Sci., USA 78: 5122, 1981.

Vafier, J. A., Javadpour, N., Worsham, G. F., and O'Connel, K. J.: Double blind comparison of T-antigen and ABO (H) cell surface antigens in bladder cancer. Urology, *23:* 348–351, 1984.

Valles, A. M., Boyer, B., Badet, J., Tucker, G. C., Barritault, D., and Thiery, J. P.: Acidic fibroblast growth factor is a modulator of epithelial plasticity in a rat bladder carcinoma cell line. Proc. Natl. Acad. Sci., *87:* 1124–1128, 1990.

Van Eyken, P., Sciot, R., and Desmet, J.: A cytokeratin immunohistochemical study of cholestatic liver disease: evidence that hepatocytes can express "bile duct-type" cytokeratins. Histopathology, *15:* 125–135, 1989.

Van Krieken, J. H. J. M.: Prostate marker immunoreactivity in salivary gland neoplasms. A rare pitfall in immunohistochemistry. Am. J. Surg. Pathol., *17:* 410–414, 1993.

Van Muijen, G. N. P., Ruiter, D. J., Franke, W. W., Achtstätter, T., Haasnoot, W. H. B., Ponec, M., and Warnaar, S. O.: Cell type heterogeneity of cytokeratin expression in complex epithelia and carcinomas as demonstrated by monoclonal antibodies specific for cytokeratins nos. 4 and 13. Exp. Cell Res., *162:* 97–113, 1986.

Van Waes, C., Kozarsky, K. F., Warren, A. B., Kidd, L.,

Paugh, D., Liebert, M., and Carey, T. E.: The A9 antigen associated with aggressive human squamous carcinoma is structurally and functionally similar to the newly defined integrin alpha 6 beta 4. Cancer Res., *51:* 2395–2402, 1991.

Vleminckx, K., Vakaet, L., Jr., Mareel, M., Fiers, W., and Van Roy, F.: Genetic manipulation of E-cadherin expression by epithelial tumor cells reveals an invasion suppressor role. Cell, *66:* 107–119, 1991.

Vojtesek, B., and Lane, D. P.: Regulation of p53 protein expression in human breast cancer cell lines. J. Cell Sci., *105:* 607–612, 1993.

Volm, M., Efferth, T., Bak, M., Ho, A. D., and Mattern, J.: Detection of the multidrug resistant phenotype in human tumors by monoclonal antibodies and the streptavidin-biotinylated phycoerythrin complex method. Eur. J. Cancer Clin. Oncol., *25:* 743–749, 1989.

Von Overbeck, J., Stähli, C., Gudat, F., Carmann, H., Lautenschläger, C., Durmüller, C., Takacs, C., Miggiano, V., Staehelin, T., and Heitz, P.: Immunohistochemical characterization of an antiepithelial monoclonal antibody (mAb lu-5). Virchows Arch. A, *407:* 1–12, 1985.

Von Wasielewsky, R., Werner, M., Nolte, M., Wilkens, L., and Georgii, A.: Effects of antigen retrieval by microwave heating in formalin fixed tissue sections on a broad panel of antibodies. Histochemistry, *102:* 165–172, 1994.

Wagner, U., Sauter, G., Moch, H., Waldman, F., and Mihatsch, M. J.: p53 and erbB-2 protein expression in normal and precancerous urothelium: association with grade of dysplasia and proliferation rate. Path. Res. Pract., *190:* 251, 1994.

Wahren, B., Esposti, P., and Zimmerman, R.: Characterization of urothelial carcinoma with respect to the content of carcinoembryonic antigen in exfoliated cells. Cancer, *40:* 1511–1518, 1977.

Wahren, B.: Cellular content of carcinoembryonic antigen in urothelial carcinoma. Cancer, *42:* 1533–1539, 1978.

Waldherr, R., and Schwechheimer, K.: Co-expression of cytokeratin and vimentin intermediate-sized filaments in renal cell carcinomas. Comparative study of the intermediate-sized filament distribution in renal cell carcinomas and normal human kidney. Virchows Arch. A, *408:* 15–27, 1985.

Warnke, R. A., Gatter, K. C., Falini, B., Hildreth, A. B., Woolston, R. -E., Pulford, K., Cordell, J. L., Cohen, B., De Wolf-Peeters, C., and Mason, D. Y.: Diagnosis of human lymphoma with monoclonal antileukocyte antibodies. N. Engl. J. Med., *309:* 1275–1281, 1983.

Waseem, N. H., and Lane, D. P.: Monoclonal antibody analysis of the proliferating cell nuclear antigen (PCNA). Structural conservation and the detection of a nuclear form. J. Cell Sci., *96:* 121–129, 1990.

Weber, G., Osborn, M., Moll, R., Wiklund, B., and Lüning, B.: Tissue polypeptide antigen (TPA) is related to the non-epidermal keratins 8, 18 and 19 typical of simple and non-squamous epithelia: Reevaluation of a human tumor marker. EMBO J., *3:* 2707–2714, 1984.

Weinberg, R. A.: Tumor suppressor genes. Science, *254:* 1138–1146, 1991.

Weinstein, R. S., Miller, A. W., and Coon, J. S.: Tissue blood group ABH and Thomsen-Friedenreich antigens in human urinary bladder carcinoma. Prog. Clin. Biol. Res., *153:* 249–260, 1984.

Weinstein, R. S., Alroy, J., Farrow, G. M., Miller, A. W., III, and Davidsohn, I.: Blood group isoantigen deletion in carcinoma in situ of the urinary bladder. Cancer, *43:* 661–668, 1979.

Weinstein, R. S., Coon, J., Alroy, J., and Davidsohn, I.: Tissue-associated blood group antigens in human tumors. *In* De Lellis, R. A. (Ed.): Diagnostic Immunohistochemistry. New York, Masson, 1981, pp. 239–261.

Weiss, S. W., Langloss, J. M., and Enzinger, F. M.: Value of S-100 protein in the diagnosis of soft tissue tumors with particular reference to benign and malignant Schwann cell tumors. Lab. Invest., *49:* 299–308, 1983.

Weiss, R. E., Liu, B. C. -S., Ahlering, Th., Dubeau, L., and Droller, M. J.: Mechanisms of human bladder tumor invasion: Role of protease cathepsin B. J. Urol., *144:* 798–804, 1990.

Wernert, N., Seitz, G., and Achtstätter, Th.: Immunohistochemical investigation of different cytokeratins and vimentin in the prostate from the fetal period up to adulthood and in prostate carcinoma. Path. Res. Pract., *182:* 617–626, 1987.

Wersto, R. P., Herz, F., Gallagher, R. E., and Koss, L. G.: Cell cycle-dependent reactivity with the monoclonal antibody Ki-67 during myeloid cell differentiation. Exp. Cell. Res., *179:* 79–88, 1988.

Wetzels, R. H., Robben, H. C., Leigh, I. M., Schaafsma, H. E., Vooijs, G. P., and Ramaekers, F. C.: Distribution patterns of type VII collagen in normal and malignant human tissues. Am. J. Pathol., *139:* 451–459, 1991.

Wiley, E. L., Mendelsohn, G., Droller, M. J., and Eggleston, J. C.: Immunoperoxidase detection of carcinoembryonic antigen and blood group substances in papillary transitional cell carcinoma of the bladder. J. Urol., *128:* 276–280, 1982.

Wilson, B. S., and Lloyd, R. V.: Detection of chromogranin in neuroendocrine cells with a monoclonal antibody. Am. J. Pathol., *115:* 458–468, 1984.

Wilson, P. D., Nathrath, W. B. J., Trejdosiewicz, L. K.: Immunoelectron microscopic localisation of keratin and luminal epithelial antigens in normal and neoplastic urothelium. Pathol. Res. Pract., *175:* 289–298, 1982.

Wolf, G. T., Carey, T. E., Schmaltz, S. P., McClatchey, K. D., Poore, J., Glaser, L., Hayashida, D. J., and Hsu, S.: Altered antigen expression predicts outcome in squamous cell carcinoma of the head and neck. J. Natl. Cancer Inst., *82:* 1566–1572, 1990.

Woods, A. L., Hanby, A. M., Hall, P. A., Shepherd, N. A., Waseem, N. H., Lane, D. P., Levison, D. A.: The prognostic value of PCNA (proliferative cell nuclear an-

tigen) immunostaining in gastrointestinal lymphomas. J. Pathol., *161:* 342, 1990.

Wright, C., Mellon, K., Johnston, P., Lane, D. P., Harris, A. L., Horne, C. H. W., and Neal, D. E.: Expression of mutant p53, c-erbB-2 and the epidermal growth factor receptor in transitional cell carcinoma of the human urinary bladder. Br. J. Cancer, *63:* 967–970, 1991.

Wu, X. -R., Manabe, M., Yu, J., and Sun, T. -T.: Large scale purification and immunolocalization of bovine uroplakins I, II, and III. J. Biol. Chem., *265:* 19170–19179, 1990.

Xu, H. J., Hu, S. -X., and Benedict, W. F.: Lack of nuclear RB protein staining in G0/middle G1 cells: correlation to changes in total RB protein level. Oncogene, *6:* 1139–1140, 1991.

Yachi, A., and Shiveley, J. E. (Eds.): The CEA antigen gene family. New York, Elsevier, 1989.

Yamamoto, T., Ikawa, S., Akiyama, T., Semba, K., Nomura, N., Miyajima, N., Saito, T., and Toyoshima, K.: Similarity of protein encoded by the human c-erbB-2 gene to epidermal growth factor receptor. Nature, *319:* 230–234, 1986.

Yamase, H. T., Powell, G. T., and Koss, L. G.: A simplified method of preparing permanent tissue sections for the erythrocyte adherence test. Am. J. Clin. Pathol., *75:* 178–181, 1981.

Yarden, Y., and Peles, E.: Biochemical analysis of the ligand for the neu oncogeneic receptor. Biochemistry, *30:* 3543–3550, 1991.

Yonemura, Y., Ninomiya, I., Ohoyama, S., Kimura, H., Yamaguchi, A., Fushida, S., Kosaka, T., Miwa, K., Miyazaki, I., and Endou, Y.: Expression of c-erbB-2 oncoprotein in gastric carcinoma. Immunoreactivity for c-erbB-2 protein is an independent indicator of poor short-term prognosis in patients with gastric carcinoma. Cancer, *67:* 2914–2918, 1991.

Young, W. W., Portoukalian, J., and Hakomori, S. -I.: Two monoclonal anticarbohydrate antibodies directed to glycosphingolipids with a lacto-N-glycosyl type II chain. J. Biol. Chem., *256:* 10967–10972, 1981.

Yu, J., Manabe, M., Wu, X. -R., Surya, B., and Sun, T. -T.: Uroplakin I: A 27-kD protein associated with the asymmetric unit membrane of mammalian urothelium. J. Cell. Biol., *111:* 1207–1216, 1990.

Zhang, D. S., and Lin, C. W.: Immunochemical and biochemical characterization of two monoclonal antibody-reacting antigens associated with human bladder carcinoma. Cancer Res., *49:* 6621–6628, 1989.

Zimmerman, I. J., Biron, R. E., and MacMahon, H. E.: Pheochromocytoma of the urinary bladder. N. Engl. J. Med., *249:* 25–26, 1953.

Zukerberg, L. R., Harris, N. L., and Young, R. H.: Carcinoma of the urinary bladder simulating malignant lymphoma: a report of 5 cases. Am. J. Surg. Pathol., *15:* 569–576, 1991.

CHAPTER 11

Molecular Biology of Common Tumors of the Urinary Tract

Bogdan Czerniak, M.D.
Fritz Herz, Ph.D.

TECHNIQUES USED IN MOLECULAR GENETIC RESEARCH

Since the mid-1970s numerous technologic developments have contributed to the understanding of many molecular aspects of cell biology and shed light on some of the events that may be responsible for the malignant behavior of human and animal cells. Although, at the time of this writing (1994), no definitive statement can be made as to which of these events are responsible for the development and progression of human cancers, significant progress has been made toward understanding malignant transformation as a biologic phenomenon. This chapter discusses some of the most promising avenues of molecular genetic research on common tumors of the urinary tract.

The principles of molecular biology cannot be discussed in this summary and the reader is referred to other sources for a comprehensive review of the current status of knowledge (Watson et al., 1987; Watson et al., 1992; Koss, 1992). Briefly, the DNA molecule located in the nucleus of a cell carries codes for formation of individual proteins (genes). These coding sequences (exons) are interrupted by segments of noncoding DNA (the introns). The functions of the introns are not fully understood but some of them perform various regulatory functions, *i.e.* provide signals for start, stop, or detachment of the transcribed message. The codes for individual proteins are transcribed into messenger RNA (mRNA). The introns are eliminated from mRNA by a multistep process known as splicing. The mRNA passes from the nucleus to the cytoplasm where the actual protein synthesis takes place. If an error in the code occurs due to substitution of a nucleotide, or deletion of one or more nucleotides, the synthesis of the correct protein is impaired. The resulting protein may have a very different function from the one intended or may not be synthesized at all. The search for such errors in genes and their regulatory elements is the basis of molecular genetic research in cancer.

Because DNA is packaged in chromosomes, abnormalities of chromosomes may be observed by cytogenetic studies of metaphases, providing the initial evidence of a genetic abnormality. More specific identification of chromosomal abnormalities requires complex strategies which involve chromosomal microdissection, mapping with hypervariable probes, and use of fluorescent chromosomal probes (FISH), collectively known as positional cloning.

The most common techniques used to elucidate some of the genetic abnormalities discussed here are based on the extraction and analysis of deoxyribonucleic acid (DNA), ribonucleic acid (RNA), or proteins. To facilitate the separation and identification of the genetic material, the long strands of DNA are usually cut with specific restriction endonucleases, a unique class of enzymes that recognizes specific nucleotide sequences and cuts the double-stranded DNA at specific points. These enzymes are used in nearly all gene reconstruction and transfection (gene transfer) experiments, collectively referred to as DNA recombinant technology or genetic engineering. The many techniques used to identify normal or altered components of the genome are typically assembled into strategies capable of identifying structural and functional aspects of the genetic element under study. They can also be used to identify new, hitherto unknown elements of the genome (gene hunting strategies). The final step in this approach—and its ultimate goal—is the identification of new genes, which involves series of DNA recombinant techniques known as gene cloning.

The techniques used to identify the normal or altered elements of the genome can be divided into three main groups: DNA hybridization techniques; polymerase chain reaction-based technologies; and genomic mapping technologies.

Hybridization Techniques

Southern Blotting

Southern blotting is used for the localization of particular sequences within genomic DNA. Traditionally, the DNA is digested with restriction endonucleases and the resulting DNA fragments are separated by size using electrophoresis through agarose gels. After in situ denaturation of the fragments by an alkaline solution or by heat, the DNA is transferred from the gel onto a solid support (*e.g.,* nylon membranes, nitrocellulose filters). The relative positions of the fragments are preserved during this transfer. Subsequently the DNA blotted to the solid support is hybridized with a known, specific, DNA or RNA probe with a radioactive label, and then is visualized by autoradiography to locate positions of bands complementary to the probe.

Northern Blotting

Northern blotting is used to determine the size and amount of specific messenger RNA (mRNA). As in Southern blotting, the RNA is separated by electrophoresis on the basis of size using denatured agarose gels and transferred to a solid support (*e.g.,* nylon membranes, nitrocellulose filters). The RNA of interest is located by hybridization with the appropriately labeled DNA or RNA probes.

Western Blotting

Western blotting is used for the immunologic identification of proteins extracted from tissues or cells. The protein extracts are separated by electrophoresis, then transferred onto a solid support and identified with labeled or unlabeled antibodies that recognize the antigenic epitopes displayed by the target protein.

When unlabeled antibodies are used, identification of the bands is done with a labeled secondary antibody to the immunoglobulin class of the animal species in which the first antibody was raised.

Dot Blotting

In dot blotting small aliquots of DNA or RNA are placed (spotted) onto filters to which labeled specific probes are added. The hybridization is visualized by autoradiography or other techniques. Dot blotting differs from Southern and Northern hybridization in that no electrophoretic separation is involved. The purpose of dot blotting is to identify the presence of given nucleotide fragments.

Polymerase Chain Reaction

Polymerase chain reaction (PCR) is an in vitro technique used to amplify a DNA segment lying between two regions of known sequences, using two oligonucleotide primers. The primers are complementary of the strand opposite to the sequence of the target template DNA and flank the DNA segment to be amplified. The reaction mixture contains the four nucleotides required for DNA synthesis in the presence of a heat-stable DNA polymerase. The procedure consists of three basic steps: heat denaturation of the template DNA, cooling and annealing of the primers to their target sequences, and extension by the DNA polymerase. Because the product generated in the first PCR round serves as template for the next and subsequent rounds, an exponential amplification of the DNA segment of interest may be obtained by repeating the cycles. The usual amplification level is of the order of 10^6 after 25 to 30 cycles. Greater amplification (10^9 to 10^{11}) of DNA copies may be achieved by repeating the cycles using the product generated in the first run as a template and fresh DNA polymerase. PCR can also be used to generate amplified DNA from mRNA following initial reverse transcription.

Genomic Mapping

The development of accurate, high-density human genome maps was possible because of the Human Genome Project. This is a multi-institutional and international effort for the study of organization and function of the human genome, and its ultimate goal is to sequence the entire human genome. The intermediate tasks are the identification of multiple loci with known chromosomal locations and distances (genetic maps), which can be related to fragments of the human ge-

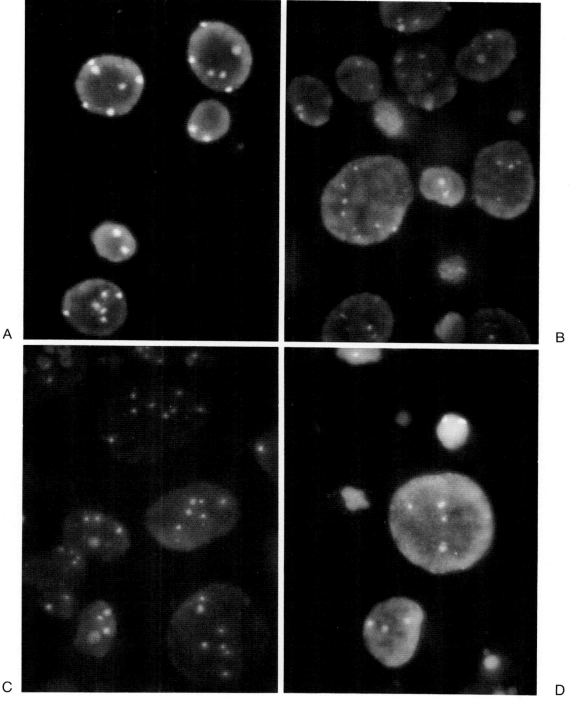

Color Plate 11-1. Fluorescence in situ hybridization (FISH) with centromeric DNA probes of urinary bladder carcinoma cells in the sediment of voided urine. (*A*) Multiple copies of chromosome 7 in a low-grade papillary urothelial carcinoma. (*B*) Multiple copies of chromosome 9 in a high-grade invasive non-papillary urothelial carcinoma. The number of chromosome 9 copies in the cancer cells varies from 3 to 9. (*C*) Chromosome 17 alterations in a high-grade papillary carcinoma. Two cell populations are present. One consists of cells with 7 to 8 copies of chromosome 17 and the other of cells exhibiting trisomy 17. (*D*) Chromosome 11 alterations in a high-grade non-papillary invasive urothelial carcinoma. Most cells exhibit trisomy 11, with individual larger cells having 4 to 5 copies of chromosome 11. (Courtesy of R. Katz, M.D., and H-Z Zhang, M.D., Department of Pathology, M. D. Anderson Cancer Center.)

nome organized in sequential order (physical maps) and stored in yeast artificial chromosomes (YACs).

The advances in genetic mapping became possible because multiple repetitive DNA sequences (microsatellites) were identified within the human genome. The repeating units are usually di-, tri-, or tetra-nucleotides that are distributed relatively evenly throughout the genome. They tend to be polymorphic and vary from one person to another. Microsatellites are unstable in some types of cancer. The instability consists of contraction or expansion of the DNA within the repeat elements. These alterations, attributed to DNA replication errors, are readily detectable by PCR. The microsatellites provide useful loci for linkage analysis and for the identification of altered loci in familial genetic disorders, including the cancer-predisposing syndromes.

Fluorescence In Situ Hybridization (FISH)

Fluorescence in situ hybridization (FISH) is applicable to archival material, to whole cells, and to metaphase chromosomes. It permits the identification of individual chromosomes and of genetic loci by hybridization with specific, labeled DNA probes. The signal is visualized by fluorescent microscopy and may be evaluated by computerized image analysis (see Color Plate 11-1). It is particularly useful in studies in which appropriate probes are used to identify numerical aberrations, as well as mapping of chromosomal deletions, numerical aberrations, and translocations that cannot be identified by the conventional banding techniques.

Allelic Loss

Allelic loss refers to the deletion of specific chromosomal loci. Allelic loss can be detected by Southern blotting or by PCR, followed by hybridization with chromosome-specific polymorphic probes.

URINARY BLADDER

Tumors of the urinary bladder represent a group of neoplasms with diverse morphology and clinical behavior (Raghavan et al., 1990). Current concepts postulate that they result from at least two distinct, but sometimes overlapping, genetic pathways (Koss et al., 1991; Koss, 1975; 1992). Approximately 80% of urothelial tumors are superficially growing exophytic papillary lesions, which may recur but usually do not invade and metastasize. The remaining 20% are solid carcinomas which at the time of diagnosis are usually invasive. Most invasive carcinomas arise from flat carcinomas in situ that develop within the bladder epithelium, either as a primary lesion or as a lesion accompanying papillary tumors (Brawn, 1982; Kaye, et al., 1982; Koss, 1975; see also Chap. 5). Consequently, urothelial tumors of the bladder can be divided into two main groups: papillary and non-papillary (solid) (Koss et al., 1991). It is very likely that tumors with such different morphology, growth patterns, and clinical behavior arise as a result of different molecular events. The search for distinctive molecular features that distinguish between papillary and solid urothelial tumors of the bladder is currently a central target of research.

Chromosomal Changes

The search for information on alterations of the human genome responsible for the malignant phenotype of urothelial cells begins at the chromosome level. Numerous attempts have been made to correlate specific chromosomal alterations with histologic tumor types, grade, invasiveness, and clinical behavior. It has been shown that aggressive high-grade tumors are usually aneuploid (Color Plate 11-1). Such tumors usually display numerous marker chromosomes. Hence, it has been postulated that the presence of marker chromosomes is one of the unfavorable prognostic factors (Falor and Ward, 1978; Burke et al., 1984). It also has been shown that urothelial tumors, classified as having a diploid DNA content as determined by flow cytometry or image analysis, frequently have numerical changes of individual chromosomes, as documented by FISH (Hopman et al., 1991; 1989; 1988). Certain chromosomes apparently are more prone to structural changes and are more likely to contribute to the formation of marker chromosomes than others. The chromosomes found to be involved frequently in a non-random fashion in bladder tumors were 1, 6, 11, and 13 (Gibas et al., 1986). In some tumors trisomy 7 or 5q deletion was seen as the sole chromosomal change (Atkin et al., 1990; Berrozpe et al., 1990). It has been postulated that trisomy of chromosome 7, when present as the sole abnormality, is associated with non-invasive growth and may represent a primary event in low-grade papillary tumors (Berrozpe et al., 1990). In situ hybridization studies also documented that trisomy of chromosome 1 is frequent in these tumors. In an in vitro transformation system, human urothelial cells developed progressive non-random deletions of chromosome regions 3p, 6q, and 18q (Wu et al., 1991). The smallest common losses were found on chromosomes 6(q21-q23) and 18(q21). Deletion of 3p and 18q apparently correlated with progression to high grade or invasive carcinomas (Wu et al., 1991). Subsequent studies have shown that deletions of 3p(21-25) and 17p(11-13) regions, containing putative tumor suppressor genes, correlate with high-grade tumors and advanced tumor stages (Presti et al., 1991). In one case report, a constitutional somatic deletion of 3p(11-21) was documented in a patient with bladder carcinoma (Barrios et al., 1986).

Some chromosomal deletions are common in urothelial cancers. For example, allelic loss of chromosome 9q is quite frequent; loss of heterozygosity occurs in more than 50% of grade I and II superficial tumors (Miyao et al., 1993). By contrast, allelic losses of chromosomes 11p and 17p are seen predominantly in high-grade invasive tumors (Olumi et al., 1990). The deletion of 17p has a strong correlation with high histologic grade and invasive growth pattern (Olumi et al., 1990).

It appears, therefore, that despite significant overlap, low-grade papillary tumors and high-grade invasive carcinomas may have some distinct cytogenetic features. Low-grade papillary lesions have fewer chromosomal changes than high-grade carcinomas and show mainly trisomies of chromosomes 1 and 7. Furthermore, investigation of chromosome 9 alterations may provide important clues on the pathogenesis of superficial low-grade papillary lesions of the bladder. On the other hand, high-grade invasive bladder carcinomas develop multiple cumulative rearrangements and deletions of chromosomes with formation of marker chromosomes, frequently involving chromosomes 3, 11, 17, and 18. Alterations of chromosome 17 in particular seem to be a common event in high-grade invasive, solid carcinomas of the bladder. The correlation of these alterations with modifications in the expression of the tumor suppressor gene p53 is discussed below.

Oncogenes and Tumor Suppressor Genes

Among the more than 100 transforming and tumor suppressor genes identified so far, only a few have been shown to play a significant role in the biology of urothelial tumors. They include the *ras* family of genes, p53 genes as well as genes of the so-called p53 regulatory pathway, and the Rb gene.

ras *Genes*

The human *ras* gene family (Ha-, Ki-, and N-*ras*) has served as a prototype of cellular genes whose mutations and/or overexpression can lead to malig-

nant transformation (Barbacid et al., 1987). These genes encode a group of closely related 21-kd proteins (p21). *ras* p21 binds guanine nucleotides with high affinity and has guanosine triphosphatase (GTPase) activity. The protein is anchored to the cytoplasmic surface of the cell membrane and serves as a transducer molecule for signals affecting cell proliferation and differentiation (Barbacid et al., 1987). Two mechanisms have been proposed to explain how *ras* genes transform cells (Bos et al., 1989; Reddy et al., 1982; Taparowsky et al., 1982). One involves a single nucleotide mutation in the coding sequence that occurs most frequently at codon 12, 13, 59, or 61. This alteration results in an amino acid substitution of the gene product p21 that affects the GTP binding domain and reduces its GTPase activity. The second possible mechanism involves overexpression of the *ras* gene product.

It has been shown that in the Ha-*ras* gene the introns play a regulatory role. The DNA sequence around nucleotide 2719 within intron D functions as an alternative splicing site (Cohen et al., 1988). It suppresses gene expression by destabilizing the transcript and causing it to enter a non-productive pathway. From the functional point of view, the intron D splicing recognition sequence acts as a negative regulatory element by suppressing gene expression and, presumably, protecting the cell from eventual transforming activity of the mutated (altered) gene product. As a result of the alternative splicing pathway, a minimal amount of a different gene product of 19 kd (p19) may be produced. This protein possibly acts as an antioncogene and protects the cell from the effects of the oncogene (Cohen et al., 1989). Hence, Ha-*ras* appears to represent a gene capable of encoding two antagonistic products: one with transforming capability and the other with anti-oncogenic (tumor suppressor gene) activity. An A→T point mutation at position 2719 of intron D abolishes the alternative splicing pathway and its regulatory role, causing overexpression of p21 and significantly increasing transforming efficiency (Cohen et al., 1988, 1989). Thus, a mutation at position 2719 of the Ha-*ras* gene intron is analogous in function to that of a strong promoter–enhancer in that it causes overexpression of the gene product. Although point mutations at coding sequences alone are not essential for transforming activity, their presence enhances the transforming efficiency of overexpressed *ras* gene products (Chakraborty et al., 1991). The exon/intron structure of the Ha-*ras* gene with frequent sites of point mutations and the function of alternative splicing site within the last intron are shown in Figure 11-1.

Mutations of coding sequences of *ras* genes are the most frequent genetic alterations seen in urothelial

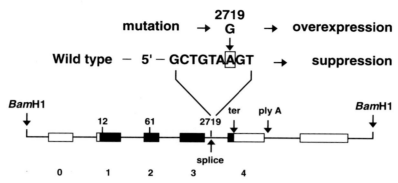

FIGURE 11-1. Exon/intron structure of the Ha-*ras* gene. The black bars indicate the translated sequences (the exons). Frequent sites of point mutation within exons 1 and 2 (codon 12 and 61) and the sequence of the alternative splicing site around nucleotide 2719 are shown. The A→G mutation at position 2719 abolishes the splicing mechanism, causing overexpression of the gene product.

cancer (Barbacid, 1987; Bos, 1989). They usually involve codon 12 and, less frequently, codon 13 or 61 of Ha-*ras*. Sporadically, the Ki-*ras* gene can be also affected. The elimination of functional mutated Ha-*ras* gene in the human urinary bladder carcinoma cell line T24 by an antisense oligonucleotide inhibits cell proliferation (Saison-Bohemaras et al., 1991). The originally reported frequency of *ras* gene mutations in human urinary bladder carcinomas was low (Feinberg et al., 1983; Fujita et al., 1984). More recently, however, with the use of highly sensitive PCR-based techniques, it has been found that the rate of mutations involving predominantly codon 12 of Ha-*ras* is much higher than originally reported (Visvanathan et al., 1988; Nagata et al., 1990). Several recent studies have shown that Ha-*ras* mutations occur in approximately 50% of urinary bladder carcinomas (Burchill et al., 1991; Czerniak et al., 1992), but in one report a much lower frequency was noted (Knowles and Williamson, 1993).

Our studies have shown that a G→T substitution in the second nucleotide of codon 12 of the Ha-*ras* gene, which results in the replacement of glycine for valine in the gene product p21, is a dominant *ras* gene mutation in human bladder carcinomas (Fig. 11-2) (Czerniak et al., 1992). This preponderance of one specific point mutation suggests that it could be related to the possible exposure of urothelial cells to very specific environmental carcinogens. Although induction of specific *ras* mutations related to a particular carcinogen has been documented in animal models, no such evidence is available for human bladder tumors. Ha-*ras* gene codon 12 mutations occur more frequently in high-grade aneuploid bladder carcinomas than in low-grade diploid papillary carcinomas, but

no definite correlation with tumor grade or invasiveness has been established (Ooi et al., 1994). Hence, mutations of coding sequences of the Ha-*ras* gene alone may not be useful as reliable prognostic indicators for individual patients.

On the other hand, the above-mentioned A→T substitution at position 2719 within the alternative splicing site in intron D was identified in approximately 10% of all bladder tumors examined (Fig. 11-3) (Czerniak et al., 1992). This relatively rare event occurs most often in high-grade invasive aneuploid carcinomas and may be responsible for the striking *ras* p21 overexpression by about 40% of these tumors (Fig. 11-4). Moreover, the mutation at position 2719 was almost invariably accompanied by a synchronous codon 12 mutation. This indicates that if the same allele carries both mutations, it may result in the overexpression of an altered *ras* p21 with enhanced transforming potential. These findings further suggest that multifocal synchronous mutations of coding and negative regulatory sequences of the Ha-*ras* gene may be responsible, at least in part, for the aggressive behavior of some human urothelial tumors. However, as the concurrent codon 12/intron D mutations were identified in only about 40% of invasive carcinomas, they cannot be the sole factor responsible for the invasive phenotype. Hence, it is evident that other molecular genetic alterations must be responsible for the aggressive behavior of bladder tumors.

During an ongoing study we addressed the question of when *ras* gene mutations become evident during tumor development and progression and how they relate to the dual track concept of bladder tumorigenesis. To answer these questions we searched for Ha-*ras* codon 12 and intron D mutations in sequential

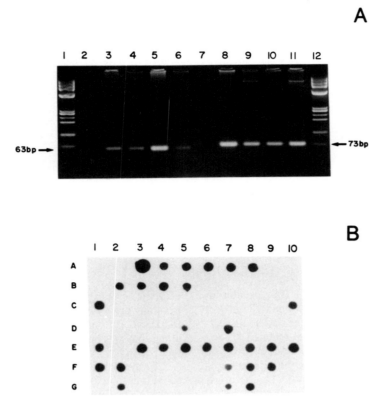

FIGURE 11-2. Identification of Ha-*ras* gene mutations in urinary bladder carcinomas by PCR and hybridization with point mutation-specific oligonucleotides. (*A*) PCR amplification of 63 (lanes 3 to 6) and 73 (lanes 8 to 11) base pair fragments of Ha-*ras*–containing codons 12 and 61, respectively. Lanes 2 and 7, reaction controls without genomic DNA; Lanes 1 and 12, size marker. (*B*) Dot blot hybridization with the value-specific oligonucleotide probe of PCR-amplified Ha-*ras* fragments containing codon 12. *1A,* no DNA; *2A,* human placental DNA (negative control); *3A,* T24 cells (positive control). The remaining dots represent 67 bladder tumors. (from Czerniak, B., Cohen, G. L., Etkind, P., et al.: Concurrent mutations of coding and regulatory sequences of the Ha-*ras* gene in urinary bladder carcinomas. Hum. Pathol., *23*, 1199–1203, 1992.)

archival samples from patients who initially presented with a low-grade papillary carcinoma and who subsequently developed high-grade invasive solid carcinomas. Multiple samples of bladder mucosa containing morphologically normal urothelium, urothelium with features of premalignant lesion (dysplasia), and carcinoma in situ were also included in the study. Our initial results indicate that synchronous codon 12/intron D mutations are detectable even in the normal mucosa of patients with non-invasive papillary carcinomas who subsequently, sometimes many years later, developed intra-urothelial flat neoplasia elsewhere in the bladder (Table 11-1). The synchronous Ha-*ras* mutations were also readily identified in premalignant flat urothelial lesions, sometimes many years before invasive cancer developed (Fig. 11-5). The subsequent invasive carcinomas almost invariably exhibited the same concurrent mutations. By comparison, the papillary non-invasive carcinomas of the same patient usually only had the codon 12 mutation. These results would indicate that aggressive solid bladder tumors are more likely to have synchronous Ha-*ras* codon 12/intron D mutations than non-invasive papillary lesions.

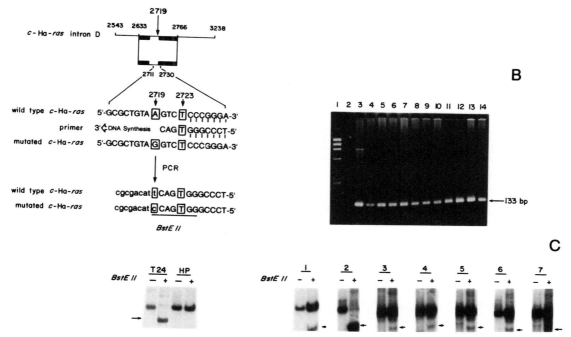

FIGURE 11-3. Screening for mutation at position 2719 of intron D of the Ha-*ras* gene. (*A*) Outline of amplification of an intron D fragment and identification of the A→G mutation at position 2719. To generate a *Bst* EII restriction site dependent on the presence of a G at position 2719, the A at position 2723 was replaced by T in the reverse primer. A positive and negative control with DNA of T24 cells and of human placenta (HP), respectively, are shown. The amplified fragment of T24 cells is cut (*arrow*) when exposed to *Bst* EII, thus demonstrating the presence of the A→G mutation. No *Bst* EII site is present in HP DNA (both cut and uncut fragments are of equal size). (*B*) Evaluation of PCR-amplified 133-bp fragments containing nucleotide 2719. Lane 1, size marker; lane 2, negative control (no template DNA added); lane 3 human placenta; lane 4, T24 cells; lanes 5 to 14 bladder carcinomas. (*C*) Identification of the A→G mutation at position 2719 in seven cases of urinary bladder carcinoma. (from Czerniak, B., Cohen, G. L., Etkind, P., et al.: Concurrent mutations of coding and regulatory sequences of the Ha-*ras* gene in urinary bladder carcinomas. Hum. Pathol., *23*, 1199–1203, 1992.)

It is of special significance for screening and monitoring of tumor progression that the modifications of the Ha-*ras* gene can be detected in DNA extracted from cells in the voided urinary sediment (Fig. 11-6). Our initial data indicate that it can be identified in approximately 25% of patients with urinary bladder carcinoma (Table 11-2). The significance of this observation remains to be established.

p53 Gene

The p53 gene has been a source of fascination since its discovery in 1979 (review in Levine et al.,

1991). The gene product was originally identified as a 53-kd nuclear phosphoprotein in cells transformed by simian virus 40 (SV40). The protein formed a complex with the large T antigen of SV40, suggesting that this interaction was important for transformation (Levine et al., 1991). It was later shown that the transforming activity of p53 is related to gene point mutations and that the mutated protein has a much longer half-life than the wild-type gene product. Moreover, it was established that the wild-type protein acts more like a tumor suppressor gene, negatively regulating the cell cycle requiring loss-of-function and/or a gain of a new function for transforming activity (Finlay et al., 1989). Because of the gain of a new function it

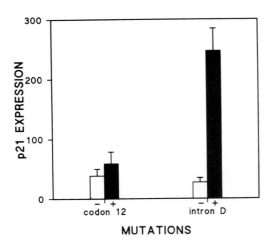

FIGURE 11-4. Expression of p21 in relation to mutations at codon 12 and at position 2719 of intron D of the Ha-*ras* gene in bladder carcinomas. Note the approximately 10-fold higher levels of p21 when position 2719 mutation is present.

can act in the heterozygous state and does not require allelic deletion for its transforming activity. p53 is a DNA-binding protein and a transcription activation factor capable of induction of the so-called p53 dependent genes (Kern et al., 1991). The recently discovered Cip-1 (WAF-1) is a prototype of this class of genes and codes for a 21-kd protein that inhibits the cyclin-dependent kinases (Cdk) responsible for the initiation of the G_1 phase of the cell cycle (Harper et al., 1993). Mutations in the p53 gene result in its failure to stimulate Cip-1, with subsequent loss of inhibition of Cdk–cyclin complexes and initiation of G_1. The discovery of p53-dependent Cdk inhibitors links this gene to the basic enzymatic mechanisms operative in negative cell cycle regulation.

The mutations that change the properties of p53 are usually missense substitutions. They are clustered in one particular region of the gene product located between amino acids 130 and 290 and mainly involve residues 117-142, 171-181, 239-258, and 270-286. These regions are highly conserved among species and are most likely of importance for the normal function of p53 (Finlay et al., 1989; Levine et al., 1991). The human p53 gene is located on chromosome 17 p13.1, and mutations have been documented in a wide range of tumors (McBride et al., 1986; Nigro et al., 1989; Hollstein et al., 1991). Loss of heterozygosity of the p53 locus has been found in many human cancers (Tisty et al., 1992). Therefore, p53 most likely contributes to human carcinogenesis when its normal allele is deleted or inactivated. The transforming activity in the heterozygous state can be due to the formation of an oligomeric complex between mutant and wild-type p53. It has been shown that in cells transformed with mutant p53 gene, the altered protein complexes with endogenous p53 and the complex remains in the cytoplasm (Martinez et al., 1991).

Mutated p53 genes can cooperate with *ras* genes to transform primary cultured fibroblasts in the presence of endogenous wild-type p53 protein (Halvey et al., 1990). Because in certain human tumors deletions of chromosome 17 loci may occur simultaneously with other chromosomal abnormalities, it has been suggested that p53 mutation is a late event during carcinogenesis. It was proposed that tumor cell aneuploidy, reflecting chromosomal instability, plays a role in the selection of tumor cells with p53 gene mutations. This may lead to a loss of the remaining wild-type allele and to inactivation of negative growth control function of the normal p53 protein. This view of the role of p53 may have to be modified, however, because p53 mutations have also been observed in premalignant lesions of esophageal and head and neck tumors. Moreover, germ-line transmission of p53 mutations has been described in certain cancer-prone

TABLE 11-1
Ha-*ras* Codon 12/Intron D Mutations in Urinary Bladder Carcinoma on Sequential Samples of 38 Patients (120 Samples) Who Progressed from Low Grade Papillary Tumor to High Grade Invasive Carcinoma

| | | | Codon 12+ | |
| | | | INTRON D | INTRON D |
Type of lesion	Total	Codon 12		
Normal urothelium	30	14(46)*	3(10)	2(6)
Dysplasia/CIS	28	22(78)	5(17)	4(14)
Papillary Ca (low grade)	34	29(85)	4(14)	4(11)
Solid Ca (high grade)	28	21(75)	9(32)	9(32)
Total	120	86(71)	21(17)	19(15)

*Numbers in parentheses represent the percentage of cases within a given category.

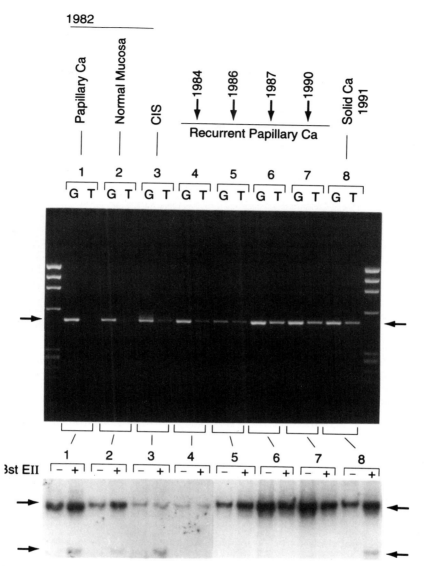

FIGURE 11-5. Chronological identification of codon 12 (*top panel*) and intron D position 2719 (*bottom panel*) mutations of Ha-*ras* in sequential samples from a patient who initially presented with a low-grade non-invasive papillary carcinoma and after 9 years, following several recurrences of low-grade non-invasive papillary tumors, developed a high-grade invasive non-papillary carcinoma. Codon 12 mutations were identified with point mutation specific primers using allele specific PCR (Ooi et al., 1994). The presence of a band in the G lane identifies the wild type (normal) codon 12. The presence of a band in the T lane identifies a G→T mutation at codon 12 of Ha-*ras*.

Intron D mutations at position 2719 were identified as described in Figure 11-3. The initial low-grade papillary carcinoma (1982) had an A→G position 2719 intron D mutation and a wild type codon 12. The initial carcinoma in situ showed a synchronous mutation in codon 12 and intron D. The subsequent recurrent papillary tumors (1984–1990) show a wild type position 2719 of intron D and a G→T mutation at codon 12. The final non-papillary invasive carcinoma exhibits synchronous codon 12 and intron D mutations that were present in a flat carcinoma in situ 9 years before the development of invasive cancer.

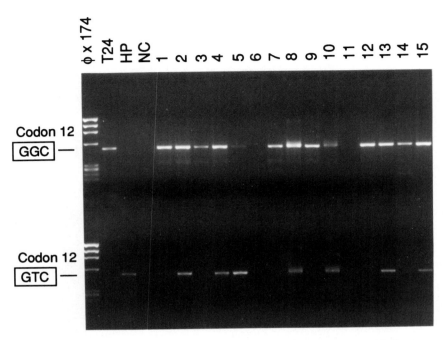

FIGURE 11-6. Identification of codon 12 Ha-*ras* mutations in voided urine. Allele-specific PCR with wild-type and codon 12, G→T mutation-specific primers was used. Presence of a band with the latter (*bottom lines*) denotes G→T mutation at codon 12. The normal triplet (GGC) coding for glycine and the mutated triplet (GTC) coding for value are shown for clarity. φ*X174*, DNA size marker; *T24*, T24 cells; *HP*, human placenta; *NC*, control without template DNA; *lanes 1–15*, DNA extracted from voided urine samples of patients with carcinoma of bladder.

families, especially those with Li-Fraumeni syndrome (Tisty et al., 1992). The functional domains of p53 and the distribution of mutation sites in human tumor are shown in Figure 11-7.

A survey of 18 invasive bladder cancers revealed the presence of p53 gene mutations in 11 of them (Sidransky et al., 1991). The most common mutations were single base-pair substitutions. Missense mutations were found in 7 and non-sense mutations in 3.

TABLE 11-2
Ha-*ras* Codon 12 G→T Mutation in Exfoliated Cells in Voided Urine Samples of Bladder Cancer Patients in Relation to Urine Cytology

Urine Cytology	*Ha*-ras *Mutations*
Negative	15/55 (27.2%)
Atypical	17/75 (22.6%)
Positive	7/20 (35.0%)
Total	39/151 (25.8%)

One tumor had a 24 base-pair deletion. The presence of p53 mutations was also detected in the urine sediments from the 3 patients tested. In another series of 25 bladder tumors from 23 patients it was shown that the incidence of p53 mutations was significantly higher in invasive (7/12) than in superficial (1/13) tumors (Fujimoto et al., 1992). The one mutated superficial tumor was a flat carcinoma in situ from a patient with multiple tumors. No other precancerous lesions were included in the study, and the authors cautioned that the reported incidence of p53 mutations in bladder cancer should be considered a minimal estimate. In a series of a variety of high-grade bladder tumors, diverse p53 mutations were identified in 36% of the cases (Cordon-Cardo et al., 1994). These molecular genetic findings are in line with immunohistochemical observations on p53 protein expression in bladder carcinomas (Sarkis et al., 1993). Esrig et al. (1993, 1994) reported that accumulation of p53 in tumor nuclei, detected by immunohistochemical methods, predicted a significant risk of recurrence and progression of bladder cancer and a decreased survival. The iden-

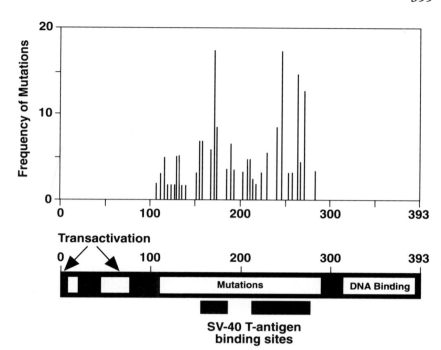

FIGURE 11-7. Functional domains of p53 protein and frequent mutation sites identified in human tumors.

Primary Amino Acid Sequence of p53

tification of alterations (mutations) of the recently discovered Cip1 and MTS1 genes in urinary bladder carcinomas and in other human neoplasms indicates that similar biologic effects, *e.g.,* lack of cell cycle inhibition, can be due to alterations of different genes that belong to the so-called p53 regulatory pathway. Moreover, the alterations of multiple genes belonging to the superfamily of negative cell cycle regulators can occur in the same tumor (Czerniak et al., unpublished data) (Table 11-3).

Retinoblastoma Gene

The retinoblastoma (Rb) gene was originally identified as a gene of retinoblastoma, a rare intraocular malignant neoplasm of childhood. It is the first gene identified as a tumor suppressor gene, *i.e.,* a gene whose loss of function leads to the development of malignant neoplasms. It was discovered as a germ cell line mutation that strongly predisposes infants to develop retinoblastomas. Rb gene codes for a 105-kd

TABLE 11-3
Alterations of Multiple Genes in Urinary Bladder Carcinomas in Relation to Histological Grade DNA Ploidy and Type of Growth

Type of lesion	Ha-ras	p53	Cip1	Alterations of all three genes
Papillary tumors grade I-II				
Diploid	0/15	0/15	0/15	0/15
Aneuploid	3/8	0/8	1/8	0/8
Papillary and solid tumors grade III				
Diploid	1/3	1/3	0/3	
Aneuploid	3/9	3/9	2/9	2/9
Total	7/35	4/35	2/35	2/35

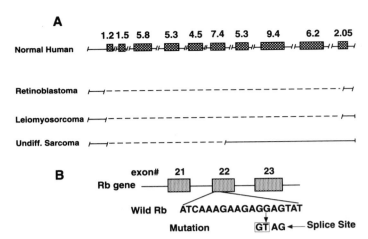

FIGURE 11-8. Main types of structural alterations of the Rb gene in human neoplasms leading to the absence of a functional gene product. (*A*) Major deletions of Rb, found predominantly in retinoblastoma and in several other human tumors. (*B*) Example of a point mutation generating an inappropriately located splicing site within exon 22 of Rb and causing translation of a truncated gene product.

protein that was shown to be a transcription regulator in all adult cells (De Caprio et al., 1989). The normal gene product suppresses the expression of genes required for cell cycle progression (Goodrich et al., 1992; Xu et al., 1991). Cyclin and cyclin-dependent kinases, known to be basic molecular regulators of cell proliferation, inactivate the Rb gene product by phosphorylation (Dowdy et al., 1993). In retinoblastoma the Rb gene is associated with tumorigenesis when both alleles are altered in retinal cells. In other types of tumors, loss of functional Rb protein can be due to similar mechanism or the Rb gene product can be inhibited by other mechanisms such as overexpression of cyclin D_1. Humans with one altered Rb allele are normal, except for increased risk to develop cancers. Their risk for the development of retinoblastoma is 36,000 times that of individuals without the mutation (Gallie, 1994). Humans with germ-line Rb mutations also have 2000 times the normal risk for osteosarcoma and an undefined, but increased, risk for other tumors, predominantly melanoma and soft tissue sarcomas (Gallie, 1994).

There are two main types of alterations of Rb gene in human cancers: deletions and mutations (Fig. 11-8). The first consists of major deletions of large segments of the gene, resulting in the absence of a properly functioning gene product (Friend et al., 1987). The second consists of nucleotide substitutions that alter gene function by creating improperly located initiation signals, splicing sites, stop codons, aminoacid substitutions, and so forth. The latter destabilizes the transcript, produces a truncated gene product, or otherwise modifies the mRNA, causing the absence of a functional Rb protein (Horowitz et al., 1990). The Rb gene alterations in human bladder carcinomas represent subtle point mutations rather than major deletions (Horowitz et al., 1990). Rb gene

is one of the major genetic factors responsible for the development and progression of high-grade, muscle-invasive bladder tumors (Cordon-Cardo et al., 1992). Loss of Rb function has been observed in several human bladder carcinoma cell lines. More importantly, the introduction of the normal Rb gene into such cells suppressed proliferation and tumorigenicity in nude mice, but the suppression was not complete. Loss of Rb function occurs in approximately 30% of high-grade papillary and non-papillary flat urothelial carcinomas (Cairns et al., 1991; Ishikawa et al., 1991). This loss appears to correlate with loss of heterozygosity at the Rb gene locus, and with high histologic grade and muscle invasion.

PROSTATE

The prostate is the major accessory organ of the male reproductive system and a common site of malignant tumors in men. Adenocarcinoma of the prostate, the second leading cause of cancer death in American males, has an exponentially increasing incidence in each successive decade of life, and clinically unapparent disease is present in most men over the age of 80 (see Chap. 7). Both incidence and mortality are significantly higher in blacks than whites. The morphology of the lesions ranges from well-differentiated to highly anaplastic tumors. Epidemiologic observation suggests that several different factors could be of etiologic importance in prostate tumorigenesis. These include genetic, hormonal, and chemical/environmental factors. However, no overall unifying concept has emerged with respect to the contribution of each of these factors to prostate cancer.

As is the case with other organs, neoplastic lesions of the prostate often contain cells with chromosomal aberrations. Theoretically, a comprehensive cytogenetic examination could provide information regarding numerical chromosome alterations. However, the technical problems with chromosome analysis of solid tumors seem to make this approach unrewarding. Nevertheless, early attempts that included the use of short-term culture have been made, but with no consistent results. With the advent of the FISH technique and its application even to fine-needle aspirates of the prostate, it seems that some of the inherent difficulties in chromosome analysis may have been overcome (Micale et al., 1993; Persons et al., 1993; see also p. 273). Moreover, the application of molecular genetic methodologies in the study of prostate tumors is of special significance for elucidating chromosomal anomalies in this disease. At the chromosomal level some prostatic adenocarcinomas show a normal chromosomal complement (Arps et al., 1993). A subset of prostate cancers is aneuploid with multiple chromosomal rearrangements (Lundgren et al., 1988). Clonal chromosomal alterations ranging from trisomy 7, loss of Y chromosomes to deletion of 10q(24) and 16q have been described (Babu et al., 1990; Micale et al., 1993; Arps et al., 1993; Carter et al., 1990). Deletion of 10q and possibly of 7q seems to be a recurring theme in prostatic carcinomas. The use of chromosome transfer techniques have shown that the metastatic phenotype of some prostatic cancer cells can be suppressed by chromosome 11 insertion. These observations suggest that the loss of a gene located on 11p11.2-13 may play a role in the metastatic behavior of these cells (Ichikawa et al., 1992). Chromosome 8 mapping studies have defined frequently deleted regions between 8p21.3-8p21.2 and overlap to a 14cM interval in this region (Bova et al., 1993). Deletions on other chromosomes were also reported, most frequently chromosomes 8, 10, 16, and 18, with the long arm of chromosome 16 having deletions in 56% of informative cases (Bergerheim et al., 1991). It has been documented that prostatic carcinomas with a diploid DNA content have a better prognosis than aneuploid tumors (see Chap. 9).

It has been reported that mutations of ras genes occur in approximately 25% of prostate cancer, but other studies have not confirmed such a frequency. The mutations occur predominantly in the Ha-ras gene and less frequently in N- or Ki-ras (Moul et al., 1992; Gumerlock et al., 1991; Pergolizzi et al., 1993). Enhanced expression of the c-myc protooncogene occurs predominantly in high-grade tumors (Fleming et al., 1986; Buttyan et al., 1987). p53 mutations occur in between 30% and 40% of prostatic carcinomas and seem to correlate with advanced stage and metastatic phenotype (Bookstein et al., 1993; Effert et al., 1992; Visakorpi et al., 1992). Loss of

heterozygosity at a locus telemetric to p53 correlates with the metastatic potential of tumor cells (Effert et al., 1992). In general, loss of chromosome 17p seems to correlate with a metastatic phenotype of prostatic carcinoma (Macoska et al., 1992). Deletions of the Rb gene leading to an aberrant short mRNA transcript were documented in some prostatic cancers, but the biologic significance of these findings has not been established (Bookstein et al., 1990; Sarkar et al., 1992).

The most important issue of prostate cancer biology is the hormonal growth dependence of these tumors, on which androgen ablation therapy is based. Unfortunately, all prostatic carcinomas eventually relapse to an androgen-independent state. The molecular events responsible for hormonal independence are still poorly understood. It is thought that changes that affect the androgen-signaling pathway, as well as other growth regulatory elements may be responsible for the androgen-independent status of prostate tumor cells. The androgen-independent cells seem to have a structurally normal androgen receptor gene, but with an altered level of expression. Since the antihormonal or hormone ablation demise of prostatic cancer cells is associated with apoptotic tumor cell death, the gene involved in programmed cell death (apoptosis) may have a role in the development of hormone independent status (Martikainen et al., 1991). Expression of the protooncogene bcl-2 in prostatic adenocarcinoma cells has been shown to be associated with the emergence of androgen independence (McDonnell et al., 1992). This supports the concept that an altered genetic cell death program may, at least in part, be responsible for androgen independence of prostatic cancer. For a recent review of molecular biologic aspects of prostatic carcinoma see Netto and Humphrey, 1994.

KIDNEY

The central issue of the molecular biology of renal carcinomas is the specific non-random abnormality of chromosome 3 present in sporadic and familial renal cell carcinomas, as well as in renal cell carcinomas in von Hippel-Lindau syndrome (Wang et al., 1984; van der Hout et al., 1988; Anderson et al., 1992; King et al., 1987; Decker et al., 1989; Gnarra et al., 1993). Although renal cell carcinomas usually have an aneuploid karyotype with complex alterations of multiple chromosomes, non-random abnormalities involving the 3p12-21 region are dominant. Restriction fragment length polymorphism studies have led to the tentative conclusion that renal cell carcinomas may arise by a double-loss mechanism similar to that of retinoblastoma and Wilms' tumors (Erlandsson et al., 1988). The epidemiologic data indicate single-hit kinetics for the age distribution of hereditary renal cell carcinoma and two-hit kinetics for sporadic tumors (Erlandsson et al., 1988). Most authors postulate that the loss of a recessive cancer gene located on the short arm of chromosome 3 plays an important role in the development of renal cell carcinoma. More detailed mapping studies indicate that the loss of heterozygosity on chromosome 3 (Anglard et al., 1991) can be documented in nearly 80% of the tumors (Bergerheim et al., 1989; Yamakawa et al., 1991). The breakpoint is not stable, and the most commonly deleted regions are 3p13-14.3 and 3p21,3, suggesting that more than one tumor suppressor gene may be involved (Yamakawa et al., 1992). The most commonly deleted region of chromosome 3 spans between 3p21 and 3p24 (loci THRB and D3S2) (van der Hout et al., 1991; LaForgia et al., 1993). The most frequently deleted locus on chromosome 3 can be identified with a D3F15S2 probe (Erlandsson et al., 1988). The common fragile site of chromosome 3 at p14 is probably a frequent site of the breakpoint causing deletions in renal carcinomas (Tajara et al., 1988). This mechanism is most likely operative in renal cell tumors with clear cell morphology (Carroll et al., 1987; Ogawa et al., 1991). The most frequently deleted regions of chromosome 3 found in human renal cell carcinomas are depicted in Figure 11-9.

Papillary renal carcinomas are genetically distinct and usually exhibit trisomy 7,17 and loss of chromosome 4 (Kovacs et al., 1989, 1991). Some papillary tumors also exhibit + (x;1) (p11.2; q21) (Meloni et al., 1993; Kovacs et al., 1992). Loss of heterozygosity of chromosome 17 at the p53 locus is present in nearly 50% of renal cell carcinomas, and mutations of the p53 gene are present in approximately 30% (Reiter et al., 1993). Most tumors with p53 mutations also exhibit loss of heterozygosity of the p53 locus, indicating that in these carcinomas an altered p53 protein acts in a homozygous state (Reiter et al., 1993). The hypermethylation at region D17S5 of chromosome 17 precedes the allelic deletion at the p53 locus. The DNA hypermethylation occurs in the early stage, whereas 17p deletion at the p53 locus occurs in the later stages of renal cell carcinoma (Makos et al., 1993). Interestingly, allelic losses at chromosome 17p in renal cell carcinomas are inversely related to 3p deletions (Ogawa et al., 1992). Overexpression of epidermal growth factor (EGF) receptor is a frequent event in renal cell carcinoma, occurring in 60% of cases, but it does not correlate with tumor stage and progression (Weidner et al., 1990; Yao et al., 1988; Ishikawa et al., 1990; Gomella et al., 1990). EGF receptor is a transmembrane glycoprotein that binds

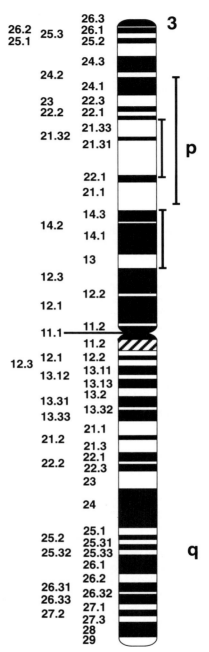

FIGURE 11-9.   Diagram of chromosome 3. The regions most frequently deleted in renal cell carcinoma are indicated by the vertical bars.

mitogenic proteins such as EGF and other related growth-transforming factors. Renal cell carcinomas are known for their particular resistance to chemotherapy. It has been postulated that resistance is mainly the result of overexpression of the multidrug resistance (MDR1) gene (Klein et al., 1989; Rochlitz et al., 1992).

Loss of heterozygosity in the Rb locus and loss of functional Rb protein are infrequent in renal cell carcinomas (Kanayama et al., 1991). Mutations of *ras* gene are also rare events in these tumors (Rochlitz et al., 1992).

SUMMARY

Common tumors of the genitourinary tract represent a heterogeneous group of neoplasms with distinct clinico-pathologic features, etiology, and pathogenesis. The exact molecular events leading to their development are still unclear, and the association between genetic abnormalities and the origin and behavior of human neoplastic cells is still based for the most part on circumstantial evidence. The tumors discussed in this chapter exemplify the three major phenomena considered important in the biology of human neoplasia: multistep carcinogenesis (urinary bladder carcinoma); involvement of a single tumor suppressor gene (renal cell carcinoma); and hormonal growth dependence and programmed cell death (prostatic carcinoma). The two main groups of urinary bladder carcinomas (papillary and solid) can serve as a model for multistep carcinogenesis, now generally accepted as the process that leads to the development of most common sporadic human cancers (see Chap. 5). The alterations of known tumor suppressor and transforming genes discussed in this chapter are probably secondary events commonly encountered in many tumors of different origin. The most intriguing aspect of multistep carcinogenesis is the question concerning the initiating event. It has been postulated that the so-called master genes, responsible for overall genomic transcriptional fidelity, are altered and consequently responsible for the cascade of genomic instabilities. The candidate genes that can initiate the process were recently discovered in lower organisms, and it was shown that they belong to the class of DNA repair genes (Kolberg, 1993). A mutated human DNA repair gene located on chromosome 2 has been linked to the predisposition for development of a nonpolyposis familial colonic carcinoma (Lynch I syndrome) (Aaltonen et al., 1993; Thibodeau et al., 1993). It has been postulated that a similar mechanism may be operative in the development of a subset of urinary bladder carcinomas occurring in a spectrum of extra-intestinal tumors in families affected by this syndrome (Linnenbach et al., 1994).

The presence of a non-random chromosomal deletion in renal cell carcinomas indicates that a particular gene is involved in the development of most of these neoplasms (see Chap. 7). Genomic mapping with hypervariable probes is used to identify the deleted segment and to locate the candidate gene on chromosome 3. Cloning of this gene in the near future can be anticipated.

The current research on prostatic carcinoma is focused on two phenomena: metastatic phenotype and hormonal dependence. The progress in clinical management of prostatic carcinoma, combining ultrasound and serum PSA measurement, allowed the identification of an ever-increasing number of small intraprostatic carcinomas. Retrospective studies indicate that only a fraction of them will progress to a clinically significant disease and to metastases (see Chaps. 7 and 9). Therefore, the identification of molecular markers that may permit the identification of a subset of clinically aggressive versus clinically indolent prostatic carcinomas is of prime importance. On the other hand, the androgen-dependent growth of prostatic carcinomas offers the opportunity to control their growth by hormonal manipulation. The development of androgen-independent growth is responsible for the ultimate failure of this approach; consequently, the elucidation of the underlying molecular mechanism is of great clinical importance.

Molecular genetic studies of human cancer have barely began. An important issue that has not been addressed as yet has to do with the sequences of genetic changes. Do these changes follow human logic—*i.e.*, does one change inexorably lead to another—or could it be that the sequence is unpredictable and chaotic? It is likely that many years of additional work will be required to answer these fundamental questions.

BIBLIOGRAPHY

Aaltonen, L., Deltomaki, P., Leach, F., Sistonen, P., Pylkkanen, L., Mecklin, Y. P., Jarvinen, H., Powell, S. M., Jen, J., Hamilton, S. R., Peterson, G. M., Kintzler, K. W., Vogelstein, B., and de la Chapelle, A.: Clues to the pathogenesis of familial colorectal cancer. Science, *260*, 812–816, 1993.

Anderson, G. A., and Lawson, R. K.: Chromosomal defects in renal cell carcinoma. Urology, *39*, 473–477, 1992.

Anglard, P., Tory, K., Brauch, H., Weiss, G. H., Latif, F., Merino, M. J., Lerman, M. I., Zbar, B., and Linehan, W. M.: Molecular analysis of genetic changes in the origin and development of renal cell carcinoma. Cancer Res., *51*, 1071–1077, 1991.

Arps, S., Rodewald, A., Schmalenberger, B., Carl, P., Bressel, M., and Kastendieck, H.: Cytogenetic survey of 32 cancers of the prostate. Cancer Genet. Cytogenet., *66*, 93–99, 1993.

Atkin, N. B., Fox, M. F.: 5q deletion. The sole chromosome change in a carcinoma of the bladder. Cancer Genet. Cytogenet., *46*, 129–131, 1990.

Babu, V. R., Miles, B. J., Cerny, J. C., Weiss, L., and Van Dyke, D. L.: Cytogenetic study of four cancers of the prostate. Cancer Genet. Cytogenet., *48*, 83–87, 1990.

Barbacid, M.: *ras* Genes. Ann. Rev. Biochem., *56*, 779–827, 1987.

Barrios, L., Miro, R., Caballin, M. R., Vayrda, J., Subias, A., and Eqozcue, J.: Constitutional del (3) (p14-p21) in a patient with bladder carcinoma. Cancer Genet. Cytogenet., *21*, 171–173, 1986.

Bergerheim, U., Nordenskjold, M., and Collins, P.: Deletion mapping in human renal cell carcinoma. Cancer Res., *49*, 1390–1396, 1989.

Bergerheim, U. S., Kunimi, K., Collins, V. P., and Ekman, P.: Deletion mapping of chromosomes 8, 10 and 16 in human prostatic carcinoma. Genes Chromosom. Cancer, *3*, 215–220, 1991.

Berrozpe, G., Miro, R., Caballin, M. R., Salvador, J., and Eqozcue, J.: Trisomy 7 may be a primary change in noninvasive transitional cell carcinoma of the bladder. Cancer Genet. Cytogenet., *50*, 9–14, 1990.

Bookstein, R., MacGrogan, D., Hilsenbeck, S. G., Sharkey, F., and Allred, D. C.: p53 is mutated in a subset of advanced-stage prostate cancers. Cancer Res., *53*, 3369–3373, 1993.

Bookstein, R., Rio, P., Madreperla, S. A., Hong, F., Allred, C., Grizzle, W. E., and Lee, W. H.: Promoter deletion and loss of retinoblastoma gene expression in human prostate carcinoma. Proc. Natl. Acad. Sci. USA, *87*, 7762–7766, 1990.

Bos, J. L.: *ras* Oncogenes in human cancer. A review. Cancer Res., *49*, 4682–4689, 1989.

Bova, G. S., Carter, B. S., Bussemakers, M. J., Emi, M., Fujiwara, Y., Kyprianou, N., Jacobs, S. C., Robinson, J. C., Epstein, J. I., Walsh, P. C., and Isaacs, W. B.: Homozygous deletion and frequent allelic loss of chromosome 8p22 loci in human prostate cancer. Cancer Res., *53*, 3869–3873, 1993.

Brawn, P. N.: The origin of invasive carcinoma of the bladder. Cancer, *50*, 515–519, 1982.

Burchill, S. A., Lunec, J., Mellon, K., and Neal, D. E.: Analysis of Ha-*ras* mutations in primary human bladder tumors. Br. J. Cancer., *63*(Suppl. 13), 62, 1991.

Burke, K., and Harbott, J.: The prognostic meaning of marker chromosomes in human urinary bladder carcinoma. Prog. Clin. Biol. Res., *162A*, 347–357, 1984.

Buttyan, R., Sawczuk, I. S., Benson, M. C., Siegal, J. D., and Olsson, C. A.: Enhanced expression of the c-myc protooncogene in high-grade human prostate cancers. Prostate, *11*, 327–337, 1987.

Cairns, P., Proctor, A. J., and Knowles, M. A.: Loss of heterozygosity at the RB locus is frequent and correlates with muscle invasion in bladder carcinoma. Oncogene, *6*, 2305–2359, 1991.

Carroll, P. R., Murty, V. V., Reuter, V., Jhanwar, S., Fair, W. R., Whitmore, W. F., and Chaganti, R. S.: Abnormalities at chromosome region 3p12-14 characterized clear cell renal carcinoma. Cancer Genet. Cytogenet., *26*, 253–259, 1987.

Carter, B. S., Ewing, C. M., Ward, W. S., Treiger, B. F., Aalders, T. W., Schalken, J. A., Epstein, J. I., and Isaacs, W. B.: Allelic loss of chromosomes 16q and 10q in human prostate cancer. Proc. Natl. Acad. Sci. USA, *87*, 8751–8755, 1990.

Chakraborty, K., Cichutek, K., and Duesberg, P. H.: Transforming function of proto-*ras* genes depends on heterologous promoters and is enhanced by specific point mutations. Proc. Natl. Acad. Sci. USA, *88*, 2217–2221, 1991.

Cohen, J. B., Broz, S. D., and Levinson, A. D.: Expression of the Ha-*ras* proto-oncogene is controlled by alternative splicing. Cell, *58*, 461–472, 1989.

Cohen, J. B., and Levinson, A. D.: A point mutation in the last intron responsible for increased expression and transforming activity for the c-Ha-*ras* oncogene. Nature, *334*, 119–124, 1988.

Cordon-Cardo, C., Dalbagni, G., Saez, G. T., Oliva, M. R., Zhang, Z. F., Rosai, J., Reuter, V. E., and Pellicer, A.: p53 mutations in human bladder cancer: genotypic versus phenotypic patterns. Int. J. Cancer, *56*, 347–353, 1994.

Cordon-Cardo, C., Wartinger, D., Petrylak, D., Dalbagni, G., Fair, W. R., Fuks, Z., and Reuter, V. E.: Altered expressions of the retinoblastoma gene product: prognostic indicator in bladder cancer. J. Natl. Cancer. Inst., *84*, 1251–1256, 1992.

Culig, Z., Klocker, H., Eberle, J., Kaspar, F., Hobisch, A., Cronauer, M. V., and Bartsch, G.: DNA sequence of the androgen receptor in prostatic tumor cell lines and tissue specimens assessed by means of the polymerase chain reaction. Prostate, *22*, 11–22, 1993.

Czerniak, B., Cohen, G. L., Etkind, P., Deitch, D., Simmons, H., Herz, F., and Koss, L. G.: Concurrent mutations of coding and regulatory sequences of the Ha-*ras* gene in urinary bladder carcinomas. Hum. Pathol., *23*, 1199–1203, 1992.

De Caprio, J. A., Ludlow, J. W., and Lynch, D.: The product of retinoblastoma susceptibility gene has properties of a cycle regulatory element. Cell, *58*, 1085–1095, 1989.

Decker, H. J., Gemmill, R. M., Neumann, H. P., Walter, T. A., and Sandbert, A. A.: Loss of heterozygosity on 3p in a renal cell carcinoma in von Hippel-Lindau syndrome. Cancer Genet. Cytogenet., *39*, 289–293, 1989.

Dowdy, S. F., Hinds, P. W., Louie, K., Ree, S. I., Arnold, A., and Weinberg, R. A.: Physical interaction of the retinoblastoma protein with human D cyclins. Cell, *73*, 449–511, 1993.

Effert, P. J., McCoy, R. H., Walther, P. J., and Liu, E. T.: p53 gene alterations in human prostate carcinoma. J. Urol., *150*, 257–261, 1992.

Effert, P. J., Neubauer, A., Walther, P. J., and Liu, E. T.: Alterations of the p53 gene are associated with the progression of a human prostate carcinoma. J. Urol., *147*, 789–793, 1992.

Erlandsson, R., Boldog, F., Sumegi, J., and Klein, G.: Do human renal cell carcinomas arise by a double-loss mechanism? Cancer Genet. Cytogenet., *36*, 197–202, 1988.

Esrig, D., Elmajian, D., Groshen, S., Freeman, J. A., Stein, J. P., Chen, S. C., Nichols, P. W., Skinner, D. G., Jones, P. A., and Cote, R. J.: Accumulation of nuclear p53 and tumor progression in bladder cancer. New Engl. J. Med., *331*, 1259–1264, 1994.

Falor, W. H., and Ward, R. M.: Prognosis of early carcinoma of the bladder based on chromosomal analysis. J. Urol., *119*, 44–48, 1978.

Feinberg, A. P., Vogelstein, B., Droller, M. J., Baylin, S. B., and Nelkin, B. D.: Mutation affecting the 12th amino acid of the c-Ha-*ras* oncogene product occurs infrequently in human cancer. Science, *220*, 1175–1177, 1983.

Finlay, C., Hinds, P., and Levine, A.: The p53 protooncogene can act as a suppressor of transformation. Cell, *57*, 1083–1093, 1989.

Fleming, W. H., Hamel, A., MacDonald, R., Ramsey, E., Pettigrew, N. M., Johnston, B., Dodd, J. G., and Matusik, R. J.: Expression of the c-*myc* protooncogene in human prostatic carcinoma and benign prostatic hyperplasia. Cancer Res., *46*, 1535–1538, 1986.

Friend, S. H., Horowitz, J. M., Gerber, M. R., Wang, X. F., Bogenmann, E., Li, F. P., and Weinberg, R. A.: Deletions of a DNA sequence in retinoblastomas and mesenchymal tumors: organization of the sequence and its encoded protein. Proc. Natl. Acad. Sci. USA, *84*, 9059–9063, 1987.

Fujimoto, K., Yamada, Y., Okajima, E., Kakizoe, T., Sasaki, H., Sugimura, T., and Terada, M.: Frequent association of p53 gene mutation in invasive bladder cancer. Cancer Res., *52*, 1393–1398, 1992.

Fujita, J., Yoshida, O., Yuasa, Y., Rhim, J. S., Hatanaka, M., and Aaronson, S. A.: Ha-*ras* oncogenes are activated by somatic alterations in human urinary tract tumours. Nature, *309*, 464–466, 1984.

Gallie, B. L.: Retinoblastoma gene mutations in human cancer. N. Engl. J. Med., *330*, 786–787, 1994.

Gibas, Z., Prout, G. R., Pontes, J. E., Connolly, J. G., and Sandberg, A. A.: A possible specific chromosome change in transitional cell carcinoma of the bladder. Cancer Genet. Cytogenet., *19*, 229–238, 1986.

Gnarra, J. R., Glenn, G. M., Latif, F., Anglard, P., Lerman, M. I., Zbar, B., and Linehan, W. M.: Molecular genetic studies of sporadic and familial renal cell carcinoma. Urol. Clin. North Am., *20*, 207–216, 1993.

Gomella, L. G., Anglard, P., Sargent, E. R., Robertson, C. N., Kasid, A., and Linehan, W. M.: Epidermal growth factor receptor gene analysis in renal cell carcinoma. J. Urol., *143*, 191–193, 1990.

Goodrich, D. W., Chen, Y., Sculley, P., and Lee, W. H.: Expression of the retinoblastoma gene product in bladder carcinoma cells associates with a low frequency of tumor formation. Cancer Res., *52*, 1968–1973, 1992.

Gumerlock, P. H., Poonamallee, U. R., Meyers, F. J., and deVere White, R. W.: Activated ras alleles in human carcinoma of the prostate are rare. Cancer Res., *51*, 1632–1637, 1991.

Halvey, O., Michalovitz, D., and Oren, M.: Different tumor-derived p53 mutants exhibit distinct biological activities. Science, *250*, 113–116, 1990.

Harper, J. W., Adam, G. R., Wei, N., Keyomarsi, K., and Elledgle, S. J.: The p21 Cdk–interacting protein. Cip-1 is a potent inhibitor of G_1 cyclin-dependent kinases. Cell, *25*, 805–816, 1993.

Hollstein, M., Sidransky, D., Vogelstein, G., and Harris, C. C.: p53 Mutations in human cancers. Science, *253*, 49–53, 1991.

Hopman, A. H., Moesker, O., Smeets, A. W., Pauwels, R. P., Vooigs, G. P., and Ramaekers, F. C.: Numerical chromosome 1, 7, 9, and 11 aberrations in bladder cancer detected by in situ hybridization. Cancer Res., *51*, 644–651, 1991.

Hopman, A. H., Poddighe, P. J., Smeets, A. W., Moesker, O., Beck, J. L., Vooijs, G. P., and Ramaekers, F. C.: Detection of numerical chromosome aberrations in bladder cancer by in situ hybridization. Am. J. Pathol., *135*, 1105–1117, 1989.

Hopman, A. H., Ramaekers, F. C., Raap, A. K., Beck, J. L., Devi-Lee, P., van der Ploeg, M., and Vooijs, G. P.: In situ hybridization as a tool to study numerical chromosome aberrations in solid bladder tumors. Histochemistry, *89*, 307–316, 1988.

Horowitz, J. M., Park, S. H., Bogenmann, E., Cheng, J. C., Yandell, D. W., Kaye, F. J., Minna, J. D., Dryia, T. P., and Weinberg, R. A.: Frequent inactivation of the retinoblastoma anti-oncogene is restricted to a subset of human tumor cells. Proc. Natl. Acad. Sci. USA, *87*, 2755–2779, 1990.

Ichikawa, T., Ichikawa, Y., Dong, J., Hawkins, A. L., Griffin, C. A., Isaacs, W. B., Oshimura, M., Barrett, J. C., and Isaacs, J. T.: Localization of metastasis suppressor gene(s) for prostatic cancer to the short arm of human chromosome 11. Cancer Res., *52*, 3486–3490, 1992.

Ishikawa, J., Maeda, S., Umezu, K., Sugiyama, T., and Kamidono, S.: Amplification and over-expression of the epidermal growth factor receptor gene in human renal cell carcinoma. Int. J. Cancer, *45*, 1018–1021, 1990.

Ishikawa, J., Xu, H-J., Hu, S-X., Yandell, D. W., Maeda, S., Kamidono, S., Benedict, W. F., and Takahashi, R.: Inactivation of the retinoblastoma gene in human bladder and renal cell carcinomas. Cancer Res., *51*, 5736–5743, 1991.

Kanayama, H., Tanaka, K., Aki, M., Kagawa, S., Miyaji, H., Satoh, M., Okada, F., Sato, S., Shimbara, N., and Ichihara, A.: Changes in expression of proteasome and ubiquitin genes in human renal cancer cells. Cancer Res., *66*, 77–85, 1991.

Kaye, K. W., and Lange, P. H.: Mode of presentation of invasive bladder cancer. Reassessment of the problem. J. Urol., *128*, 31–33, 1982.

Kern, S., Kinzler-Baker, W., and Vogelstein, B.: Identification of p53 as a sequence specific DNA binding protein. Science, *252*, 1708–1711, 1991.

King, C. R., Schimke, R. N., Arthur, T., Davoren, B., and Collins, D.: Proximal 3p deletion in renal cell carcinoma cells from a patient with von Hippel-Lindau disease. Cancer Genet. Cytogenet., *27*, 345–348, 1987.

Klein, E. A.: The multidrug resistance gene in renal cell carcinoma. Sem. Urol., *7*, 207–214, 1989.

Knowles, M. A., and Williamson, M.: Mutation of Ha-*ras* is infrequent in bladder cancer: confirmation by single-strand conformation polymorphism analysis, designed fragment length polymorphism and direct sequencing. Cancer Res., *53*, 133–139, 1993.

Kolberg, R.: Linking DNA mismatch repair to carcinogenesis. Journal of the National Institutes of Health Research, *5*, 32–34, 1993.

Koss, L. G.: Tumors of the urinary bladder. *In* Atlas of Tumor Pathology, Second Series, Fascicle 11. Washington, D.C., Armed Forces Institute of Pathology, 1975 (Suppl. 1985).

Koss, L. G., and Czerniak, B.: Biology and management of urinary bladder cancer (letter). N. Engl. J. Med., *324*, 125–126, 1991.

Koss, L. G.: How cells function: fundamental concepts of molecular biology. Chapter 2 *In*: Koss, L. G., Diagnostic Cytology and its Histopathologic Bases. 4th Ed. Philadelphia, J. B. Lippincott, 1992.

Koss, L. G.: Tumor of the urinary tract and prostate in urinary sediment. *In* Diagnostic Cytology and Its Histopathologic Bases. 4th edition. Philadelphia, J. B. Lippincott, 1992, pp. 934–977.

Kovacs, G., Fuzesi, L., Emanual, A., and Kung, H. F.: Cytogenetics of papillary renal cell tumors. Genes Chromosom. Cancer, *3*, 249–255, 1991.

Kovacs, G., Kiechle-Schwarz, M., Scherer, G., and Kung, H. F.: Molecular analysis of the chromosome 11p region in renal cell carcinomas. Cell. Mol. Biol., *38*, 59–62, 1992.

Kovacs, G., Wilkens, T. P., and DeRiese, W.: Differentiation between papillary and nonpapillary renal cell carcinomas by DNA analysis. J. Natl. Cancer Inst., *81*, 527–530, 1989.

Kovacs, G.: Papillary renal cell carcinoma: a morphologic and cytogenetic study of 11 cases. Am. J. Pathol., *134*, 27–34, 1989.

LaForgia, S., Lasota, J., Latif, F., Boghosian-Sell, L., Kastury, K., Ohta, M., Druck, T., Atchison, L., Cannizzaro, L. A., Barnea, G., et al.: Detailed genetic and physical map of the 3p chromosome region surrounding the familial renal cell carcinoma chromosome translocation, t(3;8) (p14.2;q24.1). Cancer Res., *53*, 3118–3124, 1993.

Levine, A. J., Momand, J., and Finlay, C. A.: The p53 tumor suppressor gene. Nature, *351*, 453–456, 1991.

Linnenbach, A. J., Robbins, S. L., Seng, B. A., Tomaszewski, J. E., Pressier, L. B., and Molkowicz: Urothelial carcinogenesis. Nature, *367*, 419–420, 1994.

Lundgren, R., Kristoffersson, U., Heim, S., Mandahl, N., and Mitelman, F.: Multiple structural chromosome rearrangements, including del(7q) and del(10q), in an adenocarcinoma of the prostate. Cancer Genet. Cytogenet., *35*, 103–108, 1988.

Macoska, J. A., Powell, I. J., Sakr, W., and Lane, M. A.: Loss of the 17p chromosomal region in a metastatic carcinoma of the prostate. J. Urol., *147*, 1142–1146, 1992.

Makos, M., Nelkin, B. D., Reiter, R. E., Gnarra, J. R.,

Brooks, J., Isaacs, W., Linehan, M., and Baylin, S. B.: Regional DNA hypermethylation at D17S5 precedes 17p structural changes in the progression of renal tumors. Cancer Res., *53*, 2719–2722, 1993.

Martikainen, P., Kyprianou, N., Tucker, R. W., and Isaacs, J. T.: Programmed death of non-proliferating androgen-independent prostatic cancer cells. Cancer Res., *51*, 4693–4700, 1991.

Martinez, J., Georgeff, I., and Levine, A. J.: Cellular localization and cell cycle regulation by a temperature sensitive p53 protein. Genes Dev., *5*, 151–159, 1991.

McBride, O. W., Merry, D., and Girol, D.: The gene for human p53 cellular tumor antigen is located on chromosome 17 short arm. Proc. Natl. Acad. Sci. USA, *83*, 130–134, 1986.

McDonnell, T. J., Troncoso, P., Brisbay, S. M., Logothetis, C., Chung, L. W., Hsieh, J. T., Tu, S. M., and Campbell, M. L.: Expression of the protooncogene *bcl*-2 in the prostate and its association with emergency of androgen-independent prostate cancer. Cancer Res., *52*, 6940–6944, 1992.

Meloni, A. M., Dobbs, R. M., Pontes, J. E., and Sandberg, A. A.: Translocation (X;1) in papillary renal cell carcinoma. A new cytogenetic subtype. Cancer Genet. Cytogenet., *65*, 1–6, 1993.

Micale, M. A., Sanford, J. S., Powell, I. J., Sakr, W. A., and Wolman, S. R.: Defining the extent and nature of cytogenetic events in prostatic adenocarcinoma: paraffin FISH vs. metaphase analysis. Cancer Genet. Cytogenet., *69*, 7–12, 1993.

Miyao, N., Tsai, Y. C., Lerner, S. P., Owmni, A. F., Spruck, Ch. III, Gonzalez-Zulueta, M., Nichols, P. W., Skinner, D. G., and Jones, P. A.: The role of chromosome 9 in human bladder cancer. Cancer Res., *53*, 4066–4070, 1993.

Moul, J. W., Friedrichs, P. A., Lance, R. S., Theune, S. M., and Chang, E. H.: Infrequent RAS oncogene mutations in human prostate cancer. Prostate, *20*, 327–338, 1992.

Nagata, Y., Abe, M., Kobayashi, K., Saiki, S., Kotake, T., Yoshikawa, K., Ueda, R., Nakayama, E., and Shiku, H.: Point mutations of c-*ras* genes in human bladder cancer and kidney cancer. Jpn. J. Cancer Res., *81*, 22–27, 1990.

Netto, G. J., and Humphrey, P. A.: Molecular biologic aspects of human prostatic carcinoma. Am. J. Clin. Pathol., *102*, (Suppl. 1), S57–S64, 1994.

Nigro, J. M., Baker, S. J., Preisinger, A. C., Jessup, J. M., Hostetter, R., Cleary, K., Bigner, S. H., Davidson, N., Baylin, S., Devilee, P., Glover, T., Collins, F. S., Weston, A., Modali, R., Harris, C. C., and Vogelstein, B.: Mutations in the p53 gene occur in diverse tumor types. Nature, *342*, 705–708, 1989.

Ogawa, O., Habuchi, T., Kakehi, Y., Koshiba, M., Sugiyama, T., and Yoshida, O.: Allelic losses at chromosome 17p in human renal cell carcinoma are inversely related to allelic losses at chromosome 3p. Cancer Res., *52*, 1881–1885, 1992.

Ogawa, O., Kakehi, Y., Ogawa, K., Koshiba, M., Sugiyama, T., and Yoshida, O.: Allelic loss at chromosome 3p characterizes clear cell phenotype of renal cell carcinoma. Cancer Res., *51,* 949–953, 1991.

Olumi, A. F., Tsai, Y. C., Nichols, P. W., Skinner, D. G., Cain, D. R., Bender, L. I., and Jones, P. A.: Allelic loss of chromosome 17p distinguishes high grade from low grade transitional cell carcinomas of the bladder. Cancer Res., *50,* 7081–8083, 1990.

Ooi, A., Herz, F., Ii, S, Cordon-Cardo, C., Fradet, Y., and Mayall, B. H.: Ha-*ras* codon 12 mutations in papillary tumors of the urinary bladder. A retrospective study. Int. J. Oncol., *4,* 85–90, 1994.

Pergolizzi, R. G., Kreis, W., Rottach, C., Susin, M., Broome, J. D.: Mutational status of codons 12 and 13 of the N- and K-*ras* genes in tissue and cell lines derived from primary and metastatic prostate carcinomas. Cancer Invest., *11,* 25–32, 1993.

Persons, D. L., Gibney, D. J., Katzmann, J. A., Lieber, M. M., Farrow, G. M., and Jenkins, R. B.: Use of fluorescent in situ hybridization for deoxyribonucleic acid ploidy analysis of prostatic adenocarcinoma. J. Urol., *150,* 120–125, 1993.

Presti, J. C., Jr., Reuter, V. E., Galan, T., Fair, W. R., and Cordon-Carco, C.: Molecular genetic alterations in superficial and locally advanced human bladder cancer. Cancer Res., *51,* 5405–5409, 1991.

Raghavan, D., Shipley, W. V., Garnick, M. B., Russell, P. J., and Richie, J. P.: Biology and management of bladder cancer. N. Engl. J. Med., *322,* 1129–1138, 1990.

Reddy, E. P., Reynolds, R. K., Santos, E., and Barbacid, M.: A point mutation is responsible for the acquisition of transforming properties by the T24 human bladder carcinoma oncogene. Nature, *300,* 149–152, 1982.

Reiter, R. E., Anglard, P., Liu, S., Gnarra, J. R., and Linehan, W. M.: Chromosome 17p deletions and p53 mutations in renal cell carcinomas. Cancer Res., *53,* 3092–3097, 1993.

Rochlitz, C. F., Lobeck, H., Peter, S., Reuter, J., Mohr, B., de Kant, E., Huhn, D., and Herrmann, R.: Multiple drug resistance gene expression in human renal cell cancer is associated with the histologic subtype. Cancer, *69,* 2993–2998, 1992.

Rochlitz, C. F., Peter, S., Willroth, G., de Kant, E., Lobeck, H., Huhn, D., and Herrmann, R.: Mutations in the *ras* proto-oncogene are rare events in renal cell cancer. Eur. J. Cancer, *28,* 333–336, 1992.

Saison-Bohemaras, T., Tocque, B., Rey, I., Chassignol, M., Thuong, N. T., and Helene, C.: Short modified antisense oligonucleotide directed against Ha-*ras* point mutation induce selective clearge of the mRNA and inhibit T24 cell proliferation. EMBO J., *10,* 1111–1118, 1991.

Sarkar, F. H., Sakr, W., Li, Y. W., Macoska, J., Ball, E. D., and Crissman, J. D.: Analysis of retinoblastoma (RB) gene deletion in human prostatic carcinomas. Prostate, *21,* 145–152, 1992.

Sarkis, A. S., Dalbagni, G., Cordon, C. C., Zhang, Z. F., Sheinfeld, J., Fair, W. R., Herr, H. W., and Reuter, V. E.: Nuclear overexpression of p53 protein in transitional cell bladder carcinoma: a marker for disease progression. J. Natl. Can. Inst., *85,* 53–59, 1993.

Sidransky, D., von Eschenbach, A., Tsai, Y. C., Jones, P., Summerhayes, I., Marshall, F., Paul, M., Green, P., Hamilton, S. R., Frost, P., and Vogelstein, B.: Identification of p53 mutations in bladder cancer and urine samples. Science, *252,* 706–709, 1991.

Tajara, E. H., Berger, C. S., Hecht, B. K., Gemmill, R. M., Sandberg, A. A., and Hecht, F.: Loss of common 3p14 fragile site expression in renal cell carcinoma with deletion breakpoint at 3p14. Cancer Genet. Cytogenet., *31,* 75–82, 1988.

Taparowsky, E., Suard, Y., Fasano, O., Shimizu, K., Goldfarb, M., and Wigler, M.: Activation of the T24 bladder carcinoma transforming gene is linked to a single amino acid change. Nature, *300,* 762–765, 1982.

Thibodeau, S. N., Bren, G., and Schoid, D.: Microsatellite instability in cancer of the proximal colon. Science, *260,* 816–819, 1993.

Tisty, T.: Altered cell cycle arrest and gene amplification potential accompanying loss of wild type p53. Cell, *70,* 937–948, 1992.

van der Hout, A. H., Kok, K., van den Berg, A., Oosterhuis, J. W., Carritt, B., and Buys, C. H.: Direct molecular analysis of a deletion of 3p in tumors from patients with sporadic renal cell carcinoma. Cancer Genet. Cytogenet., *32,* 281–285, 1988.

van der Hout, A. H., van der Vlies, P., Wijmenga, C., Li, F. P., Oosterhuis, J. W., and Buys, C. H.: The region of common allelic losses in sporadic renal cell carcinoma is bordered by the loci D3S2 and THRB. Genomics, *11,* 537–542, 1991.

Visakorpi, T., Kallioniemi, O. P., Heikkinen, A., Koivula, T., and Isola, J.: Small subgroup of aggressive, highly proliferative prostatic carcinomas defined by p53 accumulation. J. Nat. Cancer Inst., *84,* 883–887, 1992.

Visvanathan, K. V., Pocock, R. D., and Summerhayes, I. C.: Preferential and novel activation of Ha-*ras* in human bladder carcinomas. Oncogene Res., *2,* 77–86, 1988.

Wang, N., and Perkins, K. L.: Involvement of band 3p14 in t(3;8) hereditary renal carcinoma. Cancer Genet. Cytogenet., *11,* 479–481, 1984.

Watson, J. D., Hopkins, N. H., Roberts, J. W., Steitz, J. A., and Weiner, A. M.: Molecular Biology of the Gene. 4th Ed. Menlo Park, Benjamin/Cummings, 1987.

Watson, J. D., Tooze, J., and Kurtz, D. T.: Recombinant DNA. 2nd Ed. New York, Scientific American Books, W. H. Freeman, 1992.

Weidner, U., Peter, S., Strohmeyer, T., Hussnatter, R., Ackermann, R., and Sies, H.: Inverse relationship of epidermal growth factor receptor and HER2/neu gene expression in human renal cell carcinoma. Cancer Res., *50,* 4504–4509, 1990.

Wu, S. Q., Storer, B. E., Bookland, E. A., Klingelhutz, A. J., Gilchrist, K. W., Meisner, L. F., Oyasu, R., and Reznikoff, C. A.: Nonrandom chromosome losses in stepwise neoplastic transformation in vitro of human uroepithelial cells. Cancer Res., *51,* 3323–3326, 1991.

Xu, H. J., Hu, S. H., and Benedict, E. F.: Lack of nuclear Rb protein staining in G_0/middle G_1 cells: correlation to changes in total Rb protein level. Oncogene, *6*, 1139–1146, 1991.

Yamakawa, K., Morita, R., Takahashi, E., Hori, T., Ishikawa, J., and Nakamura, Y.: A detailed deletion mapping of the short arm of chromosome 3 in sporadic renal cell carcinoma. Cancer Res., *51*, 4707–4711, 1991.

Yamakawa, K., Takahashi, E., Murata, M., Okui, K., Yokoyama, S., and Nakamura, Y.: Detailed mapping around the breakpoint of (3;8) translocation in familial renal cell carcinoma and FRA3B. Genomics, *14*, 412–416, 1992.

Yao, M., Shuin, T., Misaki, H., and Kubota, Y.: Enhanced expression of c-*myc* and epidermal growth factor receptor (c-*erb* B-1) genes in primary human renal cancer. Cancer Res., *48*, 6753–6757, 1988.

Index

Index